PHYSIOLOGY OF THE HEART

PHYSIOLOGY OF THE HEART

Fourth Edition

Arnold M. Katz, MD, D.Med (Hon), FACP, FACC
Professor of Medicine Emeritus
University of Connecticut School of Medicine
Farmington, Connecticut;
Visiting Professor of Medicine and Physiology
Dartmouth Medical School
Lebanon, New Hampshire

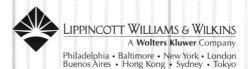

LIPPINCOTT WILLIAMS & WILKINS
A **Wolters Kluwer** Company
Philadelphia • Baltimore • New York • London
Buenos Aires • Hong Kong • Sydney • Tokyo

Acquisitions Editor: Frances R. Destefano
Managing Editor: Joanne Bersin
Marketing Manager: Kathy Neely
Project Manager: Bridgett Dougherty
Senior Manufacturing Manager: Benjamin Rivera
Design Coordinator: Holly McLaughlin
Compositor: TechBooks
Printer: Edwards Brothers

© 2006 by LIPPINCOTT WILLIAMS & WILKINS
530 Walnut Street
Philadelphia, PA 19106 USA
LWW.com

Copyright © 2001 by Lippincott Williams & Wilkins.
Copyright © 1991, 1977 by Raven Publishers.

Printed in the USA

Library of Congress Cataloging-in-Publication Data

Katz, Arnold M.
    Physiology of the heart / Arnold M. Katz.—4th ed.
        p. ; cm.
    Includes bibliographical references and index.   24312797
    ISBN-10: 0-7817-5501-8 (alk. paper) ISBN-13: 978-0-7817-5501-6
    1. Heart—Physiology. 2. Heart—Pathophysiology. I. Title.
    [DNLM: 1. Heart—physiology. 2. Heart Diseases—physiopathology. WG 202
K19p 2006] QP111.4.K38 2006 612.1′7—dc22
                                                    2005017130

Care has been taken to confirm the accuracy of the information presented and to describe generally accepted practices. However, the authors, editors, and publisher are not responsible for errors or omissions or for any consequences from application of the information in this book and make no warranty, expressed or implied, with respect to the currency, completeness, or accuracy of the contents of the publication. Application of this information in a particular situation remains the professional responsibility of the practitioner.

The authors, editors, and publisher have exerted every effort to ensure that drug selection and dosage set forth in this text are in accordance with current recommendations and practice at the time of publication. However, in view of ongoing research, changes in government regulations, and the constant flow of information relating to drug therapy and drug reactions, the reader is urged to check the package insert for each drug for any change in indications and dosage and for added warnings and precautions. This is particularly important when the recommended agent is a new or infrequently employed drug.

Some drugs and medical devices presented in this publication have Food and Drug Administration (FDA) clearance for limited use in restricted research settings. It is the responsibility of the health care provider to ascertain the FDA status of each drug or device planned for use in their clinical practice.

To purchase additional copies of this book, call our customer service department at (800) 638-3030 or fax orders to (301) 824-7390. International customers shoud call (301) 714-2324.

Visit Lippincott Williams & Wilkins on the Internet: at LWW.com. Lippincott Williams & Wilkins customer service representatives are available from 8:30 am to 6:00 pm, EST.

10 9 8 7 6 5 4 3

To my father
Louis N. Katz
1897–1973

CONTENTS

FOREWORD

The cardiovascular pandemic is now advancing at an alarming pace in many parts of the world. Epidemiologists inform us that by 2020—in a mere fifteen years—cardiovascular disease will be responsible for 25 million deaths annually, 36% of all deaths, and for the first time in the history of our species, it will be the most common cause of death. Thus, cardiovascular disease may now be considered to be humankind's most serious health threat.

On a more positive note, age-adjusted cardiovascular mortality and morbidity have been declining steadily for more than two decades in North America and Europe. Translating into the extension of useful life for millions of people, results from advances in cardiovascular science have led to both the prevention and improved treatment of cardiovascular diseases. A few examples of the latter: the impairment of conduction and of automaticity of specialized cardiac tissue, which lead to heart block and other serious bradyarrhythmias can be readily corrected with implantation of a cardiac pacemaker; fatal ventricular fibrillation can be averted with an implanted cardioverter defibrillator; asynchronous ventricular contraction in heart failure can be corrected by biventricular pacing; hypertension secondary to increased activity of the renin-angiotensin-aldosterone axis and of the adrenergic nervous system can be relieved by pharmacologic blockers; the imbalance between myocardial oxygen supply and demand that can lead to debilitating angina pectoris or fatal myocardial infarction can be relieved by increasing oxygen supply and/or reducing demand.

These landmark improvements in cardiac care result directly from the advances in cardiovascular physiology and pathophysiology that occurred during the first half of the twentieth century, an era when physiology was devoted largely to the study of the function of the intact heart. It then became clear that further understanding of cardiovascular function required a focus on progressively smaller components of the organ. Accordingly, there has been a steady march from the examination of the whole heart to strips of cardiac muscle, to individual myocytes, to organelles within the myocyte, to the proteins of which these organelles are composed, and to the genes that encode these proteins. In other words, a reductionist approach has been dominant in cardiovascular (and other biomedical) sciences for more than fifty years. An important subsequent step will be to obtain a clearer understanding of how the individual components affect the function of the whole heart in the intact human.

This magnificent fourth edition of the now classic text, Katz's *Physiology of the Heart*, considers the normal and diseased heart at all of these levels. After an incisive exposition of cellular, subcellular, molecular, and genetic processes in the first half of the book, the second half explains how these processes affect the function of the entire organ, both in health and disease.

What is, of course, so remarkable is that *Physiology of the Heart* remains a single-authored comprehensive text, probably among the last of its kind. It is a tour de force that reflects Dr. Katz's rich experience as a creative scientist, a gifted educator, and an experienced clinician. It flows smoothly without the repetition, inconsistencies, gaps, and abrupt changes in style that are characteristic of so many multi-authored texts. Dr. Katz has the rare gift of explaining complex concepts so that they can be readily understood by students and physicians without advanced training in cardiovascular science. This book will also be especially useful to fundamental cardiovascular investigators who today, more than ever before, need to understand how the brick on which they are laboring fits into and is an integral part of the total structure. *Physiology of the Heart* will excite scientists, practitioners, and trainees about the heart, and it will thereby help to move the field forward.

This book improves with every edition. I can't wait for the fifth!

Eugene Braunwald, MD
Boston, MA

PREFACE TO THE FIRST EDITION

Why write a textbook about the biophysical basis of cardiac function? Of what importance are the energetics and chemistry of myocardial contraction to anyone but a physical chemist or a biochemist? Why should electrical potentials at the surface of the myocardial cell concern those who are not basic electrophysiologists? The answers to all of these questions lie in the fact that *virtually every important physiological, pharmacological, or pathological change in cardiac function arises from alterations in the physical and chemical processes that are responsible for the heartbeat.*

Although it remains fashionable to consider the heart as a muscular pump, this organ is much more than a hollow viscus that provides mechanical energy to propel blood through the vasculature. It is an intricate biological machine that contains, within each cell, a complex of control and effector mechanisms. Both the strength of cardiac contraction and its electrical control are modulated by alterations in one or more of these cellular mechanisms, which are involved in the fundamental processes of excitability, excitation-contraction coupling, and contraction.

This text is written for medical students and graduate students in the biological sciences, and for the physician who would like to find a simplified exposition of our current understanding of the physiological and biophysical basis of cardiac function. Therefore, this book is intended to provide a synoptic view of our present knowledge in this rapidly expanding area. The major emphasis is on the relationships between the biochemical properties of individual constituents of the myocardial cell, the biophysics of cardiac muscle function, and the performance of the intact heart.

The task of relating these different aspects of cardiac function to each other has required much selectivity, and undoubtedly, an excess of simplification and speculation. There can be no doubt that much of this conceptual material will become invalid as our knowledge of cardiac function advances. This is, after all, the lesson taught to us by the history of science. The early neurophysiologists who tried to understand nerve conduction as the passage of fluid down hollow tubes were trying to explain physiological phenomena in terms of the limited biophysical knowledge of their time. With the development of an understanding of animal electricity, the focus in neurophysiology shifted to studies of the electrical properties of the nervous system, and attempts were made to explain phenomena such as neuron-to-neuron communication and memory in terms of electrical circuitry. More recently, the enormous advances in our knowledge of chemical transmitters and the potential for information storage as newly synthesized macromolecules has cast doubt on many of the theories of the great neurophysiologists of the last century.

Yet these were not unintelligent scientists. They were, however, required to interpret their observations within the framework of knowledge that existed during their lifetime. It would be presumptuous indeed for us now to assume that the evolution of new principles of science has ended. For this reason, no apology is made for the misconceptions and faulty interpretation that will inevitably accompany the present attempt to organize our knowledge of cardiac function in terms of the broad principles that are understood today.

The only true "facts" in biology are the results of individual experiments carried out under controlled conditions by a carefully defined methodology. Yet, it is not the purpose of this book to catalogue and discuss the biological "facts;" for this, the reader is referred to the large number of reviews, symposia, multi-authored texts, and, most important, individual scientific papers. Instead, the present text attempts to identify and describe the unifying themes that connect different lines of investigation of the function of the heart and, in so doing, to set out interpretations of these biological "facts." The bibliographies to each chapter are intentionally brief and generally include one or more recent reviews to which the interested student may refer for more complete lists of references. In some cases, "classic" articles are also cited.

Every effort has been made to keep this book simple—suitable for use as a text for graduate and undergraduate teaching. Achievement of this goal, however, requires the resolution, more or less arbitrarily as the case may require, of many serious conflicts, as well as the addition of speculative material to connect important biochemical, biophysical, physiological, and pathophysiological observations. It is the author's intention that these departures into the realm of speculation be clearly identified in the text. Yet the expert in these fields will undoubtedly be troubled by this attempt to provide a coherent and unified text. While the author is not laboring under the illusion that all of his interpretations will prove correct, it seems especially important to provide the student with an indication of the significance of the many biological "facts" describing the heart and its function rather than just to catalogue specific experimental findings. It is, after all, the pattern on the fabric that holds the interest of most of us, rather than the threads. For this reason, though with apologies to the protagonists of opposing viewpoints, the author has chosen the present format for this text.

Arnold M. Katz
Heidelberg, Germany
1976

PREFACE

The pace of discovery in cardiac physiology has accelerated rapidly during the 30 years since I started writing the first edition of *Physiology of the Heart*. Areas such as muscle mechanics, hemodynamics, and electrocardiography have advanced within an established framework of knowledge; although details are being filled in, these can be viewed as mature sciences. Progress has been more significant in the fields of energetics and metabolism, excitation–contraction coupling and relaxation, and cardiac electrophysiology, where new concepts are illuminating our understanding of human disease. Most dramatic—and of greatest importance clinically—have been advances in areas relating to signal transduction and regulation, which were only briefly mentioned in the first edition. In 1991, when I wrote the second edition, there seemed to be two types of regulatory mechanism, which I called *phasic* and *tonic*, that mediated short-term and long-term responses, respectively. Ten years later, in the third edition, I referred to these as *functional signaling*, which mediates transient changes in such physiological variables as blood pressure, contractility, and cardiac rhythm; and *proliferative signaling*, which by modifying protein synthesis, gene expression, cell cycling, and programmed cell death (apoptosis) bring about long-lasting changes in the size, shape, and molecular composition of the heart. During the 5 years preceding this fourth edition, abnormal proliferative signaling has emerged both as a major cause of heart disease and as a target for therapy.

The importance of abnormal proliferative signaling in heart disease cannot be overstated, as it has been implicated in the three major causes of cardiovascular death. *Myocardial infarction* ("heart attack"), in which the heart is the victim of an underlying pathophysiology in the coronary arteries, results from a lifelong process in which abnormal proliferative signaling participates in cycles of injury and healing in the vessel wall. Equally important is the role of abnormal proliferative signaling in *heart failure*, which the first edition of *Physiology of the Heart* described as a hemodynamic syndrome where pump function is impaired by reduced myocardial contractility; a brief discussion of hypertrophy focused mainly on the biochemical abnormalities that depress contractile protein interactions. During the following years, our understanding of heart failure changed dramatically when drugs that inhibit proliferative signaling were found to prolong survival; this shift in perspective was reflected in the second and third editions, which discussed how abnormal growth responses might cause the overloaded heart to deteriorate. Understanding of *cardiac arrhythmias*, the third major cause of cardiovascular death, has been enhanced by the discovery of molecular abnormalities involving cardiac ion channels that not only cause heritable arrhythmias, but when initiated by abnormal proliferative signaling provide a substrate for arrhythmias in other conditions, notably heart failure.

The clinical impact of these and other advances in the basic sciences has cast a new light on the often cited "gap" between bench and bedside. It is generally assumed that the rapid growth of molecular and clinical knowledge is widening this gap; however, the history of discovery in heart failure makes it clear that these advances are, instead, filling the gap. For the ancient Greeks and Romans, health was a balance between opposing principles (the four humors) that, because blood was believed to carry heat generated by the heart, provided the rationale for bleeding in the treatment for fever. William Harvey's description of the circulation in 1628, showing that the heart is a pump and not a furnace, made it possible for 18th-century clinician-pathologists to appreciate the hemodynamics of heart failure. This knowledge was to have little impact on patient care until the development of cardiac surgery more than three centuries later. The once prevalent view that life is governed by mysterious "vitalistic" forces was challenged in the early 19th century, when biological processes were found to obey quantifiable physical and chemical laws. Thermodynamics, one set of natural laws, provided a foundation for cardiac physiology during the 19th and most of the 20th centuries, but made few contributions to patient care aside from reinforcing the view that heart failure should be treated with bed rest, a recommendation now recognized as causing more harm than good. Ernest Starling's description of the "Law of the Heart" in 1915, which was stimulated by his efforts to apply thermodynamics to cardiac physiology, highlighted the importance of hemodynamics and set the stage for a generation of discovery that was led by Carl Wiggers. When Werner Forssmann, André Cournand, and Dickinson Richards pioneered the clinical use of cardiac catheterization in the 1940s, this hemodynamic knowledge came to play a key role in the development of cardiac surgery. In the 1950s, Stanley Sarnoff's description of "families of Starling curves" made it possible to demonstrate that contractility is depressed in failing hearts. Between the 1960s and 1980s, the gap between basic science and clinical cardiology narrowed further when Eugene Braunwald and others brought this new physiology to the bedside. In that era as well, recognition of the role of calcium in regulating cardiac contraction and relaxation stimulated development of inotropic drugs that could improve hemodynamics in patients with acute heart failure. However, experiences with these drugs in chronic heart failure began to unravel the widely held view that this syndrome is largely a hemodynamic disorder caused by a weakened heart; this occurred in the early 1990s, when clinical trials showed that although inotropic drugs improve short-term symptoms, they shorten long-term survival. At the same time, other trials demonstrated that vasodilators, which because of their energy-sparing effects are of short-term benefit in patients with heart failure, often fail to improve long-term prognosis and sometimes have serious adverse effects. Explanations for these and other unexpected findings became apparent when drugs that inhibit maladaptive proliferative signaling were found to improve survival, even though some could transiently worsen symptoms. Heart failure research began to draw on the emerging field of molecular biology, which facilitated efforts to understand how proliferative responses can be both adaptive and maladaptive in the failing heart. The resulting interplay between clinical cardiology and molecular biology, one of the major topics of this text, has not only revolutionized treatment for heart failure, but also has stimulated studies in transgenic mice that have virtually obliterated the gap between bench and bedside.

Although basic research has become increasingly relevant to clinical practice, the flood of new information is making it increasingly difficult to teach the basic sciences to medical students and other health professionals. Much as inflating a balloon separates points on its surface, the current expansion of both basic and clinical knowledge is drawing preclinical and bedside teaching away from one another. This is why it is more and more difficult to find teachers who are competent in both basic science and clinical medicine, and why students commonly complain that they are taught basic science by professors who know little about clinical medicine, and clinical medicine by professors who do not understand basic science. These difficulties are heightened by two opposing trends. On the one hand, optimal patient care is becoming more dependent on a thorough understanding of physiology without which it is difficult, and often impossible, to develop an appropriate plan for prevention and therapy. Operating against this need to know the basic mechanisms of disease is a second trend, the perceived need to simplify the basic science taught to health care professionals. In an already overcrowded curriculum, this conflict generates pressures to shorten the time allocated for teaching the mechanisms of disease, which often leaves practitioners without the foundation needed to deliver optimal care to their patients. Similarly, basic science trainees, while expert in specific areas of fields like molecular biology, may not know how these basic processes relate to human disease.

These challenges have played an important role in shaping this revision of *Physiology of the Heart*, which is now divided into four parts. Part I—which reviews the structure, biochemistry, and biophysics of the normal heart—includes seven chapters that describe the mechanisms by which the heart contracts and relaxes and how it provides energy for this mechanical activity. Part II contains three chapters on regulation that detail the functional signal transduction systems that bring about short-term responses in cardiac performance, and the proliferative signaling systems that control long-term changes in the size, shape, and composition of the heart. Part III integrates Parts I and II in describing the normal pumping of the heart and the electrical systems that control its beating. The pathophysiology of three major types of heart disease are described more fully in Part IV, which begins with a review of the electrocardiogram, and concludes with discussions of arrhythmias, ischemic heart disease, and heart failure.

Specific changes include a new chapter in Part I that brings together the material on muscle energetics and energy production and a chapter that discusses the importance of the cytoskeleton in proliferative signaling. Descriptions of the biochemical mechanisms that regulate cardiac performance are updated from the third edition. Part II provides reorganized and expanded chapters on functional and proliferative signaling, and the chapters in Part III on cardiac ion channels and the electrical activity of the heart have been updated extensively. Few changes have been made in the chapter relating to the electrocardiogram, which has been moved to Part IV, but descriptions of the arrhythmias and their clinical manifestations have been modified and combined into a single chapter that describes new discoveries regarding molecular abnormalities in the cardiac ion channels. The discussions of ischemic heart disease and heart failure that complete this text have been revised to reflect the growing impact of molecular biology on the management of these syndromes.

A major goal in preparing the fourth edition of *Physiology of the Heart* has been to return my text to the relatively simple approach used in the first, and most successful, edition. Although this has been like cleaning out a cluttered attic, I have been able to reduce the size of this book while, at the same time, adding a great deal of new material. As in previous editions, the text is designed primarily for the nonexpert, so no attempt has been made to document every detail; instead, I have included bibliographies to provide starting points for further reading. I have kept a few references to classical papers, some over 50 years old, that provide clear descriptions of important concepts. I again emphasize that this is not a reference book to be consulted to verify facts, but instead is intended to explain concepts.

This text is written for medical and dental students as well as students of nursing, physical therapy, echocardiography, and other emerging fields of cardiology. It also is intended to help physicians and other health professionals learn what has happened since the completion of their formal training and to provide an overview for scientists who would like to relate a special area of basic research to the overall physiology of the heart. Stated simply, my goal is to help the health care provider to learn more about the basic sciences, and the basic scientist to learn more about how the heart works in health and disease.

I am aware that my attempt to cover a broad range of topics, which range from molecular biology through cell biochemistry and organ physiology to clinical cardiology, might be viewed as presumptuous. Although my perspectives are based on more than 50 years of experience as a basic scientist and 40 years as a clinical cardiologist and teacher, I am certainly not an expert in all of the fields covered in this text. It is therefore likely that some of my interpretations may prove to be incorrect. However, I take comfort in a statement attributed to Dr. C. Sidney Burwell, who was Dean of Harvard Medical School in the early 1950s, to the effect that "half of what the faculty teaches to medical students is wrong, but the faculty does not know which half."

The importance of a scientific foundation in medical practice was stated with remarkable clarity by William Osler, who in 1902 wrote: "A physician without physiology practices a sort of pop-gun pharmacy, hitting now the disease and again the patient, he himself not knowing which." Osler's observation is of even greater relevance today because physicians have access to powerful physiologically based therapy that, when used properly, is of immeasurable value to the patient. However, clinical observations and randomized controlled trials have made it clear that treatment lacking a solid basis in physiology can do more harm than good. It is my hope that the material presented in the following pages will help the reader gain an understanding of the physiology of the heart and so enhance both patient care and scientific discovery.

Arnold M. Katz, MD, D.MED (HON), FACP, FACC
Norwich, Vermont

ACKNOWLEDGMENTS

It has been more than 30 years since I had planned to coauthor a textbook on cardiac physiology with my father, to whom this book is dedicated. Dad's death in 1973 made this impossible, but it is my hope that those who remember him will recognize his forthright and lucid approach while reading this text.

I began the 1st edition of this book when I was Philip J. and Harriet L. Goodhart Professor of Medicine (Cardiology) at the Mount Sinai School of Medicine of the City of New York; the text was written during a sabbatical year with Professor Wilhelm Hasselbach at the Max-Planck-Institut-für Medizinische Forschung in Heidelberg, Germany with support from the Alexander von Humboldt Stiftung. The 2nd edition was written during a sabbatical year spent at Dartmouth Medical School when I was Professor of Medicine (Cardiology) at the University of Connecticut, while the 3rd edition and this 4th edition were written on our hilltop in Norwich, Vermont, after I had retired from the University of Connecticut. I thank Dartmouth Medical School for giving me access to their superb medical library and an internet link that allowed me to work from my home. Ms. Lorraine Moseley and Ms. Georgia Willette provided illustrations for the first two editions, some of which appear in this update; however, I prepared most of the drawings in this edition using a computer system graciously provided by Lippincott Williams and Wilkins.

I warmly acknowledge the probing questions posed by the many students I have taught over the past 40 years at Columbia University, the University of Chicago, the Mount Sinai School of Medicine, the University of Connecticut, and Dartmouth Medical School. These students continue to serve as gentle but firm critics of my efforts to explain things. I also thank Dr. K. Hashimoto and his colleagues for spotting several errors in the 3rd Edition.

The understanding of my children and their families when I disappeared during their visits to work on this edition is gratefully acknowledged, as are Telemachus and Peisistratus ("Max" and "Pi"), our two Springer Spaniels, who took me away from my computer for walks in the woods that restored my circulation and recharged my intellectual batteries. Above all, I thank my wife Phyllis for her steadfast and loving support during the past 46 years, and for providing an intellectually stimulating and tranquil environment without which this text could not have been written.

Arnold M. Katz MD, D.MED. (HON), FACP, FACC
Professor of Medicine Emeritus,
University of Connecticut School of Medicine,
Visiting Professor of Medicine and Physiology,
Dartmouth Medical School

Structure, Biochemistry, and Biophysics

1

STRUCTURE OF THE HEART
AND CARDIAC MUSCLE

It has been shown by reason and experiment that blood by the beat of the ventricles flows through the lungs and heart and is pumped to the whole body . . . the blood in the animal body moves around in a circle continuously, and . . . the action or function of the heart is to accomplish this by pumping. This is the only reason for the motion and beat of the heart.

William Harvey
Exercitatio Anatomica de Moto Cordis et Sanguinis in Animalibus, 1628

William Harvey's proof that the heart is a muscular pump overthrew the view, which had dominated European thought for more than 1,000 years, that the heart is the source of the body's heat. Although this made it possible for 18th- and 19th-century anatomical pathologists to understand abnormalities in pump function (Katz, 1997, 1998), it was not until the mid 1950s that efforts to understand the heartbeat began to use new understanding of cell biochemistry and biophysics (Katz and Lorell, 2000). At the end of the 20th century, discoveries in molecular biology made it possible to understand how abnormalities involving specific proteins modify cardiac performance (Katz and Katz, 1991). These findings revealed an elaborate molecular architecture that organizes the heart's electrical activity and maximizes its mechanical efficiency (Katz and Katz, 1989).

ORGAN STRUCTURE

The heart is made up of four pumping chambers: the *right* and *left atria* and the *right* and *left ventricles* (Fig. 1-1). *Atrioventricular valves* lie between the cavities of the atria and ventricles: the *tricuspid valve* on the right and the *mitral valve* on the left. *Semilunar valves*, named for their crescent-shaped cusps, separate each ventricle from its great artery: the *pulmonic valve* between the right ventricle and pulmonary artery and the *aortic valve* between the left ventricle and aorta. All four valves lie in a plane within a connective tissue "skeleton" that separates the atria and ventricles within which the mitral, tricuspid, and

3

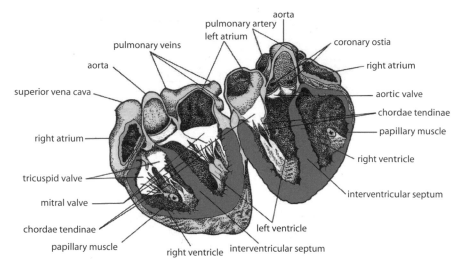

FIGURE 1-1   Major structures in a human heart opened after transection slightly anterior to the midline. (Modified from Berne and Levy, 1967.)

aortic valves surround a fibrous triangle called the *central fibrous body* (Fig. 1-2). The heart's fibrous skeleton, which can be viewed as a connective tissue "insulator" separating electrically active cardiac myocytes in the atria and ventricles, is penetrated by the *AV (atrioventricular) bundle* (also called the *common bundle* or *bundle of His*), a strand of specialized cardiac muscle that normally provides the only electrical connection between the atria and ventricles. Damage to this critical conducting structure is an important cause of AV block (Chapter 16). When the heart is viewed from the apex, the rounded margin of the left ventricle forms an obtuse angle, whereas the margin of the right ventricle is sharper, like an acute angle; this explains use of the terms *obtuse marginal* and *acute marginal* in naming branches of the coronary arteries (see below).

The semilunar aortic and pulmonary valve cusps are supported by thick tendinous margins. *Sinus of Valsalva* lie behind each of the three aortic valve cusps; the anterior and left posterior sinuses contain the orifices of coronary arteries, while the right posterior, often called the *noncoronary* sinus, does not give rise to a coronary artery (Fig. 1-2). The larger cusps of the mitral and tricuspid valves are tethered at their margins by fibrous *chordae tendinae* that attach to *papillary muscles*, which are "fingers" of myocardium that project into the right and left ventricular cavities (Fig. 1-1). Much as the strands of a parachute arise from a skydiver's harness, several chordae tendinae fan out from each papillary muscle to the valve margins. Laxity of the connective tissue supporting the mitral valve can allow the leaflets to move backward (prolapse) into the atria when intraventricular pressure rises during systole (Becker and

POSTERIOR

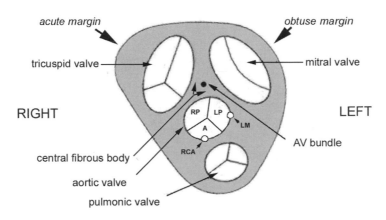

ANTERIOR

FIGURE 1-2 Schematic diagram of the fibrous skeleton of the heart, viewed from above, showing the 4 valves and the atrioventricular (AV) bundle that crosses this insulating structure through the *central fibrous body*. Sinuses of Valsalva lie behind the aortic valve cusps, two of which give rise to coronary arteries. The ostium of the left main (LM) lies in the left posterior sinus (LP) while that of the right coronary artery (RCA) lies in the anterior sinus (A); the third sinus of Valsalva, the right posterior (RP), is called the *noncoronary* sinus because it does not give rise to a coronary artery. The sharper right border of the heart forms the *acute margin*, the more rounded left border is the *obtuse margin*.

deWit, 1979). The abnormal valve opening, which can cause an audible "click," may permit blood to leak into the left atrium (mitral regurgitation), causing a late systolic murmur. This syndrome, called *mitral valve prolapse*, is often of no clinical significance, but when caused by connective tissue abnormalities, significant mitral regurgitation can occur. Rupture of a papillary muscle, which sometimes occurs after myocardial infarction (see Chapter 17), causes severe mitral regurgitation and is often fatal.

Architecture of the Walls of the Heart

The thin-walled atria, which develop relatively low pressures, contain ridges of myocardium called *pectinate muscles* that may represent preferential conducting pathways linking the sinoatrial (SA) and AV nodes; these are sometimes referred to as *internodal tracts* or *sinoatrial ring bundles* (Hayashi et al., 1982; Anderson and Ho, 1998). The ventricles develop much higher pressures than the atria and therefore have thicker muscular walls. The left ventricle, which has approximately three times the mass and twice the thickness of the right ventricle, can be viewed as a "pressure pump" whose cavity resembles an elongated cone in which inflow and outflow tracts lie side-to-side in the wider end (Fig. 1-3). The right ventricle, which pumps at lower pressure and operates as a

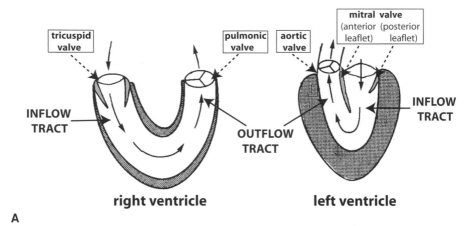

A

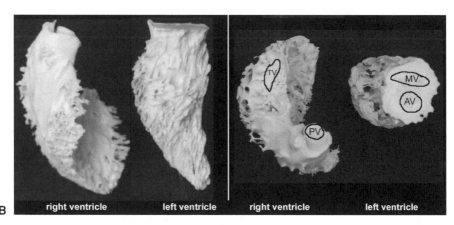

B

FIGURE 1-3 **A:** Schematic anterior views of the right and left ventricular chambers. In the U-shaped right ventricle, the inflow (tricuspid) and outflow (pulmonic) valves are widely separated, whereas in the conical left ventricle, the mitral and aortic valves lie side-by-side, where they are separated by the anterior leaflet of the mitral valve. **B:** Casts of canine right and left ventricular cavities. **Left:** Anterior view. **Right:** Superior view showing approximate locations of the pulmonic (PV) and tricuspid (TV) valves in the right ventricle, and the aortic (AV) and mitral (MV) valves in the left ventricle.

"volume pump," is shaped like a crescent with inflow through the tricuspid valve at one end and outflow through the pulmonic valve at the other (Fig. 1-3). During systole, the interventricular septum normally moves toward the left ventricular free wall and participates in left ventricular ejection. In chronic right ventricular overload—for example, in patients with pulmonary hypertension—the septum can move paradoxically away from the left ventricular cavity during systole to aid right ventricular ejection.

The heart, along with a small amount of fluid, is contained within a noncompliant fibrous sac called the *pericardium* whose inner surface, the *parietal pericardium*, is continuous with the *epicardium*, a layer of connective tissue that covers the outer surface of the heart. The cavities of the atria and ventricles, along with the valves, are lined with another connective tissue layer called the *endocardium* (Brutsaert, 1989). Because the heart is contained within the rigid pericardium (see below), the ventricles interact with one another. These interactions are especially important in diastole, when dilatation of one ventricle can impair the filling of the other (Yacoub, 1995; Santamore and Dell'Italia, 1998; Morris-Thurgood and Frenneaux, 2000).

The left ventricle, which is conical in shape during diastole, becomes more spherical as intraventricular pressure rises during systole (Hawthorne, 1969). Ejection propels blood superiorly (toward the head) so that—according to Newton's Law, *for every action there is an equal and opposite reaction*—the base of the heart moves inferiorly (toward the feet). This movement, called *descent of the base*, explains the prominent "*x* descent" in the normal venous pulse.

The muscular walls of the ventricles are made up of overlapping sheets—sometimes called *bulbospiral* and *sinuspiral* muscles—that follow spiral paths as they sweep from the fibrous skeleton at the base of the heart to its apex (Fig. 1-4) (Grant, 1965). The muscle fibers at the epicardial surface of the left ventricle tend to parallel the base-apex axis of the heart, whereas those at the endocardial surface are oriented more circumferentially (Streeter et al., 1969) (Fig. 1-5). During systole, as the ventricles empty, these muscle bundles thicken but undergo little angular distortion (Fenton et al., 1978).

Electrical Activation

The heartbeat is initiated and controlled by electrical impulses that are generated and conducted by specialized myocardial cells (Chapter 15). Activation normally begins in the *SA node* (Fig. 1-6), a band of spontaneously depolarizing cells that lies between the superior vena cava and right atrium (Oosthoek et al., 1993b; Verheijck et al., 1998; Anderson and Ho, 1998). Because of its rapid firing rate, the SA node, which is derived from the embryonic right sinus venosus, normally serves as the heart's pacemaker.

The wave of depolarization initiated by the SA node is propagated through atrial myocardium, first to the right atrium and then to the left atrium. After encountering a delay in the *AV node*, which is derived from the embryonic left sinus venosus, the wave of depolarization enters the ventricles though the *AV bundle* (Oosthoek et al., 1993a), which bifurcates at the top of the interventricular septum into *right* and *left bundle branches*. The right bundle branch crosses the right ventricular cavity within the *moderator band*, a muscular bundle that extends from the interventricular septum to the base of the papillary muscle, which supports the anterior leaflet of the tricuspid valve (Fig. 1-6). The left bundle branch is often stated to bifurcate into *anterior* and *posterior fascicles*,

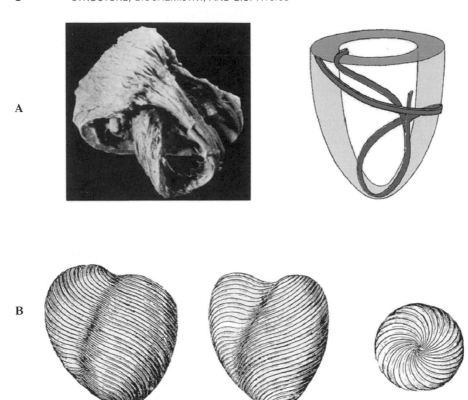

FIGURE 1-4 Spiral musculature of the ventricular walls. **A:** Spiral bundles in a dissected human heart sweep from the fibrous skeleton at the base of the heart (*above, left*) to the apex (*below*). (From Grant RP, 1965, by permission of the American Heart Association.) **B:** Schematic drawing of spiral bundles in the left ventricle. (Modified from Lower, 1669.)

but as discussed in Chapter 15, this is generally an oversimplification. Impulses transmitted via the bundle branches then enter the *His-Purkinje system*, a subendocardial network of rapidly conducting cells that synchronizes ventricular activation. The electrophysiological properties of myocardial cells in different layers of the ventricular wall are not the same;

EPICARDIUM   ENDOCARDIUM

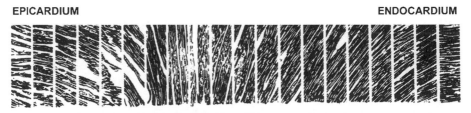

FIGURE 1-5 Reconstruction of the left ventricular wall, prepared from a series of microphotographs, showing different fiber angles between the epicardium (*left*) and endocardium (*right*). (Modified from Streeter et al., 1969, by permission of the American Heart Association.)

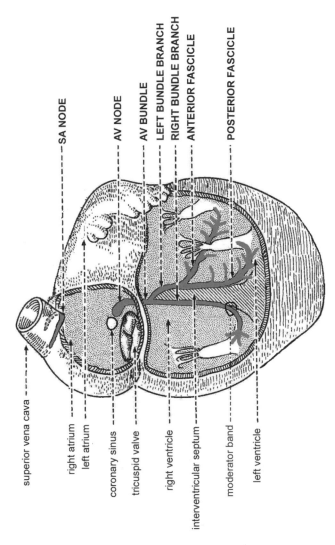

FIGURE 1-6 Conducting system of the human heart (*capitalized labels at right*) and major anatomical features (*lowercase labels at left*). (Modified from Benninghoff, 1944.)

for example, action potential duration in the endocardium is longer than that in the epicardium and is longest in *M-cells* found in the mid-regions of the ventricular wall (see Chapter 14).

THE CORONARY CIRCULATION

Major Epicardial Coronary Arteries

Large epicardial coronary arteries carry virtually all of the blood that supplies the heart. Although a few layers of endocardial myocytes are perfused from the ventricular cavities via *arteriosinusoidal* and *arterioluminal vessels*, this auxiliary blood supply is of no practical importance when a large coronary artery becomes occluded (Chapter 17). The major coronary arteries are abbreviated *LEFT MAIN* (left main coronary artery), *RCA* (right coronary artery), *LAD* (left anterior descending), *CIRC* (circumflex), and *PDA* (posterior descending) (Fig. 1-7). All lie in grooves between the heart's chambers—the RCA and CIRC between the atria and ventricles, the LAD and PDA between the left and right ventricles.

The anatomy of these vessels can be summarized by the statement *"three out of two makes four."* *Two* coronary arteries arise from the aorta

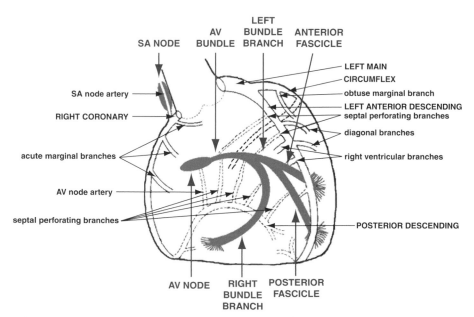

FIGURE 1-7 Major coronary arteries and their branches (*labels at right and left*) and key elements of the cardiac conduction system (*labels above and below*). AV, atrioventricular; SA, sinoatrial.

(RCA and LEFT MAIN) and continue after the LEFT MAIN divides into the LAD and CIRC as *three* vessels (RCA, LAD, and CIRC). After the PDA arises from either the RCA or CIRC, the heart is supplied by *four* large arteries (RCA, LAD, CIRC, and PDA).

The LEFT MAIN, which originates in the left posterior sinus of Valsalva (Fig. 1-2), continues as a single vessel of variable length before dividing into two major branches—the LAD and CIRC (Fig. 1-7). The LAD, which courses down the anterior interventricular groove, gives rise to *septal perforating arteries* that supply the anterior two-thirds of the interventricular septum, *diagonal branches* that supply the anterior wall of the left ventricle, and *right ventricular branches* that provide blood to the anterior wall of the right ventricle. After crossing the apex of the heart, the LAD usually turns upward to run a short distance toward the base in the posterior interventricular groove (Figs. 1-7 and 1-8). The CIRC, which courses to the left in the anterior atrioventricular groove, gives rise to *obtuse marginal branches* that supply the lateral wall of the left ventricle. The PDA, which runs inferiorly toward the apex in the posterior interventricular groove, can be supplied by the CIRC or the RCA. In most human hearts, the CIRC, after reaching the back of the

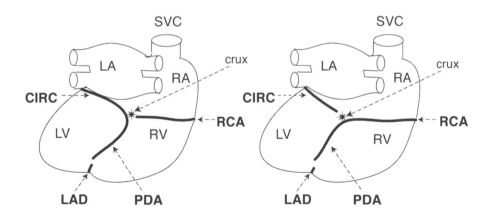

A. Left dominant   B. Right dominant

FIGURE 1-8 Posterior view of the human heart showing left dominant (A) and right dominant (B) coronary artery distribution. In the left dominant, the posterior descending artery (PDA) is a continuation of the circumflex branch of the left coronary artery (CIRC) that runs from the crux of the heart down the posterior interventricular groove; more commonly, in the right dominant distribution, the posterior descending artery is a continuation of the right coronary artery (RCA). The left anterior descending coronary artery (LAD), after wrapping around the inferior surface of the heart, usually courses upward for a short distance in the posterior interventricular groove. LA, left atrium; RA, right atrium; LV, left ventricle; RV, right ventricle; SVC, superior vena cava.

left ventricle, runs only a short distance down the posterior interventricular groove to end near the *crux of the heart*, where the plane of the interventricular septum crosses the plane of the atrioventricular groove (Fig. 1-8B). This distribution, in which the PDA is supplied by the RCA, is called *right dominant* and occurs in approximately 90% of human hearts. In the remaining 10% or so, the CIRC turns downward at the crux to supply the PDA (*left dominant*, Fig. 1-8A).

The RCA, which arises from the anterior aortic sinus, courses toward the right in the anterior atrioventricular groove, where it gives rise to *right ventricular (acute marginal) branches* that supply the free wall of the right ventricle. The RCA then crosses the acute margin of the heart, turns to the left in the posterior atrioventricular groove, and after reaching the *crux* of the heart usually continues in the posterior interventricular groove as the PDA ("right dominant" coronary circulation, Fig. 1-8B).

As already noted, the PDA, which supplies *septal perforating branches* that perfuse the posterior third of the interventricular septum, arises from the RCA in approximately 90% of human hearts and from the CIRC in about 10%.

Coronary atherosclerosis is often described as *one-vessel, two-vessel*, and *three-vessel* disease, terms that describe how many of the three major arteries (RCA, LAD, and CIRC) are narrowed. Obviously, the more vessels that are occluded, the more severe is the coronary disease. LEFT MAIN disease is especially dangerous because this vessel supplies both of the arteries that supply blood to the left ventricle (LAD and CIRC).

Collateral Vessels

The coronary arteries in humans can be viewed as "end-arteries" because there is little flow between the vascular beds supplied by the different major arteries (Factor et al., 1981). Collateral vessels, which connect arterial systems supplied by different major epicardial arteries, are not found at the level of the microcirculation, so that occlusion of a major epicardial artery generally causes an infarct whose borders are sharply demarcated from the adjacent myocardium supplied by other, nonoccluded arteries. Collateral vessels can connect larger arteries, but these are poorly developed in young individuals. However, in patients with chronic coronary atherosclerosis, these collaterals often enlarge and can play an important role in maintaining blood flow to the heart after a major coronary artery is occluded.

Blood Supply to the Ventricular Myocardium

The devastating consequences of coronary occlusion reflect the fact that cardiac contraction depends on an uninterrupted delivery of oxygen (Chapter 2). Oxygenated blood from the epicardial arteries reaches the

epicardial artery   **Epicardium**

muscular branches

muscular branches

epicardial artery

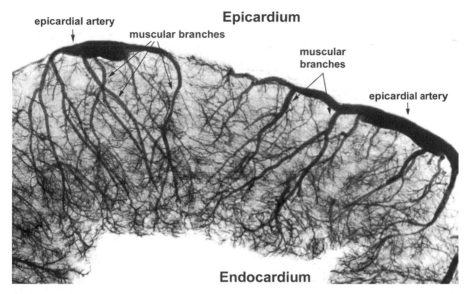

Endocardium

FIGURE 1-9 X-ray microphotograph of a heart injected with radiopaque dye showing muscular branches of large coronary arteries that penetrate the myocardium from the epicardial surface of the ventricle. (Modified from Schäper, 1979.)

myocardium via muscular branches that traverse the walls of the ventricles (Fig. 1-9). Because intramyocardial pressure compresses these vessels, the subendocardial regions of the thick-walled left ventricle are especially vulnerable to coronary artery narrowing. Normal compression of the muscular branches during systole explains why virtually all nutrient coronary flow occurs during diastole.

The *left ventricular papillary muscles* receive their blood supply from large penetrating vessels called *perforators*. The *anterolateral papillary muscle*, which supports the anterior leaflet of the mitral valve, has a dual blood supply derived from branches of the CIRC and LAD. The *posteromedial papillary muscle*, which supports the posterior leaflet, receives its blood supply from the PDA, and thus from the RCA, in the majority of human hearts that are "right dominant," and from the CIRC in those with "left dominant" coronary circulation (see above).

Blood Supply to the Conduction System

The SA node is perfused by the *SA node artery* (Fig. 1-7), which in slightly more than half of human hearts is a branch of the RCA; in the remainder, this artery arises from the CIRC. The AV node is usually supplied by an *AV node artery* that is a branch of the PDA; the blood supply to the AV node is therefore derived from the RCA in about 90% of human hearts and the CIRC in approximately 10%.

The AV bundle, along with proximal portions of both right and left bundle branches, is perfused by *septal perforators* that arise from both the LAD and PDA. Because this critical structure has a dual blood supply, damage to the AV bundle in ischemic heart disease implies that more than one major coronary artery is occluded. The anterior division of the left bundle branch and mid-portion of the right bundle branch are supplied by septal perforators arising from the LAD, while the posterior division of the left bundle branch is perfused by septal perforators supplied by the PDA.

Coronary Venous Drainage

The venous effluent of the heart is collected in veins that parallel the epicardial coronary arteries. Most venous drainage of the left ventricle enters the *coronary sinus*, which parallels the CIRC in the left posterior atrioventricular groove before emptying into the floor of the right atrium. A small portion of the venous drainage of the left ventricle, along with much of that derived from the right ventricle, enters the right atrium through *anterior cardiac veins*. A minor fraction of the venous drainage of the ventricular myocardium drains directly into the cavities of the right and left ventricles by way of *Thebesian veins*.

The ostium of the coronary sinus provides a landmark for the AV node, which lies immediately above this opening. Because the coronary sinus passes to the left behind the heart in the left atrioventricular groove, specially designed catheters can be used to record the electrical activity of the left atrium and ventricle, stimulate these structures, and perform ablation therapy on the left side of the heart.

FRACTAL ANATOMY OF THE HEART

Many asymmetrical structures in the heart, including the coronary blood vessels, chordae tendineae, and interventricular conduction system, form networks whose outwardly disorganized branching follows complex rules. These are described mathematically as *fractals*, which describe the order often found in seemingly random biological structures (Goldberger et al., 1990) and functional disorders (Goldberger et al., 2002).

LYMPHATICS

The *lymphatic vessels* that drain the heart's interstitium run alongside the coronary arteries and veins in the atrioventricular and interventricular grooves. Most cardiac lymphatic channels cross the anterior surface of the pulmonary artery to reach *pretracheal lymph nodes* that drain through a *cardiac lymph node* situated between the superior vena cava and right innominate artery. The lymph ultimately drains into the thoracic duct (Miller, 1982).

INNERVATION

The heart is richly innervated by both *sympathetic* and *parasympathetic* nerves. Postganglionic sympathetic fibers arise mainly in the fourth and fifth thoracic segments of the spinal cord and form synaptic connections in the cervical and thoracic cervical ganglia (often called *stellate ganglia*) and cardiac plexus. Postsynaptic sympathetic nerves do not form specialized junctions in the heart but instead release their neurotransmitter (norepinephrine) from varicosities that lie in plasma membrane depressions on the surface of cardiac myocytes. The heart's parasympathetic innervation originates in the dorsal efferent nuclei of the medulla oblongata and reach the heart by way of the cardiac branches of the vagus nerve. Preganglionic parasympathetic fibers impinge on postganglionic cells in the SA and AV nodes, the atria, and the heart's blood vessels, but parasympathetic innervation of the ventricular myocardium is more limited.

Sensory fibers that originate in the heart reach the brain stem by way of the cardiac plexus. Stimulation of these fibers informs patients when their heart becomes energy starved. A chest discomfort called *angina pectoris* is the most common perception caused by cardiac ischemia.

Stretch receptors located in the inferior and posterior walls of the left ventricle can evoke a powerful vagal response called the *von Bezold–Jarisch reflex* (Dawes and Comroe, 1954). This reflex, which is often activated in inferior and posterior wall myocardial infarction, can slow the SA node, inhibit conduction through the AV node, and cause blood pressure to fall (see Chapter 17).

HISTOLOGY

The outer surfaces of the atria and ventricles are covered by a layer of squamous cells and a network of fibroelastic connective tissue called the *epicardium*. The *endocardium*, which lines the heart's chambers, is also made up of squamous cells beneath which is a mesh of collagen and elastic fibers and a rudimentary layer of smooth muscle. The *myocardium*, which makes up the vast majority of the heart's thickness, contains both myocytes and connective tissue. Although cardiac myocytes represent most of the myocardial mass, approximately 70% of the cells are smaller nonmyocytes that include vascular smooth muscle, endothelial cells, and fibroblasts. The latter secrete and maintain the connective tissue fibers that contribute to the heart's tensile strength and stiffness. This connective tissue framework is organized into the *endomysium*, which surrounds individual cardiac myocytes; the *perimysium*, which supports groups of myocytes; and the *epimysium*, which encases the entire muscle (Fig. 1-10).

Several types of cardiac myocytes are found in the adult human heart (Fig. 1-11). The most numerous are *working myocytes* of the atria and ventricles that are specialized for contraction. Atrial myocytes are smaller

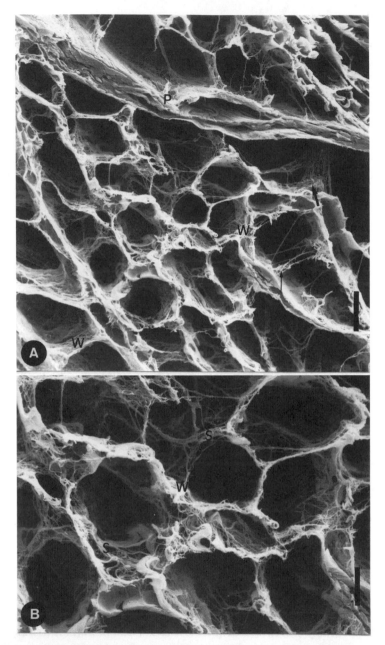

FIGURE 1-10 Connective tissue framework of the human heart, showing groups of myocytes surrounded by the perimysium (P). A weave of endomysium that surrounds the individual myocytes (W) forms lateral struts (S) that connect adjacent cells. Collagen struts also connect myocytes to microvessels (*thin arrow*) and to the perimysium (*thick arrow*). (From Rossi et al., 1998, by permission of the American Heart Association.)

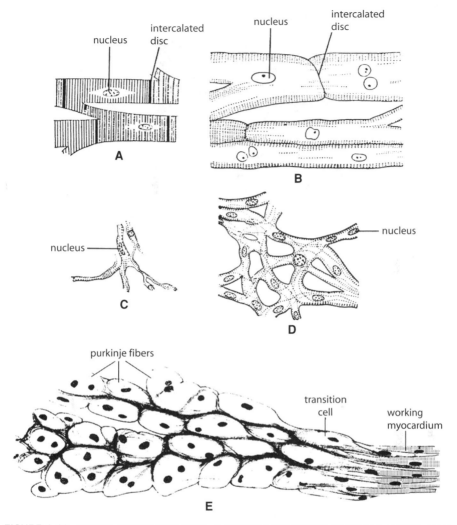

FIGURE 1-11 Human cardiac myocytes. **A:** Working ventricular myocytes contain cross striations, central nuclei, and intercalated discs. **B:** Purkinje fibers are large, poorly staining cells with sparse cross striations. The SA node **(C)** and AV node **(D)** are networks of small, sparsely cross-striated cells. **E:** Transition cells are seen where Purkinje fibers (*left*) impinge on the working myocardium (*right*). (Modified from Benninghoff, 1944.)

in diameter than those of the ventricles. *Purkinje fibers*—found in the AV bundle, bundle branches, and ventricular endocardium—are specialized for rapid conduction. *Nodal cells* in the SA and AV nodes are responsible for pacemaker activity and an atrioventricular conduction delay, respectively. Additional heterogeneity is seen at the molecular level, where histologically similar cardiac myocytes represent different molecular phenotypes that are distributed in a mosaic pattern (Fig. 1-12) (Sartore et al., 1981; Bouvagnet et al., 1984).

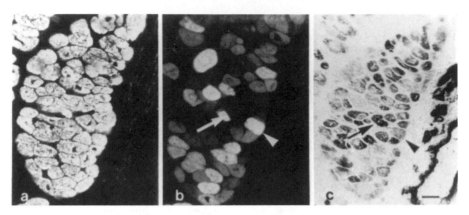

FIGURE 1-12 Microphotographs of serial sections from human right atrium incubated with two different immunofluorescent antiventricular human myosin antibodies (a, b) and stained histochemically for myosin ATPase activity (c). One antibody binds to all atrial myosin isoforms (a); the other binds more strongly to some cells (b). The arrowheads in (b) and (c) show a fiber that binds the antibody used (b) but exhibits weak ATPase activity in (c), while the arrows show a cell that binds weakly to the antibody but exhibits high ATPase activity. Bar = 20 μM. (Reprinted from Bouvagnet et al., 1984, by permission of the American Heart Association.)

The cells of the myocardium are arranged in a branched network that was once believed to represent an anatomical syncytium. However, the *intercalated discs*, which are densely staining transverse bands that characteristically appear at right angles to the long axis of the cardiac myofibers, are now known to represent specialized cell-cell junctions that contain regions of low electrical resistance (see below). While not a true anatomical syncytium, the heart functions as if all of the myocytes are in free electrical communication.

Working cardiac myocytes, which usually contain a single centrally located nucleus, are filled with cross-striated myofibers and mitochondria (Fig. 1-11A). *Purkinje fibers*, which are specialized for rapid conduction, are large pale cells that contain more glycogen but fewer contractile filaments and mitochondria (Fig. 1-11B). Cells intermediate in appearance between the Purkinje fibers and the working cardiac myocytes are called *transition cells* (Fig. 1-11E). The myocytes in the *SA node* (Fig. 1-11C) and *AV node* (Fig. 1-11D), like Purkinje fibers, are rich in glycogen and contain few contractile filaments; however, nodal cells conduct slowly because of their small size and high internal electrical resistance. Unlike the working myocytes of the atria and ventricles, which use oxidative reactions to generate ATP, the myocytes that make up the heart's conduction system rely on anaerobic energy production (Henry and Lowry, 1983).

Atrial cardiac myocytes contain granules that represent stores of the biologically active *atrial natriuretic peptide* (ANP), which is natriuretic and diuretic and relaxes vascular smooth muscle. The heart is therefore not only a pump, but also an endocrine organ. Small amounts of ANP and the structurally related *brain natriuretic peptide* (BNP) also are found in the ventricles. These peptides are released when the walls of the heart are stretched and can be viewed as "volume sensors" that help the body to defend against expanded blood volume (for a review, see Levin et al., 1998; Boomama and Van der Meiracker, 2001).

ULTRASTRUCTURE

The *contractile proteins*, which make up almost one-half of the volume of working cardiac myocytes, are organized in a regular array of cross-striated myofibrils (Figs. 1-13 and 1-14). Most of the remaining cell volume is occupied by *mitochondria* that generate the large amounts of chemical energy required for contraction (Table 1-1). Key membrane systems that regulate cardiac performance include the *plasma membrane*, which separates the cytosol from the surrounding extracellular space, and the intracellular membranes of the *sarcoplasmic reticulum* (Table 1-2). The most abundant membranes are those of the mitochondria (Page, 1978).

Myofibrils

The cross-striated pattern in working cardiac myocytes (Figs. 1-13–1-15) reflects the distribution of contractile protein filaments. The more darkly staining striations, which contain a parallel array of thick filaments (see below), strongly rotate polarized light and are anisotropic (birefringent), hence their designation *A-bands*. The more lightly staining striations, which contain only thin filaments, are the more isotropic (less birefringent) *I-bands*. Each I-band is bisected by a darkly staining *Z-line*. The fundamental morphological unit of striated muscle is the *sarcomere*, which is defined as the region between two Z-lines; each sarcomere therefore includes a central A-band and two adjacent half I-bands.

The thick filaments that extend the length of the A-band are polymers of *myosin* and a huge protein called *titin*. The central regions of the thick filaments also contain *myosin-binding protein C, M-protein, myomesin*, and the MM isoform of *creatine phosphokinase* (see Chapter 5). *Cross-bridges* that project from the thick filaments and interact with the thin filaments represent the heads of myosin molecules. The thin filaments are double-stranded *actin* polymers that include *tropomyosin* and the three proteins of the *troponin complex* (see Chapter 4). At the Z-lines, the thin filaments are interwoven with several cytoskeletal proteins, including α-*actinin, Cap Z (β-actinin), nebulette*, and *desmin*, which

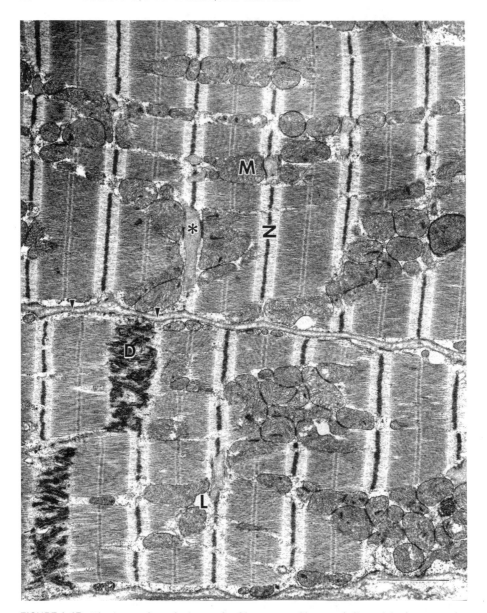

FIGURE 1-13 Electron microphotograph of two normal human left ventricular myocytes (*above and below*) that are separated by a thin band of extracellular fluid (*oriented from right to left in center of figure*). Sarcomeres are aligned within each cell. Endomysium separates the cells (*arrowheads*). M, mitochondria; Z, Z-lines; D, intercalated disc; L, lipid droplet; *, t-tubule. Scale bar = 2 μM. (Reproduced with permission from Gerdes et al., 1995.)

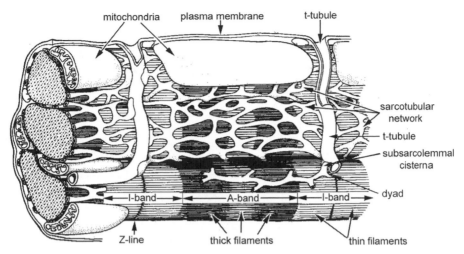

FIGURE 1-14 Ultrastructure of a working cardiac myocyte. Contractile proteins are arranged in a regular array of thick and thin filaments (*seen in cross section at left*). The A-band represents the region of the sarcomere occupied by the thick filaments into which thin filaments extend from either side. The I-band contains only thin filaments that extend toward the center of the sarcomere from Z-lines that bisect each I-band. The sarcomere, the functional unit of the contractile apparatus, lies between two Z-lines and contains one A-band and two half I-bands. The sarcoplasmic reticulum, an intracellular membrane system that surrounds the contractile proteins, consists of the sarcotubular network at the center of the sarcomere and subsarcolemmal cisternae. The latter form specialized composite structures with the transverse tubular system (t-tubules) called *dyads*. The t-tubular membrane is continuous with the sarcolemma; the lumen of the t-tubules contains extracellular fluid. Mitochondria are shown in the central sarcomere and in cross section at left. (Modified from Katz, 1975.)

TABLE 1-1 **Morphology of a Working Myocardial Cell (Rat Left Ventricle)**

Component	Percent of Cell Volume
Myofibrils	47
Mitochondria	36
Sarcoplasmic reticulum	3.5
Subsarcolemmal cisternae	0.35
Sarcotubular network	3.15
Nuclei	2
Other (mainly cytosol)	11.5

Modified from Page, 1978.

TABLE 1-2 **Membrane Areas in a Working Myocardial Cell (Rat Left Ventricle)**

Membrane	μm^2 Membrane Area per μm^3 Cell Volume
Plasma membrane	0.465
Sarcolemma	0.31
t-Tubules	0.15
Nexus	0.005
Total sarcoplasmic reticulum	1.22
Subsarcolemmal cisternae	0.19
Sarcotubular network	1.03
Mitochondria	20

Modified from Page, 1978.

attach the sarcomeres to cell adhesion molecules that link myocytes to each other and to the extracellular matrix (see Chapter 5).

The lengths of the thick and thin filaments remain constant during contraction and relaxation, so that changes in the extent of overlap between thick and thin filaments cause sarcomeres to shorten and lengthen (Fig. 1-16). During systole, changes in the orientation of the myosin cross-bridges

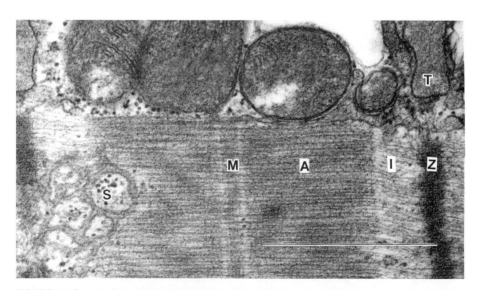

FIGURE 1-15 Electron microphotograph of a sarcomere in normal human left ventricle. A grazing section on the left side of the sarcomere shows the sarcotubular network (S) overlying the I band. Mitochondria are seen above the sarcomere. M, line in the center of the A-band (A); I, I-band; Z, Z-line; T, t-tubule. Scale bar = 2 μM. (Reproduced with permission from Gerdes et al., 1995.)

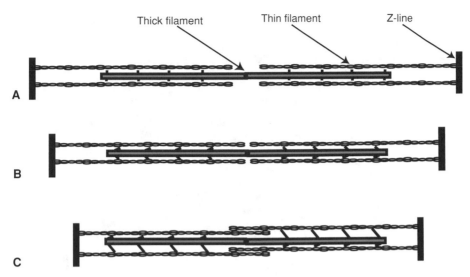

FIGURE 1-16 Schematic diagram of a sarcomere showing length-dependent changes in the overlap between thick and thin filaments. **A:** At long sarcomere lengths in resting muscle (note myosin cross-bridges at right angles to the thick filament), the thin filaments do not extend to the center of the A-band. **B:** During contraction, the thin filaments are drawn toward the center of the sarcomere (note angulated myosin cross-bridges attached to thin filaments). **C:** As the sarcomere shortens further, the thin filaments of adjacent I-bands pass in the center of the A-band ("double overlap").

draw the thin filaments toward the center of the A-band (see Chapter 4). At very short sarcomere lengths, thin filaments from the two sides of the sarcomere pass in the center of the A-band, giving rise to "double overlap" (Fig. 1-16).

In cross section, the A-band is a hexagonal array of thick filaments, each of which is surrounded by six thin filaments that lie at the trigonal points between adjacent thick filaments (Figs. 1-17 and 1-18).

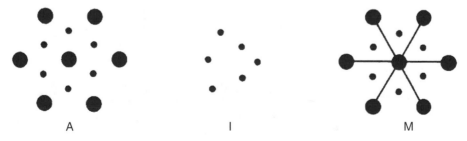

FIGURE 1-17 Schematic cross sections at different levels of the sarcomere. **A:** In the A-band, thin filaments lie at the trigonal points in a hexagonal array of thick filaments. **I:** In the I-band, where thick filaments are absent, the thin filaments are less ordered. **M:** Thin radial filaments made up of myosin-binding protein C in the M-band at the center of the A-band connect adjacent thick filaments.

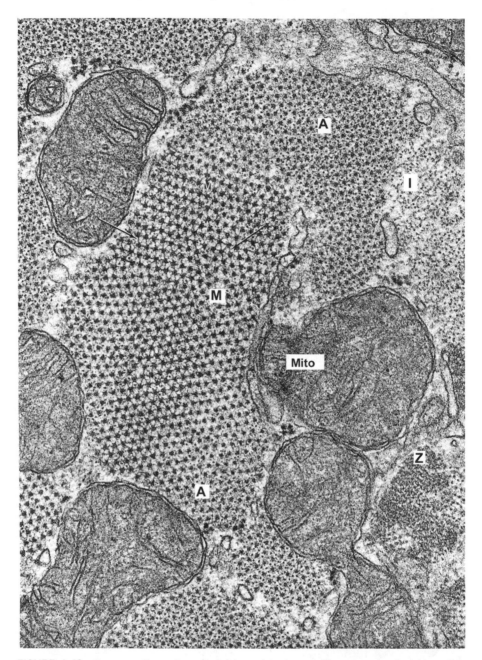

FIGURE 1-18   Cross section of a cat right ventricular papillary muscle showing mitochondria (Mito) and myofilaments cut at the level of the A-band (A), I-band (I), and M-band (M); in the latter, radial filaments link adjacent thick filaments (compare with Fig. 1-17). The Z-line (Z) appears as a dense network. (From McNutt and Fawcett, 1974.)

In the I-band, which lacks thick filaments, the thin filaments are less ordered. Radial cross-links, formed by myosin-binding protein C, link the thick filaments in a hexagonal array at the center of the A-band (Figs. 1-17 and 1-18).

The Plasma Membrane and Transverse Tubular System

The *plasma membrane* (*sarcolemma*), which separates the intracellular and extracellular spaces, forms *transverse tubules* (*t-system*) that extend into the cell (Fig. 1-14). These tubules, which contain extracellular fluid and open freely to the extracellular space, play a key role in excitation-contraction coupling by carrying action potentials deep into the cell (see Chapter 7). The plasma membrane contains channels, carriers, and pumps that regulate cell composition and function; receptors and enzymes that participate in cell signaling; and adhesion molecules that link cells to each other and to the extracellular matrix.

Intracellular Membrane Structures

Cardiac myocytes, like all eukaryotic cells, contain intracellular membrane–delimited organelles (Figs. 1-18–1-21). These include the *nucleus*, which contains the genetic material that determines cell structure, and *mitochondria*, which catalyze the oxidative reactions that generate most of the ATP used by the heart (Chapter 2). Mitochondria include an outer membrane that encircles these organelles and an inner membrane that contains infoldings called *cristae*. The latter contain key enzymes that participate in oxidative phosphorylation. When the heart is fixed under conditions that do not permit oxidative phosphorylation (e.g., low oxygen tension or low substrate concentration), the cristae appear as stacks of flat membrane sheets, whereas in hearts fixed when the mitochondria are carrying out oxidative phosphorylation, the cristae are angulated in an "energized" configuration. Phase contrast studies in living cardiac myocytes show that the mitochondria change constantly, enlarging and contracting, and branching and fusing with one another. Mitochondria contain circular DNA that is characteristic of prokaryotes; this reflects the origin of these organelles as micro-organisms that hundreds of millions of years ago crept into the cells of our progenitors (Margulis, 1970; Roger, 1999; Katz and Berger, 1999). In return for a nutrient-filled environment, these symbiotic invaders provide our hearts with a generous supply of ATP.

The *sarcoplasmic reticulum* (SR)—which takes up, stores, and releases the calcium that regulates contraction and relaxation (Chapter 7) —is a specialized form of the *endoplasmic reticulum* found in virtually every cell type. The endoplasmic reticulum in most cells includes a *rough endoplasmic reticulum* whose outer surface is studded with ribosomes that carry out protein synthesis, and *smooth endoplasmic reticulum* that participates in such processes as lipid metabolism and drug detoxification. In muscle, the major function of these internal membranes, often referred

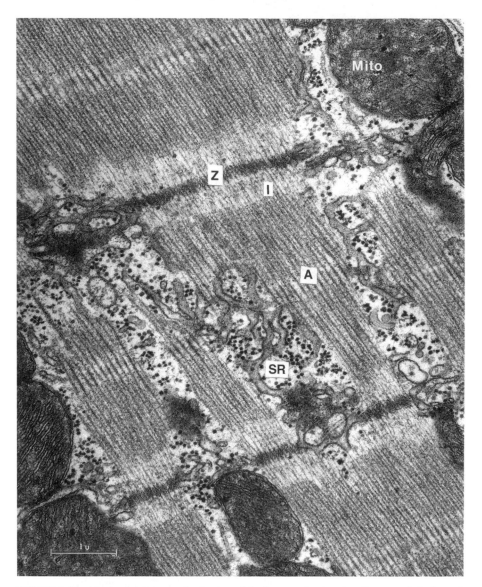

FIGURE 1-19 Electron micrograph of rat ventricular muscle showing the sarcotubular net-work (SR) in a "grazing" section overlying a sarcomere (center). The dark granules are glyco-gen. A faint linear structure, composed of two parallel lines, that crosses the sarcotubular network at the lower right is probably a microtubule. Mito, mitochondria; A, A-band; I, I-band; Z, Z-line. Scale bar = I μm. (Courtesy of Mrs. Judy Upshaw-Earley and Dr. Ernest Page.)

to as the *sarcoendoplasmic reticulum* (SERCA), is to regulate cytosolic calcium concentration.

The cardiac sarcoplasmic reticulum consists of two regions (Figs. 1-14 and 1-20). The *sarcotubular network*, which pumps calcium out of the cytosol, is a network of tubules that surrounds the myofilaments.

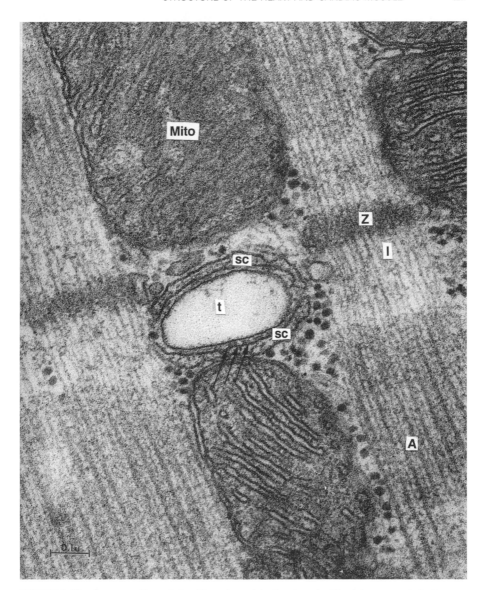

FIGURE 1-20   Cross section of dyad in rat ventricular muscle. The transverse tubular system (t), seen in cross section, lies between two subsarcolemmal cisternae (sc). Electron-dense feet (*arrows*) can be seen in the cytosol between the membranes of the t-tubule and subsarcolemmal cisterna. Mito, mitochondria; A, A-band; I, I-band; Z, Z-line. Scale bar = 0.1 μm. (Courtesy of Mrs. Judy Upshaw-Earley and Dr. Ernest Page.)

Subsarcolemmal cisternae, which release calcium from the sarcoplasmic reticulum into the cytosol in response to plasma membrane depolarization, are flattened structures that form composite structures with the plasma membrane. In the latter, called *dyad*s, the sarcoplasmic reticulum and plasma membranes approach one another but do not fuse. The

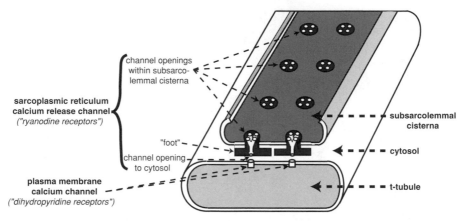

FIGURE 1-21 Schematic diagram of a dyad, showing sarcoplasmic reticulum calcium release channels ("ryanodine receptors") adjacent to plasma membrane calcium channels ("dihydropyridine receptors") in the t-tubule. The former, which form the "feet," have a single opening into the cytosol and four openings into the lumen of the subsarcolemmal cisterna.

narrow cytosolic space between these membranes contains huge electron-dense proteins, often called *feet* because they resemble the feet of a caterpillar (Franzini-Armstrong and Nunzi, 1983) (Figs. 1-20 and 1-21). These foot proteins are the calcium release channels of the sarcoplasmic reticulum (called *ryanodine receptors*) that open to initiate cardiac contraction by allowing calcium to flow out of the sarcoplasmic reticulum into the cytosol (Chapter 7). The sarcoplasmic reticulum calcium release channels differ from the L-type calcium channels (called *dihydropyridine receptors*) found in the plasma membrane.

The Cytoskeleton

Cells contain a network of filaments called the *cytoskeleton*, which maintains cellular architecture, forms mechanical linkages between cells and with the extracellular matrix, organizes enzymes that participate in integrated catalytic cycles, and maintains the proximity of membrane pumps and channels that regulate key ion fluxes. The cytoskeleton also plays an important role in cell signaling, such as allowing different types of cell deformation to initiate specific proliferative responses in response to various types of overload (see Chapter 5).

The cytoskeleton contains three fiber types: *microfilaments*, *microtubules*, and *intermediate filaments*. Microfilaments, which contain actin, are found in two structures: *sarcomeric actin filaments*, which are the thin filaments of the myofibrils described above, and *cortical actin filaments* that form a network beneath the plasma membrane. The latter link the contractile machinery to other cytoskeletal elements, anchor cells to each other, and connect the cytoskeleton to the extracellular matrix. Cortical actin filaments interact with members of an extended family of myosin molecules (see Chapter 4) to transport membrane vesicles to and from the cell surface. Microtubules, which have a tubulin backbone, form networks that transport cell organelles and participate in cell division; specialized arrays of microtubules are instrumental in the movements of cilia and flagella. Microtubular transport is analogous to muscle contraction except that the filaments are polymers of *tubulin*, rather than actin, and the "motor proteins" are *kinesins* and *dyneins*, rather than myosin. The third type of cytoskeletal fiber, the intermediate filaments, are polymers of *desmin* that form very strong rivetlike structures called *desmosomes* that help maintain cell architecture, link cells to one another, and attach cells to the extracellular matrix. Unlike microfilaments and microtubules, intermediate filaments are not motile.

The Intercalated Disc

Specialized cell-to-cell junctions called *intercalated discs* (Fig. 1-22) form mechanical and electrical connections between cardiac myocytes (Table 1-3). (For a review, see Gallicano et al., 1998; Perriard et al., 2003.) The mechanical linkages are provided by the *fascia adherens*, in which sarcomeric actin filaments are connected to networks of cytoskeletal actin filaments, and by *desmosomes* that connect intermediate filaments in adjacent cardiac myocytes. A third structure, the *gap junction*, contains large nonselective *connexin* channels that allow ions and other small molecules to diffuse freely between the cytosol of adjacent cells. By providing low-resistance connections between cells, gap junction channels allow electrical impulses to be conducted rapidly throughout the heart (see Chapter 13).

MEMBRANE STRUCTURE AND FUNCTION

Biological membranes can be viewed as barriers consisting of a central hydrophobic sheet that lies between two hydrophilic surfaces (Fig. 1-23). The barrier is provided by the lipid core, which is virtually impermeable to charged molecules, while charged phospholipid head groups on the surfaces interact with the aqueous media on the two sides of the membrane.

Membrane Lipids

Membranes contain a mixture of lipids, most of which are *amphipathic* in that they contain both hydrophilic (polar) and hydrophobic (apolar) moieties. Most membrane lipids are built upon glycerol, a 3-carbon sugar that is generally esterified to a hydrophilic "head group" and one or two hydrophobic fatty acyl chain "tails" (Fig. 1-24). Other membrane lipids include sphingolipids, in which the glycerol backbone is

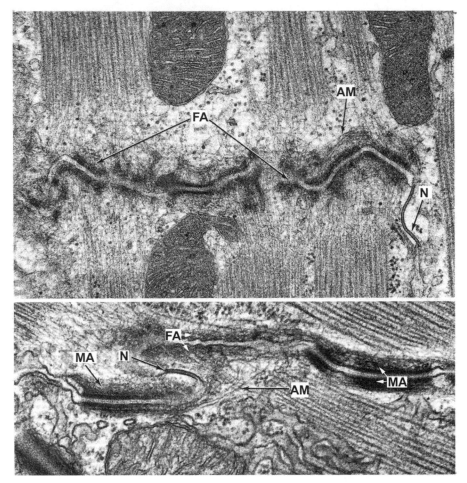

FIGURE 1-22 Electron microphotographs of the intercalated disc. **Top:** Transverse section of cat ventricular myocardium, showing insertions of *sarcomeric actin microfilaments* into the *fascia adherens* of the intercalated disc (FA), which is made up of *cortical actin microfilaments* (AM). At the right, the intercalated disc continues as a *nexus*, or *gap junction* (N). **Bottom:** Oblique section of intercalated disc in mouse ventricular myocardium showing *cortical actin myofilaments* (AM), *fascia adherens* (FA), a *nexus* (N), and two *desmosomes* or *maculae adherens* (MA). (Modified from McNutt and Fawcett, 1974.)

replaced by the 3-carbon amino acid serine. Most head groups contain charged anionic phosphate compounds, hence the term *phospholipid.* Cholesterol is found in the plasma membrane, where it reduces fluidity and "stiffens" the bilayer (Fig. 1-23).

Virtually all of the fatty acids in membrane lipids contain an even number of carbon atoms; in mammalian membranes, these are mainly palmitic and stearic acids (saturated C_{16} and C_{18}) and oleic, linoleic, and linolenic acids (unsaturated C_{18} fatty acids that contain 1, 2, and 3

TABLE 1-3 **Cell-to-Cell Communication Across the Intercalated Disc**

Structure	Type of Connection	Transmembrane Proteins	Cytoplasmic Proteins	Cellular Structure
Fascia adherens	mechanical	N-cadherin β-1D integrin	β-catenin plakoglobin vinculin	microfilament (actin, α-actinin)
Desmosome	mechanical	desmoglyein-2 desmocollin-2	desmoplakin plakophilins plakoglobulin	intermediate filament (desmin)
Gap junction	electrical	connexin 43		ion channel

double bonds, respectively). Saturated fatty acids form relatively ordered regions in membrane bilayers, whereas regions made up of unsaturated fatty acids are more fluid (Klausner et al., 1980). Natural unsaturated membrane fatty acids are *cis*-isomers, in which the fatty acyl chains adjacent to the double bond are on the same side of the molecule. *Trans*-fatty acids, which occur in artificially hydrogenated fats, modify membrane

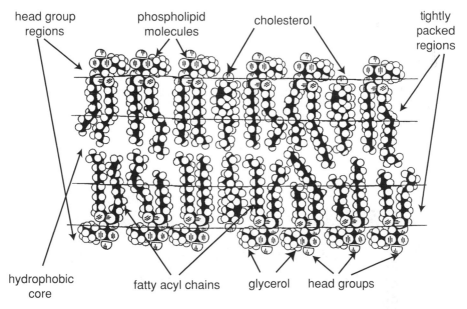

FIGURE 1-23 The membrane bilayer showing phospholipid molecules and cholesterol. The hydrophobic core, which is made up of uncharged (apolar or hydrophobic) fatty acyl chains and cholesterol, is lined by charged (polar or hydrophilic) "head groups." Tightly packed lipids lie between the head groups and hydrophobic core.

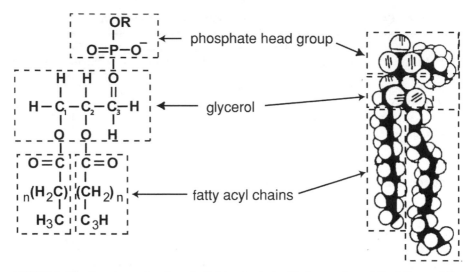

FIGURE 1-24   Structure of a phospholipid, oriented with the surface of the bilayer at the top, showing the glycerol "backbone" that is esterified to a head group and two fatty acyl chains. **Left:** Atomic structure. **Right:** Molecular model as shown in Fig. 1-23. The glycerol carbons are numbered 1, 2, and 3. The fatty acids in most phospholipids are esterified to carbons 1 and 2 and the head group, which can be linked to a variety of compounds (R), is esterified to carbon 3.

structure because the fatty acyl chains are on opposite (trans) sides of the molecule (Fig. 1-25).

Hydrolysis of membrane lipids by enzymes called *phospholipases* contributes to membrane damage in a number of diseases. *Phospholipases A_1 and A_2* hydrolyze the ester bonds linking fatty acids to glycerol carbons 1 and 2, respectively (Fig. 1-26). *Phospholipase B* is a mixture of

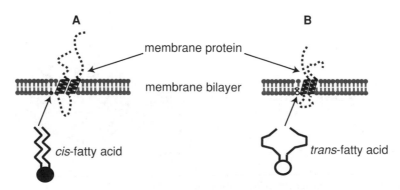

FIGURE 1-25   Schematic representation of phospholipids containing *cis-* (**A**) and *trans-* (**B**) unsaturated fatty acids. Because the conformations of the fatty acyl chains are different, trans-fatty acids can modify the conformation and function of membrane proteins.

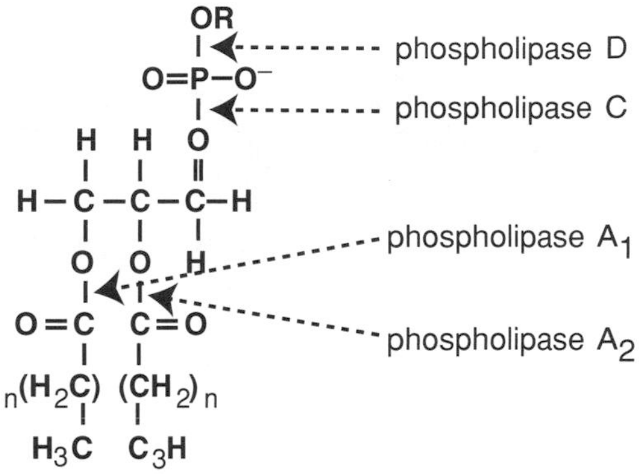

FIGURE 1-26 Phospholipases A_1 and A_2 release the fatty acids esterified to glycerol at carbons 1 and 2, respectively, while phospholipases C and D release all or part of the head groups from glycerol carbon 3. When R represents inositol, phospholipase C releases a phosphosugar that provides the precursor for inositol phosphates; the remainder of the phospholipid that remains bound within the membrane, diacylglycerol, also serves as a second messenger.

phospholipases A_1 and A_2 that hydrolyzes both of these ester bonds. *Phospholipase C* cleaves the phosphate head group from the glycerol "backbone," while *phospholipase D* removes organic structures from the head group, leaving the phosphatidic acid moiety attached to carbon 3 of glycerol.

Membrane lipids released by phospholipases often serve as signaling molecules (see Chapters 8 and 9). For example, hydrolysis of the membrane phospholipid *phosphatidylinositol 4,5-bisphosphate* by phospholipase C releases two messengers: *diacyl glycerol* (DAG) and *inositol triphosphate* (InsP$_3$). *Arachidonic* acid (unsaturated C_{20}) released from membrane phospholipids by phospholipase A_2 is the precursor of a family of extracellular messengers that includes *prostaglandins, thromboxanes*, and *leukotrienes*, while *myristic* (saturated C_{14}) and *palmitic* acids released into the cytosol can be covalently linked to proteins where they modify function (Resh, 1999; Chen and Manning, 2001; Farazi et al., 2001).

Membrane Proteins

Most of the important activities of biological membranes are mediated by *intrinsic membrane proteins* that are imbedded in one or both leaflets of the bilayer (Fig. 1-27). These proteins, which can make up more than one-half of the weight of a membrane, include receptors, enzymes, channels, carriers, pumps, and exchangers. The extracellular portions of plasma membrane proteins often contain covalently bound lipid (lipoproteins) or carbohydrate (glycoproteins).

The fluid nature of the lipid bilayer allows the membrane proteins to move in the plane of the bilayer, much as icebergs float in the sea. The lipids that surround the hydrophobic surfaces of membrane proteins, sometimes called the *boundary layer lipids* or *annulus*, play an important role in regulating the activity of these proteins (Katz and Messineo, 1981). Changes in this lipid environment have been implicated in the pathogenesis of clinical arrhythmias (Kang and Leaf, 1996; Leaf and Xiao, 2001;

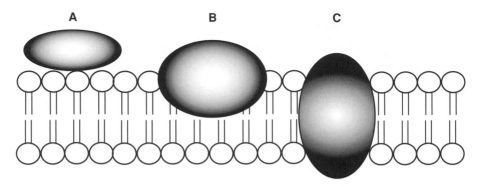

FIGURE 1-27 Membrane proteins (*shaded*) can be adsorbed to the membrane surface (**A**), incorporated into one leaflet of the bilayer (**B**), or can span the bilayer (**C**). Parts **B** and **C** represent intrinsic membrane proteins.

Katz, 2002). Many cardioactive drugs are amphipathic molecules that modify function when they enter the bilayer and interact with the hydrophobic surfaces of membrane proteins (Herbette and Mason, 1991).

Membrane Transport

Transport of materials across the membrane barrier can be effected by two fundamentally different mechanisms. The first, exemplified by the ion pumps and ion exchangers described in Chapter 7 and the ion channels discussed in Chapter 13, are generally highly selective for a given molecule. Not all membrane channels exhibit this specificity. For example, the gap junction channels in the intercalated disc allow a variety of molecules to move between neighboring cells, and anion channels in the sarcoplasmic reticulum allow several anions to cross this internal membrane.

An entirely different mechanism that transports large molecules across the plasma membrane occurs when parts of the membrane invaginate and then pinch off to form vesicles that move through the cytosol. An example is *exocytosis*, where intracellular membrane vesicles transport substances manufactured within cells to the cell surface where the vesicles fuse with the plasma membrane, which allows the substances to be released into the extracellular fluid. Bulk transport in the opposite direction occurs by *endocytosis*, in which molecules, often bound to a specific receptor, enter cells within vesicles formed by invagination of the plasma membrane. These transport processes are facilitated by "molecular motors" that are powered by interactions between cortical actin filaments and nonmuscle myosin and of tubulin with kinesins and dyneins (see above).

Endocytosis is effected by several mechanisms. In *pinocytosis*, vesicles formed from plasma membrane invaginations take up small amounts

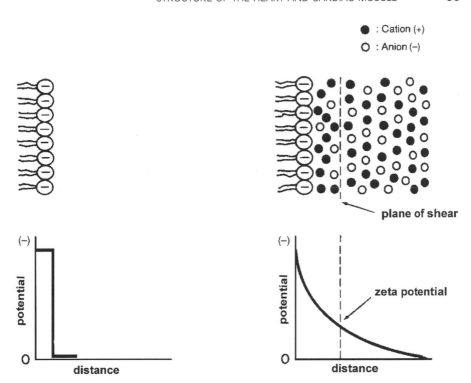

● : Cation (+)

○ : Anion (−)

plane of shear

zeta potential

FIGURE 1-28 Distribution of electrical potential at the surface of a membrane composed of phospholipids with negatively charged head groups. **Left**: Surface charge falls sharply with increasing distance from the membrane when ions are absent in the surrounding medium. **Right**: When salts are included in the medium adjacent to the membrane, attraction of the cations to the anionic surface causes a more gradual fall in surface charge. Some of these cations remain associated with the membrane when it is moved through to the surrounding medium, giving rise to a "plane of shear" outside of which ions move freely. The potential at the plane of shear is the zeta potential.

of extracellular fluid, which is then transported into the cell. *Receptor-mediated endocytosis* occurs when selected molecules in the extracellular fluid (ligands) bind to specific receptors on the outer surface of the plasma membrane; the ligand-bound receptors then stimulate the adjacent plasma membrane to invaginate. These invaginations, which are called *coated pits* because their cytosolic surfaces are lined by proteins such as *clathrin* and *caveolin*, form sealed *coated vesicles* that contain the receptor-bound ligands. These vesicles then fuse with other intracellular vesicles called *endosomes* that can be transported within cells.

Surface Charge and Transmembrane Potential

Anionic phosphate moieties in the head groups of membrane lipids give rise to a negative *surface charge* that attracts cations in the aqueous media toward the membrane surface. The result is a gradual change in surface potential as one moves away from the membrane (Fig. 1-28). The potential at the plane of shear when the membrane moves through the surrounding aqueous medium is called the *zeta potential*.

Biological membranes often separate regions of different electrical potential; cardiac Purkinje fibers, for example, have a potential difference across the resting plasma membrane of about 90 mV. Changes in the magnitude, and often the polarity, of this potential difference exert forces that modify the conformations of intrinsic membrane proteins such as *voltage-gated ion channels* (Chapter 13). Although the absolute potential differences across the plasma membrane are small, they create enormous electrical potential gradients because they occur across a very thin surface. A potential difference of -90 mV (-90×10^{-3} V viewed from within the cell) across the sarcolemma, which is approximately 30 Å (30×10^{-8} cm) thick, represents a potential *gradient* of $-300,000$ V/cm (90×10^{-3} V $\div$ 30×10^{-8} cm). During depolarization, this potential difference becomes $+30$ mV, so the gradient reverses to $+100,000$ V/cm. This means that the *change* in transmembrane potential gradient is about 400,000 V/cm! These large changes in potential gradient explain how what seem to be small changes in transmembrane potential generate powerful forces that can open and close ion channels.

BIBLIOGRAPHY

Alberts B, Bray D, Lewis J, et al. *Molecular biology of the cell*, 3rd ed. New York: Garland Publishing, Inc., 1994.

Anderson RH, Becker AE. *The heart. Structure in health and disease*. London: Gower Medical, 1992.

Cooper GM. *The cell. A molecular approach*. Washington DC: ASM Press, 2000.

Devlin TM, ed. *Textbook of biochemistry*. New York: Wiley-Liss, 1997.

Finean JB, Coleman R, Michell RH. *Membranes and their cellular functions*. Oxford: Blackwell, 1978.

Lodish H, Berk A, Zipursky SL, et al. *Molecular cell biology*, 4th ed. Basingstoke: Freeman, 1999.

McNutt NS, Fawcett DW. Myocardial ultrastructure. In: Langer GA, Brady AJ, eds. The *Mammalian myocardium*. New York: Wiley, 1974:1–49.

Quinn PJ. *The molecular biology of cellular membranes*. Baltimore: University Park Press, 1976.

Robertson RN. *The lively membranes*. Cambridge: Cambridge University Press, 1983.

Sommer JR, Dolber PC. Cardiac muscle: ultrastructure of its cells and bundles. In: de Carvalho AP, Hoffman BF, Lieberman M, eds. *Normal and abnormal conduction in the heart*. Mt Kisco, NY: Futura, 1982.

Sommer JR, Johnson EA. Ultrastructure of cardiac muscle. In: Berne RM, Sperelakis N, Geiger JR, eds. *Handbook of physiology, section 2: The cardiovascular system. vol. I, The heart. Am Physiol Soc* 1979: 113–186.

REFERENCES

Anderson RH, Ho SY. The architecture of the sinus node, the atrioventricular conduction axis, and the internodal atrial myocardium. *J Cardiovasc Electrophysiol* 1998;9:1233–1248.

Becker AE, deWit APM. Mitral valve apparatus. A spectrum of normality relevant to mitral valve prolapse. *Br Heart J* 1979;42:680–689.

Benninghoff A. *Lehrbuch der Anatomie des Menschen*. Munich: JF Lehmanns Verlag, 1944.

Berne RM, Levy MN. *Cardiovascular physiology*. St. Louis: CV Mosby, 1967.

Boomama F, Van der Meiracker AH. Plasma A- and B-type natriuretic peptides: physiology, methodology and clinical use. *Cardiovasc Res* 2001;51:442–449.

Bouvagnet P, Leger J, Dechesne C, et al. Fiber types and myosin types in human atrial and ventricular myosin. An anatomical description. *Circ Res* 1984;55:794–804.

Brutsaert DL. The endocardium. *Ann Rev Physiol* 1989;51:263–273.

Chen CA, Manning DR. Regulation of G proteins by covalent modification. *Oncogene* 1989;20:1643–1652.

Dawes GS, Comroe JH Jr. Chemoreflexes from the heart and lungs. *Physiol Rev* 1954;34:167–201.

Factor SM, Okun EM, Kirk ES. The histological lateral border of acute canine myocardial infarction. A function of microcirculation. *Circ Res* 1981;48:640–649.

Farazi TA, Waksman G, Gordon JI. The biology and enzymology of protein N-myristoylation. *J Biol Chem* 2001;276:39501–39504.

Fenton TR, Cherry JM, Klassen GA. Transmural myocardial deformation in the canine left ventricular wall. *Am J Physiol* 1978;235:H523–H530.

Franzini-Armstrong C, Nunzi G. Junctional feet and particles in the triads of a fast-twitch muscle fibre. *J Muscle Res Cell Motil* 1983;4:233–252.

Gallicano GI, Kouklis P, Christoph C, et al. Desmoplakin is required early in development for assembly of desmosomes and cytoskeletal linkage. *J Cell Biol* 1998;143: 2009–2022.

Gerdes AM, Graves JH, Settles HE, et al. Improved preservation of myocardial ultrastructure in perfusion-fixed human heart explants. In: Singal PK, Dixon IMC, Beamish RE, et al., eds. *Mechanisms of heart failure*. Boston: Kluwer, 1995;129–141.

Goldberger AL, Rigney DR, West BJ. Chaos and fractals in human physiology. *Sci Am* 1990:26243–26249.

Goldberger AL, Amaral LA, Hausdorff JM, et al. Fractal dynamics in physiology: alterations with disease and aging. *Proc Natl Acad Sci USA* 2002;9[Suppl 1]:2466–2472.

Grant RP. Notes on the muscular architecture of the heart. *Circulation* 1965;32:301–308.

Hawthorne EW. Dynamic geometry of the left ventricle. Introduction. *Fed Proc* 1969;4: 1323–1367.

Hayashi H, Lux RL, Wyatt RF, et al. Relation of canine atrial activation sequence to anatomical landmarks. *Am J Physiol* 1982;242:H421–H428.

Henry CG, Lowry OH. Quantitative histochemistry of canine Purkinje fibers. *Am J Physiol* 1983;245:H824–H829.

Herbette LG, Mason RP. Techniques for determining membrane and drug-membrane structures: a reevaluation of the molecular and kinetic basis for the binding of lipid-soluble drugs to their receptors in heart and brain. In: Fozzard H, Haber E, Katz A, et al. The heart and cardiovascular system, 2nd ed. New York: Raven Press, 1991:417–462.

Kang JX, Leaf A. Antiarrhythmic effects of polyunsaturated fatty acids. *Circulation* 1996;94: 1774–1780.

Katz AM. Congestive heart failure: role of altered myocardial cellular control. *N Engl J Med* 1975;293:1184–1975.

Katz AM. Evolving concepts of heart failure: cooling furnace, malfunctioning pump, enlarging muscle—Part I. Heart failure as a disorder of the cardiac pump. *J Cardiac Fail* 1997;3:319–334.

Katz AM. Evolving concepts of heart failure: cooling furnace, malfunctioning pump, enlarging muscle—Part II. Hypertrophy and dilatation of the failing heart. *J Cardiac Fail* 1998;4:67–81.

Katz AM. Trans-fatty acids and sudden cardiac death. (Editorial) *Circulation* 2002;105: 669–671.

Katz AM, Katz LA. What is a paradigm and when does it shift? *J Mol Cell Cardiol* 1991;23: 403–408.

Katz AM, Katz PB. Homogeneity out of heterogeneity. *Circulation* 1989;79:712–717.

Katz AM, Lorell BH. Regulation of cardiac contraction and relaxation. *Circulation* 2000;102 [Suppl IV]:IV-69–IV-74.

Katz AM, Messineo FC. Lipid-membrane interactions and the pathogenesis of ischemic damage in the myocardium. *Circ Res* 1981;48:1–16.

Katz LA, Berger JD. Parade of the little millions. *Am Nat* 1999;154:S93–S95.

Klausner RD, Kleinfeld AM, Hoover RL, et al. Lipid domains in membranes. Evidence derived from structural perturbations induced by free fatty acids and lifetime heterogeneity analysis. *J Biol Chem* 1980;255:1286–1295.

Leaf A, Xiao YF. The modulation of ionic currents in excitable tissues by n-3 polyunsaturated fatty acids. *J Memb Biol* 2001;184:263–271.

Levin ER, Gardner DG, Samson WK. Natriuretic peptides. *N Eng J Med* 1998;339:321–328.

Lower R. *Tractus de Corde*. London: Allestry, 1669.

Margulis L. *Origin of eukaryotic cells*. New Haven: Yale University Press, 1970.

McNutt NS, Fawcett DW. Myocardial ultrastructure. In: Langer GA, Brady AJ, eds. *The mammalian myocardium*. New York: Wiley, 1974:1–49.

Miller AJ. *Lymphatics of the heart*. New York: Raven, 1982.

Moncman CL, Wang K. Nebulette: a 107 kD nebulin-like protein in cardiac muscle. *Cell Motil Cytoskeleton* 1995;32:205–225.

Moncman CL, Wang K. Architecture of the thin filament-Z-line junction: lessons from nebulette and nebulin homologies. *J Muscle Res Cell Motil* 2000;21:153–169.

Morris-Thurgood JA, Frenneaux MP. Diastolic ventricular interaction and ventricular diastolic filling. *Heart Fail Rev* 2000;5:307–323.

Oosthoek PW, Virágh S, Lamers WH, et al. Immunohistochemical delineation of the conduction system. II: The atrioventricular node and Purkinje fibers. *Circ Res* 1993a;73:482–491.

Oosthoek PW, Virágh S, Mayen AEM, et al. Immunohistochemical delineation of the conduction system. I: The sinoatrial node. *Circ Res* 1993b;73:473–481.

Page E. Quantitative ultrastructural analysis in cardiac membrane physiology. *Am J Physiol* 1978;63:C147–C158.

Perriard JC, Hirschy A, Ehler E. Dilated cardiomyopathy: a disease of the intercalated disc? *Trends Cardiovasc Med* 2003;13:30–38.

Resh MD. Fatty acylation of proteins: new insights into membrane targeting of myristoylated and palmitoylated proteins. *Biochim Biophys Acta* 1999;145:1–16.

Roger AJ. Reconstructing early events in eukaryotic evolution. *Am Nat* 1999;154:S146–S163.

Rossi MA, Abreu MA, Santoro LB. Connective tissue skeleton of the human heart. A demonstration by cell-maceration scanning electron microscope method. *Circulation* 1998;97: 934–935.

Santamore WP, Dell'Italia LJ. Ventricular interdependence: significant left ventricular contributions to right ventricular systolic function. *Prog Cardiovasc Dis* 1998;40:289–308.

Sartore S, Gorza L, Pierobon Bormioli S, et al. Myosin types and fiber types in cardiac muscle. I: Ventricular myocardium. *J Cell Biol* 1981;88:226–233.

Schäper W, ed. *The Pathophysiology of Myocardial Perfusion.* Amsterdam: Elsevier/North Holland, 1979.

Schlegel A, Volonte D, Engelman JA, et al. Crowded little caves: structure and function of caveolae. *Cell Signal* 1998;10:457–463.

Streeter DD, Spotnitz HM, Patel DP, et al. Fiber orientation in the canine left ventricle during systole and diastole. *Circ Res* 1969;24:339–347.

Verheijck EE, Wessels A, van Ginneken ACG, et al. Distribution of atrial and nodal cells within the rabbit sinoatrial node. Models of sinoatrial transmission. *Circulation* 1998;97:1623–1631.

Yacoub MH. Two hearts that beat as one. *Circulation* 1995;92:160–161.

2

ENERGETICS AND ENERGY PRODUCTION

The heart functions an energy transducer that converts chemical energy to the mechanical work expended when blood is ejected under pressure into the aorta and pulmonary artery. This chapter describes the mechanisms that provide the chemical energy used by the heart, highlighting the need for an uninterrupted supply of substrates and oxygen. Because the heart beats without pause, which requires a high and sustained rate of energy expenditure, its energy supply is "at the edge" even under normal conditions. Therefore, a brief interruption of coronary flow can severely impair pump function.

CHEMICAL ENERGY SUPPLY FOR MUSCLE CONTRACTION—A HISTORY

Efforts to identify the source of the chemical energy used for muscle contraction illustrates some of the pitfalls encountered in scientific research. Berzelius, in the early 19th century, was the first to observe that an acid found in milk (*lactic acid*) appears in the muscle of a hunted stag. In 1907, Fletcher and Hopkins found that the lactate generated by fatigued muscle disappears when the muscle is allowed to recover in the presence of oxygen. Myerhof, who in the 1920s detailed the enzymatic reactions in glucose metabolism (called *glycolysis*), showed that lactic acid production in a muscle contracting under anaerobic conditions, where lactate cannot be oxidized, is proportional to the amount of work done. This suggested that glycolysis is directly coupled to muscle contraction:

$$\text{Carbohydrate} \rightarrow \text{lactic acid} + \text{mechanical energy}$$

That attractive hypothesis, although able to explain a large body of experimental data, collapsed in 1930 when Lundsgaard discovered that muscles still contract when glycolysis is blocked with iodoacetic acid. Lundsgaard subsequently observed that working muscles hydrolyze *phosphocreatine*, a labile compound composed of creatine and phosphoric acid. Eggleton and Eggleton demonstrated that the decrease in phosphocreatine is proportional to the amount of work performed during muscle contraction. These new findings led to a revised hypothesis—that energy is provided for muscle contraction when phosphocreatine is broken down to creatine and inorganic phosphate (P_i):

Phosphocreatine $\rightarrow$ creatine + P_i + mechanical energy

These observations also explained the role of glycolysis, which, instead of delivering energy directly to the contractile machinery, energizes phosphocreatine formation from creatine and P_i.

The hypothesis that phosphocreatine hydrolysis is directly coupled to muscle contraction had to be abandoned after only a few years, when *adenosine triphosphate* (ATP) was found to be essential for phosphocreatine breakdown. The discovery that ATP transfers P_i and chemical energy from phosphocreatine to energy-consuming reactions led to the concept of the *high-energy phosphate bond* ($\sim$P). The role of phosphocreatine in cellular energetics is therefore indirect and depends on two reactions—transfer of $\sim$P from phosphocreatine to *adenosine diphosphate* (ADP), which forms ATP, and hydrolysis of ATP to yield ADP, P_i, and chemical energy:

Phosphocreatine + ADP $\leftrightarrow$ creatine + ATP

and

ATP $\rightarrow$ ADP + P_i + energy

For 30 years, ATP hydrolysis was believed to be coupled directly to muscle contraction. However, ATP concentration could not be shown to decrease during contraction because muscles contain *creatine phosphokinase*, an enzyme that stabilizes ATP concentration by transferring $\sim$P from phosphocreatine to ADP. It was not until 1962 that an inhibitor of creatine phosphokinase made it possible to demonstrate that ATP hydrolysis is coupled to energy release by working muscle:

ATP $\rightarrow$ ADP + P_i + mechanical energy

The final chapter in this story was written when it was learned how the myosin cross-bridges utilize energy released by ATP hydrolysis for muscle contraction (see Chapter 4).

Adenine nucleotides are now known to participate in chemical reactions throughout cells, where ADP accepts chemical energy by incorporating $\sim$P to form ATP and ATP supplies chemical energy when the high-energy phosphate bond is hydrolyzed. Albert Szent-Györgyi likened ATP to money. Like cash, ATP can be obtained (regenerated) using energy derived from metabolism of a number of substrates, and like cash, ATP can be expended (hydrolyzed) to energize a variety of energy-consuming processes, such as muscle contraction, active transport, and biosynthesis.

According to this monetary analogy, the ~P in phosphocreatine represents a cash reserve.

"PATTERNS" OF ENERGY PRODUCTION AND UTILIZATION BY DIFFERENT MUSCLES

Adaptation of the pathways of energy production and energy utilization to the functional needs of different muscle types can be understood by examining the behavior of two long-eared mammals, the rabbit and the hare (Fig. 2-1). (Many years ago, the author was informed by a cardiology fellow from Texas that the following description, while valid for the European rabbit and hare, is not true for their American counterparts.)

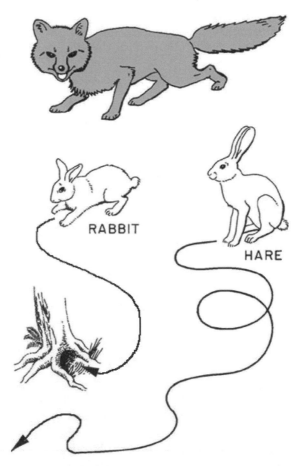

RABBIT

HARE

FIGURE 2-1 Functional specializations of the European rabbit and hare. When confronted with danger, such as a fox, the rabbit tries to escape by sprinting to its burrow, whereas the hare tries to outrun, and outlast, the pursuing fox.

European rabbits live in burrows from which they venture only a short distance in search of food and adventure. To escape predators, these rabbits rely on a rapid sprint to safety, so survival depends on their ability to accelerate quickly and run rapidly for short distances. Although excellent sprinters, rabbits are poor distance runners, tiring quickly if they cannot reach their burrow. Many species of the European hare, on the other hand, have no burrow but range widely in their habitat. Such hares are excellent distance runners, relying on their staying power to escape pursuers—indeed, the coursing of hares has been known since antiquity.

Early in the 20th century, it became clear to scientists—although this information had long been known to hunters and cooks—that the back and leg muscles of rabbits and hares differ in color; those in the rabbit are pale pink, almost white, whereas the back and leg muscles of the hare are deep red. Similar relationships between muscle color and function are found in other vertebrate species: "white" muscle is generally found where the need is for short bursts of intense activity and "red" muscle where activity is sustained. In common culinary experience, the chicken breast, which powers wings that are used only intermittently, is white meat, whereas the dark meat of the chicken leg is obtained from muscles that are used for more continuous activity, like walking around a barnyard. In birds capable of sustained flight, unlike the chicken, the breast muscles are "red" (e.g., the dark meat of duck or goose breast).

The following discussion focuses on red and white muscle, the "extremes" of biochemical specialization (Table 2-1); intermediate types exist, and there are exceptions to the generalizations described below. For clarity in describing how biochemical specializations meet functional needs, these exceptions are not considered further.

TABLE 2-1 **Biochemical Differences between Red and White Muscle**

Biochemical Characteristic	Red Muscle	White Muscle
Pathways of energy production	Aerobic	Anaerobic
Substrates	Lipid, carbohydrate	Carbohydrate
Metabolites	CO_2, H_2O	Lactic acid
Glycolytic enzymes	Sparse	Abundant
Mitochondria	Abundant	Sparse
Phosphocreatine stores	Minor	Significant
Dependence on oxygen	Marked	Little
Intrinsic ATPase of contractile proteins	Low	High

Energy Production and Utilization by Red and White Muscle

Red muscle is specialized for sustained activity, where the rate of energy production cannot exceed that of energy utilization and requires an uninterrupted supply of ATP produced by oxidative (aerobic) metabolism. The most important substrates for aerobic energy production are lipids and, to a lesser extent, carbohydrates. Although red muscle can carry out anaerobic glycolysis and have a limited reserve of high-energy phosphate in the form of phosphocreatine, these are of little functional significance because neither can provide the large amounts of ATP needed for sustained activity. The red color of these muscles is due mainly to myoglobin, a heme-containing protein that facilitates oxygen diffusion through the muscle.

Red muscles pay a threefold price for their dependence on a high rate of ATP production. First, these muscles require an uninterrupted supply of oxygen to generate the ATP consumed during sustained activity. If blood flow is interrupted, the lack of oxygen quickly brings oxidative metabolism to a halt and exhausts the phosphocreatine stores. Although anaerobic glycolysis can provide a limited supply of ATP, it cannot support sustained activity. Second, to carry out oxidative metabolism, red muscles depend on large numbers of bulky mitochondria, which, by occupying space that could otherwise contain contractile proteins, weakens the muscle. The third price—which helps to match energy utilization and energy production—is that the contractile proteins have a low intrinsic rate of ATP hydrolysis (ATPase activity), which slows intrinsic shortening velocity and reduces contractility (see Chapter 6).

In *white muscle* (Table 2-1), where specialization is for brief periods of intense activity, the rate of energy expenditure can exceed that of energy production. Although these muscles require periods of rest, they do not depend on oxidative metabolism during activity. Muscle strength is therefore increased because cell volume otherwise filled with mitochondria can be occupied by contractile proteins. During their brief bursts of activity, white muscles utilize energy stored as phosphocreatine and the limited supply of ATP regenerated by anaerobic glycolysis. Because the latter produces lactate that must eventually be oxidized to CO_2 and water, white muscles incur an "oxygen debt" that is repaid by the muscle when lactate is oxidized during periods of rest, and by the liver when the lactate enters the circulation. During their brief bursts of activity, white muscles are not required to balance the rates of energy production and energy utilization; this allows their contractile proteins to have a high ATPase activity so that these muscles can achieve a high velocity of shortening (see Chapter 6).

The physiological consequences of these biochemical specializations allow the rabbit to escape pursuit by a rapid dash to its burrow (the "jackrabbit" start); should the rabbit fail to reach safety, it soon tires because phosphocreatine stores are quickly depleted, anaerobic glycolysis ceases, and lactic acid accumulation causes the muscles to become acidotic. Once in its burrow, the rabbit requires a period of rest to replenish its phosphocreatine reserves and to repay the "oxygen debt" by oxidizing lactate—if the rabbit shown in Fig. 2-1 is caught, repaying this debt becomes the fox's problem. The hare, which relies on its staying power to elude pursuers, can run long distances because even during intense activity, its red muscles regenerate ATP at the same rate at which it is being consumed. These muscles, however, require that a continuous supply of oxygen and substrate be delivered by way of the bloodstream. Owing to the lower intrinsic ATPase of their contractile proteins and the larger volume of muscle occupied by mitochondria, the running muscles of the hare are slower and weaker than those of the rabbit. These differences were summarized by Mommaerts, who said that white muscle operates on a "twitch now, pay later" basis, whereas the *modus operandi* of red muscle is "pay as you go." In this context, of course, the heart functions like a red muscle.

Most human skeletal muscles are "mixed" in that they contain several fiber types. These include *slow oxidative* fibers, which are similar to the red muscles described above; *fast glycolytic* fibers, which are like white muscle (although the muscles are pink in color); and *fast oxidative–glycolytic* fibers, which have high ATPase contractile proteins but contain numerous mitochondria and can produce ATP by oxidative reactions (Pette and Staron, 1990).

MUSCULAR EFFICIENCY

The term *efficiency* has many meanings (Backx, 1993). Most precise is *thermodynamic efficiency*, which is the ratio between the mechanical work performed during contraction and the free energy made available by substrate metabolism. Because the free energy changes in most of the chemical reactions in muscle are not precisely known, it is more practical to estimate *mechanical efficiency*, which is the ratio between useful work and the enthalpy changes during substrate metabolism.

The mechanical efficiency of a muscle is influenced by an interplay between load and the intrinsic ATPase activity of its contractile proteins. When contracting against a light load, fast muscles with high ATPase myosin are more efficient than slow muscles, whereas heavily loaded slow muscles, whose contractile proteins hydrolyze ATP at a slower intrinsic rate, maintain tension at less energy cost than fast muscles (Awan and Goldspink, 1972). For this reason, muscles with high ATPase contractile proteins are more efficient when shortening rapidly against a light load, whereas muscles with low ATPase contractile proteins are more efficient when developing high levels of tension.

The mechanical efficiency of the working heart is readily calculated because the myocardium regenerates ATP almost entirely by oxidative metabolism, which allows enthalpy changes to be estimated by measuring cardiac oxygen consumption. Even though the amount of energy liberated by the oxidation of fat (~9 kcal/gm) is more than twice that of either carbohydrate or protein (~4 kcal/gm) (see also Table 2-4), more oxygen is needed to metabolize fat. As a result, the enthalpies of the oxidation of all three substrates, when calculated per liter of oxygen consumption, are similar: fat 4.69 kcal, carbohydrate 5.05 kcal, protein 4.60 kcal. Cardiac efficiency can therefore be calculated as the ratio between the work performed (see Chapter 12) and the energy equivalent of the oxygen consumed.

The efficiency of the heart, calculated from measurements of external work and oxygen consumption, is usually less than 20% to 25%. Some of the energy consumed by the heart is used for reactions other than contraction (e.g., active ion fluxes) and wasted as entropy, so the efficiency of the contractile process is higher. A major cause of the heart's inefficiency is heat liberation during relaxation, when energy used to stretch elasticities in the walls of the contracting ventricle is dissipated as heat (see Chapter 12). Efficiencies as high as 40% during ejection (Suga et al., 1993) compare favorably with efficiencies of approximately 30% for man-made machines, such as gasoline engines. Efficiency is reduced when the heart oxidizes fatty acid instead of carbohydrate; this effect may be significant in the energy-starved heart, where replacing fat with carbohydrate can improve cardiac performance (see below).

OVERVIEW OF ENERGY PRODUCTION BY THE HEART

Most of the energy utilized by the heart is derived from the oxidation of fats; carbohydrate metabolism makes a significant contribution, but amino acid metabolism normally contributes little to cardiac energy production. Unlike fat, which can be metabolized only in the well-oxygenated heart, carbohydrates are metabolized by glycolysis under both aerobic and anaerobic conditions. *Anaerobic glycolysis*, because of its limited capacity to regenerate ATP, cannot meet the energy needs of the beating heart, which explains why interruption of oxygen supply brings effective contraction to a halt within less than a minute. *Aerobic glycolysis* also generates only a fraction of the energy used by the normal heart but plays a key role in supplying substrate for oxidative metabolism. As noted below, ATP regenerated by glycolysis (*glycolytic ATP*) plays a special role in supplying the needs of key energy-consuming reactions.

GLYCOGEN FORMATION AND BREAKDOWN

Carbohydrate is stored in the heart as *glycogen*, a polysaccharide made up of glucose-1-phosphate subunits formed when *phosphoglucomutase* catalyzes the isomerization of glucose-6-phosphate (see below). The formation and breakdown of glycogen do not occur by a single reversible reaction, but instead utilize two separate pathways that are catalyzed by different enzymes (Fig. 2-2). The enzymes that control glycogen formation (*glycogen synthetase*) and glycogen breakdown (*phosphorylase*)

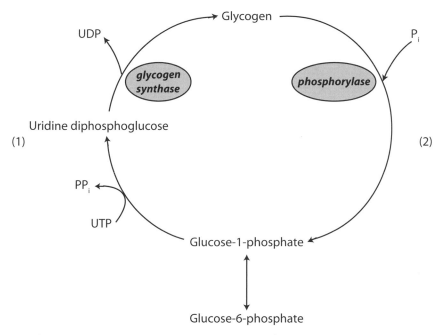

FIGURE 2-2 Pathways of glycogen formation (*left, reading upward*) differ from those of glycogen breakdown (*right, reading downward*). Glycogen synthesis involves two steps. The first step transfers uridine from uridine triphosphate (UTP) to glucose-1-phosphate. The second step, which adds uridine diphosphoglucose (UDPG) to glycogen, releases uridine diphosphate (UDP). Glycogen breakdown releases glucose-1-phosphate that, after isomerization to glucose-6-phosphate, enters the glycolytic pathway.

exist in active and inactive forms whose interconversions are regulated by sympathetic stimulation, high-energy phosphate levels, and metabolic intermediates.

Glycogen Formation: Glycogen Synthetase

Glycogen is formed from glucose-1-phosphate in a two-step reaction (Fig. 2-2, *left*). The first, which is catalyzed by *glucose 1-phosphate uridyl-yltransferase*, uses energy in uridine triphosphate (UTP) to form uridine diphosphoglucose (UDPG). The latter is added to the glycogen polymer in the second step, which releases uridine diphosphate (UDP). The second step, which is rate-limiting, is catalyzed by *glycogen synthetase*, a highly regulated enzyme that exists in two forms whose interconversions are controlled by phosphorylation and dephosphorylation reactions (Fig. 2-3).

Glycogen synthesis is slowed when sympathetic stimulation activates a *cyclic AMP–dependent protein kinase* (*protein kinase A* or *PK-A*) that converts the more active *a* (dephospho) form of *glycogen synthetase* to the less active b (phospho) form (Fig. 2-3A). Phosphorylation of glycogen synthetase a does not directly inhibit the enzyme, but instead increases the inhibitory effects of several substrates and metabolites. Most important are

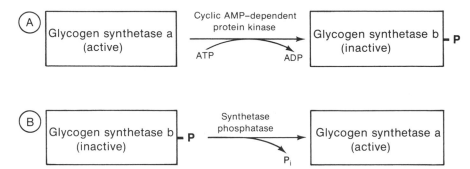

FIGURE 2-3 Phosphorylation (A) and dephosphorylation (B) reactions that modulate glycogen synthetase activity. A: Phosphorylation by cyclic AMP–dependent protein kinase converts the active, dephosphorylated glycogen synthetase a to the less active, phosphorylated glycogen synthetase b. B: Dephosphorylation by synthetase phosphatase converts phosphorylated glycogen synthetase b to the more active form.

ATP and glucose-6-phosphate which, by reducing the catalytic activity of glycogen synthetase b, promotes glycogen storage when an abundant supply of energy maintains high levels of ATP and hexose. Glycogen synthesis returns to its high basal rate when glycogen synthetase b is dephosphorylated by *synthetase phosphatase* to form the more active glycogen synthetase a (Fig. 2-3B).

Glycogen Breakdown: Phosphorylase

Glycogen breakdown, which releases glucose-1-phosphate (Fig. 2-2, *right*), is catalyzed by *phosphorylase* which, like glycogen synthetase, is regulated by phosphorylation and dephosphorylation (Fig. 2-4). In contrast to glycogen synthetase, in which the phosphorylated enzyme is less active, phosphorylated phosphorylase a is the active enzyme. The less active phosphorylase b, like glycogen synthetase a, is inhibited by ATP and glucose-6-phosphate.

Phosphorylation of phosphorylase b is catalyzed by *phosphorylase b kinase*, which when activated by sympathetic stimulation increases glycogen breakdown. However, cyclic AMP does not act *directly* on phosphorylase b kinase; instead, sympathetic stimulation phosphorylates phosphorylase b kinase by activating a cyclic AMP–dependent protein kinase called *phosphorylase kinase kinase* (Fig. 2-5). Increased levels of cytosolic calcium that increase myocardial contractility (see Chapter 10) also can mobilize glycogen by activating a *calcium/calmodulin-dependent protein kinase* that phosphorylates phosphorylase b kinase. Glycogen breakdown returns to its basal level when phosphorylase kinase is dephosphorylated by *phosphorylase kinase phosphatase* and phosphorylase a is dephosphorylated by *phosphorylase phosphatase*.

The reactions described above provide an integrated control mechanism that allows cyclic AMP to regulate the flux of glucose-1-phosphate

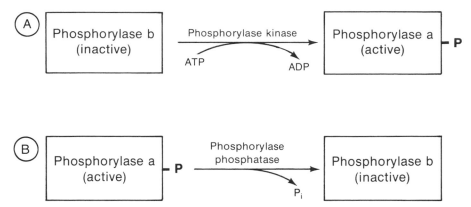

FIGURE 2-4 Phosphorylation (**A**) and dephosphorylation (**B**) reactions that modulate phosphorylase activity. **A:** Phosphorylation by phosphorylase b kinase converts the less active, dephosphorylated phosphorylase b to the more active phosphorylase a. **B:** Dephosphorylation by phosphorylase phosphatase converts phosphorylase a to the less active phosphorylase b.

into and out of glycogen stores (Fig. 2-6). Cyclic AMP–stimulated phosphorylations increase glucose supply by inhibiting glycogen synthetase and stimulating phosphorylase, while dephosphorylation of these enzymes shifts the balance toward glycogen synthesis. This allows sympathetic stimulation, which increases cardiac energy utilization, to increase energy production by inhibiting glycogen formation and stimulating glycogen breakdown.

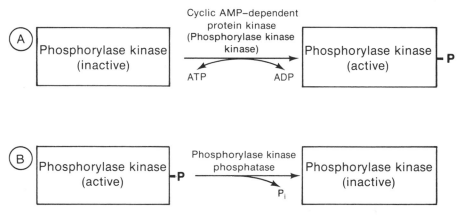

FIGURE 2-5 Phosphorylation (**A**) and dephosphorylation (**B**) reactions that control the activity of phosphorylase b kinase. **A:** Phosphorylation is catalyzed by phosphorylase kinase kinase, a cyclic AMP–dependent protein kinase, and converts the inactive, dephosphorylated form of phosphorylase to the active form. **B:** Dephosphorylation of phosphorylated phosphorylase kinase by phosphorylase kinase phosphatase forms the inactive enzyme.

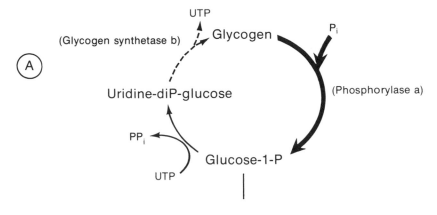

PHOSPHORYLATED ENZYMES

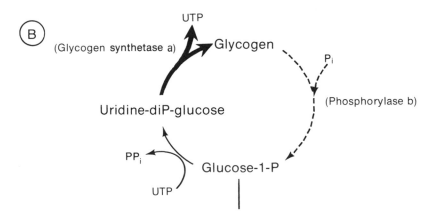

DEPHOSPHORYLATED ENZYMES

FIGURE 2-6 Integrated control of glycogen formation and breakdown by phosphorylation and dephosphorylation of glycogen synthetase and phosphorylase. **A:** Glycogen synthesis is inhibited and glycogen breakdown accelerated when phosphorylation converts glycogen synthetase to the less active b form and phosphorylase to the more active a form. **B:** Glycogen synthesis is accelerated and glycogen breakdown inhibited when both enzymes are dephosphorylated, which converts glycogen synthetase to the more active a form and phosphorylase to the less active b form.

Debranching Enzymes

Glycogen is a highly branched polysaccharide that requires special *debranching* enzymes to release glucose residues at the branch points. Although these reactions are not normally rate-limiting, molecular abnormalities in the debranching enzymes can cause *glycogen storage diseases* by preventing the complete breakdown of glycogen.

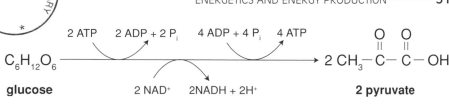

FIGURE 2-7 Overall reaction of glycolysis, which converts glucose to pyruvate.

GLYCOLYSIS

Glycolysis breaks down 1 mole of glucose to form 2 moles of pyruvate (Fig. 2-7). Two moles of ATP/mole of glucose are hydrolyzed in the initial steps to energize glycolysis, while generation of 4 moles of ATP/mole of glucose toward the end of the glycolytic pathway yields a net of 2 moles of ATP/mole of glucose. Glycolysis includes an oxidative step that reduces NAD$^+$ to NADH that, when oxidized, regenerates additional ATP (see below). In the aerobic (well-oxygenated) heart, pyruvate—the end-product of glycolysis—is oxidized and decarboxylated to form acetyl-CoA. Under anaerobic conditions, on the other hand, pyruvate is reduced to form lactate.

Enzymes, Coenzymes, and the Cytoskeleton

Glycolytic enzymes are large proteins and protein complexes that were once believed to be soluble and therefore able to diffuse freely through the cytosol. It is now clear, however, that glycolytic enzymes are organized by the cytoskeleton in a manner that delivers substrates to appropriate enzymes and releases ATP near energy-consuming structures. This structural organization explains why ATP regenerated by glycolytic pathways ("glycolytic ATP") can be used preferentially in some energy-consuming reactions (see below).

Coenzymes, which are much smaller than enzymes, play an essential role in glycolysis and other metabolic processes. These soluble organic molecules often contain moieties that cannot be synthesized by mammalian cells and must be ingested in the diet as *vitamins*.

Several coenzymes participate in redox reactions. In their oxidized form, they accept electrons from a variety of reactions to form reduced coenzymes that when oxidized in the mitochondria provide energy to regenerate ATP (see below). Coenzymes that participate in redox reactions include *nicotinamide adenine dinucleotide* (NAD), which contains *niacin*; *coenzyme Q* (*ubiquinone*), an electron carrier with a *quinone* group; and *flavine* mononucleotide (FMN) and *flavine adenine dinucleotide* (FAD), which contain *riboflavin*. *Nicotinamide adenine dinucleotide* (NADP), which is similar to NAD except that it contains an additional phosphate, generally participates in biosynthetic rather than energy-producing reactions.

Other coenzymes include *thiamine pyrophosphate*, which serves as a cofactor for decarboxylations, and *lipoic acid*, which participates in transacetylations. Thiamine deficiency causes beriberi, which can be accompanied by high output heart failure; in developed countries, this rare condition is seen mainly in alcoholics. *Coenzyme A* (CoA), which contains a vitamin called *pantothenic acid*, has a reactive sulfhydryl group (hence the abbreviation *CoA-SH*) that activates acetate and fatty acids by forming a high-energy thioester bond analogous to the high-energy phosphate bond of ATP.

Overview of Glucose Metabolism

The enzymes that catalyze glycolysis can be modified by four different types of signaling mechanism (Table 2-2). Three are *functional* in that they modify the catalytic activity of existing structures; the fourth is proliferative (transcriptional), as it alters the composition of the heart. Many enzymes are regulated by more than one type of signal.

Functional signals regulate glucose metabolism at the six numbered steps marked by asterisks in Figure 2-8. *Humoral* control allows sympathetic stimulation to increase the glycolytic rate by accelerating fructose 1,6-bisphosphate formation from fructose 6-phosphate (*3), which is the rate-limiting step for glycolysis in the normal heart. The second type of functional signal, which also operates at this step and the hexokinase reaction (*2), matches *energy production* to the rate of *energy utilization* by allowing high ATP concentrations to inhibit glycolysis, and ~P depletion, which increases ADP and AMP levels, to stimulate glycolysis. The third type of functional signal responds to changes in the *supply of oxidized coenzymes* by slowing glycolysis when NADH accumulates and NAD^+ becomes depleted in the energy-starved heart; this mechanism regulates the oxidation of glyceraldehyde 3-phosphate (*4) and conversion of pyruvate to lactate (*5 and *6).

The fourth type of control, long-term regulation by proliferative signaling, differs fundamentally from the three mechanisms described above because, instead of modifying the activity of pre-existing enzymes, transporters (*1), and other proteins, it alters their synthesis (van Bilsen et al., 1998). Proliferative signaling, which plays an important role in heart failure (Chapter 18), increases glycolytic capacity in the hypertrophied heart.

TABLE 2-2 **Signaling Mechanisms That Regulate Glycolysis**

Functional
Humoral: Hormones and neurotransmitters
Energy requirements: Levels of ATP, ADP, AMP, P_i, glucose 6-phosphate
Coenzymes: Levels of oxidized and reduced NAD and FAD
Proliferative
Gene expression: Synthesis of metabolic enzymes

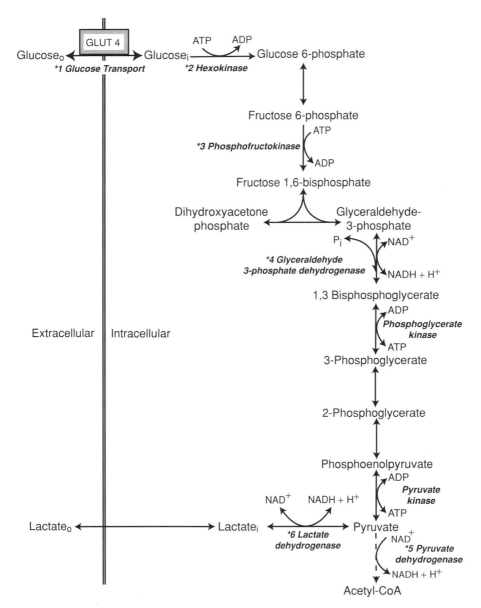

FIGURE 2-8 Major control points in glucose metabolism: glucose transport (*1); hexokinase, which catalyzes glucose phosphorylation (*2); phosphofructokinase, which catalyzes fructose-6-phosphate phosphorylation (*3); glyceraldehyde-3-phosphate dehydrogenase, which catalyzes glyceraldehyde-3-phosphate oxidation (*4); pyruvate dehydrogenase, which catalyzes acetyl-CoA formation (*5); and lactate dehydrogenase, which catalyzes pyruvate reduction (*6).

According to the monetary analogy described earlier, the mechanisms that regulate glucose metabolism are analogous to those that alter capital flow through a bank account. Expenditure (glycolytic rate) is determined by the desire to spend (neurotransmitters and hormones), by cash on hand (ATP levels), by debt (ADP and AMP levels), by short-term borrowing (supply of oxidized coenzymes), and ultimately by earning capacity (substrate supply and isoforms of key glycolytic enzymes).

Glucose Transport

Glucose enters myocardial cells (*1, Fig. 2-8) by moving down a concentration gradient from the extracellular space into the cytosol. Although glucose uptake does not require the expenditure of energy, glucose cannot cross the plasma membrane by simple diffusion. Instead, glucose uptake utilizes a transporter called *GLUT 4*, whose activity is regulated when the transporter moves between the plasma membrane and intracellular storage vesicles. Under basal conditions, most of the GLUT 4 is sequestered in the storage vesicles, where it is inactive. Insulin, ischemia, and hypoxia accelerate glucose uptake by recruiting GLUT 4 to the plasma membrane. Insulin stimulates GLUT 4 translocation by activating a complex signaling pathway, whereas ischemia and hypoxia promote GLUT 4 translocation to the plasma membrane when increased AMP levels, caused by energy starvation, activate an AMP-activated protein kinase.

Hexokinase

Before glucose can be metabolized, it must be phosphorylated by *hexokinase* in a reaction that "invests" the first of 2 moles of high-energy phosphate per mole of glucose (*2, Fig. 2-8). Hexokinase is regulated by allosteric effects of glucose-6-phosphate, ATP, ADP, AMP, and P_i. Most important is an inhibitory effect of glucose-6-phosphate that slows glycolysis when energy supplies are abundant. ATP potentiates the response of hexokinase to glucose-6-phosphate, whereas ADP, AMP, and P_i reduce the inhibition of glucose phosphorylation. Together, these responses allow the hexokinase reaction to be slowed by the high glucose-6-phosphate and ATP levels in the well-oxygenated heart and activated by the products of ATP hydrolysis in the energy-starved heart. Increased cardiac work, which lowers ATP concentration and increases ADP, AMP, and P_i levels, also stimulates hexokinase so as to help match the rates of energy production and energy utilization.

6-Phosphofructo-1-kinase

A second mole of $\sim$P is invested to phosphorylate fructose 6-phosphate, which forms fructose 1,6-bisphosphate (*3, Fig. 2-8) in the rate-limiting step of aerobic glycolysis. This reaction is catalyzed by *6-phosphofructo-1-kinase* (*phosphofructokinase* or *PFK*), a highly regulated enzyme complex that, like hexokinase, is inhibited by ATP and stimulated by the products of ATP hydrolysis. PFK is especially sensitive to stimulation by AMP, which allows a small increase in AMP to accelerate glycolysis when cardiac work is increased or the heart is deprived of oxygen. PFK activity also is increased by *fructose 2,6-bisphosphate*, which is produced from fructose-6-phosphate in a "side-reaction" catalyzed by *6-phosphofructo-2-kinase*, a cyclic AMP–dependent protein kinase that is activated by sympathetic stimulation. Calcium, which like sympathetic stimulation accelerates energy utilization by increasing myocardial contractility, also stimulates PFK. *Acidosis*, a powerful inhibitor of PFK, slows glycolysis when conversion of pyruvate to lactate releases protons; this is one reason why anaerobic glycolysis, although initially accelerated in the anaerobic heart, slows soon after coronary artery occlusion (see Chapter 17).

In 1861, Louis Pasteur found that air inhibits ethanol production by fermenting grapes. This response, called the *Pasteur effect*, is due in part to inhibition of PFK when oxidative metabolism generates large amounts of ATP and decreases ADP, AMP, and P_i levels. The Pasteur effect, which plays a key role in integrating glycolysis and oxidative phosphorylation, also occurs when PFK is inhibited by citrate, an important product of aerobic metabolism (see below).

Allosteric control of PFK by changing high-energy phosphate levels utilizes a mechanism, called *amplification*, in which small changes in ATP, ADP, and AMP concentrations exert large effects on glycolytic rate. This feature of allosteric regulation allows high-energy phosphate depletion to stimulate energy production while minimizing changes in ATP and ADP concentrations. Because the free energy available from ATP hydrolysis is proportional to the ATP–ADP ratio, minimizing a fall in this ratio is especially important for the heart, where as little as a 15% to 25% reduction can reduce the free energy available from ATP hydrolysis to an extent that impairs vital energy-dependent reactions (Kammermeier et al., 1982; Tian and Ingwall, 1996).

The effects of changing high-energy phosphate levels on PFK are amplified by *adenylate kinase* (also called *myokinase*), which catalyzes the reaction:

$$ATP + AMP \leftrightarrow 2\ ADP$$

This enzyme maintains an extremely low AMP concentration, which allows a small fall in ATP concentration to cause a proportionately large increase in the AMP–ATP ratio that stimulates PFK. The low AMP levels maintained by adenylate kinase also minimize depletion of the adenine nucleotide pool (ATP, ADP, and AMP) that can occur when AMP is dephosphorylated to form adenosine. Because adenosine is irreversibly deaminated to form hypoxanthine, adenine depletion is detrimental because this nucleoside must be replenished by *de novo* synthesis, which requires several days.

Glyceraldehyde-3 Phosphate Dehydrogenase

The next control point in glycolysis occurs after fructose 1,6-bisphosphate is hydrolyzed to form 2 moles of triose. This step, where glyceraldehyde-3-phosphate is oxidized and phosphorylated to form 1,3-bisphosphoglycerate, is catalyzed by *glyceraldehyde-3-phosphate dehydrogenase* (GAPDH) (*4, Fig. 2-8). Although GAPDH does not determine glycolytic rate in the normal heart, where PFK activity is rate-limiting, 1,3-bisphosphoglycerate formation becomes rate-limiting during hypoxia or ischemia, or when the heart is performing high levels of work. Under these conditions, where PFK is activated by lowered ATP concentration and increased ADP, AMP, and P_i levels (see above), control of glycolysis shifts "downstream" to the GAPDH reaction. In the energy-starved heart, however, this reaction is eventually slowed by depletion of NAD^+, accumulation of NADH, and 1,3-bisphosphoglycerate, and acidosis.

Phosphoglycerate Kinase and Pyruvate Kinase

The ~P used to form 1,3-bisphosphoglycerate is transferred to ATP by *phosphoglycerate kinase* in the first of two steps in glycolysis, where ATP is regenerated by substrate-level phosphorylation. *Pyruvate kinase*, which forms pyruvate and ATP from phosphoenolpyruvate and ADP (Fig. 2-8), catalyzes the second of the two substrate-level phosphorylations. Although pyruvate kinase regulates glycolysis in some tissues, this enzyme is of little regulatory importance in the heart.

PYRUVATE METABOLISM

Pyruvate stands at a metabolic "crossroads" because it can be oxidized to form acetyl-CoA or reduced to form lactate. The road taken is determined in part by the activities of two enzymes: *pyruvate dehydrogenase* (PDH) and *lactate dehydrogenase* (LDH). In the well-oxygenated heart, PDH catalyzes the conversion of pyruvate to acetyl coenzyme A (acetyl-CoA) (*5, Fig. 2-8), which can be oxidized in the citric acid cycle (see below). In the anaerobic heart, on the other hand, pyruvate is converted to lactate by LDH (*6, Fig. 2-8).

Lactate Dehydrogenase

Lactate dehydrogenase (LDH) is a tetramer made up of 2 isoforms called *M* and *H*; all combinations (H_4, H_3M, H_2M_2, H_1M_3 and M_4) are found in muscle, but the M isoform occurs mainly in skeletal muscle, while H is most prevalent in the heart. Different fates of pyruvate in cardiac and skeletal muscle are determined in part by the higher pyruvate affinity of the M subunits as compared with the H subunits. In skeletal muscles where energy production depends mainly on anaerobic glycolysis, the M subunits of LDH preferentially reduce pyruvate to lactate (*6, Fig. 2-8), whereas in the well-oxygenated heart, which has an abundant

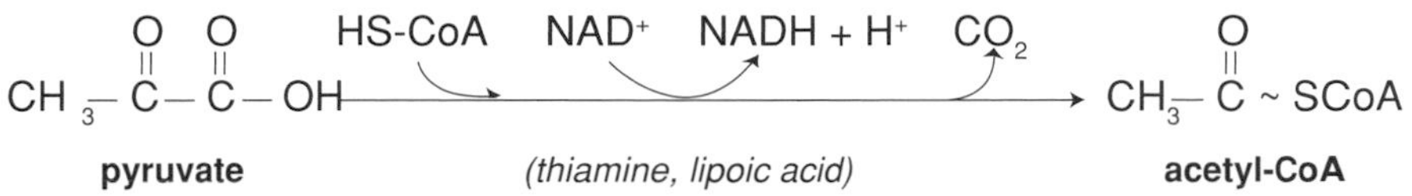

$$CH_3-\overset{\overset{O}{||}}{C}-\overset{\overset{O}{||}}{C}-OH \xrightarrow[\text{(thiamine, lipoic acid)}]{\overset{\text{HS-CoA} \quad \text{NAD}^+ \quad \text{NADH} + \text{H}^+ \quad \text{CO}_2}{\searrow \quad \searrow \quad \nearrow \quad \nearrow_2}} CH_3-\overset{\overset{O}{||}}{C} \sim \text{SCoA}$$

pyruvate   *(thiamine, lipoic acid)*   **acetyl-CoA**

FIGURE 2-9   Overall reaction by which pyruvate is oxidized and decarboxylated to form acetyl-CoA.

supply of NAD^+, the low pyruvate affinity of the H subunits of LDH favors pyruvate oxidation and decarboxylation by PDH (see below). Lactate production in the energy-starved heart provides a critical but limited supply of NAD^+.

Pyruvate Dehydrogenase

Pyruvate dehydrogenase (PDH), a huge mitochondrial enzyme complex, catalyzes an irreversible multistep reaction that oxidizes and decarboxylates pyruvate to form acetyl-CoA (*5, Figs. 2-8 and 2-9). These reactions, which require NAD^+, FAD, CoA, thiamine, and lipoic acid, are regulated by phosphorylation and dephosphorylation of PDH as well as the concentrations of substrate (pyruvate), products (acetyl-CoA and NADH), and cofactors (CoA-SH, lipoic acid, phosphorylated thiamine, and NAD^+).

PDH activity is decreased when the enzyme complex is phosphorylated by *pyruvate dehydrogenase kinase* and increased after dephosphorylation by *pyruvate dehydrogenase phosphatase* (Fig. 2-10). Pyruvate dehydrogenase kinase, which catalyzes the inhibitory phosphorylation, is activated by the products of the PDH reaction (NADH and acetyl CoA) and inhibited by pyruvate, coenzyme A, and NAD^+; together, these effects

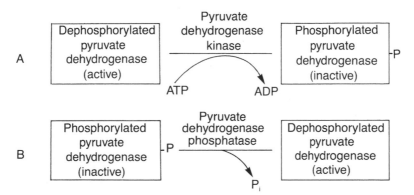

FIGURE 2-10   Phosphorylation (A) and dephosphorylation (B) reactions that modulate PDH activity. A: Phosphorylation by pyruvate dehydrogenase kinase converts active, dephosphorylated PDH to the inactive phosphorylated enzyme. B: Dephosphorylation by pyruvate dehydrogenase phosphatase converts inactive PDH to the active dephosphorylated form.

reduce PDH activity when its substrates are exhausted and the reaction products accumulate. Phosphorylation of PDH also is stimulated by NADH, which, as noted above, favors lactate production rather than formation of acetyl CoA in the energy-starved heart by inhibiting pyruvate oxidation.

Pyruvate dehydrogenase phosphatase reverses the inhibitory phosphorylation of PDH. This enzyme is inhibited by NADH, which by slowing pyruvate production favors lactate production in the energy-starved heart. Pyruvate dehydrogenase phosphatase also is inhibited by citrate, which allows this citric acid cycle intermediate to slow acetyl-CoA production from glucose; this is one reason why the high citrate levels in the well-oxygenated heart favor fatty acid oxidation rather than glucose oxidation. This effect of citrate therefore contributes to the normal "preference" of the well-oxygenated heart for lipids, rather than carbohydrates. Sympathetic stimulation and calcium, both of which increase myocardial contractility, also accelerate acetyl-CoA formation by activating this phosphatase.

Other Fates of Pyruvate

Pyruvate can be carboxylated to form 2 citric acid cycle substrates: oxaloacetate, whose formation is catalyzed by *pyruvate carboxylase*, and malate, which is formed by *malic enzyme*. Pyruvate also can be transaminated to form the amino acid alanine. The reverse of this transamination, conversion of alanine to pyruvate, allows alanine to be oxidized, but as noted above, the heart has only a limited ability to generate energy by metabolizing amino acids.

FATTY ACIDS

Fats can be viewed as "concentrated energy" whose oxidation yields 9 calories/gm substrate, compared with only 5 calories/gm for carbohydrates and proteins. After being absorbed into the bloodstream, dietary fatty acids are transported to the heart either as glycerol esters (*triacylglycerols* or *triglycerides*) or as *free fatty acids* (FFA) (Fig. 2-11). The latter is a misnomer because fatty acids bind avidly to plasma proteins, mainly albumin; FFA, therefore, are "free" only because they are not bound as esters. In order to be metabolized, fatty acids must enter myocardial cells, where they are converted to acetyl CoA that is oxidized in the mitochondria.

Hydrolysis of Triacylglycerol

Triacylglycerols cannot cross the plasma membrane until the ester bonds linking the fatty acid to glycerol are hydrolyzed by *lipoprotein lipase* (Eckel, 1989). This enzyme, located on the luminal surface of the capillary endothelium, is activated by β-adrenergic agonists so that fatty acid release from triacylglycerols, like glycolysis and glucose uptake, is under *humoral* control.

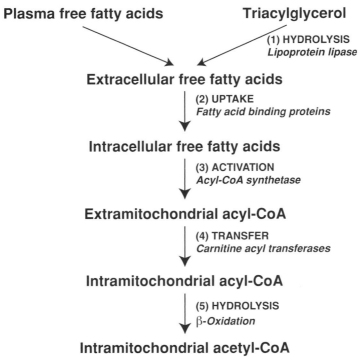

FIGURE 2-11   Transfer of long-chain fatty acids into myocardial cells and their conversion to acetyl-CoA showing key reactions (*capital letters*) and enzymes or carriers (*italics*). Hydrolysis of plasma triacylglycerols (1); uptake of plasma free fatty acids (2); activation of fatty acids by CoA (3); transfer of activated fatty acids (acyl-CoA) from the cytosol to the mitochondrial matrix (4); and hydrolysis (β-oxidation), which yields acetyl-CoA within the mitochondria (5).

Fatty Acid Uptake

Fatty acid transfer across the capillary endothelium and cardiac plasma membrane occurs by passive diffusion that is facilitated by *fatty acid binding proteins* (FABP), which include fatty acid transport proteins and fatty acid translocases. The rate of fatty acid uptake by the myocardium is determined by the law of mass action, which allows high plasma FFA and low cytoplasmic fatty acid levels to accelerate fatty acid uptake. Increased energy utilization by the working heart is therefore able to accelerate fatty acid uptake by reducing the intracellular concentration of this key substrate.

Fatty Acid Activation

Fatty acid activation, like glucose phosphorylation (see above), requires the "investment" of energy to form long-chain analogues of *acetyl-CoA* called *fatty acyl-CoA* (*acyl-CoA*). This occurs in a two-step reaction that begins when *acyl-CoA synthetase*, located on the mitochondrial outer membrane, transfers AMP derived from ATP to the fatty

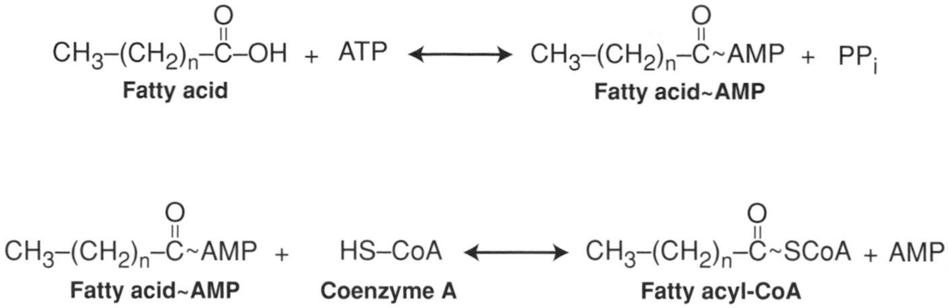

$$CH_3-(CH_2)_n-\overset{\overset{\displaystyle O}{\|}}{C}-OH + ATP \longleftrightarrow CH_3-(CH_2)_n-\overset{\overset{\displaystyle O}{\|}}{C}\sim AMP + PP_i$$

Fatty acid   Fatty acid~AMP

$$CH_3-(CH_2)_n-\overset{\overset{\displaystyle O}{\|}}{C}\sim AMP + HS-CoA \longleftrightarrow CH_3-(CH_2)_n-\overset{\overset{\displaystyle O}{\|}}{C}\sim SCoA + AMP$$

Fatty acid~AMP   Coenzyme A   Fatty acyl-CoA

FIGURE 2-12 Fatty acid activation occurs in a two-step reaction that is catalyzed by acyl-CoA synthetase. In the first step, the fatty acid binds to AMP to form an activated fatty acid~AMP complex and pyrophosphate (PP_i). In the second step, AMP is replaced by CoA to form fatty acyl-CoA, which contains a high-energy thioester bond.

acid, which forms fatty acid~AMP, a high-energy complex (Fig. 2-12). The pyrophosphate (PP_i) released in this reaction is hydrolyzed by a *pyrophosphatase* to form inorganic phosphate. In the second step, the adenylate moiety of fatty acid~AMP is replaced by CoA to form fatty acyl-CoA, which contains a high-energy thioester bond.

Fatty Acid Transfer

In order for activated fatty acids to enter the mitochondrial matrix, they must cross the inner membrane. Because this membrane is impermeable to fatty acyl-CoA, the bound CoA is replaced with *carnitine* to form *fatty acyl carnitine*, which is transferred to the matrix by an exchange-diffusion (Fig. 2-13). The heart cannot synthesize carnitine, so this essential compound must be present in the diet. Carnitine deficiency is a rare but treatable cause of heart failure (Paulson, 1998).

Fatty acid transfer begins when *carnitine acyl-transferase I*, located on the mitochondrial outer membrane, replaces the bound CoA in acyl-CoA with carnitine to form *acyl-carnitine*. A *translocase* on the inner membrane then exchanges this acyl-carnitine for carnitine in the matrix. After the cytosolic acyl-carnitine enters the matrix, *carnitine acyl-transferase II* located on the inner membrane replaces the carnitine with CoA to form acyl-CoA.

The rate of fatty acyl transfer is determined largely by the concentrations of the reactants on the two sides of the inner membrane. During periods of increased cardiac energy demand, when high rates of fatty acid oxidation consume mitochondrial acyl-CoA, both acyl-CoA formation from mitochondrial acyl-carnitine and carnitine release in the mitochondrial matrix are accelerated. Mitochondrial carnitine is exchanged for acyl-carnitine by the translocase, which provides additional cytosolic carnitine that can be exchanged for the CoA in cytosolic acyl-CoA; this provides more CoA for binding to cytosolic fatty acids, increasing fatty acid uptake by reducing free fatty acid concentration in the cytosol.

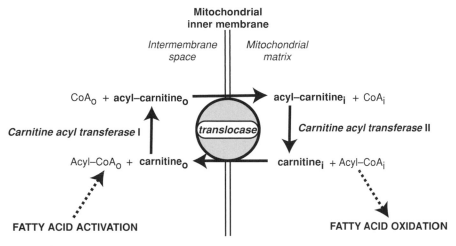

FIGURE 2-13 Carnitine-mediated exchange-diffusion of fatty acids across the mito-chondrial inner membrane. *Carnitine acyl transferases I* and *II* exchange CoA and carnitine in the mitochondrial intermembrane space (between the inner and outer membranes) and matrix, respectively. Acyl-carnitine in the intermembrane space is then exchanged for carnitine in the matrix by a translocase on the mitochondrial inner membrane. Abbre-viations: Acyl-CoA$_o$ and acyl-carnitine$_o$: activated fatty acids outside the mitochondrial matrix; acyl-CoA$_i$ and acyl-carnitine$_i$: activated fatty acids within the mitochondria.

β-Oxidation

Long-chain fatty acyl-CoA is broken down into acetyl-CoA in the mitochondria by a process called β-oxidation (Fig. 2-14). This stepwise shortening of long-chain fatty acids, most of which contain 16 or 18 carbon atoms, can be likened to a spiral in which each "turn" releases a 2-carbon acetyl-CoA through four steps—two of oxidation, one of hydration, and one of thiolysis (Fig. 2-15). The oxidations reduce NAD^+ and flavine ade-nine dinucleotide (FAD) to form NADH and $FADH_2$, respectively. Thioly-sis adds CoA to the oxidized β-ketoacyl CoA, which releases acetyl-CoA, thereby shortening the fatty acid chain by 2 carbons. Although β-oxidation does not regenerate ATP, the electrons transferred to NADH and $FADH_2$ are used to energize oxidative phosphorylation (see below).

β-Oxidation is rapid in the well-oxygenated heart, where the rate-limiting step in fat metabolism is fatty acid transfer into the mitochondria. In the energy-starved heart, where levels of oxidized NAD^+ and FAD are low, β-oxidation can become rate limiting.

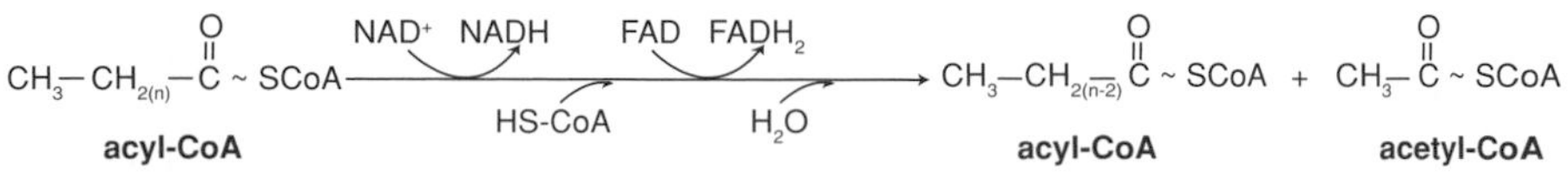

FIGURE 2-14 Overall reaction of β-oxidation, which releases acetyl-CoA from activated fatty acids (acyl-CoA).

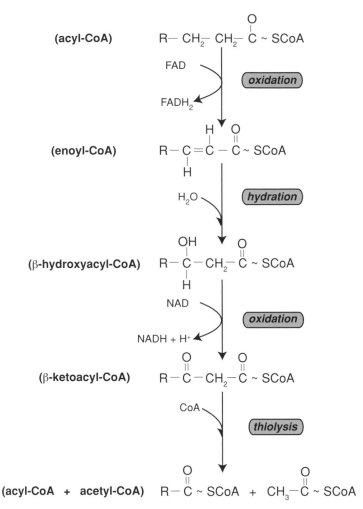

FIGURE 2-15 β-Oxidation. Each cycle in the stepwise breakdown of long-chain fatty acids involves four steps—two of oxidation, one of hydration, and one of thiolysis.

Fatty Acid Synthesis and Fat Deposition

Fat deposits, called *fatty infiltration*, are commonly found beneath the epicardium and can envelop the heart in obese individuals; these deposits, which are largely of exogenous origin, are rarely of clinical significance. In *fatty degeneration*, where fat droplets appear within myocardial cells, some of the fatty acids are synthesized by energy-starved cells. The limited capacity of the heart to synthesize fatty acids (Hillgartner et al., 1995) helps to store this important substrate and regenerates a small amount of NAD^+ and FAD. When present at high concentrations, fatty acids are incorporated into membranes, where they can have deleterious effects (Katz and Messineo, 1981).

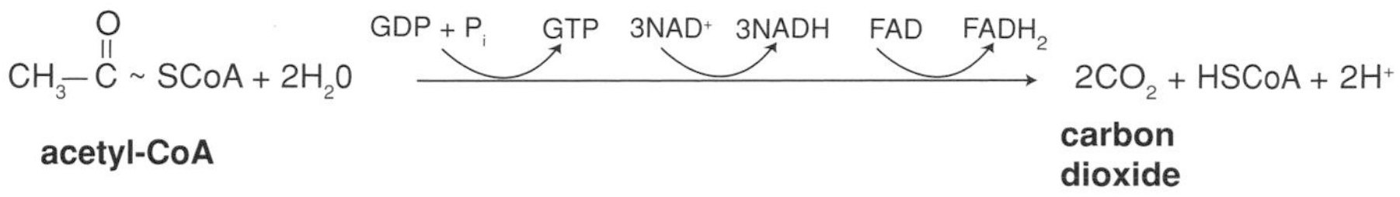

$$CH_3-\overset{\overset{\displaystyle O}{\|}}{C} \sim SCoA + 2H_2O \xrightarrow{\quad \overset{GDP + P_i \quad GTP}{\curvearrowright} \quad \overset{3NAD^+ \quad 3NADH}{\curvearrowright} \quad \overset{FAD \quad FADH_2}{\curvearrowright} \quad} 2CO_2 + HSCoA + 2H^+$$

acetyl-CoA   **carbon dioxide**

FIGURE 2-16 Overall reaction of the citric acid cycle. Oxidation and decarboxylation of each mole of acetyl CoA forms 2 moles of carbon dioxide, 1 mole of ATP, 3 moles of NADH, and 1 mole of $FADH_2$.

Fatty Acids as Regulators of Gene Expression: PPARs

Fatty acid–binding receptors called *peroxisome proliferator-activated receptors* (PPARs) regulate the transcription of many enzymes and transporters that participate in fatty acid transport and oxidation (Dyke and Lopaschuk, 2002). Regulation of gene expression by PPARs serves a number of functions in mammalian cells, including a role in mediating cardiac hypertrophy (Finck and Kelly, 2002; see Chapter 18).

ACETYL-COA OXIDATION: THE CITRIC ACID CYCLE

The acetyl-CoA formed from both pyruvate and fatty acids is oxidized within the mitochondrial matrix by the *citric acid cycle (tricarboxylic acid cycle, Krebs cycle)*. The overall reaction, which breaks down each mole of acetyl-CoA to release 2 moles of carbon dioxide, generates 1 mole of ATP by *substrate-level phosphorylation*, 3 moles of NADH, and 1 mole of $FADH_2$ (Fig. 2-16). As described below, oxidation of NADH and $FADH_2$ in the respiratory chain regenerates a much larger amount of ATP.

The citric acid cycle (Fig. 2-17) begins when acetyl-CoA condenses with oxaloacetate, a four-carbon organic acid, to form citrate and release CoA. After a configurational rearrangement that converts citrate to cis-aconitate, the six-carbon organic acid is converted to isocitrate. The latter is then oxidized and decarboxylated to form α-ketoglutaric acid, a five-carbon organic acid which, following decarboxylation and oxidation, yields succinyl-CoA, a four-carbon organic acid linked to CoA by a high-energy bond. The energy in the thiol bond is transferred to *succinyl CoA synthetase* (labeled "E" in Fig. 2-17) to form E~CoA, after which the enzyme-bound CoA is replaced by phosphate in the high-energy phosphorylated intermediate E~P (Fig. 2-17B). The ~P of E~P is transferred first to GDP, which forms GTP, and then to ADP, which regenerates ATP. This is the only reaction in the citric acid cycle where substrate-level phosphorylation forms a high-energy phosphate bond.

The citric acid cycle continues when the succinate released from succinyl-CoA is oxidized to fumarate by an FAD-containing respiratory chain enzyme complex called *succinate-coenzyme Q reductase* (labeled "E-FAD" in Fig. 2-17A; see also Fig. 2-20). Fumarate is then hydrated to form

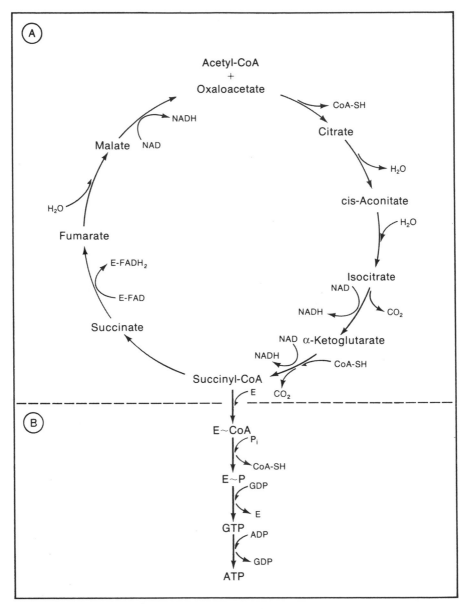

FIGURE 2-17   Citric acid cycle (A) and succinyl-CoA metabolism (B). A: Condensation of acetyl-CoA with oxaloacetate yields citrate, a six-carbon acid, which after isomerization to isocitrate is oxidized and decarboxylated to form α-ketoglutarate. The latter is oxidized and decarboxylated to form succinyl-CoA, which undergoes two steps of oxidation and one of hydration to regenerate oxaloacetate. B: Succinyl-CoA contains a high-energy thiol bond that is used to generate ATP by substrate-level phosphorylation in reactions that are catalyzed by succinyl-CoA synthase (E). This enzyme transfers the high-energy bond linking CoA to succinyl-CoA first to GTP, which forms GTP, and then to ADP to regenerate ATP.

malate, which is oxidized in a reaction that reduces NAD^+ to NADH; this reaction, which regenerates oxaloacetate, completes the citric acid cycle.

Like all important cellular processes, the citric acid cycle is highly regulated. Turnover is influenced by the supply of acetyl-CoA and oxaloacetate, high-energy phosphate levels, and the availability of oxidized NAD^+ and FAD. *Citrate synthase*, which catalyzes the first reaction in the cycle where acetyl-CoA condenses with oxaloacetate to form citrate, is inhibited by ATP and NADH. Production of α-ketoglutarate from isocitrate, which is catalyzed by *isocitrate dehydrogenase*, is inhibited by ATP and stimulated by ADP, thereby allowing increased energy consumption to accelerate energy production. The increased cytosolic calcium responsible for most increases in myocardial contractility also helps to match energy consumption and energy production by activating isocitrate dehydrogenase and α-*ketoglutarate dehydrogenase*, which catalyzes succinyl-CoA formation. In the anaerobic heart, inhibition of citrate synthetase and α-ketoglutarate dehydrogenase by NADH slows the citric acid cycle. Together, these regulatory mechanisms enable the citric acid cycle to respond to changes in substrate supply, energy requirements, and the availability of oxidized coenzymes.

TRANSPORT OF REDUCED NADH FROM CYTOSOL TO MITOCHONDRIA: THE MALATE–ASPARTATE CYCLE

Unlike NADH formed in the mitochondria, which is readily accessible to the respiratory chain, NADH produced in the cytosol must cross the mitochondrial inner membrane before it can be oxidized; furthermore, virtually all of the NAD^+ required for aerobic glycolysis is formed in the mitochondria before being returned to the cytosol. However, the inner membrane is not permeable to NADH and NAD^+ and represents a barrier to the simple transfer of reducing equivalents between the cytosol and mitochondrial matrix. NADH and NAD^+ transfer therefore depends on a complex exchange, called the *malate–aspartate cycle*, which includes the oxidations, reductions, and transaminations shown in Figure 2-18.

At first glance, the malate–aspartate cycle might seem to represent a needlessly elaborate way to move NADH from the cytosol to the mitochondrial matrix, and to deliver NAD^+ to the cytosol. The complexity of this transfer (why do the mitochondria simply not have a carrier that exchanges NADH for NAD^+?) illustrates nature's failure to adhere to Ockham's razor, written in the 14th century: "Plurality should not be posited without necessity," which can be paraphrased to mean that when choosing among competing explanations, one should start with the simplest. It is clear, however, that the overlapping layers of control that characterize biological regulation, although violating Ockham's razor, are advantageous for homeostasis. In the malate–aspartate cycle, this complexity helps to match energy production and energy utilization by adjusting the rates of anaerobic

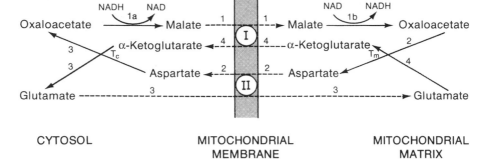

FIGURE 2-18 The malate–aspartate cycle. Four simultaneous reactions "transfer" NADH from the cytosol to the mitochondria. (1) Reduction of oxaloacetate in the cytosol oxidizes NAD^+ and forms malate (1a), after which the malate is transferred into the mitochondrial matrix by membrane carrier (I), where oxidation of the malate regenerates oxaloacetate and releases NADH (1b). (2) The oxaloacetate formed in the matrix is transaminated with glutamate (T_m) to form α-ketoglutarate and aspartate, after which aspartate is returned to the cytosol by membrane carrier (II). (3) After entering the cytosol, the aspartate is transaminated with α-ketoglutarate to form oxaloacetate and glutamate (T_c), after which the latter is returned to the matrix by membrane carrier II in exchange for the aspartate produced in reaction 2. (4) The glutamate returned to the matrix is transaminated with oxaloacetate (T_m, described in reaction 2) to yield α-ketoglutarate, after which the cycle is completed when mitochondrial α-ketoglutarate is exchanged for malate by the membrane carrier I described in reaction 1.

and aerobic energy production to changes in the supply of key substrates and cofactors.

TRANSAMINATIONS

Transfer of amino groups between organic and amino acids (e.g., between α-ketoglutarate and glutamate, oxaloacetate and aspartate, and pyruvate and glutamate) is catalyzed by enzymes called *transaminases* (*aminotransferases*). In addition to their role in the malate–aspartate cycle, transaminations enable the heart to metabolize a small amount of protein. In the anaerobic heart, transamination of pyruvate to form alanine delays the onset of acidosis by slowing lactate formation (Taegtmeyer et al., 1977).

ADENINE NUCLEOTIDE TRANSFER

The mitochondrial inner membrane is impermeable to adenine nucleotides as well as to NADH and NAD^+. For this reason, transfer of ATP and ADP between the cytosol and mitochondrial matrix requires another exchange mechanism, called the *ATP–ADP translocase* (*transferase*), that couples ATP flux in one direction to ADP flux in the opposite direction (Fig. 2-19). Because ATP has 3 negative charges and ADP only 2,

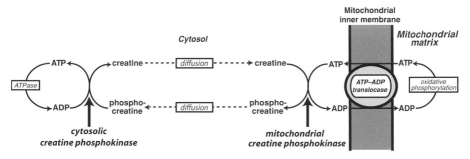

FIGURE 2-19 The phosphocreatine shuttle and ATP–ADP transferase. ATP hydrolysis by energy-utilizing structures (ATPase) in the cytosol (*left*) releases ADP that is rephosphorylated by *cytosolic creatine phosphokinase* using ~P derived from phosphocreatine. The creatine produced by this reaction diffuses to the mitochondria (*right*), where *mitochondrial creatine phosphokinase* uses ~P from ATP to regenerate phosphocreatine and release ADP. The latter is returned to the mitochondrial matrix by the *ATP–ADP translocase* in exchange for ATP. After entering the matrix, ADP is rephosphorylated by oxidative phosphorylation to form ATP, which is returned to the cytosol in exchange for ADP by the ATP–ADP translocase. The ~P in this ATP is then transferred to creatine in the reaction catalyzed by mitochondrial creatine phosphokinase (*see above*). The phosphocreatine regenerated in this reaction can then diffuse to supply energy to cytosolic ATPases (*left*).

this exchange is electrogenic, so transfer of ATP into the cytosol from the matrix adds to the negative potential generated by the proton pumps described below.

THE PHOSPHOCREATINE SHUTTLE

The high ATP concentration in myocardial cells, which is in the millimolar range, allows this high-energy compound to diffuse rapidly through the cytosol to sites where it is hydrolyzed. Diffusion of ADP through the cytosol for rephosphorylation in the mitochondria, however, is much slower because cytosolic ADP concentration is very low, ~0.02 mM (Illingworth et al., 1975; Rauch et al., 1994; Wallimann et al., 1992). Because this poses a serious problem for the heart, where energy utilization is rapid, creatine and phosphocreatine rather than ADP and ATP transfer high-energy phosphates within the cytosol (McClellan et al., 1983; Jacobus, 1985; Kammermeier, 1987). This transfer, called the *phosphocreatine shuttle* (Fig. 2-19), takes advantage of the high cytosolic concentrations of creatine and phosphocreatine, both of which diffuse rapidly, to return creatine rather than ADP to the mitochondria for rephosphorylation, and use phosphocreatine instead of ATP to carry ~P from the mitochondria to energy-consuming structures in the cytosol.

Transfer of ~P between ADP and creatine by the phosphocreatine shuttle depends on the ATP–ADP translocase described above and 2 enzymes. The first, *mitochondrial creatine phosphokinase*, is located on the mitochondrial inner membrane where it transfers ~P from ATP generated by the mitochondria to creatine, forming phosphocreatine and releasing ADP into the cytosol (Fig. 2-19, *right*). This ADP, when returned to the mitochondria in exchange for additional ATP, can be rephosphorylated by oxidative phosphorylation.

The phosphocreatine generated by mitochondrial creatine phosphokinase diffuses through the cytosol, where the second enzyme, *cytosolic creatine phosphokinase*, transfers ~P from phosphocreatine to ADP, which regenerates ATP (Fig. 2-19, *left*). The latter supplies ~P to cytosolic ATPases such as the contractile proteins and sarcoplasmic reticulum. The cytosolic creatine formed in this reaction diffuses rapidly to the mitochondria, where it can accept additional ~P (Fig. 2-19, *right*).

THE RESPIRATORY CHAIN

The ATP generated by *substrate-level phosphorylations* in glycolysis and the citric acid cycle is not sufficient to meet the energy demands of the beating heart; instead, most of this high-energy phosphate is regenerated by oxidative metabolism. The latter can be viewed as a "four-step" process (Table 2-3) that begins when electrons produced by carbohydrate and fatty acid oxidation are transferred to NAD^+ and FAD, forming NADH and $FADH_2$. The latter then transfer their electrons to the *respiratory chain* (*electron transport chain*) in the second step, after which the third step uses energy carried by these electrons to establish a proton electrochemical gradient across the mitochondrial inner membrane. The final step occurs when proton flux down this gradient releases energy to regenerate ATP by *respiratory chain-linked phosphorylations*.

I came to appreciate the large amount of energy released by oxidation of hydrogenated substances when, as a freshman in college, I set fire to a mixture of hydrogen and oxygen. I filled a rubber glove with hydrogen (generated by pouring hydrochloric acid over powdered zinc) that I ignited with a match tied to a 6-foot pole. The resulting explosion rattled windows more than 100 meters away. Oxidative phosphorylation can be viewed simply as a mechanism to retain this energy in the high-energy phosphate bonds of ATP. The "magic" of the respiratory chain is its ability to prevent the highly reactive electrons and free radicals formed during electron transfer from

---

TABLE 2-3 **Four "Steps" in Oxidative Metabolism**

Step 1: Transfer of electrons from substrates to coenzymes

Step 2: Passage of electrons from coenzymes through the respiratory chain

Step 3: Establishment of proton electrochemical gradient across mitochondrial inner membrane

Step 4: Downhill proton flux across the mitochondrial inner membrane and regeneration of ATP

interacting with structures within the cell by allowing oxygen free radicals to combine with protons to form water.

Electrons or Reducing Equivalents?

The respiratory chain uses the energy carried by the electrons in reduced NADH and $FADH_2$ in a more controlled manner than occurred in my rubber glove. One way to characterize these reactions is to view oxidation of the reduced coenzymes as the transfer of reducing equivalents and protons to oxygen, thereby forming water:

$$\text{NADH} + \text{H}^+ + \tfrac{1}{2}\text{O}_2 \rightarrow \text{NAD}^+ + \text{H}_2\text{O}$$
$$\text{(reduced)} \qquad\qquad\qquad \text{(oxidized)}$$

and

$$\text{FADH}_2 + \tfrac{1}{2}\text{O}_2 \rightarrow \text{FAD} + \text{H}_2\text{O}$$
$$\text{(reduced)} \qquad\qquad \text{(oxidized)}$$

Because each hydrogen atom (H) is a proton (H^+) plus an electron (e^-), these reactions also can be characterized as electron transfer to molecular oxygen; viewed in this manner, NADH is equivalent to ($NAD^+ - H^+ - 2e^-$) and $FADH_2$ to ($FAD - 2H^+ - 2e^-$), so that the overall reactions can be written:

$$(\text{NAD}^+ - \text{H}^+ - 2e^-) + \text{H}^+ + \tfrac{1}{2}\text{O}_2 \rightarrow \text{NAD}^+ + 2\text{H}^+ + \text{O}^{2-} \rightarrow \text{NAD}^+ + \text{H}_2\text{O}$$
$$\text{(reduced)} \qquad\qquad\qquad\qquad\qquad\qquad\qquad \text{(oxidized)}$$

and

$$(\text{FAD} - 2\text{H}^+ - 2e^-) + \tfrac{1}{2}\text{O}_2 \rightarrow \text{FAD} + 2\text{H}^+ + \text{O}^{2-} \rightarrow \text{FAD} + \text{H}_2\text{O}$$
$$\text{(reduced)} \qquad\qquad\qquad\qquad\qquad\qquad \text{(oxidized)}$$

The second pair of equations describe oxidative phosphorylation as the transfer of electrons carried by the reduced coenzymes to molecular oxygen, which forms O^{2-}, a free radical that combines with the protons to form water.

The oxidations in carbohydrate and fat metabolism also can be viewed as the transfer of electrons (along with protons) to reduced coenzymes in which the electrons become associated with nitrogen or oxygen atoms in organic ring structures:

$$-\text{N}^+ + e^- \longleftrightarrow -\text{N}$$
$$\text{(oxidized)} \qquad\qquad \text{(reduced)}$$

and

$$-\text{O} + e^- \longleftrightarrow -\text{O}^-$$
$$\text{(oxidized)} \qquad\qquad \text{(reduced)}$$

Electrons carried by respiratory chain intermediates are associated with nitrogen, oxygen, iron sulfates, the heme iron of cytochromes, and copper. The latter accept electrons according to the general reactions:

$$Fe^{3+} \quad + e^- \longleftrightarrow \quad Fe^{2+}$$
$$\text{(oxidized)} \qquad\qquad \text{(reduced)}$$

and

$$Cu^{2+} \quad + e^- \longleftrightarrow \quad Cu^+$$
$$\text{(oxidized)} \qquad\qquad \text{(reduced)}$$

All of these structures transfer electrons by a series of tightly coupled steps that prevent them from "escaping" within the cell.

Electron Transfer through the Respiratory Chain

The tightly linked oxidations and reductions that transfer electrons along the respiratory chain (Fig. 2-20) resemble the firemen in an old fashioned "bucket brigade," whose close proximity and careful handling of water-filled buckets minimizes spillage and maximizes efficiency. Structural organization of the respiratory chain electron carriers on the mitochondrial inner membrane avoids the energy loss and cell damage that would occur if the highly reactive and potentially destructive electrons were to be released into the cytosol.

The respiratory chain includes four multiprotein complexes, all of which are bound to the mitochondrial inner membrane. Three (*NADH-CoQ reductase*, *CoH₂Q-cytochrome c reductase*, and *cytochrome c oxidase*) are coupled to proton pumps that use energy released during the pass of electrons through the complexes to move H^+ uphill, out of the matrix, which generates an electrochemical gradient that energizes ATP regeneration (see below).

Electrons can enter the respiratory chain in two ways (Fig. 2-20). The electrons carried by NADH are transferred to *NADH-CoQ reductase* (Complex I) through which they are passed to flavine mononucleotide (FMN) and several iron sulfate clusters (FeS) before being transferred to *coenzyme Q (CoQH₂, ubiquinone)*. When the latter accepts an electron, it is converted to a free radical called a *semiquinone* (labeled $CoQH_2\bullet$ in Fig. 2-20). The electrons carried by the $FADH_2$ formed during β-oxidation (Fig. 2-15) and succinate oxidation (Fig. 2-17A) enter the respiratory chain in reactions that are catalyzed by *succinate-CoQ reductase* (Complex II), which transfers the electrons from $FADH_2$ first to $Fe^{3+}S$ and then to $CoQH_2\bullet$. Because electrons carried by $FADH_2$ bypass Complex I before entering the respiratory chain (Fig. 2-20), they activate only two of the three proton pumps; this "late entry" of electrons means that less ATP is generated by oxidation of $FADH_2$ than of NADH.

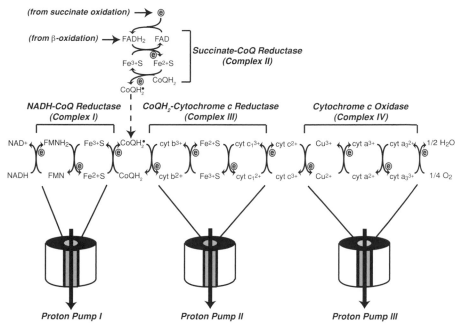

FIGURE 2-20 The respiratory chain. Reduced NADH (*left*) delivers electron pairs (*shaded circles labeled "e"*) to *NADH-CoQ reductase* (Complex I), which transfers the electrons to *CoQH₂-cytochrome c reductase* (Complex III) and *cytochrome c oxidase* (Complex IV). A decrease in the potential of the electrons as they pass along the chain energizes three proton pumps that transport H^+ uphill, out of the mitochondrial matrix. The sequence ends when the electrons interact with $\frac{1}{2}O_2$ to form an oxygen free radical (*not shown*) that combines immediately with protons to produce water (*right*). Unlike the electrons in NADH, which energize three proton pumps (*below*), the electrons in FADH₂ enter the respiratory chain by way of *succinate-CoQ reductase* (Complex II) and so bypass the first proton pump; for this reason, FADH₂ regenerates less ATP than NADH. Abbreviations: FMN, flavine mononucleotide; FeS, iron sulfate; CoQH₂, oxidized coenzyme Q (ubiquinone); CoQH₂•, semiquinone, a free radical; cyt, cytochrome; Cu, copper.

The third enzyme complex, CoH_2Q-*cytochrome c reductase* (Complex III), can accept electrons that enter the respiratory chain from both Complexes I and II. After transfer from CoQH₂, the electrons move through Complex III by way of iron atoms in cytochrome b, a ferrous sulfate-containing protein, and cytochrome c_1 before reaching cytochrome c. Electron transfer through Complex III energizes the second proton pump (Fig. 2-20). The electrons are then transferred from cytochrome c to the fourth enzyme complex, *cytochrome c oxidase* (Complex IV). The latter, which contains copper and cytochromes a and a_3, energizes the third proton pump (Fig. 2-20). Passage of electrons through the respiratory chain ends when the electrons, having lost most of their energy, are transferred to molecular oxygen in a reaction that forms a highly reactive oxygen free radical that combines immediately with protons to form H_2O.

Proton Pumps and the Proton Electromotive Force

As electrons pass through the respiratory chain, much of their energy is used to pump protons (H^+) "uphill" out of the mitochondrial matrix. The resulting proton gradient across the mitochondrial inner membrane (Fig. 2-21) provides an electromotive force that energizes ATP regeneration (see below). Transfer of the electron pair from each mole of NADH to the three enzyme complexes shown in Fig. 2-20 provides sufficient energy to regenerate approximately 3 moles of ATP, whereas the $FADH_2$ produced by succinate oxidation and β-oxidation bypasses one of the proton pumps (see above), therefore regenerating only about 2 moles of ATP.

Unlike substrate-linked phosphorylations, which transfer ~P from phosphorylated substrates directly to ADP, there is no strict stoichiometry between electron transport, proton pumping, and ATP regeneration. Nonintegral values reflect the gradual loss of energy as electrons are transferred through the respiratory chain, use of the proton gradient to transport

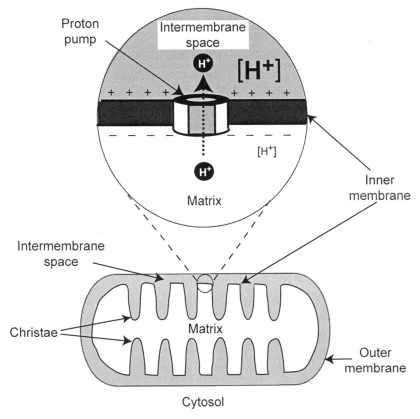

FIGURE 2-21 The proton electromotive force. Proton transport out of the mitochondrial matrix generates an electrochemical gradient across the inner membrane that causes the matrix to become electronegative and depleted of protons (alkaline). The resulting proton electromotive force allows downhill proton flux into the matrix to energize oxidative phosphorylation.

substrates and metabolites across the inner membrane, and loss of energy in "side reactions" like ATP–ADP exchange.

Calcium Fluxes Into and Out of the Mitochondria

The negative potential within the mitochondria favors calcium entry into the matrix. In the normal heart, where cytosolic calcium concentration is very low, mitochondria do not contribute to the removal of activator calcium that causes relaxation. However, under pathological conditions of cytosolic calcium overload, the mitochondria can take up calcium; when severe, calcium overload can cause calcium-phosphate to precipitate within the mitochondria. Mitochondrial calcium uptake uncouples oxidative phosphorylation by dissipating the proton electromotive force across the mitochondrial inner membrane; as a result, energy starvation can initiate a vicious cycle where low ATP levels impair active transport of calcium out of cardiac myocytes, which increases cytosolic calcium, which promotes mitochondrial calcium uptake, which uncouples oxidative phosphorylation, which worsens energy starvation. This vicious cycle can lead to cardiac myocyte necrosis in ischemic (Chapter 17) and failing hearts (Chapter 18).

OXIDATIVE PHOSPHORYLATION

Efforts to define the molecular mechanism of oxidative phosphorylation illustrate the pitfalls of extrapolating from one process to another. Much as initial theories of nerve transmission used hydraulic and electrical analogies to explain impulse conduction (see Preface), early workers in oxidative phosphorylation searched for intermediates that participate in substrate level phosphorylations like those in glycolysis. It is now clear, however, that mitochondria do not use phosphorylated intermediates to regenerate ATP; instead, a protein related to a flagellum transforms energy generated by the downhill flux of protons into a torque that transfers $\sim$P to ADP.

ATP Synthetase

A multiprotein enzyme called *ATP synthetase* regenerates ATP in the mitochondria. This membrane-spanning protein complex is made up of two connected structures: F_0, which contains a channel through which protons flow downhill into the matrix, and the F_1 *ATPase*, which projects from the inner membrane into the matrix (Fig. 2-22). ATP synthesis is energized when downhill proton flux through the F_0 channel rotates *ADP-* and *ATP-binding* sites on the F_1 complex. This rotational energy is then used to regenerate ATP by energizing formation of high-energy bonds that link P_i to ADP.

Some of the proteins in ATP synthetase are homologous to those in bacterial flagella, which use chemical energy generated by downhill proton flux to create a spinning motion that moves the prokaryotes. The ability of mitochondria to use a similar reaction to generate ATP is further evidence of the prokaryotic origin of the mitochondria described in Chapter 1.

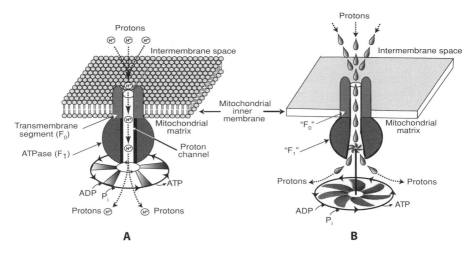

FIGURE 2-22   ATP synthetase and a hydraulic model showing its mechanism of action. **A:** ATP synthetase, a multiprotein complex that projects from the mitochondrial inner membrane into the matrix, is made up of two connected structures—a transmembrane segment, F_0, which contains a channel through which protons flow down their electrochemical gradient into the mitochondrial matrix, and F_1, which converts energy generated by this downhill proton flux to a torque that rotates the F_1 ATPase. Much as the rotation of a water-powered turbine generates electricity, the rotational energy in F_1 regenerates ATP by energizing the formation of high-energy bonds linking P_i to ADP.

Control of Oxidative Phosphorylation

The major determinant of the rate of oxidative phosphorylation in the normal heart is the availability of ADP. This is because protons cannot flow through the F_0 channel in ATP synthase unless ADP is available to allow F_1 to couple the proton flux to ATP regeneration. Normally, the tight coupling between ATP regeneration from ADP and P_i, proton flux across the inner membrane, electron flux through the respiratory chain, oxidation of NADH and $FADH_2$, and substrate metabolism bring all of these reactions to a halt in the absence of ADP. This control of oxidative energy production by ADP helps to match ATP production and utilization in the well-oxygenated heart. In the energy-starved heart, where the ability to rephosphorylate ADP is limited, control of these tightly coupled reactions shifts to the availability of oxygen, rather than of ADP.

INTEGRATION OF GLYCOLYSIS AND RESPIRATION

Although the well-oxygenated heart can metabolize both carbohydrates and lipids, the latter are the preferred substrate. This is evidenced by the ability of fatty acids to inhibit carbohydrate metabolism when the heart is presented with both substrates. Mechanisms that allow fatty acid metabolism to inhibit glycolysis include the high concentrations of ATP regenerated by oxidative phosphorylation, which along with low concentrations of

AMP and P_i slow glycogen breakdown and glycolysis by inhibiting phosphorylase b and reducing phosphofructokinase activity. The latter, by increasing glucose-6-phosphate levels, also slows the hexokinase reaction. Citrate produced when acetyl CoA generated by β-oxidation enters the citric acid cycle also slows glycolysis by inhibiting phosphofructokinase and pyruvate dehydrogenase phosphatase.

COMPARTMENTATION OF ATP IN THE HEART

The total ATP *content* (moles/weight) in the human heart is 6 to 8 mmoles/kg wet weight, so that if all of this ATP were distributed uniformly in the cell water, ATP *concentration* (moles/volume) would be 6 to 8 mM. However, ATP concentrations are not the same in all regions of myocardial cells; most important are gradients for ATP, ADP, and especially AMP across the mitochondrial inner membrane and between the cytosol and mitochondrial matrix (Illingworth et al., 1975).

Glycolytic ATP

"Compartments" created by the cytoskeleton allow many structures to utilize preferentially the ATP produced by glycolysis, often called *glycolytic ATP* (Apstein, 2000). Although there is no membrane barrier to define these cytosolic compartments, the cytoskeleton creates functional compartments by maintaining close proximity between glycolytic enzymes that regenerate ATP and energy-consuming structures that consume ATP. This structural organization allows ATP regenerated by substrate level phosphorylations to be hydrolyzed by nearby energy-consuming structures. Evidence that glycolytic ATP preserves viability in the ischemic heart can explain the reported benefits of infusing glucose, insulin, and potassium in patients following coronary artery occlusion (Opie, 1999; Apstein, 2003).

ENERGY BALANCES

Carbohydrate Metabolism

The substrate-level phosphorylations in anaerobic glycolysis yield a total of 2 moles of ATP per mole of glucose, compared with approximately 38 moles of ATP regenerated per mole of glucose under aerobic conditions (Table 2-4). Of the additional 36 moles of ATP regenerated in the presence of oxygen, only 2 moles are produced by substrate-level phosphorylation; this occurs in the citric acid cycle when the high-energy thiol bond linking CoA to succinate in succinyl CoA is used to phosphorylate GDP and then ADP. All of the remaining 34 moles of ATP are regenerated by respiratory chain-linked phosphorylation.

Aerobic glycolysis regenerates about 6 moles of ATP when electrons transferred to NADH are passed through the respiratory chain. The oxidation of each mole of triose generates one mole of NADH (during glyceraldehyde-3-phosphate oxidation), so that because glycolysis generates 2 moles of triose per mole of glucose, a total of 2 moles of NADH are produced per mole of glucose. When oxidized in the respiratory chain, each mole of NADH regenerates about 3 moles of ATP, so aerobic glycolysis, in

TABLE 2-4 Energy Balances: ATP Regeneration from Carbohydrate and Fat

Carbohydrate Metabolism (moles ATP/mole glucose)			
Reaction	Substrate-level Phosphorylation	Respiratory Chain–linked Phosphorylation	Total
Anaerobic			
Anaerobic glycolysis			
Glucose $\longrightarrow$ lactate	2	0	2
Aerobic			
Aerobic glycolysis			
Glucose $\longrightarrow$ pyruvate	2	0	
2 NADH $\longrightarrow$ 2 NAD$^+$ + 2H	0	6	
Total	2	6	8
Pyruvate oxidation			
2 pyruvate $\longrightarrow$ 2 acetyl-CoA + CO_2	0	0	
2 NADH $\longrightarrow$ 2 NAD$^+$ + 2H	0	6	
Total	0	6	6
Acetyl-CoA oxidation			
2 Acetyl-CoA $\longrightarrow$ 4 CO_2	2	0	
6 NADH $\longrightarrow$ 6 NAD$^+$ + 6H	0	18	
2 $FADH_2$ $\longrightarrow$ 2 FAD + 4H	0	4	
Total	2	22	24
Glucose oxidation (total)			
Glucose $\longrightarrow$ 6 CO_2 + 6 H_2O			
Per mole	4	34	38
Per 100 gm			~21
(MW = 180)			

TABLE 2-4   *(continued)*

Reaction	Substrate-level Phosphorylation	Respiratory Chain–linked Phosphorylation	Total
Fat Metabolism (moles ATP/mole palmitic acid)			
Fatty acid activation	−1	0	−1
β-Oxidation			
8 acyl-$CoA_{(n)} \longrightarrow$ 8 acyl-$CoA_{(n-2)}$ + 8 acetyl-CoA	0	0	
8 NADH $\longrightarrow$ 8 NAD^+ + 8H		0	24
8 $FADH_2 \longrightarrow$ 8 FAD + 16H	0	16	
Total	0	40	40
Acetyl-CoA oxidation			
8 Acetyl-CoA $\longrightarrow$ 16 CO_2	8	0	
24 NADH $\longrightarrow$ 24 NAD^+ + 24 H	0	72	
8 $FADH_2 \longrightarrow$ 8 FAD + 16 H	0	16	
Total	8	88	96
Fat oxidation (total)			
6-carbon fatty acid $\longrightarrow$ 6 CO_2 + 6 H_2O			
Per mole	7	128	135
Per 100 gm (MW = 256)			~53

Amount of ATP regenerated per mole of substrate during the metabolism of a carbohydrate (glucose) under anaerobic and aerobic conditions as well as during metabolism of a fatty acid (palmitic acid, a saturated 16-carbon fatty acid). When calculated on the basis of weight, oxidation of palmitate yields more than twice the amount of ATP as does glucose oxidation.

addition to regenerating 2 moles of ATP by substrate-level phosphorylation, provides approximately 6 moles of ATP per mole of glucose by respiratory chain-linked phosphorylation. Aerobic glycolysis therefore yields a total of approximately 8 moles of ATP per mole of glucose (Table 2-4).

Oxidation of pyruvate to form acetyl-CoA yields an additional mole of NADH that when oxidized in the respiratory chain provides about 3 moles of ATP; because each mole of glucose yields 2 moles of pyruvate, pyruvate oxidation adds about 6 moles of ATP per mole of glucose (Table 2-4).

Each mole of acetyl-CoA oxidized in the citric acid cycle generates 3 moles of NADH (one each during oxidation of isocitrate, α-ketoglutarate, and malate) and 1 mole of $FADH_2$ (generated during succinyl-CoA oxidation). Because oxidation of each mole of NADH by the respiratory chain yields nearly 3 moles of ATP, the 3 NADH produced per mole of acetyl-CoA by the citric acid cycle adds about 9 moles of ATP per mole of acetyl-CoA or about 18 per mole of glucose. $FADH_2$ oxidation yields an additional 2 moles or so of ATP per mole of acetyl-CoA or about 4 per mole of glucose. Respiratory chain-linked phosphorylation therefore regenerates nearly 11 moles of ATP per mole of acetyl-CoA, or approximately 22 per mole of glucose.

The total of about 38 moles of ATP regenerated by the complete metabolism of each mole of glucose (Table 2-4) compares to only 2 moles of ATP produced by anaerobic glycolysis.

Fat Metabolism

Most of the ATP used by the heart is regenerated by the oxidation of acetyl-CoA derived from fat which, as noted above, can be viewed as "concentrated energy." This is seen in the metabolism of palmitic acid (saturated, 16 carbons).

During β-oxidation, each mole of palmitate yields 8 moles of acetyl-CoA and 8 moles each of reduced NADH and $FADH_2$ (Table 2.4). Oxidation of the reduced coenzymes regenerates a total of about 40 moles of ATP. Subsequent oxidation of the 8 moles of acetyl-CoA regenerates an additional 96 moles of ATP: 8 moles by substrate-level phosphorylation in the citric acid cycle and 88 moles by oxidation of the reduced coenzymes (Table 2-4). After subtraction of the single mole of ATP used to activate the fatty acid, palmitate oxidation yields about 135 moles of ATP.

These calculations explain why more energy is released by the oxidation of fat than carbohydrate (see above). Palmitate oxidation, when normalized to the weight of the substrate, regenerates more than twice as much ATP per gram as does glucose oxidation (Table 2.4). The fact that lack of oxygen completely prevents ATP regeneration from fat, as well as production of almost 95% of the ATP potentially available from glucose metabolism, explains the devastating effects of coronary artery occlusion on the heart (see Chapter 17).

OVERVIEW OF THE CONTROL OF ENERGY PRODUCTION BY THE HEART

At least four types of mechanism regulate energy production by the heart. The first is *humoral*, which allows circulating hormones, neurotransmitters, and other extracellular messengers to modify both the transporters that mediate the entry of carbohydrate and fat into the myocardium and the enzymes that control the metabolism of these substrates. Most important is sympathetic stimulation, which in addition to increasing energy utilization (see Chapter 8) accelerates ATP production. The second type of control, which responds to changing *high-energy phosphate* levels, helps to match the rate of ATP production to that of ATP utilization. In the normal heart, where ADP plays a central role in determining the rate of oxidative phosphorylation, this control maintains a virtually constant level of ATP during marked changes in cardiac work. The third type of regulation responds to changing levels of oxidized and reduced coenzymes by adjusting energy production to changes in *redox state*—for example, by increasing anaerobic glycolysis when depletion of oxidized coenzymes in the energy-starved heart slows oxidative metabolism. The fourth mechanism, which is brought about by changes in proliferative signaling, plays an important role in the response to long-term challenges, such as occurs in heart failure, where cardiac myocyte hypertrophy is accompanied by increased glucose oxidation relative to fatty acid oxidation (see Chapter 18).

The interplay among these regulatory mechanisms matches substrate uptake and metabolism, allows ATP to be produced at the same rate that it is consumed, adjusts the rate of ATP regeneration to meet the changing needs of the normal heart, and maximizes energy production in diseased hearts. The words of Stephen Hales, who in 1733 first measured arterial blood pressure, seem to be especially appropriate at this point: "So curiously are we wrought, so fearfully and wonderfully are we made."

BIBLIOGRAPHY

Alberts B, Johnson A, Lewis J, et al. *Molecular biology of the cell*, 4th ed. New York: Garland, 2002.

Alpert NR, Mulieri LL, Hasenfuss G. Myocardial chemo-mechanical energy transduction. In: Fozzard H, Haber E, Katz A, et al., eds. *The heart and cardiovascular system*, 2nd ed. New York: Raven, 1991:111–128.

Balaban RS. Cardiac energy metabolism homeostasis: role of cytosolic calcium. *J Mol Cell Cardiol* 2002;34:1259–1271.

Chock PB, Stadtman ER. Superiority of interconvertible enzyme cascades in metabolic regulation: analysis of multicyclic systems. *Proc Natl Acad Sci USA* 1977;74:2766–2770.

Depre C, Vanoverschelde JL J, Taegtmeyer H. Glucose for the heart. *Circulation* 1999;99: 578–588.

Devlin TM, ed. *Textbook of biochemistry*, 4th ed. New York: Wiley, 1997.

Goodwin GW, Ahmad F, Taegtmeyer H. Preferential oxidation of glycogen in isolated working rat heart. *J Clin Invest* 1996;97:1409–1416.

Goodwin GW, Taylor CS, Taegtmeyer H. Regulation of energy metabolism of the heart during acute increase in heart work. *J Biol Chem* 1998;273:29530–29539.

Hue L, Beauloye C, Marsin AS, et al. Insulin and ischemia stimulate glycolysis by acting on the same targets through different and opposing signaling pathways. *J Mol Cell Cardiol* 2002;34:1091–1097.

Ingwall JS. *ATP and the heart*. Norwell, MA: Kluwer, 2002.

Lodish H, Berk A, Zipursky SL, et al. *Molecular cell biology*, 4th ed. New York: Freeman, 2000.

Needham DM. Machina carnis. Biochemistry of muscular contraction and its historical development. Cambridge: Cambridge University Press, 1971.

Saltiel AR, Pessin JE. Insulin signaling pathways in time and space. *Trends Cell Biol* 2002;12:65–71.

Steinberg D. Interconvertible enzymes in adipose tissue regulated by cyclic AMP-dependent protein kinase. *Adv Cyclic Nucl Res* 1977;7:157–198.

Taegtmeyer H. Metabolism—the lost child of cardiology. *J Am Coll Cardiol* 2000;36: 1386–1388.

van der Vusse GJ, Glatz JFC, Stam HCG, et al. Fatty acid homeostasis in the normoxic and ischemic heart. *Physiol Rev* 1992;72:881–940.

REFERENCES

Apstein CS. Increased glycolytic substrate protection improves ischemic cardiac dysfunction and reduces injury. *Am Heart J* 2000;139[2 Pt 3]:S107–S114.

Apstein CS. The benefits of glucose-insulin-potassium for acute myocardial infarction (and some concerns). *J Am Coll Cardiol* 2003;42:792–795.

Awan MZ, Goldspink G. Energetics of the development and maintenance of isometric tension by mammalian fast and slow muscles. *J Mechanochem Cell Motil* 1972;1:97–108.

Backx P. Efficiency of cardiac muscle: thermodynamic and statistical mechanical considerations. *Basic Res Cardiol* 1993;88[Suppl 2]:21–28.

Dyke JRB, Lopaschuk GD. Malonyl CoA control of fatty acid oxidation in the ischemic heart. *J Mol Cell Cardiol* 2002;34:1099–1109.

Eckel RH. Lipoprotein lipase: a multifunctional enzyme relevant to common metabolic disease. *N Eng J Med* 1989;320:1060–1068.

Finck BN, Kelly DP. Peroxisome proliferator-activated receptor α (PPARα) signaling in the gene regulatory control of energy metabolism in the normal and diseased heart. *J Mol Cell Cardiol* 2002;42:124–125.

Hillgartner FB, Salati LM, Goodridge AG. Physiological and molecular mechanisms involved in nutritional regulation of fatty acid synthesis. *Physiol Rev* 1995;75:47–76.

Illingworth JA, Christopher W, Ford L, et al. Regulation of myocardial energy metabolism. In: Roy PE, Harris P, eds. *Recent advances in studies on cardiac structure and metabolism*, vol. 8. Baltimore: University Park Press, 1975:271–290.

Jacobus WE. Respiratory control and the integration of heart high-energy phosphate metabolism by mitochondrial creatine kinase. *Ann Rev Physiol* 1985;47:707–725.

Kammermeier H. Why do cells need phosphocreatine and a phosphocreatine shuttle? *J Mol Cell Cardiol* 1987;19:115–118.

Kammermeier H, Schmidt P, Jüngling E. Free energy change of ATP-hydrolysis: a causal factor of early hypoxic failure of the myocardium? *J Mol Cell Cardiol* 1982;14:267–277.

Katz AM, Messineo FC. Lipid-membrane interactions and the pathogenesis of ischemic damage in the myocardium. *Circ Res* 1981;48:1–16.

McClellan G, Weisberg A, Winegrad S. Energy transport from mitochondria to myofibril by a creatine phosphate shuttle in cardiac cells. *Am J Physiol* 1983;245:C423–C427.

Opie LH. Proof that glucose-insulin-potassium provides metabolic protection of ischaemic myocardium. *Lancet* 1999;353:768–769.

Paulson DJ. Carnitine deficiency–induced cardiomyopathy. *Mol Cell Biochem* 1998;180:33–41.

Pette D, Staron RS. Cellular and molecular diversities of mammalian skeletal muscle fibers. *Rev Physiol Biochem Pharmacol* 1990;116:1–76.

Rauch B, Schultze B, Schultheiss HP. Alteration of the cytosolic-mitochondrial distribution of high-energy phosphates during global myocardial ischemia may contribute to early contractile failure. *Circ Res* 1994;75:760–769.

Suga H, Goto Y, Kawaguchi O, et al. Ventricular perspective on efficiency. *Basic Res Cardiol* 1993;88[Suppl 2]:43–65.

Taegtmeyer H, Peterson MB, Ragever VV, et al. De novo alanine synthesis in isolated oxygen-deprived rabbit myocardium. *J Biol Chem* 1977;252:5010–5018.

Tian R, Ingwall JS. Energetic basis for reduced contractile reserve in isolated rat hearts. *Am J Physiol* 1996;270:H1207–H1216.

van Bilsen M, van der Vusse GJ, Renemann RS. Transcriptional regulation of metabolic processes: implications for cardiac metabolism. *Pflügers Arch—Eur J Physiol* 1998; 437:2–14.

Wallimann T, Wyss M, Brdiczka D, et al. Intracellular compartmentation, structure and function of creatine kinase isoenzymes in tissues with high and fluctuation energy demands: the "phosphocreatine circuit" for cellular energy homeostasis. *Biochem J* 1992; 281:21–40.

3

ENERGY UTILIZATION (WORK AND HEAT)

In the early 19th century, muscle research focused on the new field of thermodynamics, notably the First Law stating that the sum of the energies in an isolated system is constant. This means that when a muscle contracts, the chemical energy provided to the contractile machinery by the metabolic reactions described in Chapter 2 appears as work and heat. Work had been quantified since the 17th century, and the first effort to measure heat production by isolated muscle was made by Helmholtz in 1848. However, it was not until the 1920s that A. V. Hill measured muscle heat with sufficient accuracy to provide insights into the energetics of the contractile process; these studies used the frog sartorius, a relatively simple skeletal muscle in which energetics could be examined during brief tetanic contractions. An early effort to measure heat production by cardiac muscle was made in 1925 by L. N. Katz, to whom this text is dedicated, but his effort proved fruitless because the heart generated too little heat to be recorded by the instruments of that time. Although subsequent research has demonstrated differences between the energetics of cardiac and skeletal muscle, Hill's studies of amphibian muscle provide important insights regarding the contractile process in the heart.

A FEW TERMS

Isometric and Isotonic Contractions

Physiologists traditionally study muscles when they contract at constant length (*isometric contraction*) or at constant load (*isotonic contraction*). In an isometric contraction, the ends of the muscle are fixed so that the muscle cannot shorten; even though tension is maximal, work (the product of force × distance) is zero because there is no change in length. In an isotonic contraction, the muscle is allowed to shorten while bearing a constant load. When the load is zero, the muscle shortens to its maximal extent, but no work is done because no force is developed. Work is maximal when the muscle shortens against an intermediate load. Contraction of the muscle fibers in the walls of the beating heart is neither isometric nor isotonic; instead, as described in Chapter 11, wall stress initially increases and then decreases as the heart empties.

Preload and Afterload

The difference between a *preload* and an *afterload* depends on when the muscle first interacts with the load. A preload stretches a relaxed skeletal muscle *before* contraction begins, whereas an afterload does not become apparent to the muscle until *after* contraction is under way. A weight hung on a resting muscle (Fig. 3-1) is a preload, while a weight that rests on a table until after contraction has begun is an afterload.

The beating heart operates with both a preload and an afterload (Chapter 11). In the left ventricle, for example, preload is determined by the pressures and volumes during diastole, while afterload is determined by the pressures and volumes after left ventricular pressure exceeds aortic pressure. Preload and afterload are important clinically because of their effects on the work of the heart and their influence on the energetics of ventricular function.

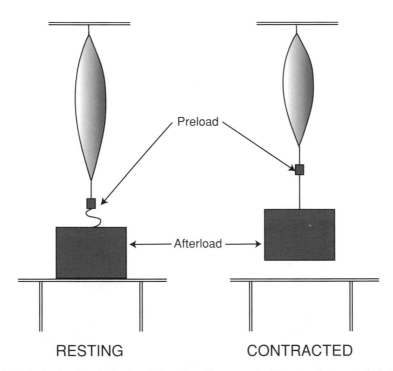

RESTING   CONTRACTED

FIGURE 3-1 Preload and afterload. A preload is supported by a resting muscle before it begins to contract (*left*). An afterload, such as a weight resting on a support, is not encountered by the muscle until developed tension exceeds its weight (*right*).

INFLUENCE OF AFTERLOAD ON MUSCLE WORK

The relationship between load (P) and work can be understood by considering a spring that is stretched by 10 cm when loaded with a 10 g weight (Fig. 3-2). If the increase in length is linearly proportional to the load (Hooke's law), tension will increase by 1 g for each centimeter of lengthening, and conversely, if an initial 10 g load is decreased in 1 g steps, the spring will shorten 1 cm for each gram removed from the load. These relationships are shown in Table 3-1, where column (a) describes the step-wise decrease in load when, after the spring had been stretched by the 10 g weight, the latter is replaced by a series of lighter weights. Column (b) describes the extent of shortening at each lighter weight, and column (c) lists the work done when the spring lifts each of the lighter weights. The

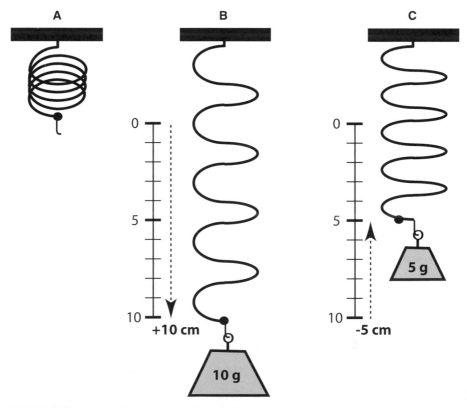

FIGURE 3-2 Effect of load on the work done by a spring that obeys Hooke's law. When the unloaded spring (A) is stretched by a 10-g weight, its length will increase by 10 cm (B). If the 10 g load is then replaced with smaller weights, the spring will shorten by 1 cm for each gram of load that is removed. For example, when the final load is 5 g, the spring will shorten 5 cm (C), and if the weight is removed completely, the spring will shorten 10 cm (A). The work done when the stretched spring in (B) is presented with a series of loads is shown in Table 3-1 and Figure 3-3.

TABLE 3-1 Relationship between Shortening and Work Performed When a Stretched Spring Is Allowed to Shorten at Various Loads

(a) Load (g)	(b) Shortening (cm)	(c) Work (g × cm)
10	0	0
9	1	9
8	2	16
7	3	21
6	4	24
5	5	25
4	6	24
3	7	21
2	8	16
1	9	9
0	10	0

work done by the spring in lifting these weights, column (c), can be calculated by multiplying each new load, column (a), by the distance shortened, column (b). When the work in column (c) is plotted as a function of load (Fig. 3-3), it is apparent that no work is done when the new weight is the same as the maximal weight (P = 10 g) because the spring does not shorten, nor when the spring is completely unloaded (P = 0) because in spite of the large extent of shortening, no force is generated. Instead, work is maximal at the intermediate loads.

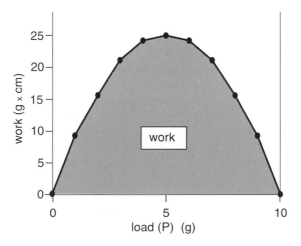

FIGURE 3-3 Work–load curve of the spring shown in Figure 3-2. Starting with the spring in its stretched state, the series of lighter loads indicated on the abscissa allows the spring to perform the amount of work indicated on the ordinate.

Work–load relationships like that for a spring also describe the influence of load on the work performed by a contracting muscle. This similarity led early physiologists to postulate that the transition from rest to activity in a muscle occurred when the latter assumed new elastic properties like those of the stretched spring. Although now known to be incorrect, this *new elastic body theory* is described at this point because correction of the fundamental error, equating active muscle to a stretched spring, provided the foundation for our modern understanding of muscle energetics.

NEW ELASTIC BODY THEORY OF MUSCLE CONTRACTION

Work–load curves such as that shown in Fig. 3-3 were initially explained by postulating that the transition from rest to activity in a muscle occurred when new elastic bonds are formed within the contractile machinery (Fig. 3-4). Contraction was therefore thought to be initiated when chemical energy is used to form springlike bonds that increase the ability of the muscle to shorten and generate tension. This explained why stretching a resting muscle (Fig. 3-4, *left*) generates only a small amount of tension (resting tension) and the greater stiffness of active muscle (Fig. 3-4, *right*). According to this theory, activation adds a fixed amount of energy that causes the muscle to become a stiffer spring—i.e., a "new elastic body."

relaxed

contracted

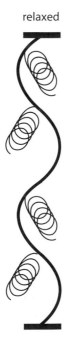
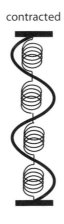

FIGURE 3-4 The new elastic body theory of muscle contraction. According to this theory, the transition from the resting state (*left*) to the active state (*right*) is caused when activation adds a fixed amount of energy to form new elastic bonds.

FIGURE 3-5 Predicted relation-ship between loading and total energy released as work plus heat in a muscle that contracts according to the new elastic body theory. Because a fixed amount of energy is added to the muscle during the transition from rest to activity, the total energy released as work and heat should be independent of load. Because the shape of the work–load curve is similar to that of a spring (Fig. 3-3), this theory predicted that heat production would decrease at intermediate loads to release a constant amount of energy.

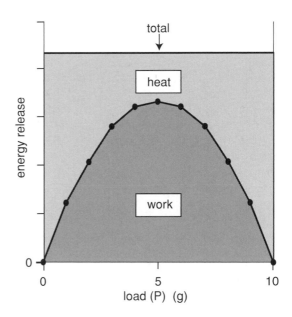

A key prediction of the new elastic body theory was that, because excitation adds a constant amount of energy to the muscle to establish the new bonds, the total energy (work + heat) available for release by the active muscle should be independent of load. This meant that curves relating load to total energy release (as work and heat) would resemble Figure 3-5. At maximum load, all of the energy added during the transition from rest to activity would appear as heat because no work is done. Similarly, all of the energy added to establish the new cross links in an unloaded muscle would appear as heat during contraction because no work is done. At intermediate loads, where the release of energy as work is maximal (see Table 3-1 and Fig. 3-3), heat liberation would be minimal (Fig. 3-5).

The new elastic body theory was generally accepted until Fenn (1923) showed that *the total energy liberated by a contracting muscle is not constant, but instead depends on load.*

FENN EFFECT

Wallace O. Fenn's decisive contribution to our understanding of muscle contraction was that the total energy released as work and heat is not constant, but increases when more work is performed (Fig. 3-6). This finding, called the *Fenn effect*, proved that the energy available for release by a contracting muscle is not determined at the time of activation, but instead depends on load because *when muscle does more work, more energy is liberated.* The finding that more energy is utilized when additional work is performed means that muscle resembles an electric motor, where electricity consumption increases when the motor is more heavily

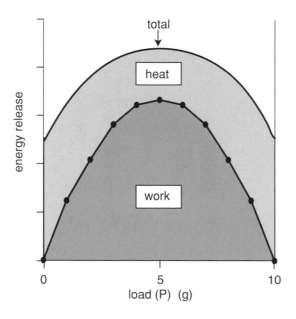

FIGURE 3-6 Relationship between load (P) and total energy released during contraction of frog sartorius muscle. Total energy release is not constant but parallels the total work performed. This increase in total energy release when a muscle does more work is the Fenn effect.

loaded. The Fenn effect was confirmed in the early 1960s, when utilization of high-energy phosphate, like energy release as work plus heat, was shown to be maximal at intermediate loads, where the highest levels of work are performed (Fig. 3-7).

It is a historical curiosity that the Fenn effect had been documented in cardiac muscle almost a decade before Fenn's report. In a paper that had been overlooked by most muscle physiologists of the time, but which

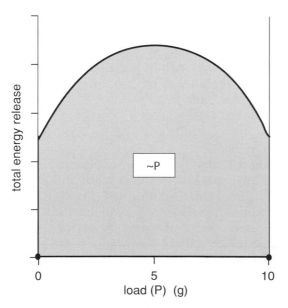

FIGURE 3-7 Influence of load (P) on high-energy phosphate breakdown ($\sim$P) during contraction of frog sartorius muscle. More chemical energy is used at intermediate loads, where the muscle performs more work, than at heavy or light loads.

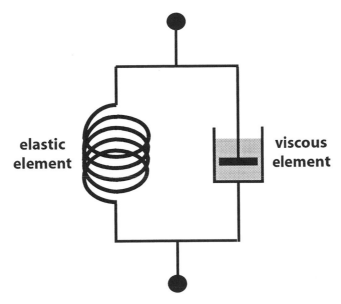

FIGURE 3-8 Representation of an active muscle as an elastic body containing an elastic element (*depicted at left as a spring*) and a viscous element (*depicted at right as a "dashpot"*).

Fenn cited in his 1923 article, Evans and Matsuoka (1914–1915) had reported that cardiac oxygen consumption increases when the heart does more work. This observation led Starling, in his Linacre lecture describing the "Law of the Heart" (1918), to equate the energetic cost of increasing cardiac work to riding a motorcycle up a hill.

FORCE–VELOCITY RELATIONSHIP

The force–velocity relationship, which plots the influence of load on the velocity of muscle shortening, provides additional evidence that contracting muscle does not behave like a stretched spring. The new elastic body theory, which viewed muscle as made up of parallel elastic and viscous elements (Fig. 3-8), predicted that shortening velocity would increase in a linear manner when load is decreased (*curve A*, Fig. 3-9). In 1935, however, Fenn and Marsh found the relationship to be hyperbolic (*curve B*, Fig. 3-9). Although this hyperbolic relationship could be explained in the context of the new elastic body theory by assuming special characteristics for muscle elasticity and viscosity, A. V. Hill demonstrated in 1938 that this shape, which is predicted by measurements of work and heat, reflects the energetic properties of the contractile machinery.

HEAT LIBERATION BY MUSCLE

Muscle liberates three types of heat (Table 3-2 and Fig. 3-10). *Maintenance (resting) heat*, the slow liberation of heat by resting muscle, is not

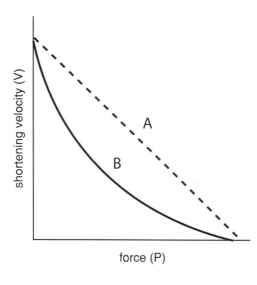

FIGURE 3-9 Force–velocity relationships. The linear relationship predicted by the model shown in Figure 3-8, in which the elastic element obeys Hooke's law and the viscous element has Newtonian characteristics (**A**, *dashed line*). The hyperbolic force–velocity relationship measured for frog sartorius muscle by Fenn and Marsh (**B**, *solid line*).

TABLE 3-2 Energy Liberated by Muscle

Heat	Some Heat-Generating Processes
I. Maintenance (resting) heat	Maintenance of ion composition, protein synthesis
II. Activity-related heat	Excitation, contraction, relaxation, recovery
A. Initial heat	Excitation, contraction, relaxation
1. Tension-independent heat	Plasma membrane depolarization and repolarization, sarcoplasmic reticulum Ca release, Ca binding to troponin, conformational changes in the thin filaments
Activation heat	Tension-independent heat at onset of contraction
2. Tension-dependent heat	Contractile protein interactions
Shortening heat	Muscle shortening, myosin–actin interactions
Tension-time heat	Cross-bridge turnover
B. Recovery heat	ATP regeneration by mitochondria during recovery, potential energy degraded to heat when a loaded muscle relaxes
Work	
External work	Load (force) times distance (shortening)
Internal work	Cross-bridge turnover [f(P,t)], internal viscosity, stretching of series elasticity

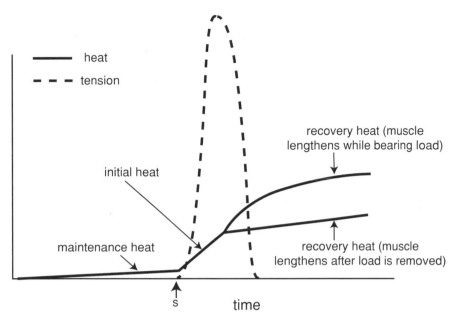

FIGURE 3-10 Heat liberation and tension development for a frog sartorius muscle. Maintenance heat is liberated by the resting muscle. Initial heat is liberated during contraction, and recovery heat is liberated during and immediately after relaxation. Recovery heat is reduced when the load is removed from the muscle prior to relaxation. s, stimulus.

related to contraction and is not considered further. The other two types of heat, called *activity-related heat*, are generated during contraction; these include initial heat and recovery heat. *Initial heat* appears during contraction, while *recovery heat* is liberated after the contraction has reached its peak.

Recovery Heat

Recovery heat, which is generated mainly by the processes that restore the state of contracted muscle to that which existed before excitation, plays an important role in determining muscle efficiency. In skeletal muscle, most of this heat is due to the oxidation of lactate produced during activity, whereas most of the recovery heat produced by cardiac muscle accompanies ATP regeneration by the mitochondria.

A large additional quantity of recovery heat appears when a muscle is allowed to relax while bearing a weight (Fig. 3-10). This extra heat, which is proportional to load, is generated by the dissipation of potential energy stored in the contracted muscle; for this reason, this component of the recovery heat disappears if the load is removed from the muscle before it begins to relax (Fig. 3-10). In the heart, dissipation of potential energy stored by elasticities in the walls of the contracted ventricle makes a major contribution to recovery heat and therefore reduces cardiac efficiency. Semilunar valve closure, which reduces wall tension at the end of systole by separating the relaxing ventricles from the blood under pressure in the aorta and pulmonary artery, decreases recovery heat. Recovery heat in the heart also is reduced because wall stress normally decreases during ejection (see Chapter 11). The energy wasted in generating recovery heat is increased by the high wall stress generally seen in dilated hearts (Chapter 12).

Initial Heat

The third form of muscle heat, which for historical reasons is called *initial heat*, is the extra heat (extra in that it exceeds maintenance heat) liberated during contraction (Fig. 3-10). Initial heat is released during activation, shortening, and tension generation and includes heat liberated during plasma membrane depolarization and repolarization, release and reuptake of activator calcium by the sarcoplasmic reticulum, and the conformational changes among the contractile proteins that are initiated when calcium binds to troponin C (Table 3-2).

TENSION-INDEPENDENT HEAT, ACTIVATION HEAT, AND TENSION-DEPENDENT HEAT. When a muscle is stimulated but the interactions between the thick and thin filaments are inhibited so that no external work can be done, a small amount of initial heat is still generated. The major sources of this heat, called *activation heat*, are calcium release from the sarcoplasmic reticulum, calcium binding to troponin, and conformational changes among the proteins of the thin filament. Following the liberation of activation heat in a "contraction-inhibited" muscle, processes that relax the muscle, notably calcium uptake by the sarcoplasmic reticulum, generate additional heat at the time when relaxation would have occurred. The latter, together with the activation heat, constitute the *tension-independent heat*.

The difference between total initial heat and tension-independent heat is the heat liberated by the contractile proteins. This heat, called the *tension-dependent heat*, is due mainly to interactions between myosin cross-bridges in the thick filaments and actin in the thin filaments.

INITIAL HEAT LIBERATION DURING ISOMETRIC CONTRACTION. Two components of initial heat are liberated in an *isometric contraction* (Fig. 3-11). The first, which appears immediately after the muscle is stimulated, is the *activation heat* (A, Fig. 3-11). Additional heat released when isometric tension is maintained ($f(P,t)$, Fig. 3-11), called *tension-time heat*, is associated with internal work (W_i) (see below). The energy released (ΔE) during an isometric contraction is therefore described by the following equation:

$$\Delta E = A + W_i \qquad\qquad \text{[3-1]}$$

Internal work is performed during an isometric contraction because although the ends of the muscle are fixed, the contractile proteins stretch the

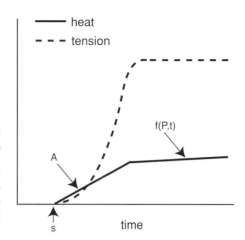

FIGURE 3-11 Liberation of initial heat and tension development by a tetanized muscle contracting under isometric conditions. The heat liberated as tension develops (A) immediately after stimulation (s) is the *activation heat*, while the slower re-lease of heat after tension reaches its peak (f(P,t)) is the *tension-time heat* [f(P,t)].

series elasticity and cause shape changes in the muscle (Chapter 12). Most of the energy associated with internal work is converted to recovery heat at the end of the isometric contraction, when tension is dissipated and the elasticities elongate. Internal work also is related to the tension-time heat, called $f(P,t)$, which is discussed below.

INITIAL HEAT LIBERATION DURING ISOTONIC CONTRACTION. The energetics of an *isotonic contraction*, where the muscle is allowed to shorten, are more complex than those of an isometric contraction because shortening releases two additional forms of energy. The first is the external work performed when a loaded muscle is allowed to shorten. The second, an additional component of initial heat, accompanies shortening itself and is called *shortening heat*.

In 1938, Hill found that a small quantity of extra heat is released during shortening of an activated muscle (labeled "ax" in Fig. 3-12). This is the shortening heat, which is independent of load but proportional to the distance that the muscle shortens (x). When a muscle presented with different loads is allowed to shorten a fixed distance, the *total amount* of shortening heat stays the same, but the *rate* at which this heat appears decreases with increasing load (Fig. 3-12). When the muscle is allowed to shorten different distances with the same load, the amount of shortening heat increases proportionately with the extent of shortening (Fig. 3-13).

To analyze these findings, Hill introduced the term a to quantify the amount of heat liberated per centimeter of shortening. This term, which is constant for a given muscle, has the dimensions of a force, so that a times x (the distance the muscle shortens) is the total amount of heat liberated during shortening:

$$\text{Shortening heat} = ax \qquad\qquad [3\text{-}2]$$

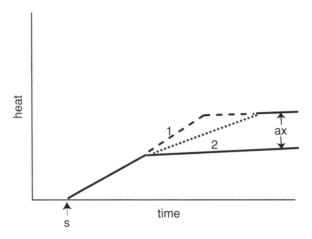

FIGURE 3-12 Liberation of initial heat by a muscle, contracting under isotonic conditions, that is allowed to shorten a constant distance while lifting a light load (*dashed line*, 1) or a heavy load (*dotted line*, 2). The time course of initial heat liberation by the muscle contracting under isometric conditions also is shown (*solid line*). The additional heat liberated when the muscle shortens is the *shortening heat* (ax), which is released more slowly when the muscle lifts the heavier load. However, the total amount of shortening heat is independent of load. s, stimulus.

Unlike the *amount* of shortening heat liberated in an isotonic contraction, which depends only on the distance shortened and is independent of load, the *rate* at which shortening heat is generated is inversely proportional to the load (see above). The velocity at which the muscle shortens also is inversely proportional to load (Fig. 3-9); for these

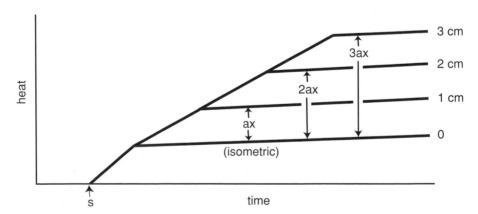

FIGURE 3-13 Liberation of initial heat when a muscle contracting under isotonic conditions with a constant load is allowed to shorten to various lengths. The shortening heat (ax) increases in direct proportion to the distance shortened, so when the muscle shortens 2 cm, it liberates twice as much shortening heat (2ax) as when it shortens 1 cm (ax); when the muscle shortens 3 cm, the shortening heat is 3ax. s, stimulus.

reasons, *the rate of total energy liberation, as work and heat, decreases at heavier loads*.

The total energy released during an isotonic contraction includes external work (W_e), activation heat (A), and shortening heat (ax). The total energy released during an isotonic contraction is therefore:

$$\Delta E = A + W_e + ax + W_i \qquad [3-3]$$

Unlike an isometric contraction, where only internal work is performed, most of the work in an isotonic contraction is the *external* work expended to lift the load (W_e).

Tension-Time Heat

Improved measurements of heat liberation during the 1960s showed that both activation heat (A) and shortening heat (ax) increase at higher loads. A simple interpretation of these findings was provided by Mommaerts (1969), who separated activation heat into two components: A and f(P,t). The first component, *A*, is the true activation heat that is described above (Table 3-2). The second term, *f(P,t)*, represents a *"tension-time heat"* whose magnitude is proportional to the tension on the muscle (P) and the length of time (t) that tension is maintained.

The major source of tension-time heat is the slow cycling of actin-bound myosin cross-bridges (see Chapter 4). Because much of the heat liberated as f(P,t) is related to internal work, this term can replace W_i in equation 3-1. The energy liberated during an isometric contraction is therefore:

$$\Delta E = A + f(P,t) \qquad [3-4]$$

And the equation for an isotonic contraction (equation 3-3) becomes:

$$\Delta E = A + W_e + ax + f(P,t) \qquad [3-5]$$

Tension-time heat [f(P,t)] plays an important role in the energetic consequences of myosin heavy chain isoform shifts that modify myosin ATPase activity. For example, the reversion to the fetal phenotype caused by chronic hemodynamic overloading, which favors the synthesis of a low ATPase myosin isoform (Chapter 18), depresses myocardial contractility. At the same time, however, the slower cycling of actin-bound myosin cross-bridges reduces the tension-time heat [f(P,t)] generated when the heart contracts against a high afterload, as occurs in hypertension and aortic stenosis. The resulting increase in efficiency represents an important adaptive mechanism because chronically overloaded hearts are often energy starved.

The tension-time heat, f(P,t) is not included in the following discussion of the Hill equation. Although this simplification introduces a small error, it clarifies the salient relationships between force, velocity, energy liberation, and the chemistry of the contractile proteins.

THE HILL EQUATION

The *Hill equation*, which describes the energetics of muscle contraction, relates the liberation of extra energy as work and heat to the chemistry of the contractile process. This equation is based on the energetics of isotonic contraction, where a muscle lifts a load (P) over a distance (x). The *amount* of extra energy liberated during shortening appears as work (Px) and shortening heat (ax), so that:

$$\text{Extra energy} = (Px) + (ax) = (P + a)x \qquad [3\text{-}6]$$

Activation heat, which appears before the muscle begins to shorten (Fig. 3-11), is not included in equation 3-6 because it not related to work performance.

The *rate* at which extra energy is liberated during shortening is readily determined by differentiating the quantity $(P + a)x$ with respect to time:

$$\text{Rate of extra energy liberation} = (P + a)dx/dt \qquad [3\text{-}7]$$

Because $dx/dt = \text{velocity (v)}$, the rate of extra energy liberation is $(P + a)v$. This allows equation 3-7 to be rewritten:

$$\text{Rate of extra energy liberation} = (P + a)v \qquad [3\text{-}8]$$

Hill found that the rate of extra energy liberation described in equation 3-8 is a direct linear function of the difference between maximal isometric tension (P_0) and the actual load (P) (Fig. 3-14). In an isometric contraction, where $P = P_0$ and the distance shortened (x) is zero, the rate of extra energy liberation is zero because there is neither shortening heat (ax) nor work (Px). The rate of extra energy release is maximal in an unloaded isotonic contraction, where $P = 0$, even though no work (Px) is done, because the distance shortened, (x) and the release of shortening heat (ax)

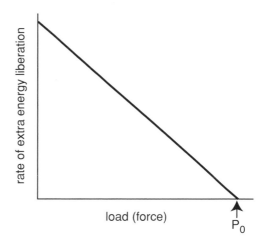

FIGURE 3-14 Relationship between load (force) and the rate of extra energy liberation (work plus heat) during isotonic contractions.

are very large. For this reason, as load (P) becomes smaller, the rate of extra energy release increases (Fig. 3-14).

The direct linear proportionality between the rate of extra energy liberation $[(P + a)v]$ and the difference between maximal isometric tension and the actual load $(P_0 - P)$ shown in Fig. 3-14 is described by the following equation:

$$(P + a)v = b\,(P_0 - P) \qquad\qquad [3\text{-}9]$$

where b is a constant of proportionality. Rearranging equation 3-9 to put all of the constants (a, b, P_0) on the right generates the Hill equation:

$$(P + a)(v + b) = (P_0 + a)b \qquad\qquad [3\text{-}10]$$

Because P and v, the only two variables, are expressed as a product on the left, and the terms on the right are all constants, equation 3-10 describes a hyperbola (x times y = constant). For this reason, a graph of the Hill equation that plots the rate of extra energy liberation $[(P + a)v]$ as an inverse function of load $(P_0 - P)$ yields a hyperbolic curve (Fig. 3-15).

The force–velocity curve based on Hill's measurements of heat and work has the same hyperbolic shape as the force–velocity relationships obtained by Fenn and Marsh (Fig. 3-9), who a decade earlier had measured the dependence of shortening velocity on load. This similarity between the Hill equation and these direct measurements demonstrates that *the hyperbolic relationship between force and velocity is an expression of the fundamental properties of muscle chemistry*!

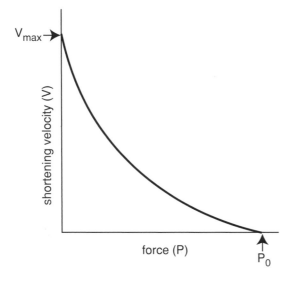

FIGURE 3-15 Hyperbolic force–velocity relationship calculated from the Hill equation (equation 3-10). This curve is similar to that observed directly during contractions of frog sartorius muscle (Fig. 3-9).

Significance of the Hill Equation

The reader who has toiled through the concepts (and algebra) described above is entitled to ask how these features of muscle physics—load, energetics, heat production, velocity, and the like—help in understanding the physiology of the heart. At this point, this question is answered in general terms; the relationship between muscle physics and muscle chemistry is discussed in more detail in Chapter 12, after cardiac contraction is described in biochemical terms.

The significance of equation 3-10 was eloquently stated by Hill (1938), who provided a remarkable prediction regarding the chemistry of the working muscle:

> The control exercised by the tension P existing in the muscle at any moment, on the rate of its energy expenditure at that moment, may be due to some such mechanisms as the following. Imagine that the chemical transformations associated with the state of activity in muscle occur by combination at, or by the catalytic effect of, or perhaps by passage through, certain active points in the molecular machinery, the number of which is determined by the tension existing in the muscle at the moment. We can imagine that when the force in the muscle is high the affinities of more of these points are being satisfied by the attractions they exert on one another, and that fewer of them are available to take part in chemical transformation. When the tension is low the affinities of less of these points are being satisfied by mutual attraction, and more of them are exposed to chemical reaction. The rate at which chemical transformation would occur, and therefore, at which energy would be liberated, would be directly proportional to the number of exposed affinities or catalytic groups, and so would be a linear function of the force exerted by the muscle, increasing as the force diminished.

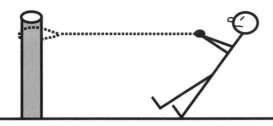

FIGURE 3-16 Anthropomorphic depiction of an active point in a muscle during an isometric contraction after the active point has become attached and has developed tension but does not liberate energy.

Hill's statement, written when virtually nothing was known of the biochemistry of the contractile proteins and a year before myosin was discovered to be an ATPase enzyme, explains the energetics of muscle contraction in terms of interactions between hypothetical "active points" within the muscle. To account for the inverse relationship between load and the rate of extra energy liberation (Fig. 3-14), Hill postulated that the active points can exist in either of two states. In one, the active points are attached and maintain tension, much as when a man pulls against a rope that is firmly anchored to a post (Fig. 3-16); in the other, the active points are free to liberate chemical energy and thus are able to move, as when the same man runs freely after the post is pulled from the ground (Fig. 3-17).

The inverse relationship between load and the rate of extra energy release (Fig. 3-14) reflects the ability of load to determine the distribution of the active points between these two states. In an isometric contraction, where load is maximal ($P = P_0$), all active points are in the state where they develop tension (Fig. 3-18); because all active points are attached, force is maximal, and the rate of energy liberation is zero. Although energy must be expended to reach this state, which accounts for the activation heat (Fig. 3-11), additional energy is not expended to maintain tension. In the unloaded contraction, where $P = 0$, the muscle shortens at maximal velocity because all of the active points are able to cycle at their maximal rate (Fig. 3-19).

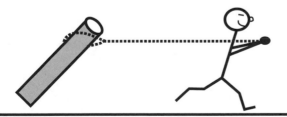

FIGURE 3-17 Anthropomorphic depiction of an active point in a muscle allowed to shorten at zero load, where the active point liberates energy at its maximal rate but does not develop tension.

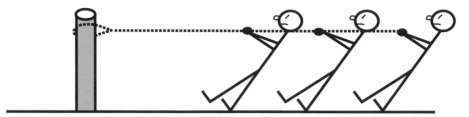

FIGURE 3-18 Anthropomorphic depiction of three active points in a muscle contracting under isometric conditions ($P = P_0$, $V = 0$). After the active points become attached and develop tension, they no longer liberate energy.

EFFICIENCY AND TENSION-TIME HEAT

The model described above is simplified because it assumes that once tension develops during an isometric contraction, all active points remain attached and do not undergo further movement. However, this is not correct; instead, a slow turnover of active points during an isometric contraction generates the tension-time heat $f(P,t)$ described in equations 3-4 and 3-5. In anthropomorphic terms, this is as if the "little men" in Figure 3-18 occasionally shifted their feet.

We now know, of course, that the active points in muscle are not little men but instead are interactions between the myosin cross-bridges and actin (Chapter 1). Tension-time heat $f(P,t)$, therefore, is caused when the cross-bridges cycle slowly between the attached and detached states, which occurs at a rate proportional to the intrinsic rate of energy turnover (ATPase activity) by purified myosin. The rate at which the tension-time heat wastes energy during an isometric contraction is greater in muscles with high myosin ATPase activity because the intrinsic turnover rate of the myosin cross-bridges *in vivo* reflects the same properties that determine myosin ATPase activity *in vitro* (Chapter 4).

Fast muscles, which contain a high ATPase myosin, are more efficient when lightly loaded than slow muscles, but less efficient in sustaining tension (Chapter 2). Slow muscles, although they shorten less rapidly, maintain tension more efficiently because the slower cross-bridge cycling

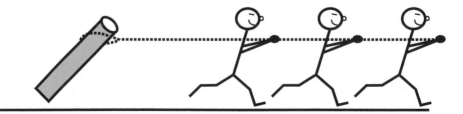

FIGURE 3-19 Anthropomorphic depiction of three active points in a muscle contracting against zero load ($P = 0$, $V = V_{max}$). All of the active points are liberating energy at their maximal rate but do not develop tension.

rate generates less tension-time heat. Returning to the analogy of the little men, a faster runner is better able to lift his feet from the ground—like the rapid cycling of a myosin cross-bridge—and is more efficient when running freely, whereas a slower athlete who keeps his feet on the ground is more efficient when pulling on a tethered rope. Simply stated, an athlete wearing lead shoes runs more slowly and less efficiently, but uses less energy when called upon to pull on a tethered rope, than a faster runner wearing Hermes's winged shoes.

P_0 and V_{max}: The Intercepts of the Force–Velocity Curve

The shortening velocity of an unloaded muscle (V_{max}) should be independent of the number of active points; this is apparent from the analogy of the little men because one runner capable of a top speed of 10 mph will pull an unloaded rope at the same speed as three (or any number) of such runners linked together (Figs. 3-17 and 3-19). For this reason, V_{max} reflects the intrinsic *velocity* of myosin cross-bridge turnover (which is proportional to myosin ATPase activity) and is independent of the number of interactions between the thick and thin filaments. The other intercept of the force–velocity curve, the maximal force generated during an isometric contraction (P_0), should be determined by the number of active points in the muscle. According to the analogy of the little men (Figs. 3-16 and 3-18), P_0 depends on the number of men pulling on the rope rather than how fast each can run when the load is zero. P_0 is therefore independent of the maximal rate of energy expenditure, reflecting instead the number of active interactions between the myosin cross-bridges and actin, which in turn is determined largely by the amount of activator calcium that is bound to the contractile proteins (see Chapter 4).

Force velocity curves, once thought to hold the key to understanding myocardial contractility, have turned out to be of little clinical value. Unfortunately, the elegant analyses of the energetics of tetanized frog sartorius muscle described earlier cannot be carried out in the heart because the active state is slow in onset and changes throughout the cardiac cycle (see Chapter 6). More important, the early view that V_{max}, but not P_0, is a valid index of contractility is not correct because changes in calcium delivery to the contractile proteins, the major mechanism regulating myocardial contractility, determines the number of interactions between the myosin cross-bridges and actin, rather than their turnover rate, and so would be expected to modify P_0 and have little or no effect on V_{max}.

BIBLIOGRAPHY

Alpert NA, Mulieri LA, Hasenfus G. Myocardial chemo-mechanical energy transduction. In: Fozzard H, Haber E, Katz A, et al., eds. *The heart and circulation*, 2nd ed. New York: Raven Press, 1991:111–128.

Bárány M. ATPase activity of myosin correlated with speed of muscle shortening. *J Gen Physiol* 1967;50[No. 6, Pt. 2]:197–206.

Curtin NA, Woledge RC. Energy changes and molecular contraction. *Physiol Rev* 1978;58:690–761.

Rall JA. Sense and nonsense about the Fenn effect. *Am J Physiol* 1982;11:H1–H6.

REFERENCES

Evans CL, Matsuoka Y. The effect of the various mechanical conditions on the gaseous metabolism and efficiency of the mammalian heart. *J Physiol (Lond)* 1914–1915;49: 378–405.

Fenn WO. The relation between the work performed and the energy liberated in muscular contraction. *J Physiol (Lond)* 1923;58:373–395.

Fenn WO, Marsh BS. Muscular force at different speeds of shortening. *J Physiol (Lond)* 1935;85:277–297.

Hill AV. The heat of shortening and the dynamic constants of muscle. *Proc R Soc (Lond.) [Biol]* 1938;126:136–195.

Mommaerts WFHM. Energetics of muscular contraction. *Physiol Rev* 1969;49:427–508.

Starling EH. *The Linacre lecture on the law of the heart.* London: Longmans, Green and Co., 1918.

4

THE CONTRACTILE PROTEINS

The work of the heart depends on the interactions among seven proteins (Table 4-1) that are organized in the thick and thin filaments discussed in Chapter 1. This chapter describes each of these proteins, how their interactions cause the walls of the heart to shorten and develop tension, and how they are regulated by calcium and by load.

MYOSIN

Myosin is one of a family of "motor proteins" that participate in cell motility, endocytosis, signal transduction, and sensory functions like hearing and vision (Hasson and Mooseker, 1996; Mermall et al., 1998). Unlike the kinesins and dyneins, other classes of motor proteins that interact with microtubules (see Chapter 1), myosin interacts with actin filaments.

Cardiac myosin, which makes up most of the thick filaments, includes six subunits: two heavy chains and four light chains (Fig. 4-1). The "tail" of this tadpole-shaped molecule is a region where the heavy chains are organized in a "coiled coil," a rigid structure made up of two α-helices wound around each other. Each heavy chain extends into one of the paired "heads," where, along with the light chains, they make up the cross-bridges. The myosin heavy chains contain an actin-activated ATPase that releases the energy used to power contraction. Interactions between the paired myosin heads play a role in regulation but are not essential for contraction.

Two fragments, called *meromyosins*, are released from myosin by the proteolytic enzymes trypsin and chymotrypsin. The smaller fragment, *light meromyosin*, is derived from the tail of the molecule, while the larger *heavy meromyosin* fragment includes the head, a small portion of the tail, and the light chains (Fig. 4-2). Further digestion of heavy meromyosin with papain, another proteolytic enzyme, removes the rest of the tail and leaves a globular protein, called *heavy meromyosin subfragment 1*, which includes the paired heads of the myosin heavy chains and the four light chains. Myosin ATPase activity and its ability to interact with actin are present in heavy meromyosin and heavy meromyosin subfragment 1.

103

TABLE 4-1 **Contractile Proteins of the Heart**

Protein	Location	Approximate Molecular Weight	Number of Components	Salient Biochemical Properties
Myosin	Thick filament	500,000	Two heavy chains, four light chains	ATP hydrolysis; interacts with actin
Actin	Thin filament	42,000	One	Activates myosin ATPase; interacts with myosin
Tropomyosin	Thin filament	70,000	Two	Modulates actin–myosin interaction
Troponin C	Thin filament	17,000	One (contains four "EF-hand" domains)	Calcium binding
Troponin I	Thin filament	30,000	One	Inhibits actin–myosin interaction
Troponin T	Thin filament	38,000	One	Binds troponin complex to thin filament

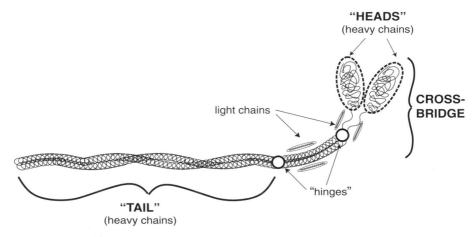

FIGURE 4-1 Each myosin molecule contains two heavy chains and four light chains. The "tail" of the elongated molecule is a coiled coil (two α-helical chains wound around each other) made up of the two heavy chains; the latter continue into the paired "heads" that, along with the light chains, form the cross-bridge. Myosin has two points of flexibility, or "hinges": One lies below the heads, the other divides the tail into two unequal lengths. The hinges represent the points at which proteolytic cleavage releases the meromyosins (Fig. 4-2).

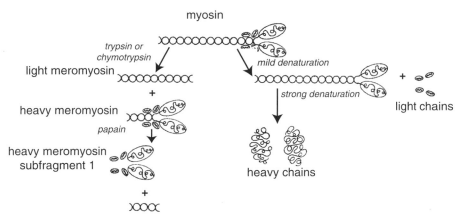

FIGURE 4-2   Myosin fragments (*left*) and subunits (*right*). Light and heavy meromyosins are fragments produced by proteolytic digestion, whereas the heavy and light chains are subunits released by denaturing agents. Mild denaturation of myosin releases the light chains, while stronger denaturing agents are needed to dissociate the heavy chains.

Myosin forms aggregates *in vitro* in which the cross-bridges project away from the center (Fig. 4-3). This arrangement, which is similar to that in the thick filaments of striated muscle, polarizes the interactions between the cross-bridges and the thin filaments that enter the A-band from each of the two adjoining I-bands. In resting muscle, where the thick and thin filaments are detached, the cross-bridges are nearly per-pendicular to the long axis of the muscle (Fig. 4-4). Following activation, the cross-bridges attach and detach from actin in a series of steps that, like the rowing of an oar, draw the thin filaments toward the center of the sarcomere. Because muscle volume remains virtually constant during contraction, the lateral distance between the thick and thin filaments increases when the sarcomeres shorten. Tension development and short-ening velocity are only minimally affected by changes in lattice spacing because "hinges" in the myosin molecule allow the cross-bridges to extend from the backbone of the thick filament to maintain contact with the thin filaments (Fig. 4-5).

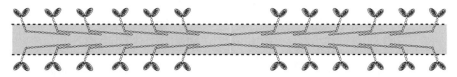

FIGURE 4-3   Myosin aggregates make up the thick filament whose "backbone," which is delineated by dashed lines, contains the tails of the individual myosin molecules whose polarities are opposite in the two halves of the filament (*left and right*). The heads of the individual myosin molecules projecting from the long axis of the thick filament are the cross-bridges. The bare area in the center of the thick filament is devoid of cross-bridges because of the "tail-to-tail" organization of the myosin molecules.

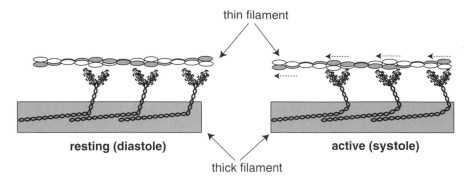

FIGURE 4-4 In resting muscle (*right*), the cross-bridges project almost at right angles to the longitudinal axis of the thick filament. In active muscle (*left*), the cross-bridges interact with the thin filaments, which are drawn toward the center of the sarcomere.

Heavy Chains

Adult human atria and ventricles contain several myosin heavy chain isoforms (Table 4-2); additional isoforms are found in fetal and neonatal hearts. The human ventricle contains mainly the low ATPase β-myosin heavy chain along with a small amount (<10%) of a higher ATPase α-myosin heavy chain. Human atria contain two atrial myosin heavy chain isoforms, both of which differ from those in the ventricles. Cells containing the α- and β-isoforms are distributed in a "mosaic" pattern, where different myosin heavy chain isoforms are found in adjacent cells (see Chapter 7).

Chronic overload induces a hypertrophic response that is accompanied by an isoform shift in which a low ATPase (fetal) heavy chain isoform replaces the high ATPase (adult) isoform (see Chapter 18). This

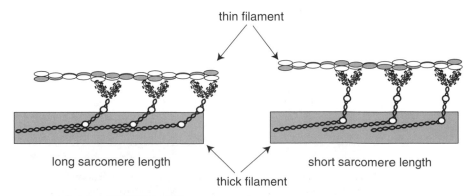

FIGURE 4-5 Relationship between the thick and thin filaments at long and short sarcomere lengths. The myosin hinges (*circles*) maintain a constant relationship between the tips of the cross-bridges and the thin filaments during changes in the lattice spacing between the thick and thin filaments.

TABLE 4-2   **Cardiac Myosin Heavy and Light Chains**

I. Heavy Chains		
Structure	**Isoform**	**Enzymatic activity**
Atria	α (atrial)	High ATPase
	β (atrial)	Low ATPase
Ventricles	α (ventricular)	High ATPase
	β (ventricular)	Low ATPase
II. Light Chains		
Structure	**Isoform**	**Characteristics**
Atria	LC_{1A}	Essential light chain
	LC_{2A}	Regulatory light chain
Ventricles	LC_{1V}	Essential light chain
	LC_{2V}	Regulatory light chain
	LC_{2V*}	Regulatory light chain

overload-induced isoform shift, which occurs in both atria and ventricles, accompanies a reversion to the fetal phenotype that weakens the heart by reducing shortening velocity. However, because low ATPase myosin develops tension with greater efficiency than high ATPase myosin (see Chapter 2), this isoform shift helps adapt the heart to the greater energy requirements associated with increased wall stress.

Light Chains

Myosin light chains are members of the family of *EF-hand calcium-binding proteins* that includes troponin C and calmodulin (see below). The light chains in the adult human heart lack key amino acids in the calcium-binding domain and so do not bind calcium; instead, they are substrates for phosphorylations that regulate myosin ATPase activity and muscle shortening velocity.

Cardiac myosins contain two pairs of light chains (Table 4-2), usually referred to as *regulatory* and *essential light chains*. The former (also called *LC_2, RLC, MLC-2, DTNB,* or *EDTA light chains*) can be removed without abolishing myosin ATPase activity, whereas extraction of the essential light chains (also called *LC_1, ELC, MLC-1,* or *alkali light chains*) inactivates myosin. Five different light chain isoforms are found in human atrial and ventricular myosin. LC_{1A} and LC_{1V} are the two essential light chains in atrial and ventricular myosin, respectively (Table 4-2). The other three isoforms are regulatory light chains, of which two are found in the ventricles (LC_{2V} and LC_{2V*}) and one (LC_{2A}) is found in the atria. In chronically overloaded ventricles, the atrial essential light chain LC_{1A}, which is normally present in developing ventricles, replaces some of the LC_{IV} and is part of the reversion to the fetal phenotype (see Chapter 18).

ACTIN

Actin, which is a highly conserved protein found in all eukaryotic cells, received its name because of its ability to activate myosin ATPase activity. Actin microfilaments, which represent one of the three types of cytoskeletal filament described in Chapter 1, make up the backbone of the thin filaments. Two isoforms are found in the human heart, α-*cardiac actin* and α-*skeletal actin*; these are encoded by separate genes but differ in only a few amino acids. Adult human ventricles contain mainly α-cardiac actin; α-skeletal actin, which is present in smaller amounts, is the fetal isoform.

Actin monomers, which are much smaller than myosin (Table 4-1), are ovoid globular proteins that are approximately 55 Å in diameter. Actin can be stabilized *in vitro* either as a monomer, called *G-actin* (G = globular), or as the filamentous *F-actin* polymer (F = fibrous). The latter is a double-stranded macromolecular helix in which two chains of actin monomers are wound around one another like two strings of beads (Fig. 4-6). Both G- and F-actin contain nucleotide- and cation-binding sites. The bound nucleotide in G-actin is ATP, while F-actin usually contains bound ADP; in both, the bound cation can be either calcium or magnesium. When G-actin polymerizes *in vitro*, the bound ATP is hydrolyzed to form ADP and P_i; it is not clear, however, whether hydrolysis of actin-bound ATP plays a role in muscular contraction.

Actomyosins reconstituted *in vitro* from highly purified actin and myosin can hydrolyze ATP and undergo physicochemical changes similar to those that occur during muscle contraction. However, these two-protein actomyosins are not regulated by calcium because they lack the regulatory proteins described below.

TROPOMYOSIN

Tropomyosin contains two α-helical peptide chains, called α- and β-*tropomyosin*, that are linked by a single disulfide bond (Fig. 4-7). The

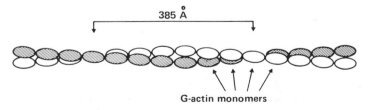

385 Å

G-actin monomers

FIGURE 4-6 The F-actin polymer, which forms the backbone of the thin filaments, is composed of two strands of G-actin monomers (*shaded and unshaded ovals*) that are wound around each other. The internodal distance is approximately 385 Å.

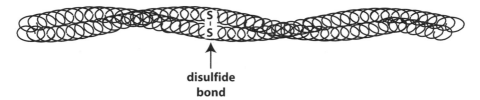

disulfide
bond

FIGURE 4-7 Tropomyosin is made up of two α-helical peptide chains wound around each other in a coiled-coil conformation. Unlike the tail of the myosin molecule (Fig. 4-1), the two polypeptide chains are linked by a single disulfide bond (-S–S-).

protein, which can be a homodimer or heterodimer made up of either or both of these isoforms, had no known function for the first 15 years after it was first purified; its structure, however, was of interest to physical chemists because, like the tail of the myosin molecule, it is a rigid coiled coil. Although tropomyosin itself has no biological activity, when incorporated into the grooves between the two F-actin chains in the thin filament (Fig. 4-8), this seemingly inert protein regulates the interactions between myosin and actin.

THE TROPONIN COMPLEX

The troponin complex includes three proteins (Table 4-1) that, along with tropomyosin, are found in the thin filaments (Figs. 4-9 and 4-10). *Troponin I*, which in concert with tropomyosin regulates the interactions between actin and myosin, was given this name because its most important effect is inhibitory. *Troponin T* binds the troponin complex to tropomyosin, while *troponin C* contains the calcium-binding sites that regulate contraction.

Troponin I

Changes in the strength of a labile bond linking troponin I and actin allow calcium to regulate cardiac contraction. In the relaxed heart, where troponin C is not bound to calcium (see below), troponin I binds tightly

tropomyosin

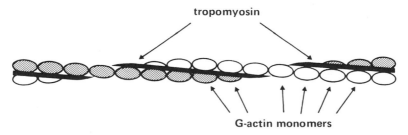

G-actin monomers

FIGURE 4-8 Tropomyosin is located in the groove between the two strands of F-actin in the thin filament.

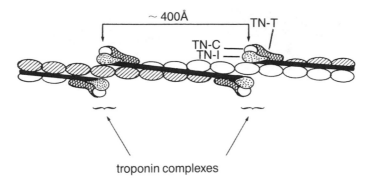

troponin complexes

FIGURE 4-9 Troponin complexes are distributed at approximately 400-Å intervals in the thin filament.

to actin in a conformation that causes tropomyosin to "block" the myosin-binding sites of actin. Calcium binding to troponin C induces an allosteric change that loosens the bond linking troponin I to actin; by favoring the dissociation of troponin I from actin, this allows active sites on actin to interact with the myosin cross bridges. Stated simply, calcium-induced changes in the actin-binding affinity of troponin I provide a molecular switch that recognizes a rise in cytosolic calcium as a signal that triggers contraction.

Different troponin I isoforms are found in cardiac, fast skeletal, and slow skeletal muscles; a fourth troponin I isoform has been identified in developing muscle. Cardiac troponin I contains sites for several regulatory phosphorylations, including one that allows sympathetic stimulation to accelerate relaxation. This phosphorylation reaction, which is catalyzed by PK-A (cyclic AMP–dependent protein kinase), reduces the calcium sensitivity of the contractile proteins, which facilitates relaxation by favoring dissociation of this activator from troponin C (see Chapter 10). Calcium, calmodulin-dependent protein kinase (CAM kinase), and protein kinase C (PK-C) also catalyze cardiac troponin I phosphorylations that facilitate relaxation and reduce contractility by inhibiting interactions between the thick and thin filaments.

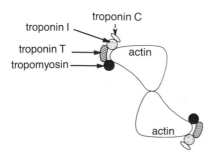

FIGURE 4-10   Cross section of the thin filament in resting muscle at the level of a troponin complex showing relationships between actin, tropomyosin, and the three components of the troponin complex.

Troponin T

Troponin T, the largest of the three troponin components, is an asymmetrical molecule that mediates allosteric effects within the thin filament that influence the calcium sensitivity of tension development. Isoform shifts involving cardiac troponin T, which result from alternate splicing of the gene that encodes this protein, modify myocardial contractility and the calcium sensitivity of the contractile process.

Troponin C and the EF-Hand Proteins

Troponin C is one of a family of *EF-hand proteins* that arose from a common ancestor some 600 million years ago, when multicellular animals evolved in the pre-Cambrian seas. This family also includes the myosin light chains, calmodulin, and other intracellular calcium-binding proteins. All contain a peptide chain of about 30 amino acids, in which two α-helical regions, designated E and F, are separated by a short nonhelical sequence (Fig. 4-11). This peptide chain is called an *EF-hand* because it resembles the extended index finger and thumb of a right hand in which

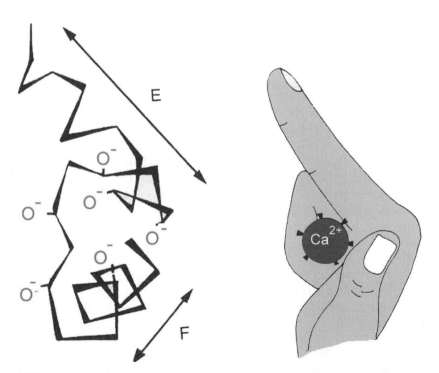

FIGURE 4-11 Structure of an EF-hand protein (*left*) showing two α-helical regions (E and F) separated by a nonhelical loop. This structure, which orients six oxygen atoms (O⁻) to form a high-affinity calcium-binding site, is called an *EF-hand* because it resembles a right hand (*right*).

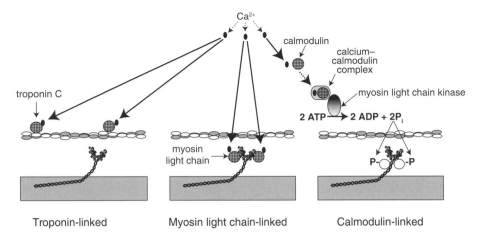

Troponin-linked   Myosin light chain-linked   Calmodulin-linked

FIGURE 4-12 Three mechanisms by which binding of calcium (*small dark ovals*) to EF-hand proteins (*cross-hatched circles*) can mediate excitation–contraction coupling. In troponin-linked regulation (*left*), the calcium-binding protein is incorporated into the thin filament, whereas in myosin light chain-linked regulation (*center*) calcium binds to an EF-hand myosin light chain in the myosin cross-bridge. The calcium receptor in vascular smooth muscle is calmodulin, a soluble EF-hand calcium-binding protein that forms a calcium–calmodulin complex that activates a protein kinase called *myosin light chain kinase* (MLCK) (*right*). This calcium–calmodulin-dependent protein kinase phosphorylates an EF-hand myosin light chain (*open circles*) that still participates in calcium-mediated signaling, although it has lost its ability to bind calcium.

the other fingers and palm correspond to nonhelical loops; proteins containing this structure are called *EF-hand proteins*. The typical EF-hand region includes several oxygen-containing amino acids in an anionic "pocket" that binds calcium ions with high affinity. Most modern calcium-binding proteins, which evolved by duplication and modification of the gene that encoded the ancestral EF-hand protein, contain two or four EF-hand regions. Amino acid substitutions in the calcium-binding regions have caused some of these proteins to lose their ability to bind calcium, while the specificity for calcium, relative to magnesium, was lost in others.

EF-hand proteins can mediate the calcium-induced signal that activates muscle contraction by three different mechanisms (Fig. 4-12). One is exemplified by cardiac troponin C, which is located on the thin filament where it binds the calcium that activates the heart. The second mechanism is seen in scallop muscle, where calcium binding to an EF-hand myosin light chain, rather than troponin C, activates contraction. In the third mechanism, which occurs in vascular smooth muscle, calcium does not interact with an EF-hand protein in the myofilaments, but instead binds to a soluble EF-hand protein called *calmodulin*. The resulting calcium–calmodulin complex activates *myosin light chain kinase* (MLCK),

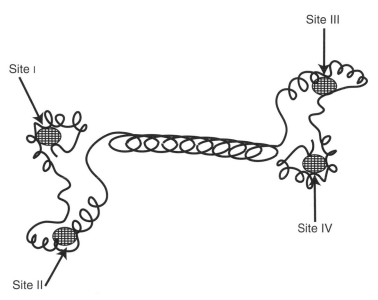

FIGURE 4-13 Schematic diagram of troponin C showing the two globular regions, each of which contains two EF-hand sites (*cross-hatched ovals*), that are separated by a nine-turn α-helix. In cardiac troponin C, Sites III and IV are calcium–magnesium sites, while Site I has lost its cation-binding properties; for this reason, only Site II is a physiological calcium receptor.

which phosphorylates a smooth muscle myosin light chain. Although it has lost the ability to bind calcium, the latter is an EF-hand protein that stimulates contraction in response to a calcium-mediated signal when it is phosphorylated by MLCK.

TROPONIN C. Troponin C is a dumbbell-shaped molecule (Fig. 4-13) that contains four EF-hand amino acid sequences, called "Sites" in Figure 4-13. Some of the latter bind only calcium and therefore are designated as *calcium-specific sites*, while others, called *calcium–magnesium sites*, also bind magnesium. Because the ionized magnesium concentration in muscle is several orders of magnitude higher than that of calcium, the calcium–magnesium sites are normally occupied by magnesium and do not play a role in excitation–contraction coupling. It is therefore the *calcium-specific sites* that serve the physiological function of recognizing a rise in cytosolic calcium concentration as a signal to activate muscular contraction.

Three troponin C isoforms are found in mammalian striated muscle: *cardiac troponin C* and *fast* and *slow skeletal troponin C*; all contain two *calcium-specific sites* (Sites I and II) and two *calcium–magnesium sites* (Sites III and IV). In cardiac troponin C, however, two negatively charged aspartic acid residues in Site I are replaced by leucine and alanine, which causes this site to lose its ability to bind calcium with high affinity. For this reason, Site II—the other calcium-specific site— serves as the physiological calcium receptor of the cardiac contractile proteins.

CALMODULIN. Calmodulin, which like troponin C is a calcium-binding protein that contains four EF-hand regions, responds to a rise in cytosolic calcium by forming a calcium–calmodulin complex in which a hydrophobic region becomes exposed on the surface of the calmodulin molecule. Once exposed, this hydrophobic surface can interact with hydrophobic domains on other proteins, including members of a family of calcium-dependent protein kinases, called *calcium–calmodulin kinases (CaM kinases)*, that participate in cell signaling by catalyzing a variety of regulatory phosphorylations. As noted above, MLCK—one of the CAM kinases—regulates contraction in vascular smooth muscle.

ACTOMYOSINS

Muscle biochemists were initially viewed with disdain because they studied insoluble actomyosin complexes rather than the soluble enzymes whose elegant kinetics once represented the "state of the art" in biochemistry. Little heed was paid to the fact that a soluble muscle would be of little use in developing tension! Although the insolubility of actomyosin made it difficult to study the kinetics of its ATPase activity, aggregates reconstituted *in vitro* from various combinations of the proteins described in Table 4-1 provided striking models of contraction. Most dramatic was an experiment by A. Szent-Györgyi, who in the early 1940s prepared actomyosin threads in which F-actin and myosin filaments were oriented parallel to one another. These actomyosin threads shortened when ATP was added, and if a load was attached, the threads could perform work and even generate hyperbolic force–velocity curves. Another fascinating observation was that addition of large amounts of ATP to gels made of these insoluble actomyosin complexes caused two different effects: at first, the milky suspensions became clear, after which the suspensions again became cloudy as smaller and denser particles reappeared. Low-speed centrifugation of the initial and final suspensions revealed that ATP had decreased the volume of the insoluble actomyosin pellet; this phenomenon was caused by shrinkage of the insoluble actomyosin particles, much as a contracting sponge might squeeze water out of itself. This experiment demonstrated that ATP has two different effects on actomyosin; at high concentrations, ATP dissociates actin and myosin, which explains why the particulate actomyosin suspensions became clearer (called *clearing*), whereas hydrolysis of the added ATP by the myosin ATPase caused actin and myosin to recombine as smaller particles. In the latter process, called *superprecipitation*, ATP provided the substrate for interactions between actin and myosin similar to those occurring in contracting muscle.

Both of the effects of ATP described above—to dissociate actin and myosin and to cause actomyosin to contract—occur in the living heart. During diastole, the normally high ATP concentration exerts a "plasticizing" effect that dissociates the thick and thin filaments by inhibiting interactions between the myosin cross-bridges and actin, whereas during systole, ATP hydrolysis by the catalytic site of myosin energizes contraction. The mechanism by which ATP is able to exert two such different effects is described below.

The discovery that calcium is the physiological activator of muscle contraction led to studies of its effects on actomyosin. However, actomyosins reconstituted from highly purified actin and myosin were found not to respond to calcium. This surprising observation stimulated a search for the missing calcium-sensitizing factor(s) that ended with the discovery of the roles of tropomyosin and the troponin complex (Katz, 1995). Unlike actomyosins reconstituted from actin and myosin, which remain active in both high and low calcium solutions, inclusion of tropomyosin and the troponin complex allows removal of calcium to inhibit the *in vitro* manifestations of contraction, an effect that is reversed by addition of calcium. These findings documented two essential features of the physiological control of the interactions between actin and myosin: first, that *the regulatory proteins are inhibitory at low calcium concentrations*; and second, that *calcium stimulates contraction by reversing this inhibitory effect*.

CALCIUM AS AN INTRACELLULAR MESSENGER

Calcium mediates a number of signals, generally serving as an activator when it binds to one of the EF-hand proteins described earlier. In muscle, calcium signaling represents the final step in *excitation–contraction coupling* (see Chapter 7), the process by which plasma membrane depolarization activates contraction. Calcium serves a similar role in *excitation–secretion coupling* and in controlling the motility of single-celled organisms by initiating cytoplasmic streaming and the motion of cilia and flagellae.

A series of hypotheses was set forth by Kretsinger (1977) to explain how calcium might have become an intracellular messenger. These hypotheses center on the very low ionized calcium concentration in the cytosol of eukaryotic cells, which is about 10,000-fold higher than that in the surrounding fluids. In the resting heart, for example, cytosolic calcium concentration is about 0.2 μM, as compared with the calcium concentration in the extracellular space that, like sea water, is in the millimolar range. Kretsinger, who noted the low solubility of calcium phosphate, suggested that calcium was initially excluded from the cytosol to allow cells to retain phosphate needed for such key molecules as phosphosugars, ATP, and nucleic acids. With the evolution of a calcium-free cytosol, the passive entry of small amounts of calcium became both a problem and an opportunity. The problem, calcium overload, was alleviated by energy-dependent ion pumps and exchangers that transport calcium out of the cell, while the opportunity arose because calcium entry through plasma membrane channels could provide a useful mechanism for signal transduction. Because calcium ions are positively charged, calcium influx generates an electrical signal that depolarizes the plasma membrane as well as a chemical signal that can be recognized by the EF-hand proteins. The latter, which might initially have protected cells from temporary calcium overload, could then have evolved into intracellular calcium sensors. While clearly speculative, this scenario is useful in understanding the signaling role of calcium flux into the cytosol and how this cation, by binding to EF-hand proteins, serves as a ubiquitous cytosolic messenger.

RESPONSE OF THE CONTRACTILE PROTEINS TO CALCIUM IONS

Calcium binding to troponin C initiates a series of cooperative interactions among the proteins of the thin filament that, by shifting the position of tropomyosin in the thin filament, exposes reactive sites on actin (Fig. 4-14). In resting muscle, where troponin C is not bound to calcium, tropomyosin lies toward the outside of the grooves in the double-stranded F-actin polymer, where it prevents actin from interacting with the myosin cross-bridges. When calcium-binding to troponin C weakens the bond connecting troponin I to actin (see above), tropomyosin is shifted away from its "blocking" position (Fig. 4-15). This conformational change allows actin to interact with the myosin cross-bridges (Fig. 4-16). The muscle relaxes when removal of calcium from troponin C returns tropomyosin to its inhibitory position in the thin filament. The spacing of troponin complexes at about 400 Å intervals along the thin filament (Fig. 4-9) allows calcium binding to each troponin complex to modify approximately seven actin monomers.

Tropomyosin and the troponin complex provide more than an "on–off" switch that recognizes a rise of cytosolic calcium as the physiological

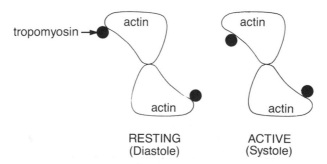

FIGURE 4-14 Cross section of a thin filament at a region that does not contain the troponin complex. Tropomyosin, which lies in the groove between the two strands of actin monomers, occupies different position at rest (*left*) and during activity (*right*).

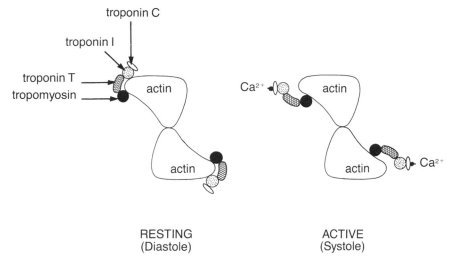

RESTING
(Diastole)

ACTIVE
(Systole)

FIGURE 4-15   Cross section of a thin filament at a region containing the troponin complex in resting (*left*) and active (*right*) muscle. At rest, the troponin complex holds the tropomyosin molecules toward the periphery of the groove between adjacent actin strands, which prevents actin from interacting with the myosin cross-bridges. In active muscle, calcium binding to troponin C weakens the bond linking troponin I to actin. Loosening of this bond rearranges the regulatory proteins so as to shift tropomyosin deeper into the groove between the strands of actin, thereby exposing active sites on actin for interaction with the myosin cross-bridges.

signal initiating contraction. For example, after actin has begun to interact with myosin, the regulatory proteins amplify tension development in the contracting muscle. Other regulatory effects include the ability of troponin I phosphorylation to reduce the calcium sensitivity of the cardiac contractile proteins (see above); troponin T phosphorylation to modify force generation; and an allosteric effect, initiated when protons bind to troponin I, that is partly responsible for the ability of acidosis to reduce

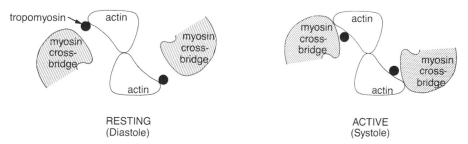

RESTING
(Diastole)

ACTIVE
(Systole)

FIGURE 4-16   Cross section at a point of potential interaction between actin and an adjacent myosin cross-bridge at rest (*left*) and during activity (*right*). The shift in the position of the tropomyosin molecules toward the center of the groove between adjacent actin strands in the thin filament (see Fig. 4-15) exposes active sites on actin for interaction with the cross-bridge.

myocardial contractility. Changes in sarcomere length have an important effect on the interactions among the contractile proteins that, by modifying their sensitivity to calcium, plays a major role in the length–tension relationship and Starling's law of the heart (see Chapter 6). Other allosteric effects result from isoform shifts involving the proteins of the thin filament that modify the performance and efficiency of hypertrophied and failing hearts (see Chapter 18).

BIOCHEMISTRY OF CONTRACTION

Is ATP Essential for Contraction or for Relaxation?

The seemingly contradictory effects of ATP both to dissociate acto-myosin suspensions and cause them to contract (clearing and superprecipitation, see above) also are seen in living muscle, where hydrolysis of the terminal high-energy phosphate bond of ATP provides the energy for contraction, whereas ATP depletion causes rigor. These and other observations led early investigators to ask whether the major function of ATP is to cause muscle to contract or to relax. One answer focused on the role of ATP in contraction:

$$\text{actin} + \text{myosin} + \text{ATP} \rightarrow \text{actomyosin} + \text{ADP} + P_i$$
$$\text{(relaxed)} \qquad\qquad \text{(active)}$$

The second, which emphasized the role of ATP in relaxation, highlighted the ability of ATP to dissociate actin and myosin:

$$\text{actomyosin} + \text{ATP} \rightarrow \text{actin} + \text{myosin–ATP}$$
$$\text{(active)} \qquad\qquad \text{(relaxed)}$$

It is now clear that both mechanisms operate when the heart contracts and relaxes. This dual role reflects the fact that ATP and its hydrolytic products, ADP and P_i, interact with the contractile proteins at several steps during the cross-bridge cycle, some during contraction, others during relaxation. For this reason, the question "Is ATP essential for contraction or for relaxation?" can be answered by analyses of the roles of ATP, ADP, and P_i during the sequence of reactions between actin and myosin that occur during each cardiac cycle. For simplicity, the following discussion considers four key steps in this reaction mechanism. Beginning with the heart in its relaxed state, when the myosin cross-bridges are bound to ATP but dissociated from actin, these are: (1) hydrolysis of myosin-bound ATP in a reaction that leaves the hydrolytic products (ADP and P_i) attached to myosin; (2) formation of an "active" complex between myosin and actin in which P_i is released but the energy of ATP remains in the cross-bridge; (3) release of ADP at the step where the myosin cross-bridge changes position; and (4) rebinding of ATP to myosin which, by dissociating actin and myosin, relaxes the heart. We begin with the simpler ATPase reaction of myosin alone, which is then contrasted with that of actomyosin to clarify the rate-limiting steps and role of actin in muscle contraction.

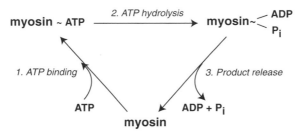

FIGURE 4-17 Simplified, three-step reaction mechanism for myosin ATPase. The sequence begins at the bottom left of the figure, where ATP binds with high affinity to myosin (*step 1*); in this step, the energy in the terminal phosphate of ATP remains in the bond linking ATP to myosin. After hydrolysis of myosin-bound ATP (*step 2*), the phosphate-bond energy remains in the myosin-bound ADP and P_i. Dissociation of these reaction products (*step 3*), which is rate-limiting, releases this energy and returns myosin to its resting state, where it can again bind ATP.

Myosin ATPase Reaction

Myosin binds with high affinity to ATP to form a myosin–ATP complex in which the chemical energy of the nucleotide remains in its terminal phosphate (*step 1*, Fig. 4-17). The next step, ATP hydrolysis by the enzymatic site of myosin (*step 2*, Fig. 4-17), does not immediately dissociate the products; instead, an energized complex is formed in which ADP and P_i remain attached to myosin. ADP and P_i then dissociate slowly from myosin, which returns to its basal state (*step 3*, Fig. 4-17). The complex between myosin and the products of ATP hydrolysis is very stable, so the slow dissociation of ADP and P_i is rate-limiting for the low ATPase activity of myosin alone.

Actomyosin ATPase Reaction—The Cross-Bridge Cycle

Actin stimulates myosin ATPase activity by interacting with myosin that is still bound to ADP and P_i at the end of step 2 in Figure 4-17. By accelerating dissociation of the reaction products from myosin, actin increases the rate-limiting step (*step 3*, Fig. 4-17) and so converts the low myosin ATPase activity to the higher ATPase activity of actomyosin.

The key reactions of the cross-bridge cycle can be summarized in four steps: two in which the myosin cross-bridges are bound to actin (*active* and *rigor* complexes), and two in which actin and myosin are detached (*relaxed* and *relaxed, energized*) (Figs. 4-18 and 4-19). In the latter, where myosin is bound either to ATP or to ADP and P_i, the muscle is relaxed because the cross-bridges are not attached to actin. The two states in which the cross-bridges are attached to actin are quite different from one another. In the *active complex*, the energy of ATP remains in the cross-bridge, whereas in forming the *rigor complex*, which is in a low-energy state, the chemical energy of the active complex is expended to shift the position of the actin-attached cross-bridge.

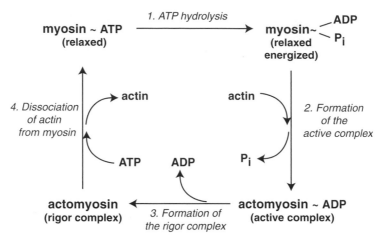

FIGURE 4-18 Simplified, four-step reaction mechanism for actomyosin ATPase. The sequence begins at the upper left, where ATP binding to myosin has caused the muscle to relax by dissociating myosin and actin. Hydrolysis of myosin-bound ATP (*step 1*) transfers the energy of the nucleotide to the cross-bridge, but because the latter is not attached to actin, the muscle remains in a relaxed, energized state (*upper right*). Interaction of the cross-bridge with actin and release of P_i (*step 2*) forms an active complex in which the energy derived from ATP remains associated with the cross-bridge. Release of ADP (*step 3*) leads to the formation of a low-energy rigor bond between the cross-bridge and thin filament; expenditure of chemical energy in this step allows the muscle to perform mechanical work. The cycle ends, and the muscle returns to its resting state, when ATP binding to the rigor complex (*step 4*) dissociates the myosin cross-bridge from actin.

In choosing where to enter the cross-bridge cycle, we follow the convention of the physiologist, who begins the cardiac cycle in diastole. This description therefore starts with the heart in the relaxed state, where ATP bound to myosin has dissociated the cross-bridge from the thin filament. The four steps that follow are: (1) hydrolysis of myosin-bound ATP; (2) release of P_i and formation of the active complex with actin; (3) release of ADP and formation of the rigor complex; and (4) dissociation of actin and myosin. In actomyosins that lack the regulatory proteins, which do not respond to calcium, the cross-bridge cycle continues as long as there is an adequate supply of ATP.

STEP 1. HYDROLYSIS OF MYOSIN-BOUND ATP. After the high ATP concentration in the resting heart dissociates the thick and thin filaments by forming a *relaxed* myosin–ATP complex (Figs. 4-18 and 4-19), the cross-bridge cycle proceeds when the bound ATP is hydrolyzed by the catalytic site of myosin. As occurs during ATP hydrolysis by myosin alone (see above), the hydrolytic products ADP and P_i remain attached to myosin. This step transfers the energy of the terminal phosphate bond of ATP to myosin, where the energy in the *relaxed–energized* complex remains in the cross-bridge and has not been used to perform work.

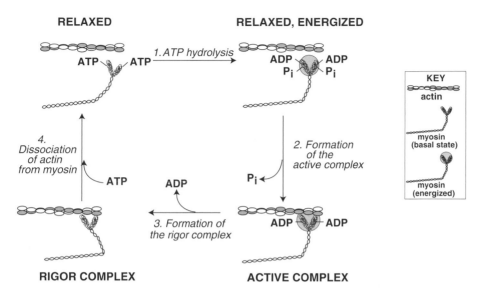

RELAXED   RELAXED, ENERGIZED

1. ATP hydrolysis

KEY

actin

myosin
(basal state)

myosin
(energized)

4.
Dissociation
of actin
from myosin

2. Formation
of the
active complex

3. Formation of
the rigor complex

RIGOR COMPLEX   ACTIVE COMPLEX

FIGURE 4-19 Four-step reaction mechanism for actomyosin ATPase depicted in Figure 4-18. The sequence begins at the upper left, where ATP binding to myosin has dissociated the cross-bridge from actin. Hydrolysis of myosin-bound ATP (*step 1*) transfers the energy of the nucleotide to the cross-bridge, which still is bound to ADP and P_i. Because the energized cross-bridge is not attached to actin, the muscle remains in a relaxed state (*upper right*). Interaction of the cross-bridge with actin and release of P_i (*step 2*) lead to the formation of the active complex in which the energy derived from ATP remains associated with the cross-bridge. Release of ADP (*step 3*) shifts the position of the myosin cross-bridge and leads to formation of a rigor bond; the chemical energy released at this step can be used to perform mechanical work. Rebinding of ATP to the rigor complex (*step 4*) dissociates the myosin cross-bridge from the thin filament, which ends the cycle and returns the muscle to its relaxed state.

STEP 2. FORMATION OF THE ACTIVE COMPLEX WITH ACTIN. Interaction of actin with the *relaxed–energized* cross-bridge in the next step forms an *active complex* between actin and myosin. Even though the myosin cross-bridge is bound to the actin in the active complex, the cross-bridge has not yet executed the "rowing" motion that pulls the thin filament toward the center of the sarcomere, which means that the energy released by ATP hydrolysis has not been expended to perform work. For this reason, the active complex contains a great deal of chemical energy. This energy is released in the next step, which energizes the cross-bridge movement that enables the heart to contract.

STEP 3. DISSOCIATION OF THE PRODUCTS OF ATP HYDROLYSIS. The heart performs mechanical work when release of the myosin-bound ADP allows the energy in the *active complex* to shift the position of the cross-bridge. This forms the *rigor complex*, in which the myosin cross-bridge, although firmly attached to actin, is in a low-energy state. ADP release from actomyosin, like ADP release from myosin (see above), is rate-limiting in the cross-bridge cycle.

The bond linking the cross-bridge to the thin filament in the *rigor complex* is quite different from that in the *active complex*, even though myosin is attached to actin in both. In the latter, this is a high-energy bond, whereas the bond linking myosin to actin in the rigor complex is of low energy because the phosphate bond energy has been expended to move the cross-bridge.

Rigor complexes persist in muscles that become severely energy-starved. In skeletal muscle, this causes *rigor mortis*, while formation of rigor bonds in the heart causes *ischemic contracture*. Prior to the development of effective cardioplegic agents, which by inhibiting actin–myosin interactions arrest the heart in a relaxed state during open heart surgery, severe ischemic contracture sometimes appeared during prolonged cardiopulmonary bypass (the "stone heart syndrome"). Less dramatic but much more common clinically is decreased diastolic compliance caused by the formation of rigor bonds in energy-starved ischemic and failing hearts.

STEP 4. DISSOCIATION OF ACTIN AND MYOSIN. Completion of the cross-bridge cycle requires that ATP again binds to myosin. This occurs in a rapid reaction, where rebinding of ATP to the rigor complex detaches the bonds linking the cross-bridge to the thin filament. Dissociation of the complex explains the "plasticizing" effect of ATP described above.

Is ATP Essential for Contraction or for Relaxation?

The reactions of the cross-bridge cycle shown in Figures 4-18 and 4-19 answer the old question as to whether ATP is essential for contraction or for relaxation. In fact, ATP participates in *both*, but in different ways. ATP *hydrolysis* by actin-activated myosin energizes contraction (*steps 1–3*), whereas ATP *binding* to myosin is essential for relaxation (*step 4*). That relaxation does not require the expenditure of energy is readily demonstrated *in vitro*, where pyrophosphate and nonhydrolyzable ATP analogues—which cannot energize the cross-bridges—are able to dissociate actin and myosin. However, hydrolysis of the high-energy phosphate bond of ATP is required to complete the cross-bridge cycle. The ATP concentration needed to dissociate the cross-bridges from actin (*step 4*) is much higher than that needed to energize the ATPase site of myosin (*steps 1–3*), so decreased ATP levels in energy-starved hearts attenuate the relaxing effect without inhibiting the formation of rigor bonds.

The rate of the cross-bridge cycle, which determines the maximal velocity of unloaded shortening in living muscle (Chapter 3), can be modified by isoform shifts involving the myosin heavy chains that alter myosin ATPase activity (see above); by isoform shifts that alter the cooperative interactions among the proteins of the thin filament; and by post-translational changes such as myosin light chain phosphorylation. The most important of the latter is the ability of tropomyosin and the troponin complex to inhibit the cycle when troponin C is bound to calcium.

REGULATION OF THE CROSS-BRIDGE CYCLE
BY CALCIUM

The role of calcium in activating cardiac contraction can be understood when two steps are added to the cross-bridge cycle shown in Figures 4-18 and 4-19. During diastole, when calcium is not bound to troponin C, the regulatory proteins prevent actin from interacting with myosin (Fig. 4-20, *right*), which halts the cycle at the step where the myosin cross-bridges are energized but not bound to the thin filaments. During systole, when calcium binds to troponin C, the cycle continues because the regulatory proteins no longer prevent the cross-bridges from interacting with actin (Fig. 4-20, *left four diagrams*).

REGULATION OF THE CROSS-BRIDGE CYCLE BY LOAD

Load plays an important role in regulating the cross-bridge cycle. As described in Chapter 3, Hill's observation that the rate of energy release by contracting muscle is inversely proportional to load suggested that load determines the distribution of "active points" between two different states: one in which they cycle freely but do not develop tension, the other where

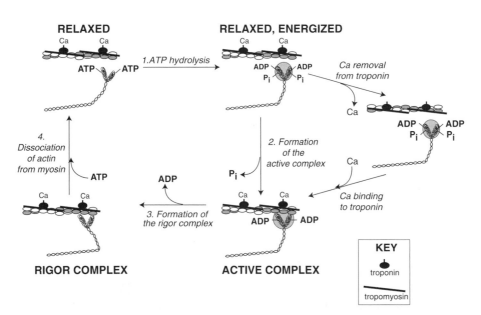

FIGURE 4-20 Role of tropomyosin and the troponin complex in regulating the cross-bridge cycle. As long as calcium is bound to troponin C, the muscle remains in its activated state (*left four diagrams*), which allows the cross-bridge cycle to continue. Calcium removal from troponin C (*right*), which shifts the regulatory proteins on the thin filament to their inhibitory state, relaxes the heart by preventing actin from interacting with the energized myosin cross-bridges. Activation occurs when calcium binding to troponin allows the cycle to resume.

they maintain tension but do not cycle. The ability of all of the active points to liberate chemical energy at zero load, and to become attached when load is increased, can be understood in terms of the cross-bridge cycle.

Active Points Liberating Chemical Energy

The biochemical basis for Hill's observation that the *rate* of energy liberation is maximal when a freely shortening muscle contracts at zero load became apparent when Bárány (1967) found that the maximal shortening velocity (V_{max}) of different muscles correlates closely with the intrinsic ATPase activity of their myosins. This indicated that the maximal speed at which the "little men" described in Chapter 3 can run at zero load (Fig. 3-17) corresponds to step 3 in the cross-bridge cycle (Figs. 4-19 and 4-20), the rate-limiting step where ADP is released from myosin. As long as the cross-bridges are allowed to cycle freely, the rate-limiting for ATP hydrolysis by myosin alone is the same as that which determines V_{max} in living muscle.

Active Points Maintaining Tension

The ability of increasing load to slow the rate of energy liberation (Chapter 3) can be explained by the ability of load to slow cross-bridge movement along the thin filaments by inhibiting the breaking of the rigor bonds linking myosin and actin. Increasing muscle tension stabilizes the rigor bonds by inhibiting the dissociation of actin and myosin (*step 4* in the cross-bridge cycle shown in Figs. 4-19 and 4-20) in the same way that tying a group of "little men" to a post prevents their feet from moving (Fig. 3-16). Because the determinants of the rate of cross-bridge cycling are not the same as those that determine the strength of the rigor bonds, this analogy helps explain why maximal shortening velocity at zero load (P_0) is not related to maximum isometric tension (V_{max}). In muscle, the number of active cross-bridges does not influence maximum shortening velocity at zero load for the same reason that increasing the number of "little men" whose top speed is unrelated to their ability to pull on a tethered rope does not increase the velocity at which they can run if the post is pulled out of the ground (Fig. 3-19).

The Force–Velocity Curve

The Hill equation suggested that the intercepts of the force–velocity curve (Fig. 3-15) are determined by different properties of the "active points." In modern terms, this means that P_0, the maximal isometric tension generated by a fully activated muscle, is determined by the *number* of rigor bonds between the cross-bridges and actin, which in turn reflects the number of troponin C molecules bound to calcium. For this reason, the amount of calcium released during excitation–contraction coupling is the major determinant of P_0. Maximal shortening velocity (V_{max}), on the other hand, is determined by the *turnover rate* of cross-bridge cycling and therefore is independent of the *number* of active cross-bridges as long as the load is zero; this means that recruiting additional actin–myosin interactions, while increasing P_0, cannot increase shortening velocity in an unloaded muscle.

In theory, this analysis indicates that two independent mechanisms can control the heart's performance: the *number* of active cross-bridges and their *turnover rate*. Together, these variables determine myocardial contractility, which can be defined as the ability of the heart to do work at any given rest length (see Chapter 10). Unfortunately, difficulties in measuring both P_0 and V_{max} in the intact heart have made it impossible to use this paradigm to define myocardial contractility (see Chapter 6).

BIBLIOGRAPHY

Bers DM. *Excitation-contraction coupling and cardiac contractile force*, 2nd ed. Dordrecht: Kluwer, 2001.

Campbell K. Rate constant of muscle force redevelopment reflects cooperative activation as well as cross-bridge kinetics. *Biophys J* 1997;72:254–262.

Cheung WY. Calmodulin: an overview. *Fed. Proc* 1982;41:2253–2257.

de Tombe PP, Solaro RJ. Integration of cardiac myofilament activity and regulation with pathways signaling hypertrophy and failure. *Ann Biomed Eng* 2000;28:991–1001.

Huxley HE, Hanson J. The molecular basis of contraction in cross-striated muscles. In: Bourne GH. *The structure and function of muscle*. Vol. 1: *Structure*. New York: Academic Press, 1960:183–227.

Kawai M, Saeki Y, Zhao Y. Crossbridge scheme and the kinetic constants of elementary steps deduced from chemically skinned papillary and trabecular muscles of the ferret. *Circ Res* 1993;73:35–50.

Kontrogianni-Konstantopoulos A, Catino DH, Strong JC, et al. Obscurin regulates the organization of myosin into A bands. *Am J Physiol* 2004;287:C209–C217.

Kretsinger RH. The informational role of calcium in the cytosol. *Adv Cyclic Nucl Res* 1979;11:1–26.

Langer GA, ed. *The myocardium*. San Diego: Academic Press, 1997.

Page E, Fozzard HA, Solaro RJ, eds. Handbook of physiology, section 2: *The cardiovascular system*. Vol. I: *The Heart*. New York: Oxford, 2002.

Schiaffino S, Reggiani C. Molecular diversity of myofibrillar proteins: gene regulation and molecular significance. *Physiol Rev* 1996;76:371–423.

Solaro RJ, Rarick HM. Troponin and tropomyosin. Proteins that switch on and tune in the activity of cardiac myofilaments. *Circ Res* 1998;83:471–480.

Taylor EW. Mechanism and energetics of actomyosin ATPase. In: Fozzard H, Haber E, Katz AM, et al., eds. *The heart and circulation*, 2nd ed. New York: Raven Press, 1991:1281–1294.

Tobacman LS. Thin filament-mediated regulation of cardiac contraction. *Annu Rev Physiol* 1996;58:447–481.

REFERENCES

Bárány M. ATPase activity of myosin correlated with speed of muscle shortening. *J Gen Physiol* 1967;50[No. 6, Pt. 2]:197–206.

Hasson T, Mooseker MS. Vertebrate unconventional myosins. *J Biol Chem* 1966;271: 16431–16434.

Katz AM. Growth of ideas: role of calcium as activator of cardiac contraction. *Cardiovasc Res* 2001;42:8–13.

Kretsinger R. Evolution of the informational role of calcium in eukaryotes. In: Wasserman RH, Corradino RA, Carafoli RH, et al., eds. *Calcium-binding proteins and calcium function.* New York: North Holland, 1977:63–72.

Mermall V, Post PL, Mooseker MS. Unconventional myosins in cell movement, membrane traffic, and signal transduction. *Science* 1998;279:527–533.

Sartore S, Gorza L, Pierobon Bormioli S, et al. Myosin types and fiber types in cardiac muscle. I: Ventricular myocardium. *J Cell Biol* 1981;88:226–233.

5

THE CYTOSKELETON

Cells are not simply fluid-filled bags in which functional elements such as myofilaments, mitochondria, and enzymes float freely in the cytosol; instead, a complex cellular architecture is maintained by a framework called the *cytoskeleton*. The latter includes structural proteins that, like the girders in a modern building, hold the cell contents in place, organize functionally related proteins within cells, and facilitate the interactions of cells with adjacent cells and the extracellular matrix. In addition to these mechanical functions, the cytoskeleton is a major participant cell signaling, where it makes a major contribution to the proliferative signal transduction pathways that modify the size and shape of the heart. The cytoskeleton, therefore, is not simply a system of girders that maintains cell shape; because of its role in cell signaling, the cytoskeleton is more accurately viewed as a structural framework that also serves as a phone system!

In cardiac myocytes, the cytoskeleton organizes spatial relationships among intracellular structures, transmits tension developed by the contractile proteins from one sarcomere to another and to the cell surface, and links cells to other cells and to the extracellular matrix. The cytoskeleton also helps the heart to adapt its architecture in response to cell deformation and changes in mechanical stress. By modifying the size, shape, and composition of the heart, cytoskeletal signaling helps adapt form to function. These responses are especially important in disease, where cytoskeletal signaling contributes to the hypertrophic response to overload. Although the initial architectural responses are generally beneficial, they often become maladaptive when the overload is sustained. It is likely, therefore, that cytoskeletal signaling plays a role in determining the prognosis in heart failure, where deleterious transcriptional signaling contributes to the progressive ventricular dilatation, called remodeling, that shortens survival in these patients (see Chapter 18).

Both the mechanical and signaling functions of the cytoskeleton are made possible by interactions among literally dozens of proteins. Classification of these proteins is difficult; some, like actin and desmin, play largely a mechanical role, whereas other proteins associated with the cytoskeleton, such as protein kinases and phosphatases, function largely in signal transduction. Many cytoskeletal proteins serve both mechanical and signaling functions, so any attempt at classification must be rather arbitrary. In many ways, these proteins resemble the wheels of an automobile, which not only connect the vehicle to the road but also participate in steering.

The cytoskeleton includes three types of intracellular fiber: *microfilaments*, which include cortical and sarcomeric actin; *intermediate filaments*, which contain desmin; and *microtubules*, which contain tubulin (see Chapter 1). The microfilaments and intermediate filaments provide the major linkages within cardiac myocytes, where they maintain sarcomere structure, connect the sarcomeres of adjacent cells, and participate in multiprotein complexes that bridge the plasma membrane to connect cells to each other and to the extracellular matrix. The most important cell–cell junctions are the fascia adherens and desmosomes in the intercalated disc (see Chapter 1), while key structures that link cells to the extracellular matrix are the dystrophin glycoprotein complex and the integrins.

CYTOSKELETAL PROTEINS ASSOCIATED WITH THE MYOFILAMENTS

In the late 1950s, extraction of myosin was found to remove the A-bands of the sarcomeres, while subsequent extraction of actin removed the I-bands (Huxley and Hanson, 1960). However, the sarcomeres did not fall apart after these proteins were removed; instead, the Z-lines retained their normal alignment within a mesh of fine filaments. The latter are now known to include a number of cytoskeletal proteins that are associated with the thick and thin filaments and with the Z-lines, where they maintain sarcomere structure and provide the mechanical linkages required to convey tension developed by the contractile proteins to adjacent sarcomeres and ultimately to other cells and the extracellular matrix.

Cytoskeletal Proteins of the Z-lines and Thin Filaments

Sarcomeric actin, the backbone of the thin filament (see Chapter 4), can be viewed as part of the cytoskeleton as well as a component of the myofilaments. Tension developed by the contractile proteins is transmitted from the thin filaments to actin microfilaments in the fascia adherens of the intercalated discs. Tension also is transmitted to desmin fibers in the Z-lines, which along with desmin-containing filaments that surround the sarcomeres, are linked to the intermediate filaments that connect to desmosomes (see Chapter 1).

A number of cytoskeletal proteins link the Z-lines to the cell surface and to the thick and thin filaments (Fig. 5-1). *Desmin*, which serves mainly a mechanical role, links the Z-lines to the intercalated discs. Proteins that bind the Z-lines to the thin filaments include α-*actinin*, which weaves the thin filaments into the Z-line, and *nebulette*, which runs alongside the thin filaments from the Z-line to the I-bands. Proteins that link the Z-lines to the thick filaments include *titin* and *t-cap* (*telethonin*). *Ankyrin* plays an

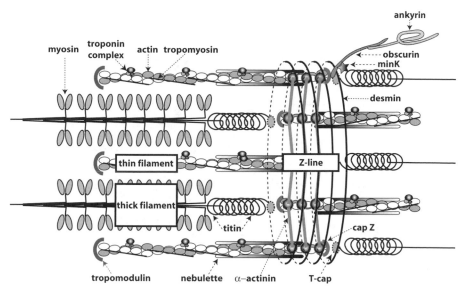

FIGURE 5-1 Cytoskeletal proteins of Z-lines and thin filaments whose major function is to provide mechanical linkages. Desmin links the Z-lines to desmosomes in the intercalated discs, while obscurin, along with ankyrin, connects the Z-lines to the sarcoplasmic reticulum. MinK appears to link the Z-lines to the t-tubules, and T-cap binds the Z-lines to titin in the thick filaments. The length of the thin filaments is regulated by two "capping" proteins: tropomodulin and cap Z; the latter, along with α-actinin and nebulette, connects the thin filaments to the Z-lines.

important role in maintaining the proximity of functionally related proteins (see below) and, in concert with *obscurin*, connects the Z-lines to the sarcoplasmic reticulum. *Titin*, *obscurin*, and *nebulette*, which are members of a class of cytoskeletal proteins associated with the contractile apparatus, contain a large number of immunoglobulin domains. A regulatory subunit of plasma membrane voltage-gated potassium channels, called *minK* (see Chapter 13), links the Z-lines to the t-tubules and may regulate the electrical potential across the t-tubular membranes.

Both ends of the thin filament are capped by cytoskeletal proteins. The ends within the Z-lines are covered by *cap Z* (β-*actinin*), while the other ends, which interdigitate with the A-bands, are capped by *tropomodulin*. In addition to regulating thin filament length and sarcomere structure, these "capping proteins" interact with a variety of signaling proteins and may participate in transcriptional regulation.

Several additional proteins that interact with the Z-line mediate intracellular signaling; these include *CARP*, *S100*, *myopalladin*, *calcineurin*, *myopodin*, *calcarcin*, *LIM proteins*, *filamin*, *cipher*, and several *protein kinases* (Fig. 5-2). Many of these proteins, in concert with other signaling proteins linked to titin (see below), participate in the hypertrophic response of the heart to overload (see Chapter 18).

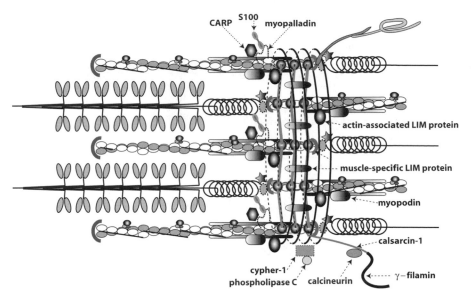

FIGURE 5-2 Cytoskeletal proteins of the Z-lines and thin filaments that participate in signal transduction. The locations of these proteins,which imply that they are linked to one or another of the proteins shown in Figure 5-1, are probably inaccurate because these signaling proteins appear able to move from one location to another.

Cytoskeletal Proteins of the Thick Filaments

The thick filaments, once thought to be composed entirely of myosin, are now known to contain several cytoskeletal proteins. *Titin*, a huge protein with a molecular weight of about 3,000,000 that extends from the Z-lines to the center of the thick filament (Fig. 5-3), supports sarcomeric structure and contributes to the high resting stiffness of the myocardium (see Chapter 6). *Myosin-binding protein C (C protein)*, which binds to both myosin and titin, forms transverse fibers that connect adjacent thick filaments near the centers of the sarcomeres. These fibers, along with *M-protein* and *myomesin*, provide lateral mechanical stability to the sarcomere and help to organize interactions between titin and the thick filaments. Other proteins, including obscurin and ankyrin, link the M-bands and the sarcoplasmic reticulum (see below).

Like the cytoskeletal proteins of the Z-bands and thin filaments, many cytoskeletal proteins associated with the thick filaments participate in cell signaling. Titin itself contains three "hot spots" that appear to participate in the proliferative responses initiated by mechanical stress (Fig. 5-3). One hot spot interacts with the signaling proteins of the Z-line (see above and Fig. 5-2), the second is located in the center of the I-band, while the third interacts with signaling proteins in the M-band (Fig. 5-4). The existence of different phenotypes of cardiac hypertrophy (see Chapter 18) can be explained in part by the ability of various types of cytoskeletal deformation to activate specific signaling pathways; this can occur because

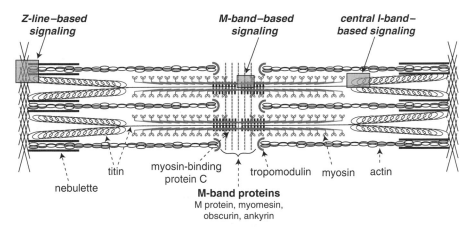

FIGURE 5-3 Cytoskeletal proteins of the thick filaments whose major function is to provide mechanical linkages. These include the giant protein *titin*, which extends from the Z-band into the thick filament, where it is connected to myosin by *myosin-binding protein C* near the center of the A-band. The portions of the titin molecule that lie within the A-band are quite rigid, while the regions in the I-band are more elastic. Several proteins make up the M-bands that link the thick filaments in the center of the A-band; these include *M-protein, myomesin, obscurin, ankyrin*, and the *MM isoform* of the enzyme creatine phosphokinase. *Nebulette* and *tropomodulin*, which are related to the thin filaments, also are shown. Regions especially active in signal transduction (*shaded rectangles*, labeled above) are labeled *Z-line–based signaling* (see Fig. 5-2), *M-band–based signaling*, and *central I-band–based signaling* (see Fig. 5-4).

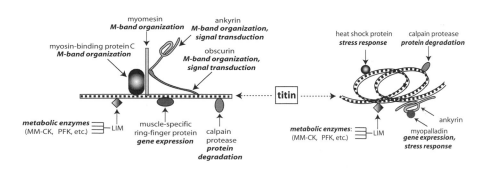

FIGURE 5-4 Signaling "hot spots" in titin. M-band–based titin signaling (*left*): The thick filaments are organized in the M-band by myomesin, myosin-binding protein C, and obscurin, which link titin and myosin. These, along with additional M-band proteins (*labeled*), also participate in cell signaling and, in the case of the LIM protein, organize energy-producing enzymes. Central I-band–based titin signaling (*right*): Titin-linked proteins in the center of the I-band also participate in cell signaling and, through the LIM proteins, organize energy-producing enzymes. For clarity, linkages with myosin are not shown.

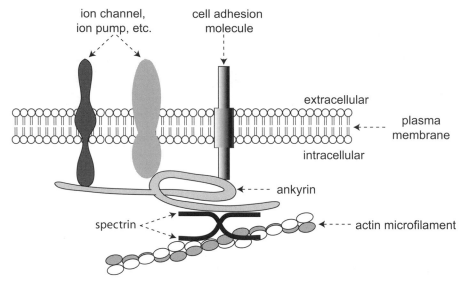

FIGURE 5-5 Ankyrin and spectrin organize functionally related membrane proteins in specific regions of membranes. They also bind actin microfilaments to cell adhesion molecules in the plasma membrane.

longitudinal and/or transverse stresses applied during systole and/or diastole can induce different rearrangements among the cytoskeletal proteins. Activation of different signal transduction pathways by systolic stress and diastolic stretch, for example, can explain the well-known ability of pressure overload to cause concentric hypertrophy (as occurs in aortic stenosis, which increases systolic stress), whereas volume overload causes eccentric hypertrophy (as occurs in aortic insufficiency, which increases diastolic stretch).

Ankyrin and Spectrin: Organizers of Membrane Proteins

Ankyrins are members of a family of adaptor proteins that link the cytoskeleton to a number of plasma membrane and sarcoendoplasmic reticulum proteins, including clathrin, and a variety of receptors, cell adhesion molecules, ion channels, ion pumps, and ion exchangers (Fig. 5-5). Actin- and membrane-binding domains in ankyrins link the actin cytoskeleton to the plasma membrane. The actin-binding domains include 24 copies of a 33–amino acid sequence called the "ankyrin repeat," while the membrane-binding domains can form linkages with a variety of structurally dissimilar membrane proteins, often in multiprotein complexes. The latter also bind adhesion molecules that link cells to the extracellular matrix.

The ankyrins play an important role in integrating the actions of functionally related proteins in specific regions of the cell; for example, by colocalizing voltage-gated sodium channels, the sodium pump ATPase, and the sodium–calcium exchanger in a complex that coordinates sodium fluxes across the plasma membrane. Ankyrins also participate in excitation–contraction coupling by organizing the interactions between plasma membrane calcium channels ("dihydropyridine receptors") and intracellular calcium release channels in the sarcoplasmic reticulum ("ryanodine receptors") (see Chapter 7).

Ankyrins participate in cell signaling, and some contain a "death domain" that may play a role in apoptosis. Mutations in the ankyrin molecule cause a long QT syndrome and lethal arrhythmias that are probably caused by disruption of interactions between membrane proteins in the t-tubules (Mohler et al., 2003).

Spectrins, which link ankyrin to the actin microfilaments (Fig. 5-5), have many similarities to α-actinin. They function as heterodimers made up of two subunits (α and β) that contain an EF-hand calcium-binding domain and an amino acid sequence similar to that found in regulatory tyrosine kinases. It is not surprising, therefore, that spectrins participate in cell signaling.

CYTOSKELETAL PROTEINS THAT LINK CELLS TO EACH OTHER

The intercalated discs contain two structures that transmit tension developed by the contractile proteins from one cardiac myocyte to another (see Chapter 1); these are the *fascia adherens* (also called *adherens junctions* or *focal adhesions*) (Fig. 5-6a), which binds to cortical actin microfilaments that are connected to sarcomeric actin, and the *desmosomes* (Fig. 5-6b), which bind to intermediate filaments that are linked to desmin. Both the fascia adherens and desmosomes contain additional cytoskeletal proteins that, like those discussed above, participate in cell signaling as well as the transmission of tension.

In both the fascia adherens and desmosomes, cells are connected to one another by *cadherins* (Fig. 5-6). The cadherins in the fascia adherens bind to cortical actin microfilaments, while other members of the cadherin family, called *desmoglein* and *desmocollin*, link the intermediate (desmin) filaments to the desmosomes. Cadherin oligomers, which are held together by calcium-dependent linkages, bind to complexes made up of α, β, and γ *catenins* (the latter is also called *plakoglobin*), which function as anchoring proteins. The cadherin-containing complexes in the fascia adherens are linked to actin microfilaments by α-*actinin* and *vinculin*. Desmocollin in the desmosomes binds to catenin γ (plakoglobin) and desmoglein in a complex that, along with a cytosolic protein called *desmoplakin*, is linked to the intermediate filaments. The adhesion molecules in the fascia adherens and desmosomes, like other cytoskeletal proteins, participate in cell signaling, in many cases by activating protein kinases.

CYTOSKELETAL PROTEINS THAT LINK CELLS TO THE EXTRACELLULAR MATRIX

The structures described above, which link cardiac myocytes to one another, differ from those that link these cells to the extracellular matrix.

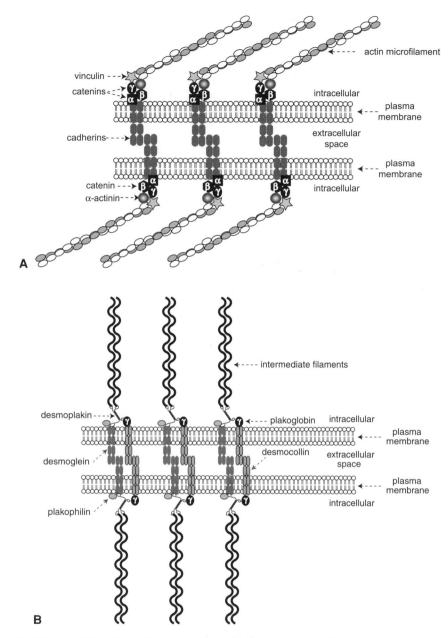

FIGURE 5-6 Structures in the intercalated disc that connect adjacent cardiac myocytes. **A:** In the fascia adherens, cadherins link actin microfilaments of adjacent cells through α, β, and γ catenins, α-actinin, and vinculin. **B:** The cadherins in the desmosomes, called *desmoglein* and *desmocollin*, are linked to intermediate microfilaments through a complex that includes plakoglobin (γ catenin), plakophilin, and desmoplakin.

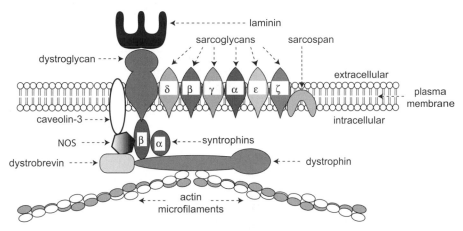

FIGURE 5-7 Major proteins of the dystrophin glycoprotein complex. Dystrophin links actin filaments to the plasma membrane through a protein complex that includes syntrophins α and β as well as dystrobrevin. The latter is bound to the plasma membrane by dystroglycan, six isoforms of sarcoglycan, and sarcospan. This complex links dystrophin to laminin in the extracellular matrix. These cytoskeletal proteins also participate in cell signaling by interacting with caveolin-3 and nitric oxide synthetase (NOS).

The latter include the dystrophin glycoprotein complex and integrins, both of which connect actin microfilaments to extracellular matrix proteins.

The Dystrophin Glycoprotein Complex

Cortical actin microfilaments are anchored to the plasma membrane by the dystrophin glycoprotein complex, which binds these intracellular filaments to the extracellular matrix (Fig. 5-7). The N-terminal region of *dystrophin* binds tightly to the actin microfilaments, while its C-terminal end is anchored to a membrane protein called *dystroglycan* that spans the plasma membrane. The extracellular domain of dystroglycan binds to several extracellular matrix proteins including *fibronectin* and *laminin*. Dystrophin and dystroglycan also bind to cytosolic proteins called *syntrophins*, which form a signaling complex that can interact with a number of intracellular signaling systems. *Dystrobrevin*, another cytosolic protein that interacts with dystrophin and dystroglycan, is a substrate for regulatory phosphorylations, contains an EF-hand (calcium-binding) domain, and regulates *nitric oxide synthetase* (*NOS*).

Dystroglycan binds to the plasma membrane through a family of membrane-spanning glycoproteins called *sarcoglycans*, whose six isoforms interact with the dystrophin glycoprotein complex (Fig. 5-7). Assembly of the sarcoglycans is regulated by *sarcospan*, another plasma membrane protein that, along with the syntrophins and dystrobrevin, links dystrophin to the plasma membrane.

The dystrophin glycoprotein complex participates in several signaling systems. Dystrobrevin, along with *caveolin-3*, regulates *nitric oxide synthetase* (*NOS*), which catalyzes nitric oxide production. Caveolin-3 is

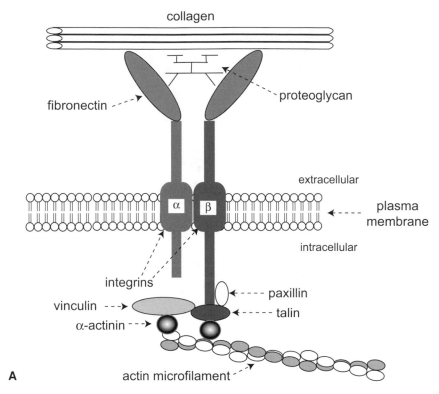

FIGURE 5-8 Integrins serve both a mechanical function that binds cells to the extracellular matrix and a signaling function that interacts with a number of intracellular signaling pathways. **A:** Integrins are heterodimers made up of α- and β-subunits, both of which can bind to fibronectin, laminin (*not shown*), proteoglycans, and other matrix proteins that link the integrins to collagen. Within the cell, the β-subunit binds to actin microfilaments through a protein complex that includes α-actin, talin, and vinculin; paxillin, which interacts with this complex, regulates cell adhesion. **B:** Integrin signaling occurs when the β subunit, in concert with talin and vinculin, activates a variety of signaling molecules including small G-proteins such a Rho, Rac, and Ras; focal adhesion–associated kinases (FAKs); and other protein kinases such as Akt, Raf, MEK, and ERK.

one family of proteins that forms mobile membrane microdomains that participate in solute uptake and integrates the activities of functionally related signaling molecules; caveolin-3 interactions with dystroglycan in the dystrophin glycoprotein complex play a role in signal transduction across the plasma membrane.

Mutations in the genes encoding several of the proteins of the dystrophin glycoprotein complex are found in patients with cardiomyopathies. Dystrophin mutations cause dilated cardiomyopathies by destabilizing cell-matrix linkages. Disruption of the linkages involving dystrophin also have been identified in other diseases that damage the heart, where they appear to exacerbate the progressive dilatation ("remodeling") commonly seen in heart failure. Mutations in dystroglycan can cause dilated cardiomyopathies as well, while a dystrobrevin mutation has been implicated in an

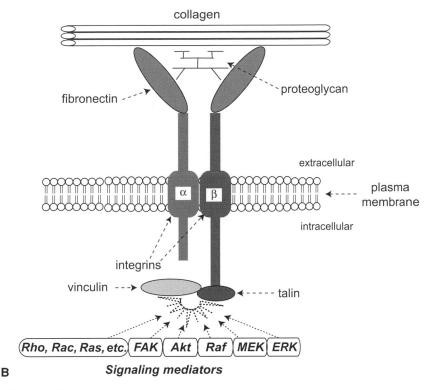

B   *Signaling mediators*

FIGURE 5-8 *(Continued)*

abnormality of the left ventricular wall, called *noncompaction*, that is associated with some forms of congenital heart disease.

Integrins

The *integrins* are members of another family of cell adhesion molecules that link cells to the extracellular matrix. These proteins form heterodimers made up of many different α- and β-subunits, whose properties determine the binding specificity and signaling effects of this cell adhesion molecule. Both the α- and β-subunits bind to extracellular matrix proteins, but only the β subunits are linked to the cytoskeleton. The intracellular domains of the β-subunits bind to actin microfilaments through adaptor protein complexes that include α-*actinin*, *vinculin*, and *talin*; *paxillin*, another intracellular protein that can bind to this complex, is a substrate for regulatory phosphorylations that influence cellular adhesion. Extracellular matrix proteins that bind to the integrins include *fibronectin*, *laminin*, and *vitronectin*, which along with *heparans* and other proteoglycans link the integrins to *collagen* (Fig. 5-8A).

In addition to their structural role, the integrins participate in a variety of signaling pathways that modify protein synthesis and cell growth in both cardiac myocytes and fibroblasts (Fig. 5-8B). Although these cell adhesion molecules lack enzymatic activity, they allow mechanical stresses to activate a number of signal transduction pathways by modifying the activity of small G-proteins like *Rho*, *Rac*, and *Ras*; *focal adhesion–associated kinases* (FAKs); and a variety of protein kinases including *Akt*, *Raf*, *MEK*, and *ERK* (see Chapter 9). These and other signaling molecules allow mechanical stresses to modify the interactions between integrins and the extracellular matrix that, by activating various signal transduction pathways, participate to the hypertrophic response of the heart to overload. The integrins also regulate the cell cycle and apoptosis, thereby allowing cell deformation to influence both cell growth and cell death.

Integrins play an important role in vascular endothelium. For example, the GPIIb/IIIa molecules that activate platelets are members of the integrin family. Other integrins participate in leukocyte migration and modify proliferative responses by the vascular endothelium.

Summary

The ability of cytoskeletal deformation to "sense" changes in the interactions among cardiac myocytes, and between cardiac myocytes and the surrounding extracellular matrix, helps to adapt cell size and shape to changing physical forces. One consequence of this local control of cell growth is the remarkable adaptation of form to function in the normal heart, whose structure allows its violent contractions to propel blood through the ventricles without causing turbulence; this explains why murmurs are not heard over the normal heart. Activation of proliferative responses by cytoskeletal deformation also contributes to the hypertrophic response in overloaded hearts and plays an important role in determining the different phenotypes of hypertrophy seen in heart disease (see Chapter 18).

BIBLIOGRAPHY

Aberle H, Schwartz H, Kemler R. Cadherin-catenin complex: protein interactions and their implications for cadherin function. *J Cell Biochem* 1996;61:514–523.

Assoian RK, Zhu X. Cell anchorage and the cytoskeleton as partners in growth factor dependent cell cycle progression. *Curr Opin Cell Biol* 1997;9:93–98.

Bennett V, Baines AJ. Spectrin and ankyrin-based pathways: metazoan inventions for integrating cells into tissues. *Physiol Rev* 2001;81:1353–1392.

Bennett V, Chen L. Ankyrins and cellular targeting of diverse membrane proteins to physiological sites. *Curr Opin Cell Biol* 2001;13:61–67.

Flashman E, Redwood C, Moolman-Smook J, et al. Cardiac myosin binding protein C. Its role in physiology and disease. *Circ Res* 2004;94:1279–1289.

Giancotti FG. Integrin signaling: specificity and control of cell survival and cell cycle progression. *Curr Opin Cell Biol* 1997;9:691–700.

Goldstein MA, Schroeter JP, Sass RL. Two structural states of the vertebrate Z band. *Electron Micros Rev* 1990;3:227–248.

Granzier HL, Labeit S. The giant protein titin. A major player in myocardial mechanics, signaling and disease. *Circ Res* 2004;94:284–295.

Gratton JP, Bernatchez P, Sessa WC. Caveolae and caveolins in the cardiovascular system. *Circ Res* 2004;94:1408–1417.

Gumbiner BM. Cell adhesion: the molecular basis of tissue architecture and morphogenesis. *Cell* 1996;84:345–357.

Heling A, Zimmermann R, Kostin S, et al. Increased expression of cytoskeletal, linkage, and extracellular proteins in failing human myocardium. *Circ Res* 2000;86:846–853.

Hillis GS, MacLeod AM. Integrins and disease. *Clin Sci* 1996;91:639–650.

Hsueh WA, Law RE, Do YS. Integrins, adhesion, and cardiac remodeling. *Hypertension* 1997;31:176–180.

Kontrogianni-Konstantopoulos A, Catino DH, Strong JC, et al. Obscurin regulates the organization of myosin into A bands. *Am J Physiol* 2004;287:C209–C217.

Kontrogianni-Konstantopoulos A, Jones EM, van Rossum DB, et al. Obscurin is a ligand for small ankyrin 1 in skeletal muscle. *Mol Biol Cell* 2003;14:1138–1148.

Lafrenie RM, Yamada KM. Integrin-dependent signal transduction. *J Cell Devel Biol* 1997;61:543–553.

Lapidos KA, Kakka R, McNally EM. The dystrophin glycoprotein complex signaling strength and integrity for the sarcolemma. *Circ Res* 2004;94:1023–1031.

Pyle WG, Solaro RJ. At the crossroads of myocardial signaling. The role of Z-discs in intracellular signaling and cardiac function. *Circ Res* 2004;94:296–305.

Ross RS, Borg TK. Integrins and the myocardium. *Circ Res* 2001;88:1112–1119.

Schlegel A, Volonte D, Engelman JA, et al. Crowded little caves: structure and function of caveolae. *Cell Signal* 1998;10:457–463.

South AP. Plakophilin1: an important stabilizer of desmosomes. *Clin Exper Dermatol* 2004; 29:161–167.

Steinberg SF. β2-Adrenergic receptor signaling complexes in cardiomyocyte caveoli/lipid rafts. *J Mol Cell Cardiol* 2004;37:407–415.

Thiery JP. The saga of adhesion molecules. *J Cell Biochem* 1996;61:489–492.

Winegrad S. Cardiac myosin binding protein C. *Circ Res* 1999;84:1117–1126.

Yap AS, Brieher WM, Gumbiner BM. Molecular and functional analysis of cadherin-based adherens junction. *Ann Rev Cell Dev Biol* 1997;13:119–146.

REFERENCES

Huxley HE, Hanson J. The molecular basis of contraction in cross-striated muscles. In: Bourne GH. *The structure and function of muscle.* Vol. 1: *Structure.* New York: Academic Press, 1960:183–227.

Mohler PJ, Schott JJ, Gramolini AO, et al. Ankyrin-B mutation causes type 4 long-QT cardiac arrhythmia and sudden cardiac death. *Nature* 2003;421:634–639.

6

ACTIVE STATE, LENGTH–TENSION RELATIONSHIP, AND CARDIAC MECHANICS

Tension development and shortening by the walls of the heart depend on the interactions between the contractile proteins (Chapter 4) and the viscoelastic properties of the cytoskeleton and matrix proteins (Chapter 5). The classical studies of these interactions were carried out in frog sartorius muscle, whose parallel fibers are ideal for analyses of muscle mechanics (see Chapter 3). Unlike this relatively simple skeletal muscle, the heart has a complex architecture in which the myocytes are branched and organized in spiral bundles (Chapter 1). An even more formidable obstacle to analyses of cardiac mechanics is the fact that the heart cannot normally be tetanized, which makes it impossible to evaluate mechanics at a steady state. Instead, these properties must be measured during the rise and fall of tension in each cardiac cycle, which creates serious problems in analyzing time-dependent and length-dependent changes in the interactions between the contractile proteins. These limitations notwithstanding, studies of the interplay between muscle chemistry and muscle energetics have provided valuable information describing the mechanics of cardiac muscle.

SERIES ELASTICITY

The importance of intrinsic elasticity in determining the rise and fall of tension in a contracting skeletal muscle twitch led early investigators to postulate that a springlike element, called the *series elasticity*, lies between the contractile element and the ends of the muscle (Fig. 6-1). When the sarcomeres shorten at the onset of a contraction, extension of the series elasticity absorbs some of the energy generated by the contractile proteins and delays the appearance of the tension developed by the contractile element at the ends of the muscle. Elongation of the series elasticity also contributes to a delay, called the *latent period*, between stimulation of a skeletal muscle and the first appearance of tension. An increase in muscle stiffness during the latent period indicates that actin and myosin begin to interact before tension appears at the ends of the muscle. The absorption of energy by elongation of the series elasticity has

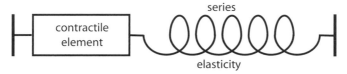

FIGURE 6-1 Simplified model of muscle showing contractile element in series with a springlike series elasticity.

important effects on the tension generated during a skeletal muscle twitch, where the contractile element is active for only a brief period of time.

TWITCH, SUMMATION, AND TETANIZATION

The response of a skeletal muscle to a single stimulus (S_1 in Fig. 6-2) is called a *twitch*. Because the skeletal muscle action potential is much briefer than the mechanical response, it is possible to restimulate the muscle before it begins to relax (Fig. 6-2); as a result, when a second stimulus is applied before relaxation is complete (S_2 in Fig. 6-2), a second contraction is superimposed on the first. The tension developed in the second contraction exceeds that developed during the twitch; this is called *summation* because the tension response to the second stimulus is added to that of the first.

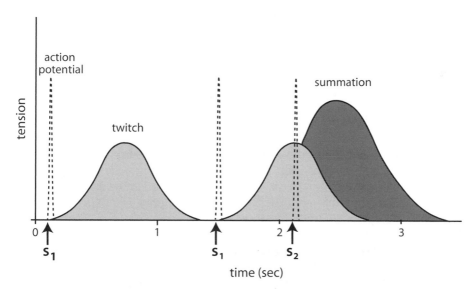

FIGURE 6-2 Twitch and summation in a skeletal muscle contracting under isometric conditions. **Left:** The contraction (*solid line*) that follows a single action potential (*dashed line*) produced by a single stimulus (S_1) is called a *twitch*. **Right:** Application of a second stimulus (S_2) during the falling phase of the twitch produces a second action potential that causes the renewed development of tension. Addition of the second tension response to the first is called *summation*.

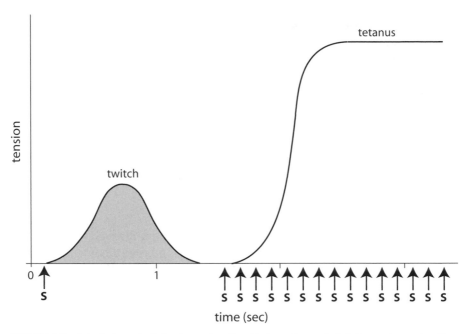

FIGURE 6-3 A twitch and a tetanic contraction (tetanus) in a skeletal muscle contracting under isometric conditions **Left:** Twitch, as shown in Figure 6-2. **Right:** Application of a train of stimuli (S) generates a series of responses that cause tension to rise to a much higher level than that developed during the twitch. Tension remains at this level until the train of stimuli is ended or the muscle fatigues.

Skeletal muscle can be stimulated so rapidly that each successive stimulus arrives before the muscle can begin to relax. Under these conditions, tension continues to rise until it reaches a new steady state (Fig. 6-3). The strong sustained contraction is called a *tetanus*, and the new level of tension is called *tetanic tension*. In a muscle contracting under isometric conditions, tetanic tension exceeds twitch tension approximately threefold and corresponds to P_0 of the force–velocity curve described in Chapter 3. The reason that twitch tension is less than that in a tetanus is that not all of the force developed by the sarcomeres can be transmitted to the ends of the muscle during the brief twitch because energy is absorbed by the stretched series elasticity (see below).

Tetanic contraction, tetanus, and tetany are not the same. Although the term *tetanus* is used to describe both a tetanic contraction and the disease caused by the endotoxin of the bacteria *Clostridium tetani*, the distinction is obvious. *Tetany*, which differs from both, is a hyperexcitable state that occurs when the threshold of the motor endplate to physical and chemical stimuli is lowered, which allows muscle contractions to appear in response to what are normally subthreshold stimuli. This pathological condition can be caused by systemic alkalosis or hypocalcemia.

The Series Elastic Element

The drawing in Figure 6-1 follows a custom that shows the *series elastic element* as distinct from the contractile element. This is largely correct in skeletal muscle, where a great deal of elasticity is in the tendinous ends of the muscle. An artifact arising from damaged regions adjacent to the clamps used to hold isolated muscles adds to this elasticity, as does asynchrony of contraction caused by incomplete or inhomogeneous stimulation. (Inhomogeneity of activation, described in Chapter 18, has recently emerged as an important cause of death and disability in patients with diseased hearts.) However, even when all of these elasticities are eliminated or compensated for, significant elasticity remains in the muscle cell itself. Much of the latter is attributable to elasticities in the cross-bridges and especially to titin and other cytoskeletal components.

ACTIVE STATE IN SKELETAL MUSCLE

The tension recorded at the ends of a muscle during a twitch is less than that generated by interactions between the myosin cross-bridges and actin because the series elasticity absorbs much of the mechanical energy released by the contractile proteins. One way to eliminate the influence of this elasticity is to apply a "quick stretch" or a "quick release" to the ends of the muscle. In a skeletal muscle twitch, these experiments reveal the surprisingly rapid development of an *active state* caused by actin–myosin interactions. Similar studies pertaining to cardiac muscle, however, yield results that are quite different from those in skeletal muscle (see below).

Quick-Stretch Experiments

One way to compensate for the absorption of mechanical energy by the series elasticity is to stretch the muscle early during a twitch. The key to understanding these quick-stretch experiments is to realize that the rapid increase in muscle length can equalize tension at three places: the ends of the muscle, within the contractile element, and across the series elasticity. When this occurs, the tension recorded at the ends of the muscle will be the same as the tension developed by the contractile element, which is, the active state.

The tension developed at the ends of a muscle that is stretched immediately after stimulation depends on how much it is stretched. This is depicted in Figure 6-4, which shows the tension recorded after a skeletal muscle is stretched to three different lengths. If the stretch "is" so small that the tension across the series elasticity is less than that developed by the contractile element, the muscle will continue to shorten and tension will rise because the contractile element remains able to shorten (curve 1 in Fig. 6-4). If, on the other hand, the muscle is stretched to a length so long that the tension across the muscle exceeds that developed by the contractile element, the muscle will lengthen and tension will decrease until it

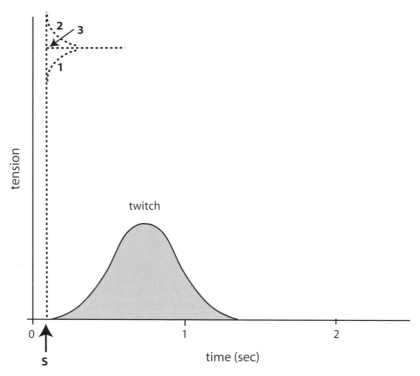

FIGURE 6-4 Measurement of the active state by application of quick stretches to a skeletal muscle contracting under isometric conditions. **Solid line:** Twitch, as shown in Figures 6-2 and 6-3. **Dashed lines:** (1) When the muscle is quickly stretched a relatively short distance immediately after stimulation, the tension at the end of the quick stretch is less than that produced by the contractile element; as a result, tension continues to increase. (2) When the muscle is quickly stretched a relatively long distance immediately after stimulation, the tension at the end of the quick stretch exceeds that developed by the contractile element; as a result, tension declines after the stretch. (3) When the muscle is quickly stretched to a length at which tension is the same as that developed by the contractile element (active state), tension remains at a plateau that equals the active state.

equals the tension developed by the contractile element (curve 2 in Fig. 6-4). If the quick stretch brings muscle tension to exactly the same level as that developed by the contractile element, the muscle will neither lengthen nor shorten; instead, tension will remain at a level equal to that of the contractile element (curve 3 in Fig. 6-4); this is the active state.

The time course of active state development can be estimated by applying a series of quick stretches at different times during tension development (Fig. 6-5). When such experiments are done with skeletal muscle, active state is found to develop very rapidly, reaching a brief plateau well before the time that twitch tension reaches its peak, after which the active state begins to decline before twitch tension reaches its maximum. Energy stored in the series elasticity is returned to the ends of the muscle during relaxation, which explains why muscle tension exceeds active state tension at the end of the twitch (Fig. 6-5, inset). Some of this energy can therefore be used to perform external work. This is especially important in the heart, where the balance between energy supply and energy demand is precarious even under normal conditions (see Chapter 2). One reason that lowering arterial blood pressure increases the efficiency of the left ventricle (see Chapter 12) is that reduction in wall tension allows more of this elastic energy to be used to pump blood.

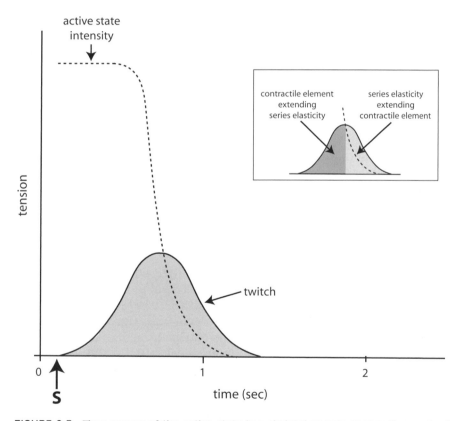

FIGURE 6-5   Time course of the active state in a skeletal muscle contracting under isometric conditions. The tension developed by the contractile element (active state), measured by a series of quick stretches, greatly exceeds the tension that appears at the ends of the muscle during the isometric twitch because energy is absorbed by the series elasticity. Storage of energy in the series elasticity explains why, at the end of the twitch, muscle tension exceeds the active state; this is shown in the inset, where the more darkly shaded area indicates where the active state exceeds the tension on the series elasticity, and the lightly shaded region shows when the tension on the series elasticity is greater than that developed by the contractile element.

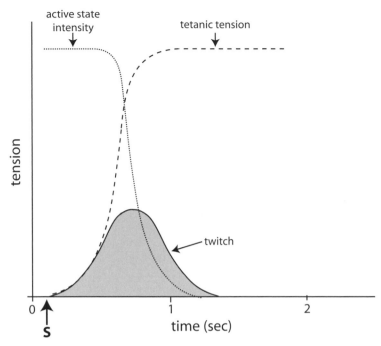

FIGURE 6-6 Relation of tetanic tension (*dashed line*) to active state intensity (*dotted line*). By maintaining the contractile element in a constant state of activity, repeated stimulation allows the full intensity of the active state to appear at the ends of the muscle in a tetanic contraction.

The differences between maximal twitch tension and that of the active state are due to the damping effect of the series elasticity, which also explains why more tension is developed during a tetanus than during a twitch. Maximum active state intensity in a skeletal muscle is the same as the tension developed during a tetanus (Fig. 6-6), in which repeated stimulation prevents the active state from declining. The tetanic tension recorded at the ends of the muscle, which equals the active state, therefore provides a measurement of the tension developed by the contractile element.

Quick-Release Experiments

We have already seen that the ability of a muscle to develop tension and to shorten reflect two different properties of the contractile process (Chapter 3). One is the *number* of rigor bonds, which determines the active state, and P_0, the maximum tension that the muscle is able to generate. Quick stretches, however, cannot measure the other property of the contracting muscle, which is the velocity of contractile element shortening (V_{max}). To evaluate the latter, an index of the rate of cross-bridge turnover, the contracting muscle can be subjected to "quick releases."

When a skeletal muscle that has been tetanized under isometric conditions is suddenly presented with a series of new, reduced loads, the shortening which follows the abrupt fall in tension occurs in two phases (Fig. 6-7). The first is a very rapid decrease in length that is caused by shortening of the series elasticity (*dashed line* in Fig. 6-7). The velocity of

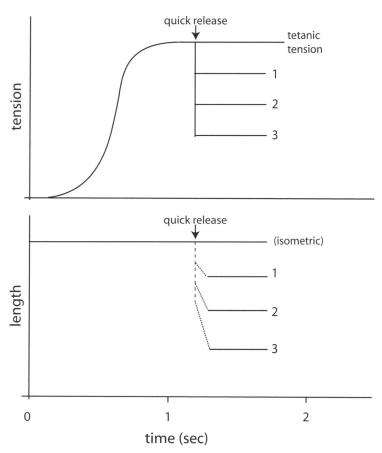

FIGURE 6-7 Quick releases to different loads in a tetanized skeletal muscle contracting under isometric conditions. **Top:** The tension developed during the tetanic contraction falls abruptly when the muscle is quickly released to a slightly reduced load (1), to a moderately reduced load (2), and to a markedly reduced load (3). **Bottom:** The quick releases allow the muscle to shorten to new lengths that are inversely proportional to the amount of the load. The initial, rapid length changes (*dashed line*) are due to shortening of the series elasticity, while the slower rates of shortening (*dotted lines*) represent the shortening velocities of the contractile element at each new load. The velocity of the second phase of shortening increases when the muscle is presented with progressively lighter loads.

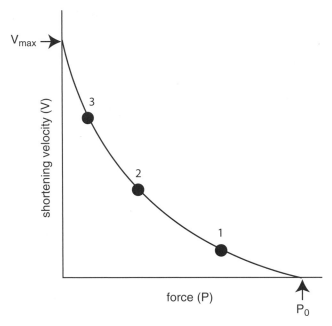

FIGURE 6-8 Force–velocity curve constructed from the quick-release experiment shown in Figure 6-7. The forces recorded by points 1, 2, and 3 are the tensions achieved after the quick releases to the new lengths in the upper part of Figure 6-7, while the shortening velocities are the rates of the length change shown by the dotted lines in the lower part of Figure 6-7. This hyperbolic curve is similar to that shown in Figure 3-15.

the second, slower phase of shortening (*dotted lines* in Fig. 6-7) increases when the quick releases are made to progressively lighter loads (1, 2, and 3 in Fig. 6-7, going from heaviest to lightest). Plots of the load dependence of the shortening velocities in this second phase yield hyperbolic curves (Fig. 6-8) that are similar to the force–velocity relationship described in Chapter 3 (Fig. 3-15). Quick-release experiments in skeletal muscle therefore provide measurements of V_{max}, an index of the rate of cross-bridge cycle, as well as P_0, an index of the number of active force-generating sites. In cardiac muscle, however, the results of quick-release experiments are quite different from those shown in Figure 6-7.

THE LENGTH–TENSION RELATIONSHIP

A major determinant of the ability of a skeletal or cardiac muscle to develop tension is its resting length. Curves describing this *length–tension relationship* (Fig. 6-9) are customarily scanned from left to right, so the increase in developed tension that occurs when a muscle is stretched at shorter sarcomere lengths is called the *ascending limb*, while the decline of tension when the muscle is stretched at high sarcomere lengths is called the *descending limb*. The tension developed during tetanic contractions,

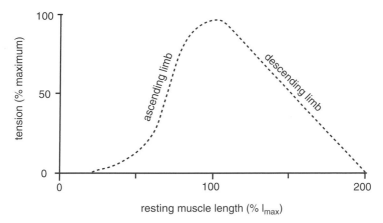

FIGURE 6-9 Length–tension curve for tetanic contractions by a skeletal muscle contracting under isometric conditions. Resting length is expressed as percent of l_{max}, the
length at which developed tension is maximal. Curves of this sort are conventionally
scanned from left to right; as such, the ascending limb is to the left, where tension rises
with increasing muscle length, and the descending limb is to the right, where tension
decreases with increasing muscle length.

which in a skeletal muscle measures the intensity of the active state, is
maximal at intermediate muscle lengths (l_{max} or l_0).

Unlike most skeletal muscles, where resting length is determined by
the angles between the bones to which the muscle is attached, resting
length in the heart is proportional to the volume of blood contained in its
cavities. Because the extent of ejection is a major determinant of cavity
volume at the start of the next cardiac cycle, reducing the amount of blood
ejected increases resting length for the next beat.

Shortly after the sliding filament hypothesis of muscular contraction
became widely accepted, attempts were made to explain the length–tension
relationship in terms of the number of myosin cross-bridges on the thick
filaments that could interact with actin on the thin filaments (Gordon
et al., 1966). Although, this *ultrastructural mechanism* can explain the
descending limb, there is still no universally accepted explanation for the
ascending limb.

Ultrastructural Mechanism

The key to understanding the length–tension relationship in skeletal
muscle was provided by measurements of length–tension curves generated
by a single sarcomere (Fig. 6-10); these curves are narrower than those in
the whole muscle because of damage to the ends of the muscle that were
attached to the recording device and inhomogeneities within the muscle.
These "sarcomere length–tension relationships" are not only narrower, but
demonstrate sharp changes in tension not seen in studies of whole muscles (B and C in Fig. 6-10).

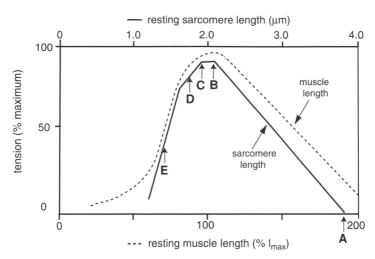

FIGURE 6-10   Length–tension curve for a single sarcomere in a frog semitendinosus muscle (*solid line*) compared with that for the whole muscle shown in Figure 6-9 (*dashed line*). Sarcomere length is shown as the upper abscissa; muscle length is below. At a sarcomere length of about 3.65 μm (A), no tension is developed. Developed tension increases to a maximum as the sarcomere shortens to around 2.2 μm (A $\rightarrow$ B), but as sarcomere length decreases to nearly 2.0 μm (B $\rightarrow$ C), tension remains constant. As sarcomere length decreases below about 2.0 μm, tension decreases (C $\rightarrow$ D). At sarcomere lengths below approximately 1.65 μm (D $\rightarrow$ E), tension declines rapidly, and contraction bands appear.

In examining the sarcomere length–tension curve, it is simplest to begin at the right, at the end of the descending limb where developed tension is zero (A, Fig. 6-10). At this point, where sarcomere length is approximately 3.65 μm, there is no overlap between the thick filaments (whose length is about 1.65 μm) and the two thin filaments (whose combined length is about 2.0 μm) (Fig. 6-11). Because there is no overlap, no myosin cross-bridges are able to interact with actin, and no tension can be developed.

When sarcomere length is reduced (A $\rightarrow$ B, Fig. 6-10), tension increases, reaching a maximum at about 2.2 μm (B, Fig. 6-10). At this sarcomere length, which corresponds to l_{max} (see above), all of the myosin cross-bridges in the two halves of the sarcomere are adjacent to one of the thin filaments (Fig. 6-12). A small, nearly 0.2 μm gap that remains between the ends of the thin filaments corresponds to the bare area in the center of the thick filament that is devoid of cross-bridges (see Chapter 4; Fig. 4-3).

Further reduction in sarcomere length, from about 2.2 μm to 2.0 μm (B $\rightarrow$ C, Fig. 6-10), does not change active tension because changing sarcomere length neither increases nor decreases the number of potential interactions between the thick and thin filaments. This is because as the thin filaments lose potential interactions with cross-bridges when they

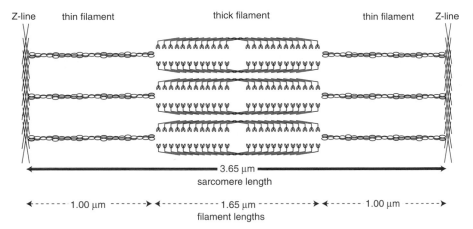

Z-line   thin filament   thick filament   thin filament   Z-line

3.65 μm
sarcomere length

◄------ 1.00 μm ------► ◄----------- 1.65 μm -----------► ◄------ 1.00 μm ------►
filament lengths

FIGURE 6-11 At a sarcomere length of about 3.65 μm (A, Figure 6-10), there is no over-lap between the thick and thin filaments, so no interactions are possible between the myosin cross-bridges and actin. The lengths of the thick and thin filaments are shown below (*dashed arrows*).

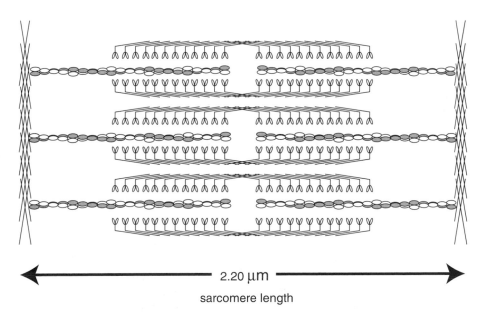

2.20 μm
sarcomere length

FIGURE 6-12 At a sarcomere length of about 2.2 μm (B, Figure 6-10), all myosin cross-bridges are adjacent to the thin filaments, so the number of potential interactions between the contractile proteins is maximal.

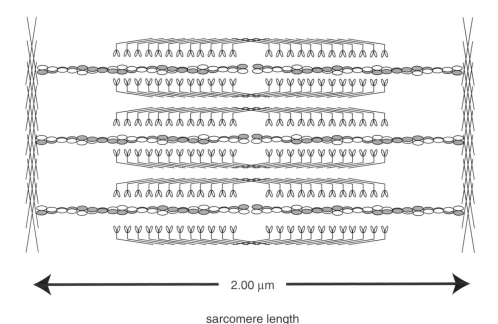

2.00 μm

sarcomere length

FIGURE 6-13   Between sarcomere lengths of approximately 2.2 μm and 2.0 μm (C, Figure 6-10), the potential cross-bridge interactions lost at the ends of the thin filaments in the center of the sarcomere are matched by a gain at the ends of the thick filaments; as a result, all myosin cross-bridges remain able to interact with the thin filaments.

enter the bare area in the center of the sarcomere, new potential interactions with cross-bridges are gained at the ends of the thick filament (Fig. 6-13).

The fall in tension at sarcomere lengths below 2.0 μm (C → D, Fig. 6-11) cannot be explained by a change in the number of potential interactions between the thick and thin filaments because, as is true for sarcomere length changes between from about 2.2 μm to 2.0 μm, potential interactions lost in the center of the thick filament are matched by gains at its ends. The fall in tension with decreasing sarcomere length was initially attributed to mechanical interference between the thin filaments in the region of "double overlap" (Fig. 6-14). This seemed logical because the thin filaments from the opposite halves of the sarcomere have crossed into the domains of the "wrong" halves of the thick filament, where the polarities of the cross-bridges and actin do not allow interactions between adjacent thick and thin filaments (see Chapter 4). It now appears, however, that neither mismatched polarities nor mechanical interferences in the region of double overlap explain the fall in tension when sarcomere length is decreased below l_{max}. Instead, changes in tension developed along the ascending limb are probably due to other length-dependent factors that influence the interactions between the contractile proteins (see below).

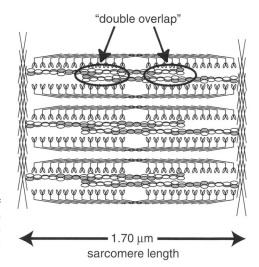

"double overlap"

1.70 μm
sarcomere length

FIGURE 6-14 At a sarcomere length of around 1.7 μm (C → D, Figure 6-10), the central ends of the thin filaments have crossed in the middle of the sarcomere ("double overlap").

The steep decline in tension as muscle length decreases at very short sarcomere lengths, below 1.65 μm (D → E, Fig. 6-10), is caused by "collisions" between the Z-lines and the ends of the thick filaments. The latter, whose length is about 1.65 μm, begin to "crumple" when they impinge on the Z-lines, which causes *contraction bands* to appear (Fig. 6-15). The latter are seen when the heart is severely calcium-overloaded, where the active state can become so intense as to tear the myocytes apart. This phenomenon can occur when the heart is reperfused following prolonged ischemia, where plasma membrane damage allows large amounts of calcium to enter the cytosol, causing "contraction band necrosis" (see Chapter 17).

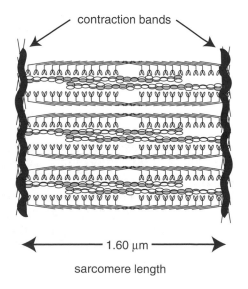

contraction bands

1.60 μm
sarcomere length

FIGURE 6-15 At a sarcomere length less than 1.65 μm (D → E, Figure 6-10), the Z-lines "collide" with the ends of thick filaments, causing the latter to "crumple" (thick, wavy lines), which gives rise to contraction bands at the periphery of the A-band. Interactions between the thick filaments and the Z-lines explain the precipitous fall of tension as the sarcomere shortens further on this nonphysiological portion of the sarcomere length–tension curve.

Length-Dependent Variations in Excitation–Contraction Coupling

The mechanism(s) responsible for the ascending limb of the length–tension curve in the heart remains controversial. Suggested explanations include changes in the lateral distances between thick and thin filaments caused by altered lattice-spacing of the myofilaments (Fuchs and Wang, 1995; Konhilas, 2002), and length-dependent changes in calcium release from the sarcoplasmic reticulum (Fabiato and Fabiato, 1975) and the calcium-sensitivity of the contractile proteins (Hibberd and Jewell, 1982). Length-dependent changes in the cardiac action potential do not appear to represent a likely mechanism (Hennekes et al., 1981). It also has been suggested that the radial force exerted by titin decreases when sarcomere length is increased on the ascending limb of the length–tension relationship (Carzola et al., 1999). Unfortunately, a consensus has not been reached regarding the mechanism that underlies this classical relationship.

DIASTOLIC PROPERTIES OF THE MYOCARDIUM

The heart has a low resting compliance, or high stiffness (Table 6-1); therefore, its resting length–tension curve is very steep (Fig. 6-16). [These and other terms used to describe the passive properties of the heart are reviewed by Mirsky and Parmley (1973).] This low diastolic compliance distinguishes the heart from skeletal muscle, where resting tension is nearly zero at l_{max}, although the relationships between sarcomere length and active tension are similar in skeletal and cardiac muscle. The high

TABLE 6-1 Terms Used to Describe the Passive Properties of the Myocardium

Tension: Force along a line
Stress: Force per unit of cross-sectional area; for example, dynes/cm^2
Strain: Deformation of a material; for example, the fractional, or percent, change in dimension caused by the application of stress
Compliance or distensibility: The change in volume of a hollow structure that accompanies a change in pressure: dV/dP or (dP/dV)$^{-1}$.
Stiffness: Often equated to the change in pressure that accompanies a change in volume: dP/dV or (dV/dP)$^{-1}$—the reciprocal of compliance
Elasticity: A property defining the recovery of a material from a stressed state to its original conformation when the stress is removed
Elastic stiffness: The slope of a stress–strain curve—for instance, the amount of stress needed to cause a given strain; in nonphysical terms, this can be viewed simply as *stiffness*, the tendency of the myocardium to resist stretching (a strain) in response to an increase in tension (a stress)

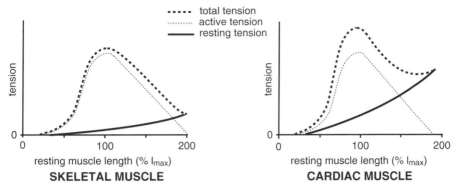

FIGURE 6-16 Isometric length–tension curves in skeletal and cardiac muscle. Active tension (*dotted line*), which is the tension developed during contraction, equals total tension after stimulation (*dashed line*) minus the tension in the resting muscle prior to stimulation (*solid line*). Although the active length–tension curves are similar for the two muscle types, the resting tension in cardiac muscle is much higher and, unlike skeletal muscle, is significant at lengths below l_{max}.

resting tension in the heart helps to prevent the ventricles from moving onto the descending limb of their length–tension curves, which can establish a dangerous vicious cycle (see below).

The exact cause of the high diastolic stiffness of cardiac muscle is not fully understood. Some of the heart's resistance to stretch can be attributed to the extracellular matrix, notably collagen (Weber, 1989). Recent evidence also implicates the cytoskeletal proteins, notably titin, as a major cause of the high diastolic stiffness of the myocardium (see Chapter 5). Spontaneous oscillations in sarcomere length caused by cyclic release and reuptake of calcium by the sarcoplasmic reticulum represent a dynamic mechanism for the low compliance of the myocardium (Lakatta et al., 1985), as do residual interactions between the thick and thin filaments during diastole; the latter, which are exacerbated by calcium overload, can represent an important cause of increased diastolic stiffness in energy-starved hearts.

The importance of the high resting stiffness of the myocardium lies in its ability to minimize chamber dilatation, which by increasing wall stress is energetically costly ("The Law of Laplace," see Chapter 11). More important is the requirement that the heart *must* respond to an increase in filling with a greater ability to eject (Chapter 10). This is because a ventricle can function at a steady state only on the ascending limb of its length–tension curve (Katz, 1965). Were the ventricle to operate on the descending limb, an increase in venous return would reduce ejection, increasing the "residual" volume remaining in the ventricle at the end of systole. The resulting increase in cavity volume would reduce ejection further, thereby establishing a vicious cycle that is probably an important cause of acute pulmonary edema (see Chapter 18). The likelihood of this potentially fatal catastrophe is reduced by the low compliance of the myocardium, which makes it difficult—and normally impossible—to stretch the heart's sarcomeres onto the descending limb of their length–tension curves.

ACTIVE STATE IN THE HEART: CARDIAC MECHANICS

Efforts to quantify myocardial function in the late 1960s were stimulated when advances in cardiac surgery made it clear that prolonged hemodynamic overloading could irreversibly damage the myocardium. It was quickly recognized that measuring hemodynamic variables, such as cardiac output and atrial pressures, cannot define the contractile state of the myocardium. This is especially true in patients with damaged cardiac valves, where hemodynamic abnormalities are determined by the severity of the valve abnormality as well as by the state of the heart muscle. Equally difficult was the challenge of distinguishing between impaired pump function caused by abnormal contractile properties and abnormalities caused by altered sarcomere length (length–tension relationship). These considerations stimulated the emergence of a new field, called *cardiac mechanics*, which was based on the work in isolated skeletal muscle described in Chapter 3. It was hoped that estimates of such variables as P_0 and V_{max} would allow cardiologists to select the optimal time for palliative procedures like valve replacement before myocardial deterioration passed a "point of no return," but not so early as to expose patients prematurely to the complications of prosthetic valves.

Initial studies of cardiac mechanics also offered promise that the intrinsic contractile properties of the heart, called *myocardial contractility* (see Chapter 10), could be quantified. This approach was based on studies of frog sartorius muscle, where fibers are parallel to each other, and the active state is rapid in onset and can be stabilized in tetanic contractions; studies of mechanics using these muscles provided an excellent way to quantify energetics and contractile performance. However, it soon became clear that the relatively straightforward time-dependent and length-dependent features of skeletal muscle mechanics described in Chapter 3 are not seen in the heart. One reason is the slow onset of the active state in cardiac muscle, which cannot ordinarily be tetanized, making it impossible to achieve the steady state needed to study cardiac mechanics. Another problem is created by the spiral arrangement of the heart's muscle bundles (see Chapter 1), which adds to the elasticities in the walls of the heart that permit sarcomeres to shorten even when ventricular volume remains constant. The inability of skeletal muscle mechanics to describe the contractile performance of the heart became especially clear when the results of quick-stretch and quick-release studies in cardiac muscle were compared with those in skeletal muscle. These studies revealed an entirely unexpected type of regulation that helps to maintain homogeneity of tension development in the walls of the heart.

Quick Stretch in Cardiac Muscle

Unlike quick-stretch experiments in skeletal muscle, which demonstrate that active state tension rapidly reaches a steady state following stimulation (Fig. 6-4), tension does not reach a plateau after a quick stretch in cardiac muscle (Fig. 6-17). A quick stretch that initially exceeds the ability of cardiac muscle to hold tension, as evidenced by a fall in tension immediately after the stretch, is followed by a slow rise in tension that initially follows a time course similar to tension development by the unstretched muscle (A in Fig. 6-17). Increasing the quick stretch to a longer length causes an even greater initial drop in tension before a similar slow rise in tension (B in Fig. 6-17).

Even more striking differences between cardiac and skeletal muscle are seen when quick stretches and quick releases are applied at different times during tension development. In cardiac muscle, the increase in tension after a quick stretch does not reach a plateau (see Fig. 6-4) but instead follows a time course that is virtually independent of the time when stretch is applied (A and B in Fig. 6-18). In fact, the increase in tension after cardiac muscle is stretched *during* the period of tension development is the same as that seen when the muscle is stretched to the same new length *before* stimulation (X in Fig. 6-18). This means that the increased tension developed after a quick stretch in cardiac muscle (Figs. 6-17 and 6-18) is

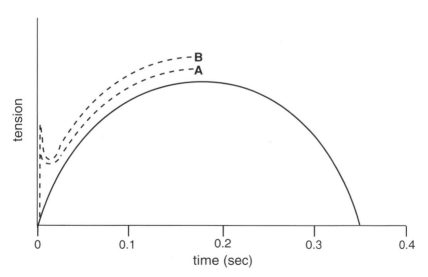

FIGURE 6-17 Results of a quick-stretch experiment in cardiac muscle. Tension developed during isometric contraction (*solid line*). Tension developed after quick stretches to two different lengths (B is stretched to a longer length than A) (*dashed lines*). Even though the quick stretches cause the muscle to reach a length that causes total tension to exceed that developed by the contractile element—as evidenced by a transient fall in tension—total tension resumes its rise. Unlike the analogous experiment in skeletal muscle (Fig. 6-4), no plateau of tension is seen.

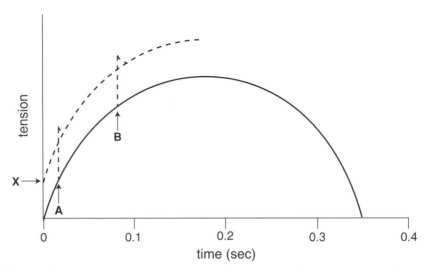

FIGURE 6-18   Results of a quick-stretch experiment in cardiac muscle where the same stretch is applied at two times after stimulation (A and B). Although the tension developed after each stretch initially exceeds that developed by the contractile element—as evidenced by a transient fall in tension—total tension resumes its rise so that both curves become superimposed as tension approaches its peak. The increment in tension following the stretches is the same when the muscle is stretched to the same length prior to stimulation (X).

simply a manifestation of the length–tension relationship caused by increased sarcomere length!

These experiments show that unlike skeletal muscle, where active state develops rapidly and is sustained, the active state in cardiac muscle is slow in onset. The increase in tension following quick stretches in cardiac muscle (Figs. 6-17 and 6-18) therefore is simply due to the effects of the new, longer length on the length–tension relationship.

Effects of Changing Muscle Length on Active State in Cardiac Muscle

Analysis of quick stretches and quick releases applied at different times after the onset of contractions in heart muscle have proved especially surprising because changes in muscle length have major effects on the time course of subsequent tension development (Brutsaert and Sys, 1989).

The immediate effect of stretching the heart early during contraction, as noted above (Figs. 6-17 and 6-18), is to increase tension by pulling the sarcomeres to a longer length along the ascending limb of the length–tension curve. If, however, the time course of tension is followed for a longer time, stretch is seen also to prolong contraction (A in Fig. 6-19). Conversely, unloading the heart during shortening has the opposite effect—to abbreviate the contraction (B and C in Fig. 6-19). The earlier during the

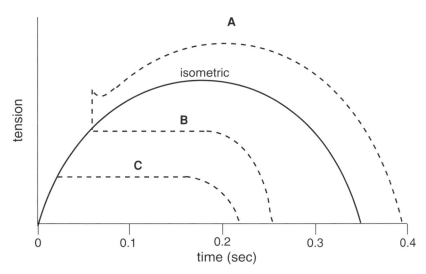

FIGURE 6-19 Effects of length changes in cardiac muscle on the subsequent development of tension. When an isometrically contracting muscle (*solid line*) is stretched early during systole, tension is increased, and systole is prolonged (A). Releasing the muscle to lower tensions not only allows the muscle to shorten (B and C), but also shortens the duration of the contraction. The earlier the tension on the muscle is reduced, the greater the abbreviation of systole.

contraction that the muscle is allowed to shorten, the greater is the abbreviation of systole (compare B and C in Fig. 6-19).

These effects of changing length during systole are very important in the heart, in which branched myocytes of different dimensions are connected in series (see Chapter 1). This architecture makes it difficult to achieve the homogeneous tension within the walls of the heart that is needed to maximize efficiency (Katz and Katz, 1989). Energy would be wasted (as heat) if two myocytes of unequal strength were linked in series because the stronger myocyte would stretch the weaker myocyte (B in Fig. 6-20). However, cardiac muscle has a remarkable ability to reduce these inequalities because when a stronger myocyte stretches a weaker myocyte, contraction of the latter is not only stronger, but also is prolonged (A in Fig. 6-19). At the same time, shortening of the stronger myocyte reduces both the tension that it develops and the duration of its contraction (B and C in Fig. 6-19), both of which lessen the extent to which it can stretch the weaker myocyte. The considerations apply not only when myocytes linked in series have different abilities to develop tension, but also when they are not activated simultaneously. In the latter situation, shortening would weaken the contraction of the myocyte that is activated earliest (which, like the stronger myocyte, would shorten more) and strengthen the contraction of the myocyte that is activated later (which, like the weaker myocyte, would be stretched).

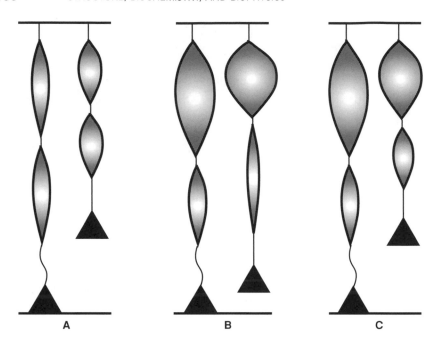

A   B   C

FIGURE 6-20 Drawings showing the shortening of two muscles that are connected in series. The situation at rest is at the left of each drawing, that after contraction has lifted the load (solid triangles) is at the right. **A:** When the two muscles are identical and develop the same tension, both shorten to the same extent. **B:** If the upper muscle is stronger than the lower, when the two muscles lift a load, the greater extent of shortening by the stronger muscle would stretch the weaker muscle. **C:** The same pair of muscles shown in **(B)**, except that, as occurs in cardiac muscle, shortening weakens contraction and stretch causes the contraction to become stronger. Together, these responses reduce shortening by the stronger muscle and increase shortening by the weaker muscle, which tends to equalize the shortening of the two mismatched muscles.

These remarkable mechanisms operate to equalize the tension developed by the millions of myocytes in the walls of the intact heart. It is striking that nature developed these adaptive mechanisms long before the human intellect realized the serious problem caused by heterogeneity of contraction, and human ingenuity made it possible to develop "cardiac resynchronization therapy," which uses electrical stimulation to accomplish the same effect—to maintain homogeneity of contraction in the walls of the heart (see Chapter 18).

BIBLIOGRAPHY

Brady AJ. Time and displacement dependence of cardiac contractility: problems in defining the active state and force velocity relations. *Fed Proc* 1965;24:1410–1420.

Brady AJ. Mechanical properties of isolated cardiac myocytes. *Physiol Rev* 1991;71:413–428.

Lakatta EG. Starling's Law of the Heart is explained by intimate interaction of muscle length and myofilament calcium activation. *J Am Coll Cardiol* 1987;10:1157–1164.

Moss RL, Fitzsimons DP. Frank–Starling relationship. Long on importance, short on mechanism. *Circ Res* 2002;90:11–13.

REFERENCES

Brutsaert DL, Sys SU. Relaxation and diastole of the heart. *Physiol Rev* 1989;69:1228–1315.

Carzola O, Vassort G, Granzier D. Length modulation of active force in rat cardiac myocytes: is titin the sensor? *Circ Res* 1999;2001:1028–1035.

Fabiato A, Fabiato F. Dependence of the contractile activation of skinned cardiac cells on the sarcomere length. *Nature* 1975;256:54–56.

Fuchs F, Wang YP. Sarcomere length versus interfilament spacing as determinant of cardiac myofilament Ca^{2+} sensitivity and Ca^{2+} binding. *J Mol Cell Cardiol* 1995;28:1375–1383.

Gordon AM, Huxley AF, Julian FG. The variation in isometric tension with sarcomere length in vertebrate muscle fibers. *J Physiol (Lond)* 1966;184:170–192

Hennekes R, Kaufmann R, Lab M. The dependence of cardiac membrane excitation and contractile ability on active muscle shortening (cat papillary muscle). *Pflüger's Archiv* 1981;392:22–28.

Hibberd MG, Jewell BR. Calcium- and length-dependent force production in rat ventricular muscle. *J Physiol (Lond)* 1982;329:527–540.

Katz AM. The descending limb of the Starling Curve and the failing heart. *Circulation* 1965;32:871–875.

Katz AM, Katz PB. Homogeneity out of heterogeneity. *Circulation* 1989;79:712–717.

Konhilas JP, Irving TC, de Tombe PP. Myofilament calcium sensitivity in skinned rat trabecula: role of interfilament spacing. *Circ Res* 2002;90:59–65.

Lakatta EG, Capogrossi MC, Kort AA, et al. Spontaneous myocardial Ca oscillations: an overview with emphasis on ryanodine and caffeine. *Fed Proc* 1985;44:2977–2983.

Mirsky I, Parmley WW. Assessment of passive elastic stiffness for isolated heart muscle and the intact heart. *Circ Res* 1973;33:233–243.

Weber KT. Cardiac interstitium in health and disease: the fibrillar collagen network. *J Am Coll Cardiol* 1989;13:1637–1652.

7

EXCITATION–CONTRACTION COUPLING: EXTRACELLULAR AND INTRACELLULAR CALCIUM CYCLES

It is quite . . . impossible to explain the rapid development of full activity in a [skeletal muscle] twitch by assuming that it is set up by the arrival at any point of some substance diffusing from the surface: diffusion is far too slow. Either we must suppose that [the muscle is stimulated by] excitation (natural or artificial) throughout the interior, not merely at the surface: or we must look for some physical or physico-chemical process which is released by excitation at the surface and then propagated inwards.

A. V. Hill, 1949

Hill's observation that diffusion is too slow to allow a substance entering a muscle from the cell surface to activate the contractile machinery (see above) provided the key to understanding *excitation–contraction coupling*, which describes how plasma membrane depolarization initiates contraction. Along with changing rest length (see Chapter 6), this process called *excitation–contraction coupling* provides the basis for understanding myocardial contractility and its regulation.

DIFFUSION

To appreciate how calcium is delivered to its binding site on troponin C to activate cardiac contraction (see Chapter 4), it is useful to compare the myocytes of primitive and embryonic hearts with those of the adult heart. The latter, which are larger and contain more myofilaments, develop higher tension and contract more rapidly (Fig. 7-1). Hill (1949), writing before calcium was discovered to activate the contractile proteins, noted that diffusion of an activator from the cell surface is too slow to account for the rapid onset of the active state in the large, rapidly contracting cells of the frog sartorius muscle; this led him to predict that activation must depend either on a process that is more rapid than

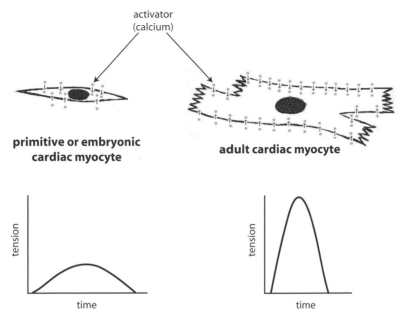

FIGURE 7-1 Primitive and embryonic cardiac myocytes (*left*) are smaller and contain fewer myofilaments than adult myocytes (*right*). Calcium influx from the extracellular space can deliver enough of this activator to explain the more slowly developing, weaker contractions of these primitive myocytes, whereas diffusion of calcium across the plasma membrane from the extracellular space is too slow to activate the more rapidly developing, stronger contractions of adult cardiac myocytes.

diffusion, or that a diffusible activator is released within the myocytes. We now know that excitation–contraction coupling involves *both* of these mechanisms.

Excitation–contraction coupling in the adult mammalian heart depends on interactions between two membrane systems that together overcome the limitations caused by the slowness of diffusion. The first is the *transverse tubular system* (*t-system* or *t-tubules*), which is made up of plasma membrane extensions that propagate action potentials to the interior of the myocytes. The second, called the *sarcoplasmic reticulum*, is a specialized region of the endoplasmic reticulum found within eukaryotic cells (Fig. 7-2). In small, slowly contracting primitive embryonic myocytes, which lack these specialized membranes, excitation–contraction coupling can be effected by an *extracellular calcium cycle* in which activator calcium derived from the extracellular fluid enters and leaves the cytosol across the plasma membrane. The larger, more rapidly contracting myocytes of the adult mammalian heart, on the other hand, utilize an *intracellular calcium cycle* in which action potentials transmitted down the t-tubules trigger the release of activator calcium from stores within the sarcoplasmic reticulum.

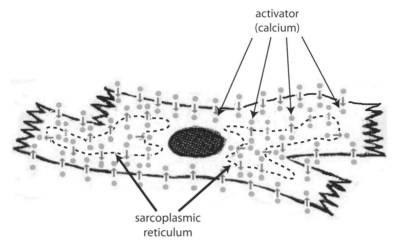

FIGURE-7-2   The solution to the problem caused by slow diffusion of activator from the extracellular space into the cytosol lies in an intracellular calcium store within the membranes of the sarcoplasmic reticulum.

ROLES OF THE SARCOPLASMIC RETICULUM AND TRANSVERSE TUBULAR SYSTEM

The first part of the question raised by Hill, how plasma membrane depolarization can activate the contractile machinery with sufficient rapidity to explain the large contractions of skeletal muscle, was answered in the early 1960s. At that time, sarcoplasmic reticulum (also called the *sarcoendoplasmic reticulum* or SERCA) (Fig. 7-3) was discovered to store calcium within muscle cells. Calcium release from these internal stores means that this activator does not have diffuse to the contractile proteins from the cell surface.

The discovery of the sarcoplasmic reticulum has an interesting history. In the 1950s, it was found that supernatants obtained after low-speed centrifugation of muscle minces relaxed actomyosins *in vitro* (see Chapter 4). This relaxing effect, which required the presence of ATP and could be abolished by calcium, was initially believed to be caused by a "soluble relaxing factor" (Gergely, 1959). However, Hasselbach and Makinose (1961) and Ebashi and Lipmann (1962) found independently that the relaxing effect of these supernatant fractions depends on tiny membrane vesicles (called *microsomes*), derived from the sarcoplasmic reticulum, that use energy from ATP to pump calcium into their interior. The concurrent discovery that actin–myosin interactions are activated under physiological conditions by micromolar ionized calcium concentrations (Weber and Winicur, 1961) made it clear that muscle relaxation is not caused by a soluble factor, but instead occurs when calcium is taken up by the sarcoplasmic reticulum. Within a few years, it was possible to show that the cardiac sarcoplasmic reticulum contains a calcium pump with both sufficient capacity

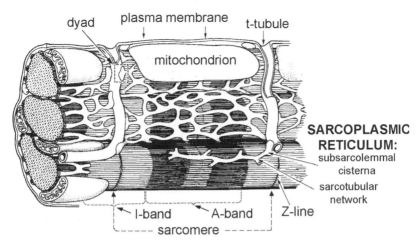

FIGURE 7-3 Ultrastructure of a working myocardial cell. Contractile proteins are arranged in a regular array of thick and thin filaments. The A-band contains the thick filaments and the ends of the thin filaments that extend from the adjoining Z-lines, while the I-band is occupied only by thin filaments that extend toward the center of the sarcomere from the Z-lines. The sarcoplasmic reticulum includes the subsarcolemmal cisternae, which form composite membrane structures with the plasma membrane called *dyads*, and the sarcotubular network, which surrounds the contractile proteins. The lumens of the t-tubules open to the extracellular space, which allows these structures to propagate action potentials into the cell. Mitochondria are shown in the central sarcomere and in cross section at the left side of the figure. (Modified from Katz, 1975.)

and calcium affinity to relax the heart (Katz and Repke, 1967; Harigaya and Schwartz, 1969).

The answer to the second part of Hill's question, how a signal generated by activation at the cell surface reaches the interior of the myocytes, was provided when t-tubules were discovered to be extensions of the plasma membrane whose lumens open into the extracellular space, and that the t-tubular membranes propagate action potentials into the interior of the muscle cells. The role of the t-tubules in activating contraction was documented by Huxley and Taylor (1958) who, in one of the classic experiments in skeletal muscle physiology, demonstrated that applying a very small electrical stimulus through a microelectrode placed at the mouth of a t-tubule induces a contraction that is limited to the sarcomeres adjacent to the point of stimulation. Further evidence that the t-tubules are essential for excitation–contraction coupling was obtained when disruption of the connections between the t-tubules and the plasma membrane was found to make it impossible to activate contraction (Eisenberg and Eisenberg, 1968). This and other evidence that transmission of a wave of depolarization down the t-tubules into the cell interior, which is much more rapid than diffusion of an activator substance, completed the answer to Hill's question.

EXTRACELLULAR AND INTRACELLULAR CALCIUM CYCLES

There are two possible sources of the calcium needed to activate contraction: the extracellular fluid (extracellular calcium cycle) and the sarcoplasmic reticulum (intracellular calcium cycle). Different muscles use these two potential sources of calcium in different ways; as noted above, most of the calcium that activates the small, slowly contracting myocytes of the embryonic heart enters the cytosol from the extracellular fluid, whereas the larger, more rapidly contracting myocytes of the adult mammalian heart depend mainly on calcium derived from intracellular stores. In both cases, the fluxes of activator calcium are passive (downhill) because the ionized calcium concentration in the extracellular fluid and within the sarcoplasmic reticulum is more than 1,000-fold higher than cytosolic calcium concentration in resting muscle (see Chapter 4).

There are two important differences between these calcium cycles. The first is that the electrochemical gradient driving calcium across the plasma membrane into the cytosol in the extracellular calcium cycle is increased by the electronegativity within resting cardiac myocytes. The second is that both calcium influx and calcium efflux across the plasma membrane (extracellular calcium cycle) are accompanied by depolarizing currents (see below); these depolarizing currents are important clinically because they represent a major cause of sudden cardiac death (see Chapter 14). In contrast, the calcium fluxes into and out of the sarcoplasmic reticulum (intracellular calcium cycle) do not influence the potential across the plasma membrane.

The amount of calcium released from the sarcoplasmic reticulum during a skeletal muscle twitch is generally sufficient to bind to virtually all of the troponin C; as a result, the active state is normally at its maximum. In adult mammalian cardiac myocytes, where under basal conditions a lower content of sarcoplasmic reticulum provides only enough calcium to bind approximately 40% of the troponin C, the intensity of the contractile response can be regulated by interventions that alter calcium release from the sarcoplasmic reticulum, the calcium affinity of troponin C, or both. This allows cardiac performance to be altered by changes in the activity, content, and molecular makeup of many of the structures that regulate calcium fluxes into and out of the cytosol (Table 7-1).

THE EXTRACELLULAR CALCIUM CYCLE

Calcium Influx across the Plasma Membrane

Excitation–contraction coupling is normally initiated when an action potential depolarizes the plasma membrane. In the heart, these action potentials are generated by a sequence of changes in membrane potential that result from sodium, calcium, and potassium fluxes through voltage-gated ion-specific channels in the plasma membrane (see Chapter 14). The

TABLE 7-1 **Structures that Participate in Cardiac Excitation–Contraction Coupling and Relaxation**

Structure	Excitation–Contraction Coupling	Relaxation
Plasma membrane		
Sarcolemma		
Na channel	Depolarization Open plasma membrane Ca channels	
Ca channel	Action potential plateau Open intracellular Ca release channels	
Ca pump (PMCA)		Ca removal
Na–Ca exchanger	Ca entry	Ca removal
Na pump		Establish Na gradient
Transverse tubule		
Na channel	Propagate action potential into cell	
Ca channel	Open intracellular Ca release channels	
Sarcoplasmic reticulum		
Subsarcolemmal cisternae		
Ca release channel	Ca release for binding to troponin C	
Calsequestrin	Ca storage, regulation	
Sarcotubular network		
Ca pump (SERCA)		Ca removal
Myofilaments		
Actin and myosin	Contraction	
Troponin C	Ca receptor	
Tropomyosin, troponins I and T	Regulation of actin-cross- bridge interactions	

following discussion highlights the depolarizing calcium currents in cardiac myocytes.

The opening of plasma membrane calcium channels allows a small amount of this activator to diffuse down its large electrochemical gradient into the cytosol. The most important calcium channels in the heart are the *L-type calcium channels*, named because of their relatively long openings (L-long-lasting); these channels also are called *dihydropyridine receptors* because they bind to this class of calcium channel–blocking drugs with

TABLE 7-2 Major Functions of Calcium Entry through L-Type Calcium Channels in the Heart

Role of Calcium	Functional Consequence
Electrical	
Carries positive charge into the cell	Depolarization
Working cells (atria and ventricles)	Action potential plateau
His–Purkinje system	Action potential plateau
Sinoatrial node	Pacemaker activity
Atrioventricular node	Atrioventricular conduction
Chemical	
Triggers calcium release from sarcoplasmic reticulum	Calcium-triggered calcium release
Provides calcium for binding to troponin	Activates contraction
Fills calcium stores in sarcoplasmic reticulum	Maintains contractility
Activates potassium channels	Initiates repolarization

high affinity. Calcium influx thorough the L-type calcium channels participates in both electrical and chemical signaling (Table 7-2). In the atria, ventricles, and His–Purkinje system, where the initial depolarizing current that causes the action potential upstroke is carried by sodium, the influx of positively charged calcium ions across the plasma membrane contributes to the action potential plateau, while in the sinoatrial (SA) and atrioventricular (AV) nodes, these calcium currents are responsible for impulse propagation and participate in pacemaker activity (see Chapter 14).

Calcium influx through L-type calcium channels also provides an important chemical signal. In smooth muscle and the embryonic heart, this calcium influx represents the major source of activator calcium. However, in the working myocytes of the adult mammalian heart, calcium influx from the extracellular space provides only enough of the activator to bind to about 5% of the troponin C; the remainder or so is released from intracellular stores in the sarcoplasmic reticulum (see below). In the heart, the most important chemical function of this calcium influx is to trigger the release of a much larger amount of calcium from the sarcoplasmic reticulum. Some of the calcium that enters the cytosol from the extracellular space is taken up and stored by the sarcoplasmic reticulum, where it can be added to the calcium released in *subsequent* contractions. For this reason, calcium entry by way of the extracellular calcium cycle helps to determine the strength of the heartbeat. Calcium that enters the cell though L-type calcium channels also opens calcium-activated potassium channels that generate a repolarizing current.

Calcium Efflux across the Plasma Membrane

The small amount of calcium that enters the cell through the L-type calcium channels during each action potential must be pumped out of the cell to maintain the composition of the cytosol at a steady state. In the heart, two mechanisms remove this calcium from the cytosol: a plasma membrane calcium pump and a sodium–calcium (Na–Ca) exchanger; the latter, which has a greater capacity than the plasma membrane calcium pump, is responsible for most of this calcium efflux.

P-TYPE ION PUMPS: THE PLASMA MEMBRANE CALCIUM PUMP ATPASE (PMCA). The *plasma membrane calcium pump ATPase* (PMCA) is one of a large family of *P-type ion pumps* that couple energy derived from ATP hydrolysis to active cation transport. Other members of this family include the calcium pump of the sarcoplasmic reticulum, the sodium pump, and proton pumps (Fig. 7-4). Active transport by the P-type ion pumps resembles a boat moving upstream through a series of locks (Fig. 7-5). During these reactions, the ions that are transported become "occluded," which means that they become unable to exchange with ions in the aqueous solutions on either side of the membrane—this is analogous to holding the boat in a closed lock. Transfer of chemical energy from ATP to an occluded ion increases the activity of the ion, much as pumping water into the lock raises the boat.

The turnover of the plasma membrane calcium pump is activated when calcium binds to a transport site on its cytosolic side. Increased cytosolic calcium also stimulates the pump indirectly because in its basal state, when cytosolic calcium is low, the pump is inhibited by a portion of the C-terminal region that lies within the cytosol (Fig. 7-6). This inhibition is reversed when the C-terminal region binds to the calcium–calmodulin complex. By allowing increased cytosolic calcium concentration to increase calcium efflux, this response helps to avoid calcium overload.

THE SODIUM–CALCIUM EXCHANGER. The second mechanism that removes calcium from cardiac myocytes is the *Na–Ca exchanger* (NCX), an antiport that uses the energy of the sodium gradient across the plasma membrane to energize uphill calcium transport. The discovery of this exchanger has an interesting history that began in the 1940s, when the strength of cardiac contraction was found to be proportional to the ratio between extracellular calcium and sodium (Wilbrandt and Koller, 1948). This suggested that these two ions compete for binding to a plasma membrane exchanger that could transport either ion into the cytosol (Lüttgau and Niedergerke, 1958); when the exchanger binds calcium, increased calcium influx causes the heart to contract more strongly, while increasing extracellular sodium weakens contraction by causing the exchanger to carry sodium, rather than calcium, into the cell. The concept of an exchanger was supported by the observation that contractility does not change when extracellular sodium and calcium concentrations are varied at a constant ratio. Calcium

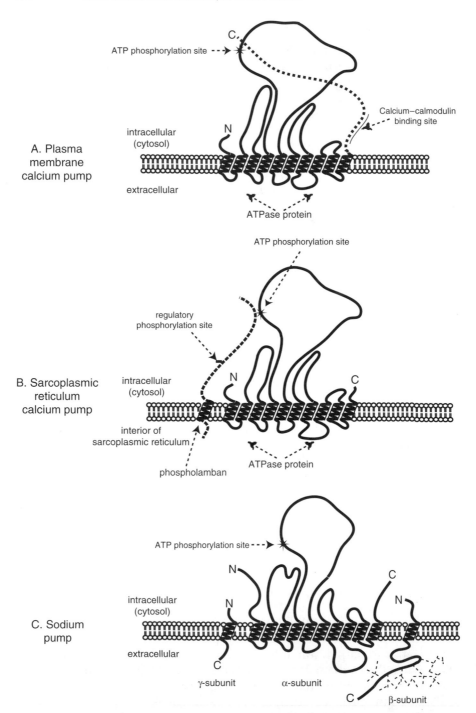

FIGURE 7-4 Molecular structure of three P-type ion pump proteins. The plasma membrane calcium pump (A), sarcoplasmic reticulum calcium pump (B), and the major α-subunit of the sodium pump (C). All contain ten membrane-spanning α-helices and a large cytosolic domain that includes an ATPase site that provides energy for active transport.

efflux also was found to be less sensitive to changing temperature than most ATPases, and metabolic inhibitors that lower ATP levels were observed to stimulate, rather than inhibit, calcium efflux from the heart. All of these findings are now known to be explained by the Na–Ca exchanger. Metabolic inhibitors stimulate calcium efflux because inhibition of ATP-dependent calcium transport into the sarcoplasmic reticulum increases cytosolic calcium, which by favoring the binding of calcium, rather than sodium, to the intracellular site of the Na–Ca exchanger, increases calcium transport out of the poisoned cell. The quantitative importance of Na–Ca exchange was established by Reuter and Seitz (1968), who found that approximately 80% of the calcium efflux from the myocardium occurs via this exchanger. Na–Ca exchange also provided the key to understanding the positive inotropic effect of digitalis, which in the 1950s had been discovered to inhibit the sodium pump (Schätzmann, 1953). The mechanism centers on the increased intracellular sodium caused by sodium pump inhibition, which by favoring sodium efflux reduces calcium efflux; the latter, by retaining calcium in intracellular stores, increases contractility (Repke, 1964).

The Na–Ca exchanger is an intrinsic membrane protein that includes nine membrane-spanning α-helices and a large cytosolic domain, called the *f-loop* (Fig. 7-7). The membrane-spanning helices, along with intervening amino acid sequences within the membrane bilayer, are organized into two groups that participate in the cation transport across the plasma membrane. The f-loop contains phosphorylation and other regulatory sites that alter the turnover of the exchanger in response to protein kinase–mediated phosphorylations, an allosteric effect of ATP, and changing intracellular levels of sodium and calcium.

A simple way to understand the Na–Ca exchanger is to view this antiport as a negatively charged carrier that, after binding either sodium or calcium both within and outside the cell, functions as a shuttle that moves these ions in opposite directions across the membrane (Fig. 7-8). The major driving force for calcium efflux is the normal sodium gradient across the plasma membrane, so the ultimate source of the energy that allows the Na–Ca exchanger to transport calcium uphill out of the cell is the ATP used by the sodium pump to establish the sodium gradient (see below).

The Na–Ca exchanger generates an ionic current because it transports three sodium ions in exchange for one calcium ion. The current, defined as the flux of positive charge, flows in the same direction as the

---

The ions that are transported bind within the plane of the bilayer to several of the membrane-spanning α-helices. In the plasma membrane calcium pump, a portion of the C-terminal peptide chain provides a regulatory site that binds the calcium–calmodulin complex. Phospholamban, which regulates calcium transport into the sarcoplasmic reticulum, is homologous to the C-terminal portion of the plasma membrane calcium pump. The sodium pump contains three subunits: the larger α-subunit contains the sodium-, potassium-, ATP-, and cardiac glycoside–binding sites, while a glycosylated β-subunit and a small γ-subunit regulate pump activity.

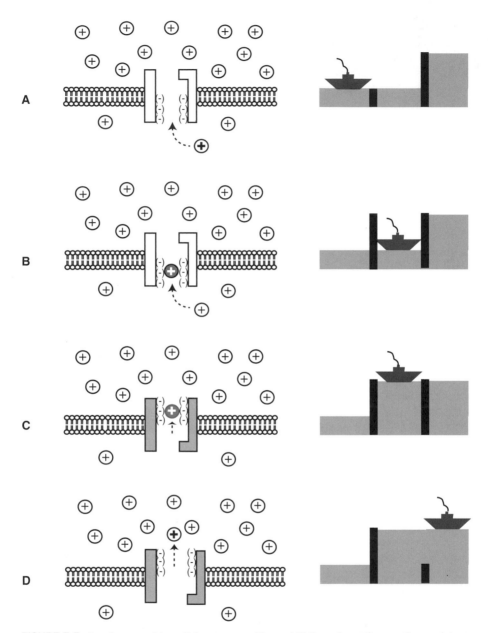

FIGURE 7-5 Ion transport by a P-type pump. The uphill flux of a cation, such as calcium, across the plasma membrane (*left*) resembles the passage of a boat up a river through a series of locks (*right*). A cation in its low-energy state approaches the channel (A) and binds to negatively charged sites in the channel where, like the boat in the lock, it becomes "occluded" (B). Energy supplied to the occluded ion within the channel (*shaded*) "raises" its activity in a process analogous to the pumping of water into the lock that lifts the boat to the higher level on the upstream side (C). After its activity is increased, the ion ceases to be occluded and, like the boat after the upstream gate is opened, is free to move into the region of high activity (D).

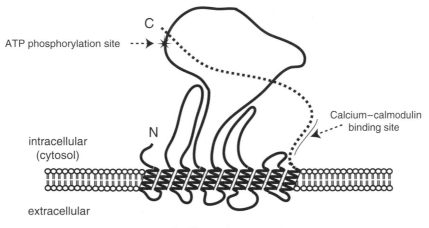

ATP phosphorylation site --->

C

Calcium–calmodulin
binding site

N

intracellular
(cytosol)

extracellular

A. Basal state

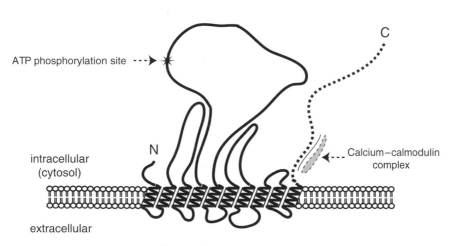

ATP phosphorylation site --->

C

intracellular
(cytosol)

N

Calcium–calmodulin
complex

extracellular

B. Activated state

FIGURE 7-6 Regulation of the plasma membrane calcium pump by the calcium–calmodulin complex. **A:** In the basal state, where low cytosolic calcium concentration prevents formation of the calcium–calmodulin complex, a portion of the C-terminal peptide chain interacts with a regulatory site to inhibit calcium transport. **B:** Binding of the calcium–calmodulin complex to this C-terminal peptide activates the pump by abolishing its inhibitory effect.

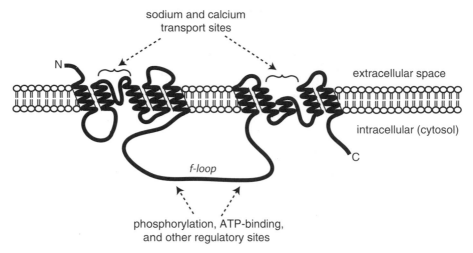

sodium and calcium
transport sites

N

extracellular space

intracellular (cytosol)

C

f-loop

phosphorylation, ATP-binding,
and other regulatory sites

FIGURE 7-7 The sodium–calcium exchanger contains nine membrane-spanning α-helices organized into two groups that are linked by a large intracellular peptide chain. The sodium and calcium transport sites include regions of both groups along with hydrophobic amino acids that lie in the plane of the bilayer. The intracellular peptide chain includes a large *f-loop* that contains sites that allow the exchanger to be regulated by an allosteric effect of ATP, phosphorylations, and changes in cytosolic sodium and calcium concentrations.

sodium flux and is opposite to the movement of calcium (Fig. 7-8); this can be remembered by the statement "current follows sodium." Although the currents generated by the exchanger are small, contributing only a few millivolts to membrane potential in the heart, they can be important clinically. This is especially true in calcium-overloaded hearts, where the depolarizing current associated with increased calcium efflux can cause transient depolarizations and lethal arrhythmias (see Chapter 14).

The electrogenicity of Na–Ca exchange allows membrane potential to influence the direction of ion transport by the exchanger. In the resting heart, the negative intracellular potential favors sodium influx across the plasma membrane and therefore increases calcium efflux during diastole. Reversal of membrane potential during systole, when the inside of the cell becomes positively charged, has the opposite effect to favor calcium influx. These effects of membrane potential allow the Na–Ca exchanger to operate in a manner that, whether the heart is relaxed or contracting, it favors calcium flux in whatever direction that helps to maintain that state. Calcium efflux, which relaxes the heart, is favored by the intracellular negativity during diastole, while calcium influx, which increases contractility, is favored during systole.

A regulatory effect of elevated intracellular calcium that increases the turnover of the exchanger helps to prevent calcium overload. Although the overall reaction of the Na–Ca exchanger does not require the expenditure of energy, its turnover is stimulated by an allosteric effect of ATP.

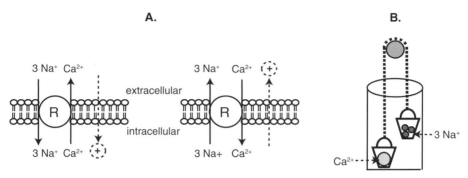

FIGURE 7-8 Overview of Na–Ca exchange. **A:** The exchanger can be depicted as a carrier (R) that can transport three Na$^+$ in either direction across the plasma membrane in exchange for a single Ca^{2+}. The exchanger generates an ionic current (*dashed arrow*) whose direction (defined as the movement of positive charge) is the same as that of sodium. Calcium efflux is therefore accompanied by a depolarizing current and calcium influx by a repolarizing current; in both cases, current follows sodium. **B:** The exchanger can be viewed as a well with two buckets—one containing a single calcium ion, the other three sodium ions.

This is one example of the general ability of ATP to accelerate ion fluxes by exchangers, channels, and pumps. In the heart, the exchanger can be activated when it is phosphorylated by protein kinases A and C as well as by calcium-calmodulin–dependent protein kinase (CAM kinase).

Other Ion Fluxes across the Plasma Membrane

In addition to the ion transport systems that participate directly in the extracellular calcium cycle (see above), two other transporters—the sodium pump and sodium–hydrogen exchanger—indirectly regulate contraction and relaxation by the heart.

THE SODIUM PUMP. The sodium pump (also called the *sodium–potassium ATPase* or *Na-K–ATPase* because its ability to hydrolyze ATP is stimulated when sodium and potassium are present together) transports sodium out of the cytosol in exchange for potassium that enters the cell. The exchange of potassium ions for sodium ions reduces the electrochemical work of the sodium pump because both sodium efflux and potassium influx are uphill processes and require energy derived from ATP hydrolysis. Its energetic importance is apparent in nonmotile tissues like the kidneys, where the sodium–potassium ATPase accounts for 20% to 30% of the ATP consumed under basal conditions.

The major function of the sodium pump in working cardiac myocytes is to exchange the small amount of sodium that enters the cytosol during each action potential with potassium that is lost during repolarization. The electrochemical gradients established by the sodium pump also are essential for excitability because they provide the driving force for the depolarizing sodium currents that activate atrial and ventricular myocytes

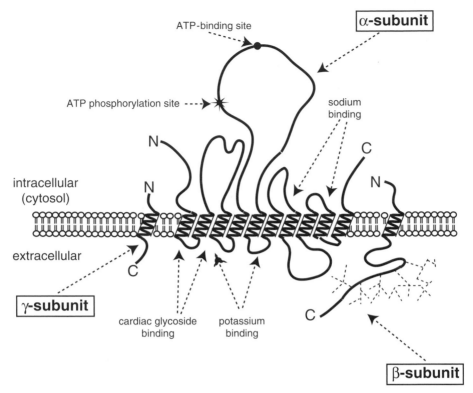

FIGURE 7-9 The sodium pump. The large cytoplasmic domain of the α-subunit contains a site that, when phosphorylated by ATP, provides the energy needed for active ion transport. The extracellular portions of several membrane-spanning α-helices bind potassium and cardiac glycosides, while sodium binds to membrane-spanning helices from the intracellular side of the membrane. Several sites on the intracellular domain along with the glycosylated β-subunit and small γ-subunit regulate sodium pump activity.

and Purkinje cells as well as the repolarizing potassium currents that maintain resting potential in all regions of the heart (Chapter 13). The sodium gradient across the plasma membrane also energizes calcium efflux by the Na–Ca exchanger (see above) and proton efflux by the Na–H exchanger (see below) as well as the active transport of several substrates and metabolites across the plasma membrane.

The sodium pump includes three subunits (Fig. 7-9). The largest, the α-subunit, is a P-type ion pump ATPase (see Fig. 7-4) whose intracellular domain contains a phosphorylation site that transduces chemical energy of ATP to osmotic work, along with several regulatory sites. Sodium and potassium bind to different regions of the α-subunit; sodium on the cytosolic side, potassium on the extracellular side. Cardiac glycosides, which inhibit the sodium pump, also bind to the extracellular side of the α-subunit, which allows changes in extracellular potassium concentration to modify the sensitivity of the sodium pump to these drugs. The smaller

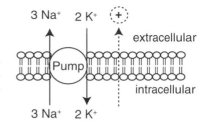

FIGURE 7-10 Overview of ion transport by the sodium pump. Because three sodium ions are exchanged for two potassium ions, the pump generates an ionic current; as is true of Na–Ca exchange, current follows sodium.

β-subunit, which is essential for normal transport activity, is a glycoprotein that includes a single membrane-spanning domain and a number of carbohydrate residues bound to its extracellular surface. Less is known about the γ-subunit, which like the β-subunit regulates interactions between sodium, potassium, and the sodium pump (Therien et al., 2001).

The sodium pump is *electrogenic* because it transports three sodium ions out of the cell in exchange for two potassium ions that enter the cytosol (Fig. 7-10). The movement of positive charge by the sodium pump, like that by the Na–Ca exchanger (Fig. 7-8), is in the same direction as the flux of sodium ions, which provides another example where "current follows sodium." The contribution of the sodium pump to membrane potential is small, usually less than 10 mV, although under some circumstances, this outward current can be of considerable functional importance. In injured cells, for example, where resting potential is reduced and sodium "leak" into the cell is increased, the outward current generated by the sodium pump helps to maintain intracellular electronegativity. The arrhythmogenic effects of sodium pump inhibition, often seen in patients who are given high doses of cardiac glycosides, are due in part to reduction of this repolarizing current; however, the major cause of arrhythmias following sodium pump inhibition is the resting depolarization that results from decreased intracellular potassium concentration (see Chapter 16).

The sodium pump forms several reaction intermediates between the protein (or enzyme, designated as "E" in the following discussion) and its substrates (Fig. 7-11). E_1, E_2, $E_1{\sim}P$, and E_2-P represent different nonphosphorylated and phosphorylated states of the enzyme. The two nonphosphorylated states, E_1 and E_2, have different reactivities to ATP and bind differently to cations: Sodium binds to the intracellular side of E_1, while potassium binds to the extracellular side of E_2. The two phosphorylated intermediates, $E_1{\sim}P$ and E_2-P, contain acyl phosphate bonds but differ in their energetics: $E_1{\sim}P$ is the high-energy intermediate, while the low-energy intermediate, E_2-P, is formed when energy is expended during the active transport of sodium and potassium. These phosphorylated intermediates resemble those formed during the cross-bridge cycle (Chapter 4), but unlike myosin, where the chemical energy liberated from ATP causes tension development and shortening by shifting the angle of the cross-bridges, the sodium pump uses energy to perform osmotic work.

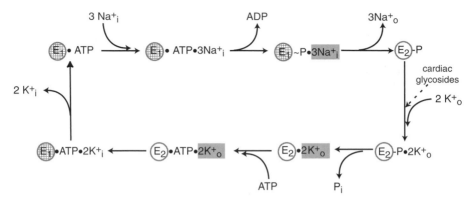

FIGURE 7-11 Reaction scheme for the sodium pump ATPase reaction. The pump (*labeled* E) can be in a high-energy E_1 state (*shaded circles*) or a low-energy E_2 state (*open circles*). Enzyme-bound ions can be "occluded" (*shaded rectangles*) or exchangeable (*no rectangles*). High- and low-energy bonds are indicated by tildes (~) and dashes (-), respectively, and the positions of the ions are shown by the subscripts i (intracellular) and o (extracellular). The reaction, described in the text, begins when sodium binds to the intracellular side of the energized pump (*upper left*).

The reaction shown in Figure 7-11, which requires magnesium, begins when three sodium ions bind to the intracellular (cytosolic) side of the sodium pump (E), which is in a high-energy state:

$$E_1 \bullet ATP + 3\ Na^+_i \longleftrightarrow E_1 \bullet ATP \bullet 3Na^+_i \qquad [7\text{-}1]$$

Release of ADP then transfers energy to the bound sodium, which becomes occluded (indicated by braces).

$$E_1 \bullet ATP \bullet 3Na^+_i \longleftrightarrow E_1 \sim P \bullet 3\{Na^+_o\} + ADP \qquad [7\text{-}2]$$

The activity of the occluded sodium is then raised to the higher activity of the extracellular fluid (Na^+_o), after which it is released into the extracellular fluid and the pump returns to the low-energy state, E_2-P. (Sodium release occurs in two steps that, for simplicity, are combined equation 7-3 below and later in Fig. 7-13.)

$$E_1 \sim P \bullet 3\{Na^+_o\} \longleftrightarrow E_2\text{-}P + 3Na^+_o \qquad [7\text{-}3]$$

The next steps in this reaction, which transport potassium into the cytosol, begin when potassium at its low activity in the extracellular space (K^+_o) binds to E_2-P.

$$E_2\text{-}P + 2K^+_o \longleftrightarrow E_2\text{-}P\bullet2K^+_o \qquad\qquad [7\text{-}4]$$

This is the step where cardiac glycosides inhibit the sodium pump by binding to the extracellular side of the enzyme. Release of inorganic phosphate in the next step causes the bound potassium, still at its low activity in the extracellular fluid, to become occluded.

$$E_2\text{-}P\bullet2K^+_o \longleftrightarrow E_2\bullet2\{K^+_o\} + P_i \qquad\qquad [7\text{-}5]$$

Binding of ATP to the $E_2\bullet2\{K^+_o\}$ complex begins the transfer of energy that raises the activity of the occluded potassium to that in the cytosol. However, most of the chemical energy of ATP initially remains in the nucleotide, so the activity of the enzyme-bound potassium remains low.

$$E_2\bullet2\{K^+_o\} + ATP \longleftrightarrow E_2\bullet ATP\bullet\{2K^+_o\} \qquad\qquad [7\text{-}6]$$

Transfer of energy from ATP to the $E_2\bullet ATP\bullet2K^+_o$ complex brings the pump to a high-energy state (E_2) and increases the activity of the occluded potassium to the higher level within the cell (K^+_i).

$$E_2\bullet ATP\bullet2\{K^+_o\} \longleftrightarrow E_1\bullet ATP\bullet2K^+_i \qquad\qquad [7\text{-}7]$$

Further transfer of energy to the pump completes the reaction by releasing potassium into the cytosol.

$$E_1\bullet ATP\bullet2K^+_i \longleftrightarrow E_1\bullet ATP + 2K^+_i \qquad\qquad [7\text{-}8]$$

The overall reaction of the sodium pump (see also Fig. 7-10) can be written:

$$3\,Na^+_i + 2\,K^+_o + ATP \longleftrightarrow 3\,Na^+_o + 2\,K^+_i + ADP + P_i \qquad [7\text{-}9]$$

This reaction can run in reverse in a sequence of steps that couple downhill ion fluxes to the synthesis of ATP from ADP and P_i; however, pump reversal is strongly inhibited by ATP and therefore does not occur under physiological conditions.

The sodium pump is regulated by several protein kinases—for example, phosphorylation by PK-A allows sympathetic activation to stimulate the pump. Pump activity also is regulated by acylation of the α-subunit and glycosylation of the β-subunit, and by an allosteric effect of high ATP concentrations that stimulates the pump. Long-term changes in pump activity are effected by isoform shifts and changes in the density of pump molecules within the plasma membrane.

The *cardiac glycosides*, the first class of drugs found to be useful in treating heart disease, have four major actions, all of which are due to sodium pump inhibition. The first action, their ability to increase myocardial contractility—traditionally viewed as the desired effect—occurs when sodium pump inhibition increases intracellular sodium concentration near a region of the plasma membrane that is rich in Na–Ca exchanger molecules. Because the higher sodium concentration at the cytosolic side of the membrane inhibits calcium efflux by way of the Na–Ca exchanger (see above), less calcium leaves the cell, which by increasing calcium stores explains the positive inotropic effect (Chapter 10). Resting membrane depolarization, the second action, results from the fall in intracellular potassium concentration and is responsible for many of the arrhythmogenic effects of these drugs (see Chapter 16). The third action, reduction of the small repolarizing current generated by the sodium pump, increases this depolarizing effect. It now appears likely, however, that many of the beneficial effects of the cardiac glycosides in heart failure are due to the fourth action, which results from central effects caused by sodium pump inhibition in the brainstem. This central action increases vagal activity and reduces sympathetic tone which, by decreasing heart rate, contractility, and peripheral resistance has an energy-sparing effect that may be beneficial in some patients with heart failure.

The cardiac glycosides, like potassium, bind to the extracellular surface of the pump, leading to an interaction where increased extracellular potassium reduces the potency of these drugs by displacing them from their extracellular binding site. This interaction also explains the dangerous potentiation of the effects of cardiac glycosides by low serum potassium levels.

MAINTENANCE OF INTRACELLULAR pH: THE SODIUM–HYDROGEN EXCHANGER. Intracellular pH is normally about 7.2, which is more alkaline than would be expected if protons were distributed according to their electrochemical gradient. Because energy production in the heart is accompanied by the generation of protons, mechanisms are needed to prevent intracellular acidosis, which has several deleterious effects that include a negative inotropic effect caused when protons compete with calcium for binding to the troponin complex. Intracellular alkalinity is maintained by one symport and three antiports; the symport is a sodium–bicarbonate transporter, while the three antiports are a chloride–bicarbonate exchanger, a chloride–hydroxyl exchanger, and most important, a sodium–hydrogen exchanger.

Sodium–hydrogen (Na–H) *exchangers* (NHE) use the energy of the sodium gradient for the uphill transport of protons out of the cell; because the stoichiometry between proton efflux and sodium influx is 1:1, Na–H exchange is electrically neutral. Na–H exchangers are members of a large and ancient superfamily of transporters that are found in both prokaryotes and eukaryotes; this family includes uniports (one ion, one direction), symports (two ions, one direction), and antiports (two ions, two directions) (Marger and Saier, 1993; Reithmeier, 1994).

NHE1, the major Na–H exchanger isoform in the heart, is a large glycoprotein that contains twelve membrane-spanning α-helices, an N-terminal portion that participates in the ion exchange reaction, and a large intracellular C-terminal domain that contains a number of regulatory sites (Fig. 7-12). The latter also links NHE1 to the actin cytoskeleton through a cytoskeletal "organizer" called *ezrin*, which is one of a family of ezrin-radixin-moesin (ERM) proteins providing regulated linkages between membrane proteins and the cytoskeleton that participate in signal transduction (Bretscher et al., 2002). NHE1 is concentrated in the intercalated discs and t-tubules, which suggests that the exchanger regulates pH around the gap junctions and intracellular calcium release channels, whose opening is inactivated by acidosis. Because the Na–H exchanger couples sodium influx to proton efflux, acidosis increases intracellular sodium, which reduces calcium efflux by the Na–Ca exchanger. This effect is especially important in energy-starved hearts, where the production of protons during anaerobic glycolysis, by activating NHE1, can worsen calcium overload.

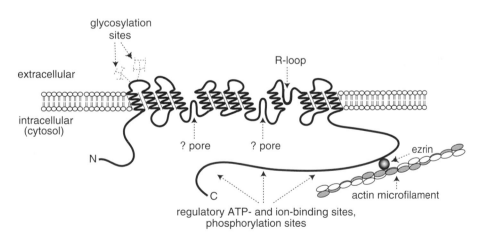

FIGURE 7-12 The sodium–hydrogen exchanger. This highly regulated protein contains twelve membrane-spanning α-helices and a glycosylated region between the first and second helices. The N-terminal region, including the adjacent membrane-spanning helices, are involved in ion transport, while the large C-terminal peptide chain contains phosphorylation sites along with ion-binding, ATP-binding, and calcium-calmodulin–binding sites that regulate the exchanger. Turnover of the exchanger is increased when protons bind to its intracellular surface in the acidotic heart. Ezrin, a cytoskeletal organizer that links the exchanger to actin microfilaments, allows NHE1 to participate in signal transduction.

The Na–H exchanger is stimulated in two ways by intracellular acidosis: a direct response to the increased concentration of the protons that participate in the exchange and an indirect effect that occurs when the protons bind to an intracellular pH "sensor" that increases the turnover of the antiport. The exchanger also is activated by an allosteric effect of ATP. Other regulators include the calcium–calmodulin complex, several regulatory proteins, and protein kinases. The latter can be activated by G-protein–coupled receptors, receptor tyrosine kinases, and integrins. The complexity of this interlocking control attests to the importance of the Na–H exchanger, which in addition to regulating intracellular pH serves additional roles such as a stimulator of cell growth and cell death.

THE INTRACELLULAR CALCIUM CYCLE

The calcium that enters the working myocytes of the mammalian heart from the extracellular fluid cannot activate more than a small fraction of the potential actin–myosin interactions, so most of the calcium that binds to troponin is derived from the sarcoplasmic reticulum (see Chapter 1). Because the ionized calcium concentration within the sarcoplasmic reticulum is several orders of magnitude higher than that in the cytosol, calcium release is a passive, downhill flux, whereas the calcium uptake into this internal membrane system that relaxes the heart requires the expenditure of energy.

The sarcoplasmic reticulum includes two regions (Fig. 7-3): the *subsarcolemmal cisternae*, which contain the calcium release channels that control the calcium efflux that initiates systole, and an extensive *sarcotubular network* that contains a densely packed array of calcium pump ATPase proteins that relax the heart. The membranes of the subsarcolemmal cisternae form composite structures with the plasma membrane and t-tubules called *dyads* (see Chapter 1), which provide a vital functional link between plasma membrane depolarization and calcium release from the sarcoplasmic reticulum. These membranes contain two different types of calcium channel: *L-type calcium channels* in the plasma membrane and t-tubules that regulate calcium flux into the cytosol from the extracellular fluid, and *calcium release channels* in the subsarcolemmal cisternae that regulate the calcium flux out of the sarcoplasmic reticulum that activates contraction. The intracellular calcium cycle is completed by the calcium pump proteins in the sarcotubular network, which transport calcium uphill into the sarcoplasmic reticulum.

Calcium Release from the Sarcoplasmic Reticulum

SIGNALS GENERATED BY PLASMA MEMBRANE DEPOLARIZATION. Three different mechanisms were initially proposed to explain how an action potential might initiate calcium release from the sarcoplasmic reticulum (Fig. 7-13). The first is that depolarization of the t-tubular membrane generates an

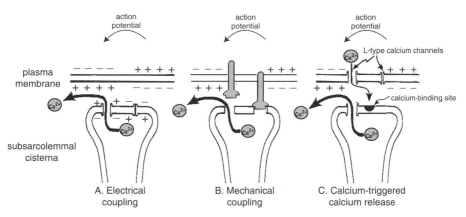

FIGURE 7-13 Three mechanisms by which an action potential, propagated across the plasma membrane or t-tubule, was proposed to release calcium from the sarcoplasmic reticulum. **A:** *Electrical coupling.* Calcium release is initiated when the sarcoplasmic reticulum membrane is depolarized by charge movements in the adjacent plasma membrane. **B:** *Mechanical coupling.* Plasma membrane depolarization shifts a voltage-regulated peptide so as to "unplug" a sarcoplasmic reticulum calcium release channel. **C:** *Calcium-triggered calcium release.* A small amount of calcium that enters the cytosol through an L-type plasma membrane calcium channel binds to and opens an intracellular channel that releases a much larger amount of calcium from within the sarcoplasmic reticulum.

electrical signal that opens voltage-sensitive calcium channels in the sarcoplasmic reticulum (A, Fig. 7-13). Although this mechanism seemed logical because of the well-known ability of a change in transmembrane potential to open ion channels in the plasma membrane (see Chapter 13), it is now clear that plasma membrane depolarization does not cause potential changes across the sarcoplasmic reticulum membrane. The second mechanism postulated a mechanical coupling in which depolarization of the t-tubule moves a voltage-sensitive "plug" to open a calcium channel in the adjacent subsarcolemmal cisternae (B, Fig. 7-13); this has been called irreverently the *plumber's helper model* because the plug can be pictured to resemble the device used to open blocked drains. This mechanism operates in fast skeletal muscle, where membrane depolarization causes a conformational change in an L-type plasma membrane calcium channel that, by moving an occluding region of the channel, unplugs the adjacent intracellular calcium release channel. According to the third mechanism, called *calcium-induced calcium release*, a small amount of calcium that crosses the plasma membrane from the extracellular fluid induces the release of a much larger amount of activator calcium from within the sarcoplasmic reticulum (C, Fig. 7-13). This is analogous to the firing mechanism of a flintlock musket, where the small primer charge explodes when the flint strikes the primer pan–like calcium entry through the L-type calcium channels—and ignites the larger amount of powder within the barrel of the musket—which is analogous to the larger quantity of calcium released from within the sarcoplasmic reticulum. It is now clear that the third mechanism operates in the adult mammalian heart (Fabiato, 1983).

The signal initiated by plasma membrane depolarization in both mechanical coupling (B, Fig. 7-13) and calcium-triggered calcium release (C, Fig. 7-13) is mediated by a voltage-dependent conformational change in the voltage sensor of an L-type plasma membrane calcium channel (see Chapter 13). In skeletal muscle, the conformational change unplugs the intracellular channel, whereas in the heart, a similar voltage-dependent conformational change opens the L-type channel to allow the small influx of "trigger" calcium that opens the intracellular calcium channel. This ability of different L-type calcium channels to activate contraction—by removing a plug in skeletal muscle, and by supplying a small amount of trigger calcium in the heart—is one of many examples of how homologous structures can use different mechanisms to bring about similar responses.

CALCIUM RELEASE CHANNELS. The amount of calcium released by the skeletal sarcoplasmic reticulum provides enough of this activator to bind to virtually all of the troponin C, which accounts for the fact that the active state in skeletal muscle is generally at its maximum. In the heart, the smaller amount of calcium released from the sarcoplasmic reticulum is not sufficient to saturate the troponin C, which allows interventions that alter calcium release by the cardiac sarcoplasmic reticulum to vary the heart's contractile response (see Chapter 10).

The intracellular calcium release channels, along with plasma membrane L-type calcium channels in the dyads, are grouped in functional clusters that include the Na–Ca exchanger and sodium pump (Stern et al., 1999; Franzini-Armstrong et al., 1999). Calcium is released in small amounts from these clusters, which causes localized areas of increased calcium concentration called *calcium sparks* (Wang et al., 2004).

The electron-dense "feet" that lie between the plasma membrane and the membrane of the subsarcolemmal cisternae in the dyad (see Chapter 1) are the intracellular calcium release channels (often called *ryanodine receptors* or *RyR* because they bind to this plant alkaloid). These large membrane proteins are made up of four subunits (Fig. 7-14), each of which includes a large cytosolic domain (the foot) and at least four α-helical membrane-spanning segments (Fig. 7-15). In the open channel, a central pore in the transmembrane region within the subsarcolemmal cisternae membrane is connected to radial channels in each of the four subunits, whereas when the channel is closed, the central pore and radial channels are not connected (A, Fig. 7-16). Calcium binding to the foot opens these channels by causing the foot to rotate so as to align the pores in the four subunits with the central pore (B, Fig. 7-16).

The cardiac calcium release channels, which are highly regulated, can be phosphorylated by several protein kinases, including a calcium–calmodulin kinase (CAM kinase), which by inhibiting channel opening at high cytosolic calcium concentrations exerts a protective effect that

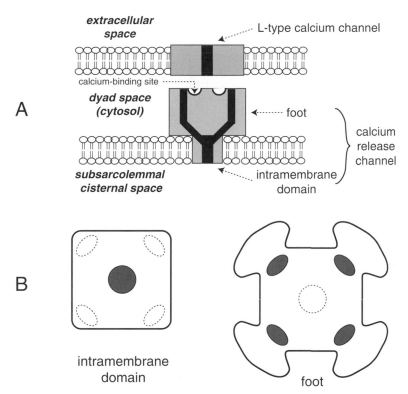

FIGURE 7-14 Schematic representation of a dyad showing the relationship between an L-type calcium channel and a calcium release channel. **A:** View across the plane of the bilayer showing the plasma membrane (*above*) and subsarcolemmal cisternal membrane (*below*). The former contains an L-type calcium channel that delivers calcium to binding sites on the sarcoplasmic reticulum calcium release channel, which contains an intramembrane domain and a large "foot" that projects into the cytosolic space. The dark areas represent the pores through which calcium crosses the membrane when these channels are in the open state. **B:** The intracellular calcium release channel showing the intramembrane domain as seen from within the subsarcolemmal cisterna (*left*), and from the cytosolic space within the dyad (*right*). The intramembrane domain contains a central pore that when the channel is open is connected to radial channels within each of the four cytosolic domains that make up the foot.

reduces calcium release from the sarcoplasmic reticulum. Phosphorylation of these channels by protein kinase A, which increases calcium release, participates in the inotropic response to sympathetic stimulation. Interactions among the four subunits of the cardiac calcium release channels are regulated by a protein, called *FKBP12* or *calstabin2*, that binds to immunosuppressive drugs related to cyclosporine. One of these FK-binding proteins stabilizes and facilitates opening of calcium release channels by coordinating the gating of the channel subunits.

The calcium release channels in cardiac and skeletal sarcoplasmic reticulum are members of a family that includes *inositol trisphosphate–*

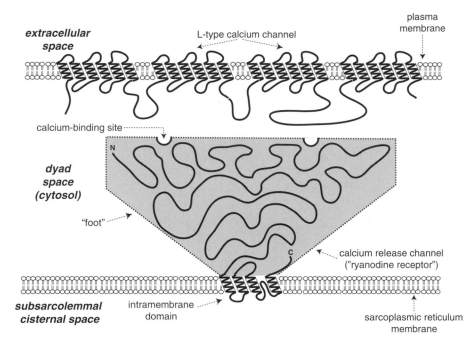

FIGURE 7-15 Structure of one subunit of the calcium release channel (*below*) showing its relationship to the plasma membrane L-type calcium channel (*above*). The cytosolic domain ("foot") contains binding sites that allow calcium to open the channel. The intramembrane domain includes at least four α-helical membrane-spanning segments.

gated calcium channels (*InsP₃* receptors). The latter, which are smaller and open and close more slowly than the skeletal and cardiac calcium release channels, play a major role in delivering the calcium that activates smooth muscle contraction. The function of the small numbers of InsP₃-gated calcium channels found in the heart is not clearly understood; they may help to regulate resting tension, but the slow release of calcium by InsP₃-gated calcium release channels also is suitable for mediating the pro-liferative signals that regulate such processes as protein synthesis, cell cycling, and apoptosis (Berridge, 1997).

Calcium Uptake by the Sarcoplasmic Reticulum

Because the calcium that activates the adult mammalian heart is derived largely from intracellular stores, at a steady state most of the calcium removed from the cytosol during diastole must be pumped back into this internal membrane system. This is effected by the *sarcoplasmic retic-ulum calcium pump* [also called the *sarco(endo)plasmic reticulum cal-cium pump ATPase* or SERCA], which is one of the P-type ion pumps (see Fig. 7-4). These proteins, which span the membrane so as to contact the aqueous spaces on either side of the bilayer, form a densely packed array within the membranes of the sarcotubular network (Fig. 7-17). There

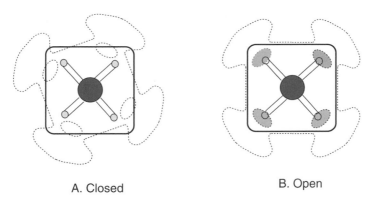

A. Closed

B. Open

FIGURE 7-16 Depiction of the rotation that opens the calcium release channel. **A:** In its closed state, the four radial channels do not connect with the central pore. **B:** The channel opens when the radial channels become aligned with the central pore.

are many isoforms of SERCA. The cardiac isoform (SERCA 2a), like the plasma membrane calcium pump ATPase described above, contains a large intracellular domain with an ATP phosphorylation site and several regulatory sites as well as a calcium-transport site made up of several of the α-helical membrane-spanning segments (see below).

Coupling of calcium transport to ATP hydrolysis by the calcium pump ATPases is similar to the coupling of alkali metal ion transport to ATP hydrolysis by the sodium pump, except that the calcium pump does

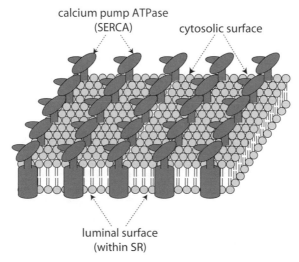

calcium pump ATPase
(SERCA)

cytosolic surface

luminal surface
(within SR)

FIGURE 7-17 Three-dimensional depiction of the membrane of the sarcotubular network; the cytosolic surface is above and the lumen below. The calcium pump ATPase molecules are packed into the bilayer, with most of their mass projecting into the cytosol. SERCA, sarco(endo)plasmic reticulum calcium pump ATPase; SR, sarcoplasmic reticulum.

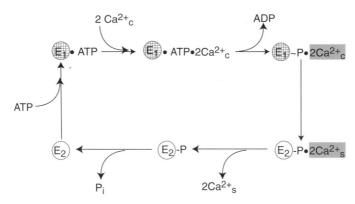

FIGURE 7-18 Reaction scheme for the calcium pump ATPase reaction. The pump (*labeled* E) can be in a high-energy E_1 state (*shaded circles*) or a low-energy E_2 state (*open circles*). Enzyme-bound calcium can be "occluded" (*shaded rectangles*) or exchangeable (*no rectangles*). High- and low-energy bonds are indicated by tildes ($\sim$) and dashes (-), respectively, and the positions of the calcium are shown by the subscripts c (*within the cytosol*) and s (*within the sarcoplasmic reticulum*). The reaction, described in the text, begins at the upper left, when ATP binds to the enzyme.

not exchange calcium for a counter-ion. Unlike ion fluxes across the plasma membrane, which cause physiologically important changes in membrane potential, movements of positively charged calcium ions into and out of the sarcoplasmic reticulum do not generate electrical currents. This is because the sarcoplasmic reticulum membrane contains nonspecific anion channels that allow fluxes of chloride and phosphate anions to neutralize the charge movement accompanying calcium fluxes across the intracellular membrane (Beil et al., 1977).

Active transport by the calcium pump (Fig. 7-18), like that of the sodium pump (Fig. 7-11), uses energy derived from ATP to "transport" cations against their concentration gradients. The designations E_1 and E_2 in the following discussion refer to nonphosphorylated states with different reactivities to ATP and calcium, while the two phosphorylated states, $E_1\sim P$ and E_2-P, are high- and low-energy intermediates, respectively. The subscripts refer to calcium activity in the cytosol (Ca^{2+}_c) and within the sarcoplasmic reticulum (Ca^{2+}_s).

The reaction begins when two calcium ions at low activity within the cytosol bind to the pump that, because it is bound to ATP, is in a high-energy state:

$$E_1 \bullet ATP + 2\ Ca^{2+}_c \longleftrightarrow E_1 \bullet ATP \bullet 2Ca^{2+}_c \qquad [7\text{-}10]$$

In the next step, release of ADP transfers energy to the complex to form $E_1\sim P \bullet 2Ca^{2+}_c$ in which the bound calcium, although still at its low cytosolic activity, becomes occluded and therefore is unable to exchange with cytosolic calcium (indicated by braces).

$$E_1 \bullet ATP \bullet 2Ca^{2+}_c \longleftrightarrow E_1 {\sim} P \bullet 2\{Ca^{2+}_c\} + ADP \qquad [7\text{-}11]$$

The activity of the occluded calcium is then raised to the high level within the sarcoplasmic reticulum in a reaction that uses energy in $E_1{\sim}P$, which returns to the low energy state in $E_2\text{-}P$:

$$E_1 {\sim} P \bullet 2\{Ca^{2+}_c\} \longleftrightarrow E_2\text{-}P \bullet 2Ca^{2+}_s \qquad [7\text{-}12]$$

Calcium is then released into the region of higher calcium activity within the sarcoplasmic reticulum,

$$E_2\text{-}P \bullet 2Ca^{2+}_s \longleftrightarrow E_2\text{-}P + 2\ Ca^{2+}_s \qquad [7\text{-}13]$$

after which the low-energy phosphoenzyme $E_2\text{-}P$ is dephosphorylated to form E_2.

$$E_2\text{-}P \longleftrightarrow E_2 + P_i \qquad [7\text{-}14]$$

Binding of ATP to E_2, by transferring energy to the pump, converts the latter to the high energy E_1:

$$E_2 + ATP \longleftrightarrow E_1 \bullet ATP \qquad [7\text{-}15]$$

One consequence of the addition of energy to E_2 is to increase the affinity of the calcium-binding site, which allows the $E_1 \bullet ATP$ complex to bind two calcium ions at their low activity within the cytosol shown in equation 7-11.

The overall reaction of the calcium pump ATPase can be written:

$$2\ Ca^{2+}_c + ATP \longleftrightarrow 2\ Ca^{2+}_s + ADP + P_i \qquad [7\text{-}16]$$

All of the steps in the calcium pump ATPase reaction, like those of the Na-K–ATPase, are reversible so that under special conditions *in vitro*, the pump can be made to run backward. When this occurs, the energy of the calcium gradient across the sarcoplasmic reticulum is coupled to the synthesis of ATP from ADP and P_i. However, to run the calcium pump in reverse, Ca^{2+}_s, ADP, and P_i levels must be high and Ca^{2+}_c and ATP levels must be low. Because these conditions are not normally found in cardiac myocytes, the pump does not ordinarily mediate a net flux of calcium out of the sarcoplasmic reticulum. However, the pump can cycle between brief phases of calcium uptake and calcium release under physiological conditions *in vitro* (Takenaka et al., 1982), which might allow this oscillatory behavior to contribute to the cyclic variations in cytosolic calcium that are associated with transient depolarizations and lethal arrhythmias in calcium-overloaded hearts (see Chapter 14).

The most important regulator of calcium pump activity is the level of cytosolic calcium, which reflects the fact that binding of cytosolic calcium is a prerequisite for pump turnover (equation 7-10). High cytosolic calcium levels also stimulate the calcium pump indirectly by forming a calcium–calmodulin complex that activates a CAM kinase that phosphorylates a regulatory site on the pump. CAM kinase and protein kinase A (PKA) also stimulate calcium transport by phosphorylating phospholamban, a regulatory protein described below. Slowing of calcium uptake is one of the most important consequences of energy starvation; this is due largely to the lower ATP concentration and the increased concentration of ADP that reduce the free energy available from ATP hydrolysis $(-\Delta G)$ (Tian and Ingwall, 1996). ATP at the high concentrations found in the heart's cytosol also has an allosteric effect that stimulates the calcium pump so that attenuation of this allosteric effect, along with the fall in free energy from ATP hydrolysis, can slow relaxation in ischemic and failing hearts (see Chapters 17 and 18).

Phospholamban, a small membrane protein that contains a single α-helical membrane-spanning segment, forms pentamers that in the dephospho form inhibit calcium transport by the cardiac sarcoplasmic reticulum (Fig. 7-19). This inhibitory effect is reversed when PKA phosphorylates phospholamban, which by accelerating relaxation is an important component of the heart's response to sympathetic stimulation (see Chapter 10). Phospholamban phosphorylation also increases calcium stores within the sarcoplasmic reticulum because the more rapid uptake of calcium into the intracellular membrane system reduces calcium efflux into the extracellular space. This allows sympathetic stimulation to increase the amount of calcium available for release during excitation–contraction coupling, which increases contractility. Phosphorylation of phospholamban by CAM kinase, which also stimulates calcium uptake into the sarcoplasmic reticulum, helps to protect the heart in situations of calcium overload.

Comparison of the stimulation of calcium transport by the calcium-calmodulin–binding domain of the plasma membrane calcium pump (Fig. 7-6) with that of phospholamban (Fig. 7-19) provides a fascinating example of the way that homologous structures can cause similar responses in different systems. Although the inhibitory action and amino acid sequence

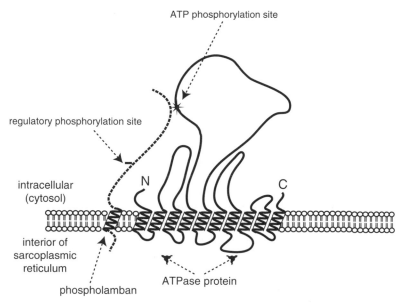

ATP phosphorylation site

regulatory phosphorylation site

intracellular
(cytosol)

N

C

interior of
sarcoplasmic
reticulum

phospholamban

ATPase protein

A. Basal State

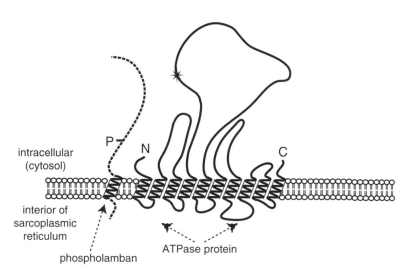

intracellular
(cytosol)

P

N

C

interior of
sarcoplasmic
reticulum

phospholamban

ATPase protein

B. Activated State

FIGURE 7-19 Regulation of the cardiac sarcoplasmic reticulum calcium pump by phospholamban. **A:** In the basal state, phospholamban inhibits calcium transport when it interacts with the phosphorylation and calcium–binding sites of the intracellular regulatory domain. **B:** Phosphorylation of phospholamban accelerates calcium transport by reversing these inhibitory effects.

of the C-terminal domain of the plasma membrane calcium pump resembles that of phospholamban, in the former, this regulatory peptide is an integral part of the pump protein, whereas in the sarcoplasmic reticulum, phospholamban is separate from the calcium pump. This suggests that a regulatory peptide in the ancestral calcium pump evolved in two different ways: In the plasma membrane calcium pump, it remained a part of the pump where it responds to a calcium-activated signal, while in the sarcoplasmic reticulum, the homologous peptide became a separate protein that mediates a signal initiated by cyclic AMP.

Calcium-Binding Proteins within the Sarcoplasmic Reticulum

Much of the calcium taken up by the sarcoplasmic reticulum is associated with calcium-binding proteins found in the subsarcolemmal cisternae. The most important of the latter is *calsequestrin*, each molecule of which contains between 18 and 50 calcium-binding sites. Other calcium-binding proteins found in smaller amounts include a *histidine-rich calcium-binding protein*, *sarcalumenin*, and possibly *calreticulin*. Binding of calcium to these proteins maintains a low calcium concentration within the sarcoplasmic reticulum, which is important because increasing intraluminal calcium inhibits the calcium pump.

Two additional proteins, *triadin* and *junctin*, which bind calsequestrin to the calcium release channels, interact with calsequestrin to regulate the opening of these channels. The histidine-rich calcium-binding protein and sarcalumenin also regulate calcium release from the sarcoplasmic reticulum. All of these effects are controlled by phosphorylation reactions that are catalyzed by a number of protein kinases and, in the case of calsequestrin, by an intrinsic protein kinase activity. The finding that a clinical syndrome characterized by dangerous ventricular arrhythmias is associated with calsequestrin mutations (Lahat et al., 2001) may reflect an action of the abnormal protein to modify calcium release from the sarcoplasmic reticulum.

MITOCHONDRIA

Mitochondrial calcium uptake and release have been suggested to play a role in cardiac excitation–contraction coupling, but the low calcium affinity and slow turnover of the mitochondrial calcium pump make it unlikely that these energy-producing structures participate in the rapid changes of cytosolic calcium that occur during each cardiac cycle. Under abnormal conditions, however, the mitochondria can buffer cytosolic calcium so as to protect the myocardium from the detrimental effects of calcium overload. However, the ability of mitochondrial calcium uptake and storage to blunt some of these adverse effects in the energy-starved heart occurs at the cost of the impaired oxidative phosphorylation that accompanies calcium accumulation by mitochondria.

OVERVIEW OF THE TWO CALCIUM CYCLES THAT PARTICIPATE IN EXCITATION–CONTRACTION COUPLING AND RELAXATION

The calcium fluxes in the extracellular and intracellular calcium cycles (Fig. 7-20) involve five pools, or compartments; the *extracellular space, sarcoplasmic reticulum, cytosol, contractile proteins*, and *mitochondria* (Fig. 7-20A). The major calcium fluxes in the adult mammalian heart are shown in Figure 7-20B, where upward arrows represent active fluxes and downward arrows passive fluxes; the thickness of each arrow is roughly proportional to the amount of the calcium flux.

The Extracellular Calcium Cycle

As shown in Figure 7-20B, calcium influx across the plasma membrane is mediated by voltage-gated L-type calcium channels (arrow A), while active calcium efflux is effected by the plasma membrane calcium pump (arrow B1) and Na–Ca exchanger (arrow B2). The most important role of the calcium that enters the cytosol by way of the external calcium cycle is to open calcium release channels in the sarcoplasmic reticulum (calcium-triggered calcium release); only a small fraction binds directly to the contractile proteins (arrow A1).

The Intracellular Calcium Cycle

Also shown in Figure 7-20B, the calcium fluxes out of (arrow C), into (arrow D), and within (arrow G) the sarcoplasmic reticulum are much greater than those of the extracellular calcium cycle (arrows A, B1, and B2). The contractile proteins are activated when calcium binds to troponin C (arrow E), while the heart relaxes when lowering of cytosolic calcium concentration causes the activator to dissociate from the high-affinity EF-hand calcium binding sites on this protein (arrow F). The ability of mitochondria to buffer high cytosolic calcium levels is shown by the double arrow H, which is narrow because these calcium fluxes do not normally play an important role in excitation–contraction coupling.

IMPLICATIONS OF THE ENERGETICS OF CALCIUM CHANNELS AND CALCIUM PUMPS ON EXCITATION–CONTRACTION COUPLING AND RELAXATION IN THE HEART

Downhill ion flux through an ion channel is much more rapid than active transport by an ion pump; this is apparent when the velocity at which calcium ions pass through an intracellular calcium release channel is compared with that of calcium uptake by the calcium pump of the sarcoplasmic reticulum (Table 7-3). The downhill calcium flux can be calculated from the calcium conductance of the intracellular calcium release channels ($\sim$75 pS; Bers, 1991), which is about ten times faster than through an L-type calcium channel (5–9 pS; Tsien and Tsien, 1990). As the latter can carry approximately 75,000 calcium ions per second when extracellular calcium is 1 mM (calculated from data provided by Tsien, 1983), calcium flux into the cytosol through a single intracellular calcium release channel is nearly 750,000 ions per second, assuming that calcium concentration within the sarcoplasmic reticulum is also 1 mM.

The velocity of calcium uptake by each sarcoplasmic reticulum calcium pump, which has been measured directly, is only about 30 ions per

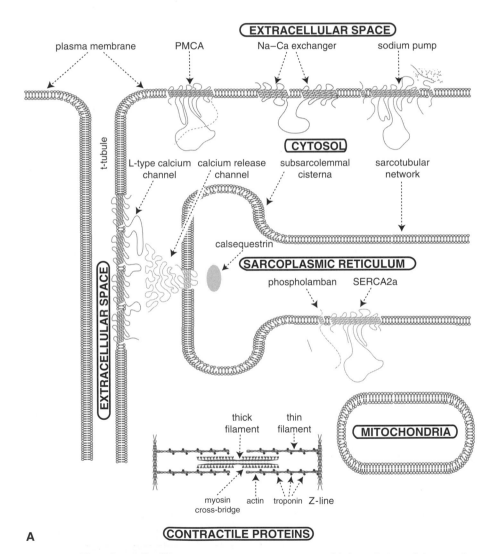

A

FIGURE 7-20 Schematic diagram showing extracellular and intracellular calcium cycles that control cardiac excitation–contraction coupling and relaxation. **A:** Major structures and calcium "pools" (*bold capital letters*).

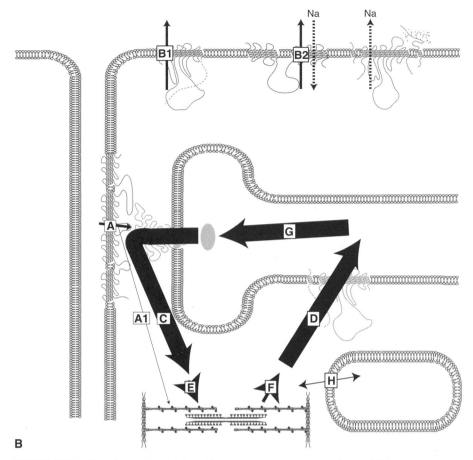

B

FIGURE 7-20 *(Continued)* **B:** Calcium fluxes, shown as arrows whose thickness indicates their magnitude and the vertical orientations describe their "energetics": *downward arrows* represent passive calcium fluxes, and *upward arrows* represent energy-dependent active calcium transport. Most of the calcium that enters the cell from the extracellular fluid by way of L-type calcium channels (*arrow* A) triggers calcium release from the sarcoplasmic reticulum; only a small portion directly activates the contractile proteins (*arrow* A1). Calcium is actively transported from the cytosol to the extracellular fluid by the plasma membrane calcium pump ATPase (PMCA, *arrow* B1) and exchanged for sodium by the Na–Ca exchanger (*arrow* B2). The sodium that enters the cell in exchange for calcium (*dashed line*) is pumped out of the cytosol by the sodium pump. Much larger calcium fluxes involve the sarcoplasmic reticulum. Most of the calcium that activates the contractile proteins crosses the subsarcolemmal cisternae calcium release channels (*arrow* C) and is taken up into the sarcotubular network by the sarco(endo)plasmic reticulum calcium pump ATPase (SERCA, *arrow* D). Calcium diffuses within the sarcoplasmic reticulum from the sarcotubular network to the subsarcolemmal cisternae (*arrow* G), where it is stored in a complex with calsequestrin and other calcium-binding proteins. Calcium binding to (*arrow* E) and dissociation from (*arrow* F) high-affinity calcium-binding sites of troponin C activate and inhibit the interactions of the contractile proteins. Calcium movements into and out of mitochondria (*arrow* H) buffer cytosolic calcium concentration. The extracellular calcium cycle is described by *arrows* A, B1, and B2, while *arrows* C, E, F, D, and G describe the intracellular calcium cycle.

TABLE 3 Comparison of Maximum Calcium Fluxes Rates Into and Out of Cardiac Sarcoplasmic Reticulum

Maximum calcium flux rates (ions/sec)	
Intracellular calcium release channel[a]	750,000
Sarcoplasmic reticulum calcium pump[b]	30
Maximum release rate per channel/Maximum uptake rate per pump	25,000
Content of pump and channel molecules (nmol/kg wet weight)[c]	
Sarcoplasmic reticulum calcium pump ATPase	6,000
Intracellular calcium release channels	36
Calcium pump ATPase molecules per calcium release channel	170
Maximum calcium flux ratio	
Maximal rate of calcium entry during systole/Maximal rate of calcium removal during diastole	~150

[a]Calculated from the calcium conductance of 0.025 pA for an L-type plasma membrane channel in 1 mM extracellular calcium, where a single channel current of 1 pA is equivalent to a flux of 3,000,000 divalent cations per second (Tsien, 1983) and the relative conductances of plasma membrane and intracellular calcium channels (Tsien and Tsien, 1990; Bers, 1991).
[b]Shigekawa et al., 1976.
[c]Bers, 1991.

second at 37° (Shigekawa et al., 1976). Even though the number of sarcoplasmic reticulum calcium pump molecules is nearly 170-fold greater than that of the intracellular calcium release channels in the heart (Bers, 1991), the large difference in maximum flux rates means that for the intracellular calcium cycle, the maximum rate of calcium delivery into the cytosol during systole is approximately 150 times faster than the maximum rate of calcium uptake into the sarcoplasmic reticulum during diastole (Table 7-3). This difference is much greater in the intact heart because cytosolic calcium concentration falls as the heart relaxes, which causes calcium uptake into the sarcoplasmic reticulum to slow significantly throughout diastole.

The differences between the rates of passive calcium diffusion into the cytosol and active calcium transport out of the cytosol illustrate the well-established precept that it is easier to get into trouble than out of trouble. One reason that it is "harder" for the heart to relax than to contract is that active transport is much slower than diffusion. Even the densely packed calcium pump proteins (Fig. 7-17), which resemble the army of terra-cotta soldiers in the underground tombs of Xian, cannot compensate for the much greater rate at which calcium diffuses into the cytosol through the smaller number of calcium release channels. These calculations are useful in understanding the rapid impairment of relaxation in the energy-starved heart.

Because increased cytosolic calcium concentration accelerates energy-consuming reactions, most important of which are the interactions between the contractile proteins, it is not difficult to understand how energy starvation can establish a vicious cycle that literally destroys the myocardium. These considerations explain why conditions that cause energy demand to exceed energy supply, such as those that occur in ischemia and heart failure, are so devastating to the cardiac patient.

BIBLIOGRAPHY

Beard NA, Laver DR, Dulhunty A.F Calsequestrin and the calcium release channel of skeletal and cardiac muscle. *Prog Biophys Mol Biol* 2004;85:3369.

Berridge MJ, Bootman MD, Rederick HL. Calcium signalling: Dynamics, homeostasis and remodelling. *Mol Cell Biol* 2003;4:517–529.

Bers DM. "Excitation-contraction coupling and cardiac contractile force, 2nd ed. Dordrecht: Kluwer, 2001.

Blanco G, Mercer RW. Isozymes of the Na-K-ATPase: heterogeneity in structure, diversity in function. *Am J Physiol* 1998;275:F633–F650.

Carafoli E. Biogenesis: plasma membrane calcium ATPase: 15 years of work on the purified enzyme. *FASEB J* 1994;8:993–1002.

DiPolo R, Beaugé L. Metabolic pathways in the regulation of invertebrate and vertebrate Na^+/Ca^{2+} exchange. *Biochim Biophys Acta* 1999;1422:57–71.

Egger M, Niggli E. Regulatory function of Na-Ca exchange in the heart: milestones and outlook. *J Memb Biol* 1999;168:107–130.

Fill M, Copello JA. Ryanodine calcium receptor calcium release channels. *Physiol Rev* 2002;82:893–922.

Fliegel L, Wang H. Regulation of the Na^+/H^+ exchanger in the mammalian myocardium. *J Mol Cell Cardiol* 1997;29:1991–1999.

Kaplan JH. Biochemistry of Na,K-ATPase. *Annu Rev Biochem* 2002;71:511–535.

Karmayzn M, Gan XT, Humphreys RA, et al. The myocardial Na^+/H^+ exchange. Structure, regulation, and its role in disease. *Circ Res* 1999;85:777–786.

MacLennan DH, Kranias EG. Phospholamban: a crucial regulator of cardiac contractility. *Nat Rev Mol Cell Biol* 2003;4:566–577.

Langer GA, ed. *The myocardium*, 2nd ed. San Diego: Academic Press, 1997.

Lehnart SE, Wehrens XHT, Kushnir A, et al. Cardiac ryanodine receptor function and regulation in heart disease. *Ann NY Acad Sci* 2004;1015:144–159.

Levi AJ, Boyett MR, Lee CO. The cellular actions of digitalis glycosides on the heart. *Prog Biophys Molec Biol* 1994;62:1–54.

Lingrel JB, Croyle ML, Woo AL, et al. Ligand binding sites of Na,K-ATPase. *Acta Physiol Scand* 1998;163[Suppl. 643]:69–77.

Orlowski J, Grinstein S. Diversity of the mammalian sodium/proton exchanger SLC9 gene family. *Pflugers Arch* 2004; 447:549–565. E-pub 2003.

Putney LK, Denker SP, Barber DL. The changing face of the Na^+/H^+ exchanger, NHE1: structure, regulation, and cellular actions. *Annu Rev Pharmacol Toxicol* 2002;42:527–552.

Rossi D, Sorrentino V. Molecular genetics of ryanodine receptors $Ca2^+$-release channels. *Cell Calcium* 2002;32:307–319.

Sachs G, ed. Symposium on ion motive ATPases. *Acta Physiol Scand* 1998;163. Suppl. 643.

Schillinger W, Fiolet JW, Schlotthauer K, et al. Relevance of $Na^+–Ca^{2+}$ exchange in heart failure. *Cardiovasc Res* 2003;57:921–933.

Wakabayashi S, Shigekawa M, Pouyssegur J. Molecular physiology of vertebrate Na^+/H^+ exchangers. *Physiol Rev* 1997;77:51–74.

Wang SQ, Wei C, Zhao G, et al. Imaging microdomain Ca2$^+$ in muscle cells. *Circ Res* 94: 1011–1022.

REFERENCES

Beil FU, von Chak D, Hasselbach W, et al. Competition between oxalate and phosphate during active calcium accumulation by sarcoplasmic vesicles. *Z Naturforsch* 1977;32:281–287.

Berridge M. The AM and FM of calcium signaling. *Nature* 1997;386:759–760.

Bers DM. *Excitation–contraction coupling and cardiac contractile force.* Dordrecht: Kluwer, 1991.

Bretscher A, Edwards K, Fehon RG. ERM proteins and merlin: integrators at the cell cortex. *Nat Rev Mol Cell Biol* 2002;3:586–599.

Ebashi S, Lipmann F. Adenosine triphosphate–linked concentration of calcium ions in a particulate fraction of rabbit muscle. *J Cell Biol* 1962;14:389–400.

Eisenberg B, Eisenberg RS. Transverse tubular system in glycerol-treated skeletal muscle. *Science* 1968;160:1243–1244.

Fabiato A. Calcium-induced release of calcium from the cardiac sarcoplasmic reticulum. *Am J Physiol* 1983;245:C1–C14.

Franzini-Armstrong C, Protasi F, Ramesh V. Shape, size, and distribution of Ca^{2+} release units and couplons in cardiac muscles. *Biophys J* 1999;77:1528–1539.

Gergely J. The relaxing factor of muscle. *Ann NY Acad Sci* 1959;81:490–504.

Harigaya S, Schwartz A. Rate of calcium binding and uptake in normal and failing human cardiac muscle. *Circ Res* 1969;25:781–794.

Hasselbach W, Makinose M. Die calciumpumpe der "ershlaffungsgrana" des muskels und ihre abhangigkeit von der ATP-spaltung. *Biochem Z* 1961;333:518–528.

Hill AV. The abrupt transition from rest to activity in muscle. *Proc Roy Soc B* 1949;136: 399–420.

Huxley AF, Taylor RE. Local activation of skeletal muscle fibres. *J Physiol (Lond)* 1958;44: 426–441.

Katz AM. Congestive heart failure: role of altered myocardial cellular control. *N Engl J Med* 1975;293:1184–1191.

Katz AM, Repke DI. Quantitative aspects of dog cardiac microsomal calcium binding and calcium uptake. *Circ Res* 1967;21:153–162.

Lahat H, Pras E, Olender T, et al. A missense mutation in a highly conserved region of CASQ2 is associated with autosomal recessive catecholamine-induced polymorphic ventricular tachycardia in Bedouin families from Israel. *Am J Hum Genet* 2001;69: 1378–1384.

Lüttgau HC, Niedergerke R. The antagonism between Ca and Na ions on the frog's heart. *J Physiol (Lond)* 1958;143:486–505.

Marger MD, Saier MH Jr. A major superfamily of transmembrane facilitators that catalyse uniport, symport and antiport. *Trends Biochem Sci* 1993;18:13–20.

Reithmeier RAF. Mammalian exchangers and co-transporters. *Curr Opin Cell Biol* 1994;6: 583–594.

Repke K. Über den biochemischen Wirkungsmodus von Digitalis. *Klin Wochschr* 1964;41: 156–165.

Reuter H, Seitz N. The dependence of calcium efflux from cardiac muscle on temperature and external ion composition. *J Physiol (Lond)* 1968;195:451–470.

Schätzmann HJ. Herzglykoside als hemmstoffe für den aktiven Kalium- und Natriumtransport durch die Erythrocytenmembran. *Helv Physiol Acta* 1953;11:346–354.

Shigekawa M, Finegan J AM, Katz AM. Calcium transport ATPase of canine cardiac sarcoplasmic reticulum. A comparison with that of rabbit fast skeletal muscle sarcoplasmic reticulum. *J Biol Chem* 1976;251:6894–6900.

Stern M, Song LS, Cheng H, et al. Local control models of cardiac excitation-contraction coupling. A possible role for allosteric interactions between ryanodine receptors. *J Gen Physiol* 1999;113:469–489.

Takenaka H, Adler PN, Katz AM. Calcium fluxes across the membrane of sarcoplasmic reticulum vesicles. *J Biol Chem* 1982;257:12649–12656.

Therien AG, Pu HX, Karlish SJD, et al. Molecular and functional studies of the gamma subunit of the sodium pump. *J Bioenerg Biomembr* 2001;33:407–414.

Tian R, Ingwall JS. Energetic basis for reduced contractile reserve in isolated rat hearts. *Am J Physiol* 1996;270 [*Heart Circ Physiol* 39]:H1207–H1216.

Tsien RW. Calcium channels in excitable cell membranes. *Ann Rev Physiol* 1983;45:341–358.

Tsien RW, Tsien RY. Calcium channels, stores, and oscillations. *Ann Rev Cell Biol* 1990;6:715–760.

Wang SQ, Wei C, Zhao G, et al. Imaging microdomain Ca^{2+} in muscle cells. *Circ Res* 2004;94:1011–1022.

Weber A, Winicur S. The role of calcium in the superprecipitation of actomyosin. *J Biol Chem* 1961;236:3198–3202.

Wilbrandt W, Koller H. Die Calcium-Wirkung am Froschherzen als Funktion des Ionengleichgewichts zwischen Zellmembran und Umgebung. *Helv Physiol Acta* 1948;6:208–221.

Signal Transduction and Regulation

8

SIGNAL TRANSDUCTION: FUNCTIONAL SIGNALING

The mechanisms that regulate cardiac function, like the pattern on a finely woven carpet, include intricacies and redundancies that help the body avoid the consequences of Murphy's Law, which states: "If anything can go wrong, it will; and at the worst possible time." However, failure of one or more of the body's components often produces few ill effects, and sometimes none, because in nature, Murphy's Law is balanced by another law: "If something is worth doing, many different mechanisms will see to it that this is done correctly." This law is well known to engineers, as seen in the construction of a modern airplane, where elaborate design and built-in redundancies prevent failure of any critical system from causing a crash. Similar redundancies, along with systems that integrate and fine-tune biological responses, operate in the heart.

Regulation of cardiac function depends on communications between the heart, the rest of the body, and the external environment. These communications are made possible by signaling systems that inform the heart that its function must be modified, and then enable the heart to mount an appropriate response. Biological signaling systems collect information from many sources to ensure smooth and appropriate responses that can be turned on when needed, operate at an appropriate intensity, and turn off when the need is over. These safeguards are made possible by interlocking controls that amplify signals, adjust responses to compensate for changes in signal intensity, and integrate one response with another. Although most biological responses are beneficial, at least initially, they can become deleterious when sustained.

Two different types of response adjust cardiovascular function to the changing needs of the body (Fig. 8-1). The first are the short-term *functional* responses to stimuli such as exercise and blood loss that develop rapidly, over a few seconds or minutes, and generally last no longer than a few minutes or hours. More prolonged *proliferative* (*transcriptional*) responses appear when the heart is overloaded—for example, by hypertension, an abnormality of a heart valve, or when myocardial infarction irreversibly damages part of the left ventricle. These responses, which evolve over a period of weeks, months, and often years, are mediated by

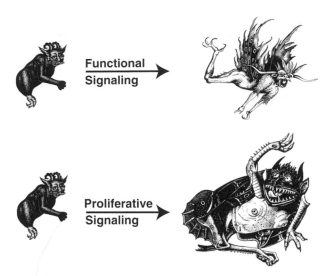

FIGURE 8-1 Functional and proliferative signaling. Functional signaling, which alters the properties of pre-existing structures by post-translational mechanisms, aids survival by modifying such responses as fight and flight. Proliferative signaling, on the other hand, allows the organism to grow out of trouble.

changes in gene expression and protein synthesis that alter the composition of myocardial cells and the structure of the heart.

FUNCTIONAL SIGNAL TRANSDUCTION

The most familiar cardiovascular response occurs during exercise, when the autonomic nervous system activates functional signaling pathways that act on the heart and blood vessels to maintain arterial blood pressure and increase blood flow to the exercising muscles. This response is due largely to increased sympathetic activity, which along with decreased parasympathetic activity, increases ventricular ejection and filling, accelerates heart rate, and causes peripheral vasoconstriction. Norepinephrine, which mediates these sympathetic responses, does not act directly to modify cardiovascular function, but instead activates multistep signaling cascades that resemble an old-fashioned bucket brigade (Fig. 8-2). However, unlike the bucket brigade, where a single substance (water) is passed from fireman to fireman, the steps in biological signaling cascades are mediated by different chemical reactions and signaling molecules (Fig. 8-2).

The first step in the response to sympathetic stimulation that increases myocardial contractility is norepinephrine release from sympathetic nerve endings at the surface of the heart (Fig. 8-2). The second step, binding of norepinephrine to the β-receptor, also takes place in the extracellular space, after which all of the remaining steps occur within the myocardial

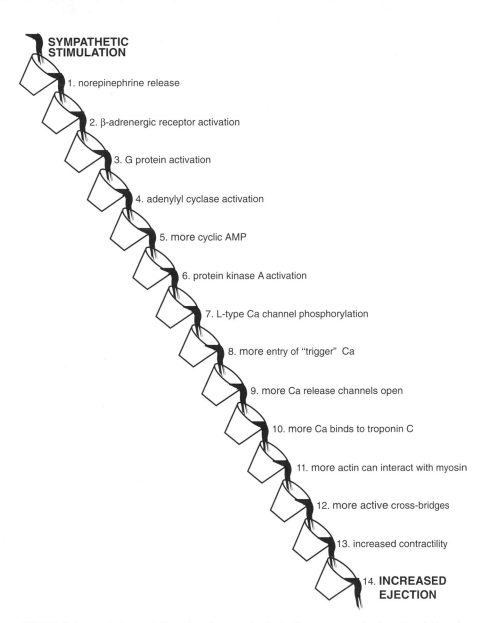

SYMPATHETIC STIMULATION

1. norepinephrine release

2. β-adrenergic receptor activation

3. G protein activation

4. adenylyl cyclase activation

5. more cyclic AMP

6. protein kinase A activation

7. L-type Ca channel phosphorylation

8. more entry of "trigger" Ca

9. more Ca release channels open

10. more Ca binds to troponin C

11. more actin can interact with myosin

12. more active cross-bridges

13. increased contractility

14. **INCREASED EJECTION**

FIGURE 8-2 Depiction of the signal cascade that allows sympathetic stimulation to increase ejection. The drawing shows fourteen steps as a series of buckets where, in each step, the incoming signal causes the bucket to pour its contents into the next bucket, thereby transmitting the signal down the cascade. The response begins when sympathetic stimulation releases norepinephrine from nerve endings at the surface of cardiac myocytes (step 1), after which this neurotransmitter binds to and activates β-adrenergic receptors (step 2). The remaining steps, which all take place within the myocardial cell, include activation of a G protein (step 3), activation of adenylyl cyclase activity (step 4), increased production of cyclic AMP (step 5), activation of a cyclic AMP–dependent protein kinase (step 6), phosphorylation of plasma membrane L-type calcium channels (step 7), increased calcium entry into the cell (step 8), increased opening of calcium release channels (step 9), increased calcium binding to troponin C (step 10), increased availability of actin in the thin filaments for interaction with myosin (step 11), participation of more cross-bridges in contraction (step 12), increased contractility (step 13), and a greater extent of ejection (step 14).

cell. These include G protein activation (step 3), which increases the catalytic activity of adenylyl cyclase (step 4), which generates cyclic AMP (3', 5'-cyclic adenosine monophosphate) (step 5), which activates a cyclic AMP– dependent protein kinase (PK-A, step 6), which catalyzes the phosphorylation of L-type calcium channels (step 7), which increases the entry of "trigger" calcium into the cytosol (step 8), which increases the opening of intracellular calcium release channels (step 9), which releases more calcium for binding to troponin C (step 10), which increases the number of exposed actin molecules in the thin filaments (step 11), which increases the number of actin-myosin interactions (step 12), which increases contractility (step 13), which increases the volume of blood ejected by the heart (step 14). Cascades similar to that in Figure 8-2, although different in detail, mediate virtually every signal that modifies cardiac function.

Why Are There So Many Steps in a Signal Transduction Cascade?

One might ask why there are so many steps between a challenge, like exercise, and a physiological response, like that depicted in Figure 8-2. The answer lies in the ability of biological signal transduction cascades, whose many steps might at first glance seem almost perverse, to enhance regulatory control. These cascades can amplify, inhibit, and fine-tune responses; integrate signal transduction cascades with one another; and prevent responses from going out of control ("runaway signaling") by allowing signals to turn themselves off automatically. In fact, the sequence of reactions depicted in Figure 8-2 is actually an oversimplification because most biological signaling pathways are not linear cascades, where each step is coupled to a single downstream reaction, but instead branch, loop forward and backward, interconnect with other pathways, and generate multiple signals at many steps. These intricacies organize responses that meet the needs of the organism by providing many options for amplification, fine-tuning, and negative feedback that integrate each step of the response with other steps in the cascade and with additional signaling systems. This fine-tuning would not be possible if cells generated only "all-or-none" responses.

One mechanism that regulates signal transduction is the allosteric effect ATP, which as noted in Chapter 7 generally accelerates ion fluxes through channels, pumps, and exchangers. This effect is important in the energy-starved heart, where a fall in ATP concentration inhibits several steps in the signaling cascade shown in Figure 8-2; these include the opening of L-type calcium channels in the plasma membrane (step 8), calcium release channels in the sarcoplasmic reticulum (step 9), and the interactions between actin and myosin (step 12). These and other allosteric effects of decreased ATP levels help match the rates of ATP production and ATP consumption by inhibiting contraction, the most expensive energy-consuming reaction in the heart. Acidosis, which occurs in the energy-starved heart (Chapter 2), also reduces energy consumption by inhibiting many steps in this cascade. A third example, which illustrates how a reaction near the "top" of a signaling pathway can respond to changes further down the cascade, occurs when increased calcium release into the cytosol (step 9) inhibits adenylyl cyclase (step 4); this negative feedback, by slowing the cascade, helps prevent calcium overload. Additional mechanisms that avoid calcium overload include regulatory effects of increased cytosolic calcium that accelerate calcium transport out of the cytosol by plasma membrane and sarcoplasmic reticulum calcium pumps and the sodium–calcium exchanger (Chapter 7).

Biological signal transduction cascades often allow a single stimulus to evoke an integrated, multifaceted response. For example, the elevated level of cyclic AMP (step 5 in Fig. 8-2) increases the rate and extent of relaxation when phosphorylation of phospholamban accelerates calcium uptake into the sarcoplasmic reticulum (Chapter 7). Another example of signal diversification occurs at step 3 in Figure 8-2, where norepinephrine binding to a single β_1-receptor activates both $G_{\alpha s}$ and $G_{\beta \gamma}$, each of which can modify a different downstream target (see below).

Control of cell function is further enhanced by the large number of isoforms of many signaling molecules. For example, binding of norepinephrine to β_1- and β_2-receptors in the heart evokes different responses, while in vascular smooth muscle, binding to α_1-receptors causes vasoconstriction, whereas β-receptor activation has a relaxing effect.

NEUROHUMORAL RESPONSES AND THE HEMODYNAMIC DEFENSE REACTION

Adaptation to changes in the external world is made possible by neurohumoral responses that stabilize the environment within our bodies, which Claude Bernard called the *milieu intèrieur*. Among of the most important of these responses is a *hemodynamic defense reaction* that evokes regulatory responses that compensate for a fall in arterial blood pressure by modifying the function of the heart, blood vessels, and kidneys. As detailed in a brilliant essay by Peter Harris (1983), exercise, hemorrhage, and chronic heart failure all evoke a similar response (Table 8-1). In *exercise*, where arterial blood pressure falls because vasodilatation in the active muscles reduces peripheral resistance, the hemodynamic defense reaction restores blood pressure by stimulating the heart and constricting the arterioles supplying nonexercising tissues such as the gut and kidneys. In *shock*, whose most obvious manifestation is a marked fall in arterial pressure, cardiac stimulation and selective vasoconstriction also help maintain blood pressure; in this case, the response is supplemented by thirst and fluid retention by the kidneys. In *heart failure*, a chronic condition where impaired cardiac pumping reduces arterial blood pressure, the hemodynamic defense reaction also stimulates the heart and causes vasoconstriction and fluid retention. Most features of these regulatory responses are adaptive when called upon to meet a short-term

TABLE 8-1 Three Conditions That Evoke the Hemodynamic Defense Reaction

Condition	Duration	Challenge	Response
Exercise	Minutes/hours	Increased blood flow to exercising muscles	Cardiac stimulation, selective vasoconstriction
Shock	Hours	Loss of vascular volume (e.g., hemorrhage, fluid loss	Cardiac stimulation, vasoconstriction, fluid retention
Heart failure	Lifetime (progressive)	Impaired pumping by a damaged or overloaded heart	Cardiac stimulation, vasoconstriction, fluid retention

challenge like exercise or hemorrhage, but become maladaptive in heart failure, where the problem is a long-term reduction in the output of the heart (Table 8-2).

Exercise

At least four mechanisms allow exercise to initiate a neurohumoral response (Table 8-3). Most important is the *baroreceptor reflex* that increases sympathetic activity and reduces parasympathetic tone when vasodilatation in the exercising muscles causes arterial blood pressure to fall. This reflex is initiated when reduced stretch on the walls of baroreceptors located at the bifurcation of the common carotid artery and in the

TABLE 8-2 The Hemodynamic Defense Reaction

Mechanism	Short-Term Adaptive Effects	Long-Term Maladaptive Effects
Increased cardiac adrenergic drive	↑ Contractility ⎱ *Increase* ↑ Relaxation ⎰ *cardiac* ↑ Heart Rate ⎰ *output*	↑ Cytosolic calcium ↑ Cardiac energy demand

Vasoconstriction	Arteriolar constriction
	  ↑ Blood pressure
	Venous constriction
	  ↑ Blood flow to the heart
	  ↑ Cardiac output
		↓ Cardiac output
		↑ Cardiac energy demand
		↑ Cardiac energy demand

Fluid retention	↓ Sodium and water excretion
	  ↑ Blood flow to the heart
	  ↑ Cardiac output
		Edema, pulmonary congestion

TABLE 8-3 Mechanisms by Which Exercise Activates Neurohumoral Responses

Baroreceptor reflex (carotid and aortic sinus reflexes): reduced baroreceptor stretch
Brain stem: autonomic center activation by exercising muscle
Cerebral cortex: anticipation of exercise
Metabolic: chemoreceptor stimulation by hypercapnia and acidosis

aortic arch stimulates autonomic centers in the *brain stem*. These autonomic centers also are stimulated by nerve impulses that arise in the exercising muscles. A third response, which is mediated by the *cerebral cortex*, often begins before the start of exercise—for example, when a trained dog on a treadmill sees the experimenter's hand move to the switch that turns on the machine, or when a sprinter hears the starter's gun. The fourth mechanism, *chemoreceptor stimulation*, increases sympathetic outflow when CO_2 and lactic acid released by the exercising muscles are sensed by chemoreceptors near the carotid sinuses and aortic arch.

CARDIAC STIMULATION AND VASOCONSTRICTION. The short-term neurohumoral response evoked by exercise is mediated largely by the heart and blood vessels (Table 8-1). Cardiac output (the volume of blood ejected by the heart per minute) is increased by an inotropic effect that increases systolic ejection, a lusitropic effect that augments diastolic filling, and a chronotropic effect that accelerates heart rate (Table 8-2) (see Chapter 10). The inotropic and lusitropic effects operate together to increase stroke volume (the volume of blood ejected during each heart beat), while the chronotropic effect increases heart rate (the number of beats per minute). Sympathetic stimulation also causes vasoconstriction; in arterial resistance vessels, this response increases resistance in vascular beds not dilated by exercise, which helps maintain blood pressure, while constriction of the large veins increases the return of blood to the heart.

Shock

Shock is a clinical syndrome, usually lasting no more than a few hours, in which the most obvious abnormality is low blood pressure; however, the major pathophysiological consequence of this syndrome is inadequate tissue perfusion. This syndrome has several causes (Table 8-4); the easiest to understand is *hypovolemic shock*, which occurs when the volume of blood in the systemic arteries becomes drastically reduced—for example, after hemorrhage or when the capillary endothelium becomes leaky because of extensive burns, vasculitis, or an endotoxin. Hypovolemic shock also can be caused by fluid loss in patients with severe diarrhea or cholera. Another type of shock is *distributive shock*, which can be caused by extensive vasodilatation; in these patients, there is enough blood in the vasculature,

TABLE 8-4 **Causes of Shock**

Hypovolemic Shock: too little blood in the vascular system

Blood loss: hemorrhage

Fluid loss: endothelial damage (burns, vasculitis, endotoxin), excessive fluid loss (diarrhea)

Distributive Shock: enough blood in the vascular system but in wrong place; veins not arteries

Sepsis: vasodilator actions of endotoxins (toxic shock, gram negative septicemia)

Reflex: vasovagal syncope (swoon), von Bezoldt–Jarisch reflex (inferior myocardial infarction)

Cardiogenic Shock: acute failure of the left ventricle

Acute myocardial infarction: left ventricular damage

Other: arrhythmias, valve rupture, pulmonary embolus, pericardial tamponade, acute myocarditis

but it is in the wrong place (i.e., the veins rather than the arteries). Distributive shock can be caused by vasodilator actions of endotoxins (e.g., toxic shock, gram negative septicemia), reflex vasodilatation (vasovagal syncope, which is the old fashioned "swoon"), and the von Bezoldt–Jarisch reflex, which can be activated in patients with inferior or posterior myocardial infarction (Chapter 17). A third type of shock, *cardiogenic shock*, also is seen after myocardial infarction, but in this case, the cause is reduced ejection that occurs when the left ventricle is severely damaged. Other causes of cardiogenic shock include arrhythmias, valve rupture, pulmonary embolus, pericardial tamponade, and acute myocarditis.

Most patients can recover from shock if the underlying cause is reversible and appropriate treatment is started promptly. Unfortunately, shock can become irreversible if treatment is delayed; these patients are doomed to die, even if blood pressure is restored, because of severe tissue damage.

FLUID RETENTION. Prolonged underfilling of the arteries causes fluid retention by the kidneys, the third major component of the hemodynamic defense reaction. Although this response is of little importance during exercise, except to reduce the need to void urine that would slow a runner, it is adaptive in patients with shock because it helps maintain cardiac output by restoring blood volume. In patients with heart failure, on the other hand, fluid retention becomes a serious problem because increased return of blood to a diseased heart can do little to increase its output; instead, the increased blood volume only adds to the already elevated systemic and pulmonary venous pressures, which increase fluid transudation into the lungs, peripheral tissues, and body cavities (Chapter 18).

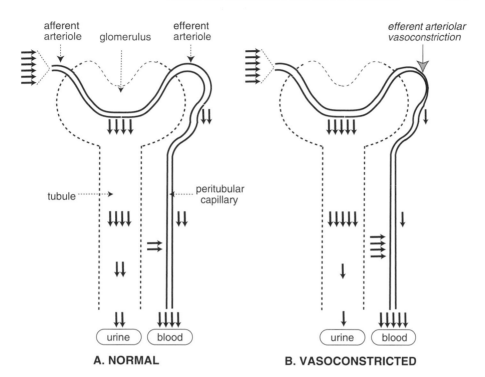

A. NORMAL   **B. VASOCONSTRICTED**

FIGURE 8-3 Effect of renal efferent artery constriction on fluid excretion. **A:** Under normal conditions, much of the salt and water (*heavy arrows*) that enters the afferent arterioles supplying the glomeruli is filtered into the glomerulus and excreted in the urine. **B:** Vasoconstriction of the efferent arterioles leading out of the glomeruli increases the amount of salt and water filtered by the glomeruli. Although this causes more fluid to enter the tubules, a greater fraction of this fluid is reabsorbed because the increased glomerular filtration reduces oncotic pressure in the fluid within the tubules and increases oncotic pressure in the peritubular capillaries. Fluid resorption from the tubules also is increased by increased hydrostatic pressure in the tubules and decreased hydrostatic pressure in the peritubular capillaries. Together, these changes in oncotic and hydrostatic pressures cause salt and water retention. Heavy arrows indicate fluid movements.

The major causes of fluid retention in the hemodynamic defense reaction are renal artery constriction, increased sodium reabsorption by the renal tubules, and increased water reabsorption by the collecting ducts. Selective constriction of the renal efferent arterioles increases glomerular filtration rate (GFR) by increasing the pressure within the glomeruli (Fig. 8-3). Because the glomerular membrane is impermeable to the proteins that maintain plasma oncotic pressure, increased glomerular filtration promotes fluid retention from the tubules by reducing the oncotic pressure of the fluid that enters the renal tubules and increasing the oncotic pressure of the blood leaving the glomeruli to perfuse the peritubular capillaries. Efferent arteriolar constriction also increases fluid resorption by raising the hydrostatic pressure transmitted from within the glomeruli to the tubular lumen, and lowering the hydrostatic pressure in the peritubular capillaries.

TABLE 8-5 **Regulatory and Counterregulatory Neurohumoral Responses**

A. Regulatory Responses
Functional responses
Increased myocardial contractility, accelerated relaxation, faster heart rate
Vasoconstriction
Fluid retention by the kidneys
Proliferative responses
Stimulate cell growth and proliferation
B. Counterregulatory Responses
Functional responses
Decreased myocardial contractility, slowed relaxation, slower heart rate
Vasodilatation
Diuresis
Proliferative responses
Inhibit cell growth and proliferation

REGULATORY AND COUNTERREGULATORY RESPONSES

The signaling systems that participate the neurohumoral responses to a fall in blood pressure evoke complex and often opposing responses. These include the *regulatory responses* described above, which help restore blood pressure, and *counterregulatory responses*, whose effects on the heart and blood vessels oppose the dominant regulatory responses (Table 8-5). This apparent paradox, which reflects the ability of many extracellular messengers to activate different receptor subtypes that generate opposing responses, illustrates the principle that biological signaling systems often include mechanisms that avoid runaway signaling limiting responses.

EXTRACELLULAR SIGNALING MOLECULES

The ability of chemical mediators to regulate cardiovascular function was discovered in 1894, when Oliver and Schäfer found that injection of adrenal extracts increased heart rate in anaesthetized cats. A decade later, Elliott suggested that the response to sympathetic nerve stimulation, whose effects resemble those of adrenal extracts, might also be mediated by a chemical messenger. However, it was not until 1921 that Otto Loewi carried out a remarkable but simple experiment which proved conclusively that a chemical can mediate a neural response—in this case, to vagal stimulation. Earlier efforts to isolate a chemical mediator had proven fruitless because, as is now known, the neurotransmitter released by vagal stimulation is inactivated very rapidly. Loewi overcame this problem by placing two frog hearts a short distance apart in a slowly moving stream of Ringer's solution. When he stimulated the vagus nerve supplying the upstream heart, not only did this heart slow, but the rate of beating also decreased in the unstimulated downstream heart. In contrast, stimulation of the vagus nerve supplying the downstream heart had no effect on the upstream heart. This elegant experiment proved that vagal stimulation releases a chemical that slows the heart; Loewi, who initially called this chemical *vagusstoff*, subsequently identified the mediator as *acetylcholine*.

In the 1930s, Cannon and Rosenblueth showed that sympathetic stimulation, whose effects resemble those caused by adrenal extracts, also releases a chemical mediator. This was subsequently shown to be a *catecholamine* similar to *epinephrine* (adrenaline), which had previously been isolated from the adrenal medulla. Shortly after World War II, von Euler showed that the sympathetic neurotransmitter was *norepinephrine*, which differs from epinephrine only in the absence of a methyl group.

A large and diverse group of signaling molecules is now known to regulate the heart and blood vessels; these include peptides, amines, steroid hormones, fatty acid derivatives, and even a highly reactive gas. Because these chemical mediators originate outside of cells, they can be viewed as *extracellular messengers*.

INTERACTIONS BETWEEN EXTRACELLULAR MESSENGERS AND THEIR RECEPTORS

Extracellular messengers are frequently called *ligands* because they bind tightly and with high specificity to *receptors* that recognize their presence as a signal to modify cell function. Most physiological ligands, as well as the majority of clinically useful drugs, contain hydrophilic moieties that prevent these molecules from crossing the lipid barrier in biological membranes (Chapter 1). For this reason, their cellular actions depend on interactions with receptors on the extracellular surface of the plasma membrane. Exceptions include steroid and thyroid hormones, which are hydrophobic molecules that can enter the cytosol to interact with intracellular receptors.

The concept of specific receptors originated when Ahlquist (1948) found that epinephrine can be a vasodilator at low concentrations and a vasoconstrictor at high concentrations, whereas norepinephrine is almost always a powerful vasoconstrictor. These and other observations led Ahlquist to postulate that the response to an extracellular messenger is determined when it is recognized by a specific receptor. To explain why low concentrations of epinephrine relax blood vessels and high concentrations cause vasoconstriction, Ahlquist suggested that it could bind to two types of receptor: one, which he called the α-receptor, mediates the constrictor action seen at high epinephrine concentrations; the other, which he called the β-receptor, was postulated to have a higher affinity for epinephrine and therefore would be responsible for the vasodilator response to low concentrations of this catecholamine. Elucidation of the structures

TABLE 8-6 **Routes by Which Extracellular Messengers Reach Cells**

Endocrine (hormonal) signaling: The extracellular messenger is generated by a distant cell and delivered via the bloodstream to the cell whose function is altered.
Neurotransmitter signaling: The extracellular messenger is generated by a nerve that releases the ligand at the surface of the cell whose function is altered.
Paracrine signaling: The extracellular messenger is generated by a nearby cell and reaches the cell whose function is altered by diffusion through the extracellular fluid.
Autocrine signaling: An extracellular messenger is released into the extracellular fluid by the cell whose function is altered.

of these and other receptor molecules, and the demonstration that different signal transduction pathways are activated when an extracellular messenger interacts with different receptors, have proven Ahlquist's hypothesis to be correct.

Routes by Which Ligands Gain Access to Their Receptors

Extracellular messengers were initially believed to reach their target cells through the bloodstream (*endocrine* or *hormonal signaling*) or from nearby nerve endings (*neurotransmitter signaling*) (Table 8-6). It is now clear, however, that these signaling molecules commonly reach their receptors by shorter routes; in *paracrine signaling*, an extracellular messenger released by one cell diffuses to a receptor on a nearby cell, while in *autocrine signaling*, a cell modifies its own function by releasing a ligand that binds to a receptor on its surface. Signaling by *cytoskeletal proteins*, which allows cells to respond to interactions with neighboring cells or the surrounding extracellular matrix (Chapter 5), resembles paracrine signaling, even though the signal is not transmitted when a small molecule binds to a receptor. This reflects the fact that many cytoskeletal proteins contain signaling modules that are homologous to those found in receptor proteins.

Most extracellular messengers, as well as the majority of clinically useful drugs, are amphipathic molecules that contain both hydrophilic and hydrophobic moieties. Because of the latter, these molecules have a high *partition coefficient*, a variable that quantifies their distribution between the lipid bilayer and the surrounding aqueous medium. For example, when cells in an aqueous medium encounter 10,001 molecules with a partition coefficient of 10,000, 10,000 of the latter will enter the membrane bilayer, leaving only one in the aqueous medium. Because of their hydrophobicity, many extracellular messengers and drugs gain access to plasma membrane receptors by first dissolving in the lipid bilayer and then diffusing to their receptors (Herbette and Mason, 1991). Utilization of this lipid pathway explains why the ligand- and drug-binding sites of many intrinsic membrane proteins include hydrophobic regions of the membrane-spanning α-helices within the lipid core of the bilayer.

Characterization of Receptors: Ligand-Binding Affinity and Number

The interactions between a ligand and its receptor can be characterized in terms of the *number* of receptors and the *affinity* of the receptor for the ligand. Receptor number can be quantified by measuring B_{max}, the maximal amount of ligand that binds specifically to a membrane receptor. The simplest index of the affinity of a receptor for its ligand is the *dissociation constant* (k_d), which is the ligand concentration at which 50% of receptors are bound to the ligand, so the greater the affinity of the receptor for the ligand, the lower will be the k_d. K_d also is a measure of the ratio between the rate of ligand dissociation from its receptor (the "off-rate") and the rate of binding of the ligand (the "on-rate"). The affinity of the receptor for a ligand also can be expressed as an *association (binding) constant* (k_b), the reciprocal of the dissociation constant (k_d), which is the ratio between the on-rate and the off-rate. Affinities for different ligands vary widely; some peptides bind to their receptors at concentrations below 10^{-12} M, while most neurohumoral transmitters and drugs occupy their receptors at concentrations between 10^{-8} and 10^{-6} M. A few compounds, like ethanol, interact with membranes at much higher concentrations (Table 8-7).

Binding affinity is an important determinant of the specificity of the response to a drug; as would be expected, a drug that binds to its receptor at low concentrations (high affinity) usually evokes a specific response that is accompanied by few side effects. This is easily understood because the high-binding affinity allows low concentrations of the drug to be

TABLE 8-7 Ligand-Binding Affinities of Some Cardiac Plasma Membrane Receptors

Ligand	Receptor	Approximate K_d[a]
Tetrodotoxin[b]	Sodium channel	10^{-12} M
Nitrendipine[c]	Calcium channel	10^{-10} M
Epinephrine	β-adrenergic receptor	10^{-8} M
Ouabain[d]	Sodium pump	10^{-6} M
Ethanol	Nonspecific	10^{-3} M

[a]K_d, the dissociation constant, is the ligand concentration at which one-half of the receptors are occupied, so a lower K_d means that the ligand binds more tightly to its receptor.
[b]A peptide toxin from puffer fish.
[c]A dihydropyridine calcium channel blocker.
[d]A cardiac glycoside.

recognized by the receptor, thereby minimizing drug interactions with other components of the cell. Drugs that act only at high concentrations, and so bind to their receptors with low affinity, often have additional, non-specific actions. Except for side effects caused by allergic or sensitivity reactions (which generally depend little on the concentration of the ligand), the toxic effects of clinically useful drugs occur at concentrations higher than are needed to produce the desired therapeutic effects. This can be described as a "toxic–therapeutic ratio," which is the ratio of the drug concentrations at which these two effects appear; the greater this ratio, the less likely is the drug to cause side effects at doses that yield desirable therapeutic effects.

The affinity of a receptor for its ligand sometimes decreases when the ligand binds to its receptor. This change results from an allosteric effect that, by blunting the response to the ligand, allows activation of the signaling pathway to inhibit the ability of the receptor to bind the ligand.

Receptor Blockade

Characterization of specific receptors made it possible to design drugs that could inhibit their ability to interact with their ligands. Such inhibitors, often called *antagonists* or simply *blockers*, usually have structures similar to those of the physiological extracellular messengers. The inhibitory effects of these drugs exhibit competitive kinetics and can be reversed by high concentrations of the physiological ligand. A few drugs inactivate a signal transduction system completely and permanently; aspirin, for example, irreversibly acetylates *cyclooxygenase*, an enzyme that generates a thrombogenic prostaglandin (see below).

The difference between a receptor blocker (antagonist) and the physiological ligand (agonist) is not where these molecules bind, but what happens after binding has occurred. Unlike an agonist, which activates the subsequent steps in a signal transduction cascade (e.g., after step 1 in Fig. 8-2), antagonists occupy the receptor but do not generate an intracellular signal. The clinical value of an antagonist (e.g., a β-blocker) therefore reflects the fact that once bound to the receptor, it inhibits its ability to bind to, and thus to be activated by, the physiological ligand (e.g., norepinephrine).

Not all drugs that interact with receptors can be classified simply as agonists and antagonists. Some drugs, called *partial agonists*, bind to a receptor where they cause a weak activation of its signal transduction cascade, while at the same time blocking the ability of the receptor to interact with the more potent physiological agonists. In the case of the β blockers, the weak stimulatory effect of a partial agonist is referred to as *intrinsic sympathomimetic activity* (ISA). By blocking the more potent effects of norepinephrine, partial β-adrenergic agonists inhibit the response to surges of sympathetic activity while providing a low level of adrenergic stimulation in the basal state. Unfortunately, many partial agonists have turned out to be less advantageous clinically than this description might suggest.

TABLE 8-8 Receptors and Extracellular Messengers That Modify Cardiac Function

G Protein–Coupled Receptors	Enzyme-Linked Receptors
Catecholamine	*Tyrosine kinase receptors*
Epinephrine and norepinephrine	Fibroblast growth factor (FGF)
Dopamine	Platelet-derived growth factor (PDGF)
Peptide	Insulinlike growth factor (IGF)
Angiotensin II	Vascular endothelial growth factor (VEGF)
Bradykinin	
Arginine vasopressin (ADH)	*Serine–threonine kinase receptors*
Endothelin	Transforming growth factor-β (TGF-β)
Neuropeptide Y	
Other	*Receptor guanylyl cyclases*
Acetylcholine	Natriuretic peptides
Adenosine	*Cytokine receptors*
Prostaglandins	Tumor necrosis factor α (TNF-α)
Nuclear Receptors	Interleukins
Aldosterone	Growth hormone
Thyroxin	**Direct Binding to an Intracellular Target**
Ion Channel–Linked Receptors	
Agmatine	Nitric oxide (NO)
	Agmatine

Types of Receptor

Many different types of receptor allow a variety of ligands to modify cardiovascular function (Table 8-8). Most functional signals are mediated by *G protein–coupled receptors*, which are named for the heterotrimeric GTP-binding proteins that mediate their cellular actions (see below). *Enzyme-linked receptors* contain an intracellular enzyme whose activity is modified when the receptor binds to its ligand; these receptors usually mediate proliferative responses, although some participate in functional signaling. *Cytokine receptors*, which are sometimes included among the enzyme-linked receptors, lack intrinsic catalytic activity but form aggregates with intracellular enzymes whose activity is modified when the receptor binds to a cytokine. *Ion channel–linked receptors* contain channels that are opened when the receptor binds its ligand, while *nuclear receptors*, which are found within cells, bind to hormones like aldosterone and thyroxin, whose hydrophobic structure allows them to cross the plasma membrane. The responses to nitric oxide, a gas that readily crosses the plasma membrane, are not mediated by a receptor; instead, this signaling molecule binds directly to guanylyl cyclase, its target enzyme.

TABLE 8-9 Some Important G Protein–Coupled Receptors in the Cardiovascular System

Ligand	Receptor	"Target"	G_α Isoform	Second Messenger/ Effector
α-Agonists	α-adrenergic	phospholipase C	$G_{\alpha q}$	diacylglycerol, InsP$_3$ (↑)
β-Agonists	β-adrenergic	adenylyl cyclase (↑)	$G_{\alpha s}$	cAMP (↑)
Acetylcholine	muscarinic	K channel	$G_{\alpha o}$	outward K current (↑)
Acetylcholine	muscarinic	adenylyl cyclase (↓)	$G_{\alpha i}$	cAMP (↓)
Adenosine	purinergic (P$_1$)	K channel	$G_{\alpha o}$	outward K current (↑)
Adenosine	purinergic (P$_1$)	adenylyl cyclase (↓)	$G_{\alpha i}$	cAMP (↓)
Angiotensin II	angiotensin (AT$_1$)	phospholipase C	$G_{\alpha q}$	diacylglycerol, InsP$_3$ (↑)
Endothelin	endothelin	phospholipase C	$G_{\alpha q}$	diacylglycerol, InsP$_3$ (↑)

InsP$_3$, inositol 1,4,5-trisphosphate; ↑, increased; ↓, decreased.

G PROTEIN–COUPLED RECEPTORS. The most important regulators of cardiovascular function are members of the family of *G protein–coupled receptors* (GPCR) (Table 8-9) that interact with the heterotrimeric *guanyl nucleotide–binding proteins* (*G proteins*) described below. This family, which includes sensory receptors such as rhodopsin, is among the largest in biology and includes more than 1,000 different proteins; approximately one in 80 human genes is estimated to encode members of this class of receptors (Clapham and Neer, 1997).

G protein–coupled receptors contain seven membrane-spanning α-helices (Fig. 8-4). The ligand-binding sites, which face the extracellular surface of the plasma membrane, include hydrophobic regions of these helices. The G protein–binding sites that lie within the cytosol include the large intracellular loop and portions of the membrane-spanning α-helices.

ENZYME-LINKED RECEPTORS. Binding of an *enzyme-linked receptor* to its ligand activates an intracellular enzyme, usually a protein kinase, that is part of the receptor molecule. This family of receptors includes *tyrosine kinase receptors*, which contain a catalytic site that phosphorylates tyrosine moieties in a variety of proteins; *serine–threonine kinase receptors*, whose catalytic site phosphorylates serine or threonine; *receptor guanylyl cyclases* that synthesize cyclic GMP (guanosine monophosphate); and *phosphatases*, which catalyze dephosphorylations. *Cytokine receptors*, which as noted above generally lack enzymatic activity, form aggregates

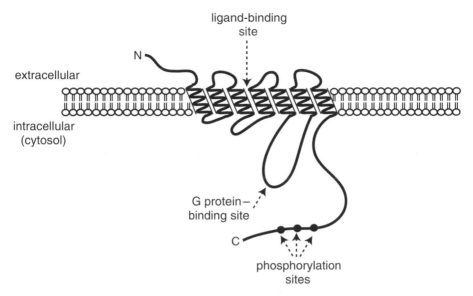

FIGURE 8-4 A G protein–coupled membrane receptor showing the seven membrane spanning α-helices, portions of which contribute to the ligand-binding site. Sites that bind the heterotrimeric G proteins are located on the intracellular peptide chain that links the fifth and sixth membrane-spanning helices. Phosphorylation of the C-terminal intracellular peptide chain participates in receptor desensitization.

with proteins whose latent tyrosine kinase activity is activated when the receptor binds to a cytokine.

ION CHANNEL–LINKED RECEPTORS. Some receptors include channels that are opened when the receptor binds to its ligand. These *ion channel–linked (ionotropic) receptors* include the nicotinic receptors found at the neuromuscular junction in skeletal muscles, where binding of acetylcholine generates a depolarizing sodium current that activates the motor end-plate (this receptor differs from the muscarinic receptors that mediate the effects of acetylcholine on the heart and vasculature, which are G protein–coupled receptors). Ion channel–linked receptors also mediate central responses to a variety of small molecules including agmatine, glutamine, serotonin, and γ-amino butyric acid.

NUCLEAR RECEPTORS. Lipophilic hormones, such as thyroxin and aldosterone, modify cardiovascular function after they bind to nuclear receptors within cells. When bound to their ligand, these receptors are transported to the nucleus, where they participate in proliferative signaling.

The following discussion highlights the G protein–coupled receptors, which are the most important mediators of functional signals in the heart and blood vessels; the enzyme-linked and nuclear receptors, whose major role is in proliferative signaling, are described in Chapter 9.

G PROTEIN–COUPLED RECEPTORS AND HETEROTRIMERIC GTP-BINDING PROTEINS (G PROTEINS)

When bound to their ligands, G protein–coupled receptors activate pathways whose cellular "targets" include enzymes that synthesize intracellular second messengers, protein kinases, and voltage-gated potassium channels (Table 8-9). The responses to these receptors are mediated by members of a family of heterotrimeric *GTP-binding proteins* (*G proteins*) that include one member of each of three protein families: G_α, which contains a bound guanine nucleotide; G_β; and G_γ. These *coupling proteins* generate two G protein–mediated signals when an extracellular messenger binds to the receptor; one signal is carried by G_α, the other by the $G_{\beta\gamma}$ dimer. The rich signaling diversity made possible by this coupling system reflects the hundreds of G protein–coupled receptors that interact with at least 23 G_α subunits, 6 G_β subunits, and 12 G_γ subunits.

There are four families of G_α subunits: $G_{\alpha s}$, $G_{\alpha i/o}$, $G_{\alpha q/11}$, and $G_{\alpha 12/13}$. Three are important in cardiovascular regulation: $G_{\alpha s}$ is involved in stimulatory responses such as activation of adenylyl cyclase by norepinephrine; $G_{\alpha o}$ and $G_{\alpha i}$ mediate potassium channel activation and inhibition of cyclic AMP production by muscarinic and purinergic agonists; and $G_{\alpha q}$ participates in signaling cascades that activate phospholipase C (Table 8-9).

Many ligand-bound G protein–coupled receptors interact with only one G_α to generate a tightly focused signal, but a single receptor can often activate several G_α subtypes as well as a $G_{\beta\gamma}$ dimer to activate several signal transduction cascades. Ligand binding to a single receptor can activate as many as ten different G_α subunits, including members of all four families (Laugwitz et al., 1996).

Interactions Between G Protein–Coupled Receptors and Heterotrimeric G Proteins

The interactions between a G protein–coupled receptor, its ligand, and the heterotrimeric G proteins can be described by the five-step sequence depicted schematically in Figure 8-5.

STEP 1: Binding of the ligand to its receptor and activation of G_α: Free (inactive) receptors, whose ligand-binding sites are unoccupied (Fig. 8-5A), are bound to the G protein trimer ($G_{\alpha\beta\gamma}$), which increases the affinity of the unoccupied receptor (R) for its ligand (L). Binding of the ligand to the receptor initiates the first step in the activation sequence (Fig. 8-5B):

$$R\text{-}G_\alpha\text{-}GDP\text{-}G_{\beta\gamma} + L \rightarrow R\text{-}L\text{-}G_\alpha\text{-}GDP\text{-}G_{\beta\gamma}$$

STEP 2: Formation of G_α-GTP and dissociation of $G_{\beta\gamma}$: After the ligand binds to the receptor–G protein complex, the guanosine diphosphate (GDP) bound to G_α is exchanged for GTP, which forms the activated G_α-GTP complex and releases activated $G_{\beta\gamma}$ (Fig. 8-5C), which can interact with its targets ($T_{\beta\gamma}$).

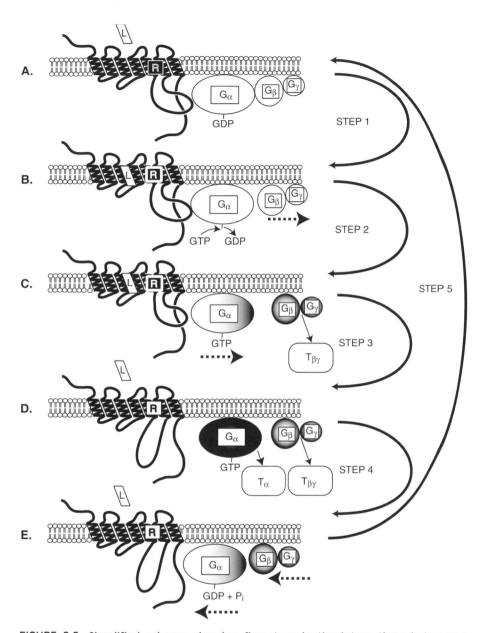

FIGURE 8-5 Simplified scheme showing five steps in the interactions between a G protein–coupled receptor, its ligand, and the heterotrimeric G proteins. Active states of these proteins are shaded. **A:** In the basal state, where the receptor (R) is not bound to its ligand (L), G_α is bound to GDP, the $G_{\beta\gamma}$ dimer, and the receptor in a R-L-G_α-GDP-$G_{\beta\gamma}$ complex. The $G_{\alpha\beta\gamma}$ trimer in this complex increases the ligand-binding affinity of the receptor. **B:** Binding of the ligand to the receptor causes G_α to bind GTP, which begins the dissociation of G_α from $G_{\beta\gamma}$. **C:** Dissociation activates $G_{\beta\gamma}$, which interacts with its targets ($T_{\beta\gamma}$). **D:** Dissociation of the G_α-GTP complex from the receptor further activates G_α (*increased shading*), which interacts with its targets (T_α). Dissociation of G_α also reduces the ligand-binding affinity of the receptor, which releases the ligand. **E:** Dissociation of G_α activates its intrinsic GTPase activity, which dephosphorylates the bound GTP to form the inactive G_α-GDP complex. The latter then rebinds both the receptor and $G_{\beta\gamma}$, which increases the ligand-binding affinity of the former and inactivates the latter, thereby returning these signaling proteins to the basal state depicted in **A.**

$$R\text{-}L\text{-}G_\alpha\text{-}GDP\text{-}G_{\beta\gamma}+GTP \rightarrow R\text{-}L\text{-}G_\alpha\text{-}GTP + GDP + G_{\beta\gamma}(T_{\beta\gamma})$$

STEP 3: Dissociation of G_α-GTP from the receptor: G_α-GTP becomes dissociated from the R-L-G_α-GTP complex (Fig. 8-5D), which allows free G_α-GTP to activate its own targets (T_α); this also reduces the ligand-binding affinity of the receptor, which releases the ligand.

$$R\text{-}L\text{-}G_\alpha\text{-}GTP \rightarrow R + L + G_\alpha\text{-}GTP(T_\alpha)$$

STEP 4: Dephosphorylation of G_α-bound GTP: Dissociation of the G_α-GTP complex from the receptor stimulates the intrinsic GTPase activity of G_α which dephosphorylates the GTP bound to G_α, which forms G_α-GDP (Fig. 8-5E). This returns G_α to its basal state (G_α-GDP), in which it no longer participates in signal transduction. G_α-GDP then rebinds and inactivates $G_{\beta\gamma}$ released in step 2, which ends signal transduction by $G_{\beta\gamma}$.

$$G_\alpha\text{-}GTP + G_{\beta\gamma} \rightarrow G_\alpha\text{-}GDP\text{-}G_{\beta\gamma} + P_i$$

The rate of GTP hydrolysis, which is key to turning off both G_α- and $G_{\beta\gamma}$-mediated signals, is the major determinant of the duration of the response to the ligand. This dephosphorylation, which is rate-limiting for the G protein cycle, is regulated by *GTPase-activating proteins* (GAPs) that accelerate GTPase activity and *guanine nucleotide exchange factors* (GEFs) that release the GDP bound to G_α. The latter effect is inhibited by *guanine nucleotide dissociation inhibitors* (GDIFs) that accelerate the cycle by preventing GEFs from inhibiting GDP release.

STEP 5: Rebinding of G_α, $G_{\beta\gamma}$, and the receptor to form the receptor-bound $G_{\alpha\beta\gamma}$ complex: The system returns to the basal state when the $G_{\alpha\beta\gamma}$ complex formed by G_α-GDP and $G_{\beta\gamma}$ rebinds the free receptor and increases its affinity for the ligand (Fig. 8-5A).

$$R + G_\alpha\text{-}GDP\text{-}G_{\beta\gamma} \rightarrow R\text{-}G_\alpha\text{-}GDP\text{-}G_{\beta\gamma}$$

Overview of the G Protein Cycle

The reactions between the heterotrimeric G proteins and their receptors allow a single ligand to generate two intracellular signals, one carried by G_α-GTP and the other by $G_{\beta\gamma}$, each of which can activate its own downstream targets. At the same time, these reactions help avoid runaway signaling by allowing the cycle to turn itself off more or less automatically; this negative feedback reflects the instability of the G_α-GTP complex, which spontaneously hydrolyzes the bound nucleotide to form the inactive G_α-GDP that rebinds and inactivates $G_{\beta\gamma}$. G protein–mediated signals also are turned off when dissociation of activated G_α-GTP from the ligand-bound receptor reduces the affinity of the receptor for its ligand. A different type of regulation reflects the dependence of the cycle on a continuing supply of GTP, which can slow G protein–coupled signaling when the GTP/GDP ratio decreases in energy-starved cells.

Desensitization of G Protein–Coupled Receptors

Patients who have used nasal sprays containing a β-adrenergic agonist often note that repeated use causes the spray to lose its efficacy. This phenomenon, once referred to as "tachyphylaxis" and now generally called *desensitization* or *downregulation*, occurs when prolonged exposure to an extracellular messenger decreases the number of receptors available to bind to the ligand. An important clinical example of desensitization is a decrease in the number of β-receptors caused by sustained adrenergic stimulation in patients with heart failure (see Chapter 18).

Desensitization of G protein–coupled receptors occurs by a three-step process: uncoupling, internalization, and digestion (Fig. 8-6). A similar mechanism can reduce the responses to other members of this family of receptors.

UNCOUPLING (PHOSPHORYLATION). The first step in β-receptor desensitization occurs when the ligand-bound receptor is phosphorylated by a protein kinase called βARK (β-adrenergic receptor kinase) (Fig. 8-6B), which is one of a family of protein kinases, called *G protein receptor kinases* (GRK), that catalyze the phosphorylation of ligand-bound receptors. These phosphorylations prevent the receptor from activating its G protein and so provide a negative feedback that inactivates the receptor. This action of βARK is mediated by a cofactor called β-*arrestin*, which binds to the phosphorylated C-terminal intracellular peptide chain of the receptor. This step in receptor desensitization can be reversed by a process called *resensitization*, which occurs when the receptor is dephosphorylated by a *G protein–coupled receptor phosphatase*.

INTERNALIZATION (SEQUESTRATION). The second step in desensitization, called *internalization*, removes the phosphorylated receptor from the plasma membrane. This occurs when the β-arrestin–bound receptor (which has already been uncoupled from its G protein) is transferred to a clathrin-coated pit within the cell, where it can no longer interact with its ligands (Fig. 8-6C). The internalized receptors initially remain structurally intact so that this step, like phosphorylation, is reversible. However receptors that remain internalized for long periods become susceptible to proteolytic digestion, the final and irreversible step in desensitization.

DIGESTION (DEGRADATION). After prolonged internalization, the receptor is digested by proteolytic enzymes (Fig. 8-6D). This process, unlike uncoupling and internalization, is irreversible, so that restoration of receptor function requires that new receptors be synthesized.

One of the more fascinating features of receptor inactivation is the ability of desensitized β_2 receptors to activate proliferative signaling; this occurs when the internalized complex between the β_2 receptor and

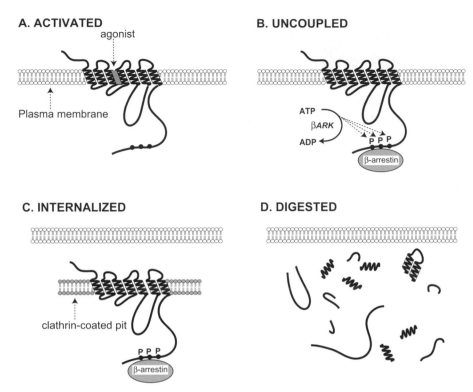

FIGURE 8-6 β-Adrenergic receptor desensitization. **A:** Activated, ligand-bound receptor. **B:** Prolonged binding of the receptor to its agonist stimulates a G protein receptor kinase (GRK) called βARK (β-adrenergic receptor kinase) to phosphorylate the C-terminal intracellular peptide chain, which then binds a cofactor called β-arrestin that inactivates the receptor. **C:** Transfer of the phosphorylated receptors from the plasma membrane to clathrin-coated pits within the cell internalizes the receptors which, although structurally intact, can no longer interact with either their agonists or G proteins. Dephosphorylation (*not shown*), by allowing the internalized receptors to return to the plasma membrane, can resensitize the receptors. **D:** Receptors that remain internalized for long periods are digested by intracellular proteolytic enzymes. This mechanism, unlike uncoupling and internalization, is irreversible.

β-arrestin forms a "platform" that activates mitogen-activated protein (MAP) kinases (Luttrell et al., 1999). This remarkable effect allows inactivation of a functional signaling pathway to activate a proliferative signaling pathway.

Enhanced Sensitivity of G Protein–Coupled Receptors: Denervation Sensitivity

The responses to β-adrenergic agonists can be increased when sympathectomy prevents the release of norepinephrine (*denervation sensitivity*) or after prolonged administration of β-blockers. This can have fatal consequences when β-blockers are used to treat patients with heart failure, which is accompanied by a hyperadrenergic state that ordinarily desensitizes the heart's β-receptors (see Chapter 18). Because prolonged β-blocker therapy increases the number of available β-receptors, sudden discontinuation of these drugs allows the high levels of norepinephrine generally seen in these patients to interact with a greater number of β-receptors. When these β-receptors interact with $G_{\alpha s}$, they can generate enough cAMP to cause sudden cardiac death (Eichhorn, 1999).

INTRACELLULAR SECOND MESSENGERS

Although some G proteins modify cell function directly—for example, when vagal stimulation activates a $G_{\beta\gamma}$ that accelerates membrane repolarization by activating plasma membrane potassium channels (Fig. 8-7A)—most G proteins transmit signals by stimulating the synthesis of an intracellular *second messenger*. The latter are small molecules that include nucleotides, lipids, and phosphosugars (Table 8-10). Cyclic AMP (cAMP), the first of these second messengers to be discovered, is generated when norepinephrine-bound β-receptors activate $G_{\alpha s}$, which stimulates *adenylyl cyclase* to synthesize cAMP from ATP (Fig. 8-7B). A more complex signal is generated when norepinephrine binds to α_1-receptors; in this case, the activated G protein is $G_{\alpha q}$, which stimulates *phospholipase C (PLC)*, a family of enzymes that hydrolyze a membrane phospholipid called *phosphatidylinositol 4,5-bisphosphate (PIP$_2$)* to generate two intracellular messengers, *inositol trisphosphate (InsP$_3$)* and *diacyl glycerol (DAG)* (Fig. 8-7C).

The concentrations of most intracellular second messengers are regulated by their rates of production and the rates at which they are broken down (Table 8-10); cAMP, for example, is synthesized by *adenylyl cyclase* and degraded by *phosphodiesterases*. This allows cAMP levels to be increased when β-adrenergic agonists activate adenylyl cyclase, when cAMP breakdown is slowed by phosphodiesterase inhibitors, or both. *Calcium*, another important intracellular messenger that participates in both functional and proliferative signaling, obviously cannot be synthesized within cells, but instead enters the cytosol from regions of high concentration in the extracellular space and sarcoplasmic reticulum (Chapter 7).

Cyclic AMP

Cyclic AMP mediates most of the important regulatory functional responses to sympathetic stimulation (Fig. 8-8). In the heart, activation of $G_{\alpha s}$ increases cardiac output by increasing contractility, accelerating relaxation, and increasing heart rate; cAMP also helps provide substrates needed for the increased energy expenditure by accelerating glycogen breakdown and fatty acid metabolism (Chapter 2). Cyclic AMP also participates in proliferative responses (Chapter 9). Parasympathetic stimulation, whose effects generally oppose those of the sympathetic nervous system, activates $G_{\alpha i}$, which inhibits adenylyl cyclase (Fig. 8-8).

A. DIRECT (MEMBRANE-DELIMITED) COUPLING

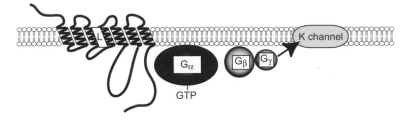

B. INDIRECT (ADENYLYL CYCLASE–MEDIATED) COUPLING

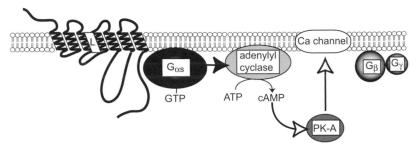

C. INDIRECT (PHOSPHOLIPASE C–MEDIATED) COUPLING

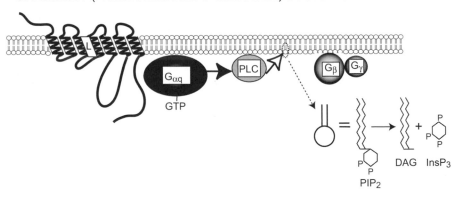

FIGURE 8-7 Three mechanisms by which ligand-binding to a G protein–coupled receptor can modify cell function. **A:** Direct coupling, where an activated G protein interacts directly with a target that alters cell function. This occurs when acetylcholine binding to muscarinic receptors activates a $G_{\beta\gamma}$, which then activates a plasma membrane potassium channel. **B** and **C:** Second messenger–mediated coupling, where G protein–coupled receptors modify the production of one or more intracellular messengers. **B:** Activation of adenylyl cyclase by a $G_{\alpha s}$ increases cAMP production, which increases calcium entry by activating a cAMP-activated protein kinase that phosphorylates plasma membrane L-type calcium channels. **C:** Activation of phospholipase C by $G_{\alpha q}$ stimulates the hydrolysis of phosphatidylinositol, a membrane phospholipid that generates two second messengers: diacylglycerol (DAG) and inositol trisphosphate ($InsP_3$).

TABLE 8-10 **Major Intracellular Messengers**

Second Messenger	Initiation of Signal	Termination of Signal
Cyclic AMP	Synthesized from ATP by adenylyl cyclase	Degraded to AMP by phosphodiesterases
Cyclic GMP	Synthesized from GTP by guanylyl cyclase	Degraded to GMP by phosphodiesterases
$InsP_3$	Synthesized from PIP_2 by phospholipase C	Dephosphorylated by phosphatases
Diacylglycerol	Synthesized from PIP_2 by phospholipase C	Phosphorylated to form a phosphatide or hydrolyzed to form monogylceride
Calcium	Diffuses into cytosol from regions of high concentration	Pumped out of cytosol

PIP_2, phosphatidylinositol 4,5-bisphosphate; $InsP_3$, inositol 1,4,5-trisphosphate.

Cyclic GMP

Nitric oxide (NO) and natriuretic peptides evoke counter-regulatory responses, whose effects generally oppose those caused by cAMP, by increasing *cyclic GMP* (cGMP) production. Nitric oxide increases cGMP levels when it binds directly to the active site of soluble guanylyl cyclases, whereas atrial and brain natriuretic peptides (ANP and BNP) increase cGMP production when by activating plasma membrane receptors called *receptor guanylyl cyclases*. Cyclic GMP levels, like those of cAMP, are determined by a balance between guanylyl cyclases and cGMP

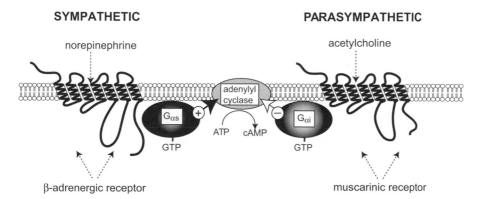

FIGURE 8-8 Opposing effects or sympathetic (*left*) and parasympathetic (*right*) on cAMP production. Norepinephrine binding to β_1 receptors on the heart activates $G_{\alpha s}$, which stimulates adenylyl cyclase to increase cAMP production, whereas acetylcholine binding to muscarinic receptors activates protein $G_{\alpha i}$, which inhibits adenylyl cyclase.

phosphatases, and most responses, like those initiated by cAMP, are mediated when cGMP activates a cGMP-dependent protein kinase.

Cyclic GMP was once believed to mediate the inhibitory responses to parasympathetic stimulation; it is now clear, however, that most inhibitory effects of acetylcholine on the heart occur when $G_{\alpha i}$ decreases cAMP production or activates repolarizing potassium currents that terminate excitatory action potentials. However, cGMP has an important *indirect* effect that allows parasympathetic stimulation to cause vasodilatation; this occurs when acetylcholine binding to muscarinic receptors on endothelial cells releases nitric oxide that, when it diffuses to adjacent vascular smooth muscle cells, activates guanylyl cyclase.

Inositol 1,4,5-trisphosphate and Diacylglycerol

Inositol 1,4,5-trisphosphate ($InsP_3$) and diacylglycerol (DAG), the second messengers produced by phospholipase C (Fig. 8-7C), activate different intracellular signal transduction pathways. The most important effect of $InsP_3$ is to cause calcium release from internal stores by opening $InsP_3$-gated intracellular calcium release channels (Chapter 7). In the heart $InsP_3$ is of little importance in generating functional responses but can participate in proliferative signaling; $InsP_3$ plays a central role in causing the calcium release that constricts vascular smooth muscle. DAG has a weak effect to increase myocardial contractility, but its major function is to catalyze serine and threonine phosphorylations that participate in proliferative signaling (Chapter 9).

Calcium

Calcium, which is among the most important of the intracellular messengers, generally serves as an activator (Chapter 7). In general, a rapid rise in cytosolic calcium modifies functional responses, whereas slower increases in cytosolic calcium, which is caused by calcium entry through T-type calcium channels (see Chapter 13) and $InsP_3$-induced calcium release, participate in proliferative signaling (Chapter 9).

SECOND MESSENGER–ACTIVATED SIGNALING ENZYMES

Many extracellular messengers activate signaling enzymes that modify other proteins in a signal transduction cascade, such as another signaling enzyme or an effector protein. In Figure 8-2, for example cAMP activates *cyclic AMP–dependent protein kinase* (a signaling enzyme) that phosphorylates a plasma membrane calcium channel (an effector protein). In a few cases, a second messenger binds directly to an effector protein; for example, acceleration of heart rate by cAMP is due in part to a direct effect caused when this second messenger binds to a cAMP-binding site on a pacemaker channel in the sinoatrial node (Chapter 13).

TABLE 8-11 **Major Intracellular Protein Kinases**

Protein Kinase	Activated by (Second Messenger)
Cyclic AMP–dependent (*protein kinase A*)	cAMP
Cyclic GMP–dependent(*protein kinase G*)	cGMP
Phospholipid-dependent (*protein kinase C*)	diacyl glycerol
Calcium–calmodulin-dependent (*CAM kinase*)	calcium

The most important signaling enzymes are protein kinases, which transfer phosphate from ATP to serine, threonine, or tyrosine (Table 8-11); other enzymes transfer moieties, such as myristate or palmitate, to effector proteins.

Most of the protein kinases that participate in functional signaling are serine–threonine kinases, a large and diverse family of enzymes that include protein kinases A (cAMP-activated), G (cGMP-activated), C (phospholipid-activated) and CAM kinase (calcium-calmodulin activated). (Protein kinase B, more commonly called Akt, is discussed in Chapter 9.) Tyrosine kinases, the other major family of protein kinases, are commonly activated by peptides and participate in proliferative signaling. Signals generated by protein kinases are turned off by *phosphoprotein phosphatases* that remove the attached phosphate (Table 8-10).

Cyclic AMP–dependent protein kinases are tetramers made up of two *catalytic subunits*, which transfer the terminal phosphate of ATP to the effector protein, and two *regulatory subunits*, which contain cAMP-binding sites that inhibit protein kinase activity under basal conditions. Binding of cAMP to the regulatory subunits dissociates the catalytic subunits from the former, which stimulates protein kinase activity according to the reaction:

$$R_2C_2 + 4 \; CAMP \rightarrow CAMP_4 \bullet R_2C_2 \rightarrow CAMP_4 \bullet R_2 + 2 \; C^*$$

where C and C* are the inactive and active states of the catalytic subunit, and R the regulatory subunit. Activation of the protein kinase ends when a fall in cytosolic cAMP levels dissociates the nucleotide from the regulatory subunits, which again form the inactive R_2C_2 complex.

MAJOR MEDIATORS OF THE HEMODYNAMIC DEFENSE REACTION

The following discussion briefly reviews several of the key extracellular messengers, receptors, second messengers, and signaling enzymes that participate in the hemodynamic defense reaction. These responses to these mediators are discussed in the chapters that describe the individual effector systems.

Epinephrine and Norepinephrine

The most important responses to a fall in blood pressure occur when norepinephrine released by sympathetic stimulation binds to β_1-receptors in the heart and α_1-receptors in the blood vessels (Table 8-12). The former causes an inotropic response that increases contractility, a lusitropic effect that accelerates relaxation, and a chronotropic effect that increases heart rate (Chapters 10 and 16), while the latter constricts arterial resistance vessels and veins and promotes fluid retention by the kidneys (see Table 8-2).

α-ADRENERGIC RECEPTORS. The cardiovascular responses to α_1- and α_2-receptors differ markedly; α_1-receptors on blood vessels mediate a vasoconstrictor response, whereas α_2-receptors in central nervous system and postsynaptic adrenergic neurons inhibit sympathetic outflow. This rather confusing arrangement allows both peripheral α_1-adrenergic blockers and central α_2-adrenergic agonists to cause vasodilatation. In the human heart, norepinephrine binding to α_1-receptors causes a weak positive inotropic effect, but this response is not seen in all species. α_1-Receptor agonists also

TABLE 8-12 Major Receptor Subtypes That Mediate Cardiovascular Actions of Norepinephrine

α_1-**Adrenergic Receptors**
Functional responses
Increased myocardial contractility (minor)
Smooth muscle contraction—vasoconstriction
Sodium retention by the kidneys
Proliferative responses
Stimulation of protein synthesis, cell growth and proliferation
α_2-**Adrenergic Receptors**
Functional responses
Central inhibition of sympathetic activity
Vasodilatation
Cardiac inhibition
β_1-**Adrenergic Receptors**
Functional responses
Cardiac stimulation—positive inotropy, lusitropy, and chronotropy
Proliferative responses
Stimulation of protein synthesis, cell growth and proliferation
β_2-**Adrenergic Receptors**
Functional responses
Increased myocardial contractility
Smooth muscle relaxation—vasodilatation

have a proliferative effect that is prominent in neonatal cardiac myocytes (Chapter 9).

β-ADRENERGIC RECEPTORS. Of the three known β-receptor subtypes, $β_1$-receptors and $β_2$-receptors play an important role in cardiovascular regulation, while $β_3$-receptors act mainly to regulate gastrointestinal motility and lipolysis. $β_1$-Receptors, the major subtype in the human heart, activate $G_{αs}$, which by increasing cAMP levels initiates powerful inotropic, lusitropic, and chronotropic responses. The effects of norepinephrine binding to cardiac $β_2$-receptors, which are coupled to both $G_{αi}$ and $G_{αs}$, are weaker and may be mediated in part by cytoskeletal proteins. In vascular smooth muscle, $β_2$-receptors mediate a counterregulatory vasodilator effect that is normally overwhelmed by the vasoconstrictor effects of $α_1$-receptor activation.

Dopamine

Dopamine, a precursor of norepinephrine in its biosynthesis from tyrosine, acts both centrally and in peripheral tissues. At low concentrations, dopamine interacts with peripheral DA_1 receptors to exert a physiological counterregulatory effect that relaxes vascular smooth muscle. When higher concentrations are administered to patients, dopamine activates $β_1$-receptors and stimulates norepinephrine release from sympathetic nerve endings in the heart, both of which have regulatory effects. At still higher concentrations, dopamine cross-reacts with peripheral $α_1$-receptors to cause vasoconstriction.

Muscarinic and Purinergic Agonists

The cardiovascular responses to both parasympathetic and purinergic stimuli are normally counterregulatory. Acetylcholine binds to at least five muscarinic receptor subtypes, called M_1 to M_5; the M_2 and M_3 receptors mediate the major cardiovascular responses to vagal stimulation. M_2-receptor activation shortens the atrial action potential (which reduces atrial contractility) by direct coupling of activated $G_{βγ}$ to potassium channels (see above). Acetylcholine binding to M_2-receptors also activates $G_{αi}$, which slows sinus node depolarization, inhibits conduction through the atrioventricular node, and causes a slight decrease in ventricular contractility. Binding of acetylcholine to M_3 receptors in vascular smooth muscle cells activates phospholipase C to produce $InsP_3$, which causes vasoconstriction; however, this response is normally outweighed when acetylcholine binds to M_3 receptors on endothelial cells, which stimulate the release of NO, a powerful vasodilator. Endothelial damage in patients with coronary atherosclerosis can impair the counterregulatory response and therefore allows acetylcholine, along with other neurotransmitters like serotonin, to evoke an abnormal vasoconstrictor response that can cause coronary vasospasm.

The dominant effects of purines such as adenosine and ATP, like those of acetylcholine, are counterregulatory. Adenosine can bind to four P_1 receptor subtypes, A_1, A_{2A}, A_{2B}, and A_3, which mediate different responses.

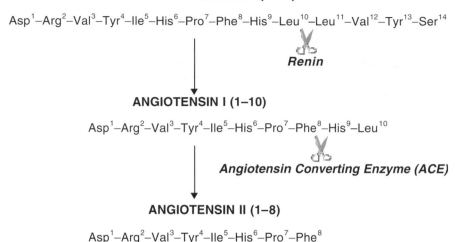

ANGIOTENSINOGEN (1–14)

$Asp^1–Arg^2–Val^3–Tyr^4–Ile^5–His^6–Pro^7–Phe^8–His^9–Leu^{10}–Leu^{11}–Val^{12}–Tyr^{13}–Ser^{14}$

Renin

ANGIOTENSIN I (1–10)

$Asp^1–Arg^2–Val^3–Tyr^4–Ile^5–His^6–Pro^7–Phe^8–His^9–Leu^{10}$

Angiotensin Converting Enzyme (ACE)

ANGIOTENSIN II (1–8)

$Asp^1–Arg^2–Val^3–Tyr^4–Ile^5–His^6–Pro^7–Phe^8$

A. THE RENIN–ANGIOTENSIN SYSTEM: "CLASSICAL" VERSION

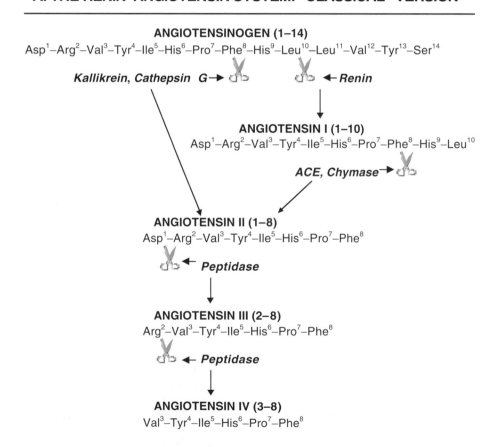

ANGIOTENSINOGEN (1–14)

$Asp^1–Arg^2–Val^3–Tyr^4–Ile^5–His^6–Pro^7–Phe^8–His^9–Leu^{10}–Leu^{11}–Val^{12}–Tyr^{13}–Ser^{14}$

Kallikrein, Cathepsin G →   ← *Renin*

ANGIOTENSIN I (1–10)

$Asp^1–Arg^2–Val^3–Tyr^4–Ile^5–His^6–Pro^7–Phe^8–His^9–Leu^{10}$

ACE, Chymase →

ANGIOTENSIN II (1–8)

$Asp^1–Arg^2–Val^3–Tyr^4–Ile^5–His^6–Pro^7–Phe^8$

← *Peptidase*

ANGIOTENSIN III (2–8)

$Arg^2–Val^3–Tyr^4–Ile^5–His^6–Pro^7–Phe^8$

← *Peptidase*

ANGIOTENSIN IV (3–8)

$Val^3–Tyr^4–Ile^5–His^6–Pro^7–Phe^8$

B. THE RENIN–ANGIOTENSIN SYSTEM: "MODERN" VERSION

The A_1 receptors activate $G_{\alpha i}$, which by inhibiting cAMP production causes the dominant counterregulatory effects. However, A_{2A} and A_{2B} receptors are coupled to $G_{\alpha s}$ and so evoke regulatory responses; activation of A_{2B} receptors also can cause vasoconstriction by $G_{\alpha q}$-mediated stimulation of phospholipase C. The major counterregulatory responses caused when adenosine binds to P_1 (purine) receptors occur when activation of $G_{\alpha i}$ inhibits cAMP production; a similar response is generated when ATP and other nucleotides bind to P_2 receptors.

ATP breakdown in energy-starved cells generates adenosine that can evoke a vasodilator response by activating A_1 receptors on nearby vascular smooth muscle. This paracrine effect provides one stimulus for *autoregulation*, a local vasodilatory response that increases blood flow to metabolically active tissues such as exercising muscles.

Imidazoline Agonists

A central imidazoline-mediated signaling system is activated by agmatine, a derivative of arginine that binds to I_1 and I_2 receptors, both of which evoke counterregulatory responses. The I_1 receptor has been suggested to be monoamine oxidase, an intracellular enzyme that inactivates catecholamines, while the I_2 receptor appears to be an ion channel–linked receptor. The counterregulatory effects of I_2 receptor activation are similar to those of central α_2-adrenergic activation in that both reduce sympathetic outflow. The ability of α_2-receptor agonists to activate central imidazoline receptors highlights the parallels between these counterregulatory systems.

The Renin–Angiotensin System

The renin–angiotensin system, which is among the most important regulatory mediators, causes vasoconstriction and decreases fluid excretion by the kidneys. The extracellular messenger responsible for most of these responses is *angiotensin II*, an octapeptide formed by a cascade of proteolytic reactions that hydrolyze *angiotensinogen*, an inactive 14-carbon precursor (Fig. 8-9). In the "classical" pathway (Fig. 8-9A), angiotensinogen is hydrolyzed by *renin*, a proteolytic enzyme that releases *angiotensin I*, a decapeptide that when digested further by *angiotensin-converting enzyme* (ACE) generates angiotensin II. Angiotensin II also can be released directly from angiotensinogen by the proteolytic enzymes *kallikrein* and *cathepsin G*, or from angiotensin I by *chymase* (Fig. 8-9B). Further proteolysis of angiotensin II generates the biologically active peptides angiotensin III and angiotensin IV.

FIGURE 8-9 Generation of signaling peptides by the renin–angiotensin system. **A:** The pathway as originally described uses two proteolytic cleavages, catalyzed by renin and angiotensin-converting enzyme (ACE), to form angiotensin II from angiotensinogen, the inactive precursor. **B:** Proteolytic reactions catalyzed by chymase, cathepsin G, and kallikrein also can form angiotensin II as well as two additional active peptides, angiotensins III and IV. (Modified from Katz, 2000.)

Angiotensin II can be generated by both circulating and tissue enzymes. Attention was initially focused on the circulating system, in which renin released into the bloodstream from the *kidneys* acts on circulating angiotensinogen made in the *liver* to form circulating angiotensin I, which is hydrolyzed by *lung* ACE to form *circulating* angiotensin II. More recently, two local systems were found to produce angiotensin II; in one, *tissue* ACE produces the extracellular messenger, while in the other, angiotensin II is formed by chymase-catalyzed proteolysis of angiotensinogen. Angiotensin II generated by circulating and tissue enzymes appear to serve different functions: The circulating system is probably most important in regulating vasomotor tone, while angiotensin II produced in the tissues participates in proliferative signaling.

The effects of angiotensin II are mediated by two angiotensin II receptor subtypes, designated AT_1 and AT_2, that mediate opposing responses (Fig. 8-10). Both AT_1 and AT_2 receptors are found in the adult human heart, where the former predominate (Haywood et al., 1997). The regulatory AT_1 receptors mediate the vasoconstrictor response, stimulate cardiac myocyte hypertrophy, and have a weak effect to increase cardiac contractility, whereas AT_2 receptors generally mediate counterregulatory effects such as vasodilatation and growth inhibition.

Endothelin

Endothelins (ET), a family of peptide vasoconstrictors first isolated from endothelial cells, are now known to be released by many cell types. Production of endothelins is regulated in part by the rate of synthesis of

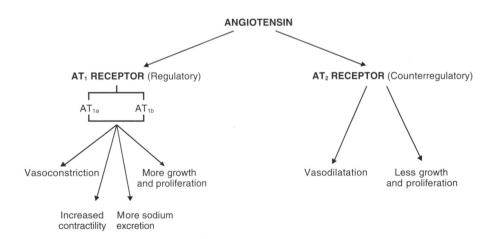

ANGIOTENSIN II RECEPTOR SUBTYPES

FIGURE 8-10 Angiotensin II receptor subtypes. The responses to these two subtypes differ and in many cases oppose one another. The AT_1 receptors, which include the AT_{1a} and AT_{1b} subtypes, exert regulatory effects, while AT_2 receptor stimulation generally evokes counterregulatory responses. (Modified from Katz, 2000.)

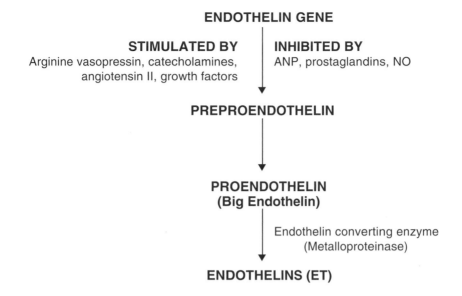

ENDOTHELIN PRODUCTION

FIGURE 8-11 Endothelin production. Endothelin gene expression produces preproendothelin that is processed by proteolytic reactions that generate proendothelin and endothelin. (From Katz, 2000.)

the protein precursors, called *preproendothelins*, and by posttranslational processing (Fig. 8-11). Preproendothelins, which are encoded by at least three genes, are processed by a series of proteolytic reactions that first release *proendothelins* (also called *big endothelins*) that are then hydrolyzed by *endothelin converting enzyme*, a metalloproteinase that forms *endothelin*. Chymases also can hydrolyze proendothelins to form endothelins.

In addition to their powerful vasoconstrictor effects, endothelins have both regulatory and counterregulatory actions on the heart and kidneys that are determined by the ET isoform and ET receptor that is activated (Fig. 8-12). ET-A receptors mediate the major regulatory cardiovascular responses that include vasoconstriction, increased myocardial contractility, and a proliferative effect; in contrast, ET-B receptors mediate counterregulatory responses by stimulating the release of NO and prostacyclin.

Bradykinin and Related Peptides

Kinins are vasodilators that are released from inactive protein precursors (*kininogens*) by proteolytic enzymes (*kallikreins*); different kinins are formed from high– and low–molecular weight kininogens (Fig. 8-13). Because bradykinin breakdown is catalyzed by converting enzymes, like

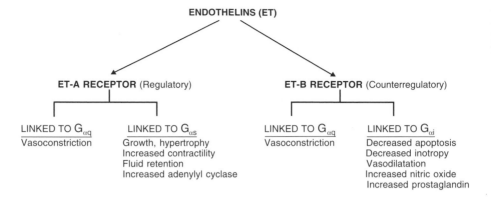

ENDOTHELIN RECEPTOR SUBTYPES

FIGURE 8-12 Endothelin receptors. ET-A and ET-B receptor subtypes have different affinities for various endothelin isoforms, activate different coupling proteins that mediate a variety of responses, and often generate opposing responses because ET-A, which activates $G_{\alpha s}$, usually exerts regulatory effects, while most responses to ET-B, which activates $G_{\alpha i}$, are counterregulatory. However, both cause vasoconstriction by activating $G_{\alpha q}$. (Modified from Katz, 2000.)

ACE, which also release angiotensin II (see above), these enzymes have a "dual" regulatory effect that generates a vasoconstrictor (angiotensin II) and inactivates a vasodilator (bradykinin). Bradykinin can cause a troublesome cough, which is occasionally noted by patients who receive ACE inhibitors, and angioneurotic edema, a rare but potentially fatal side effect.

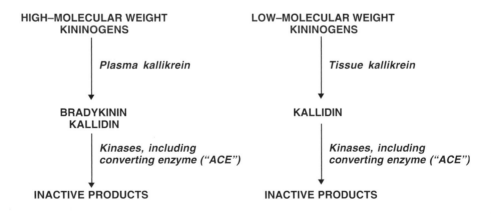

KININ PRODUCTION

FIGURE 8-13 Kinin production. Kinins are produced from high- and low-molecular weight kininogens by plasma and tissue systems, respectively. Activation of the plasma system begins when hydrolysis of high-molecular weight kininogens yields bradykinin and kallidin, while the tissue system produces kallidin from lower-molecular weight kininogens. (Modified from Katz, 2000.)

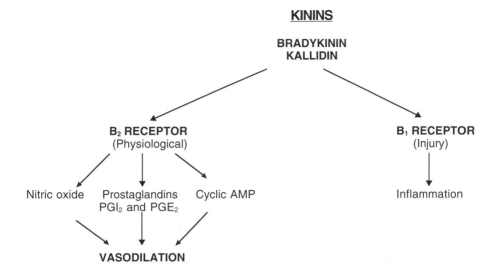

KININ RECEPTOR SUBTYPES

FIGURE 8-14   Kinin receptor subtypes. The B_2 receptors are involved in physiological regulation of the circulation, while the B_1 receptors mediate inflammatory responses. (Modified from Katz, 2000.)

The biological actions of bradykinins are mediated by bradykinin (B) receptors (Fig. 8-14). Most cardiovascular responses are initiated by the ligand-bound B_2 receptors, whose vasodilator effect is mediated by activation of a constitutive nitric oxide synthetase (see below), as well as increased production of prostacyclin and prostaglandin E_2. Activation of B_1 receptors by bradykinin induces the synthesis of an inducible nitric oxide synthetase which releases the high concentrations of NO that participate in inflammation.

Arginine Vasopressin (Antidiuretic Hormone)

Vasopressin is an octapeptide synthesized in the supraoptic and paraventricular nuclei of the hypothalamus and transported to the posterior pituitary, where it is stored and released. As indicated by its name, vasopressin was first identified as a powerful vasoconstrictor; however, this peptide also increases the water permeability of the renal collecting ducts. The latter effect inhibits diuresis by increasing water reabsorption, which is why vasopressin is also called *antidiuretic hormone* (ADH). Vasopressin also increases thirst, a physiological response that drives water-deprived individuals to seek water. The human isoform, which contains an arginine residue in position 8 is called *arginine vasopressin*.

The responses to vasopressin are mediated by V_1, V_2, and V_3 receptors that activate different intracellular signaling systems (Fig. 8-15). The vasoconstrictor effect is mediated by V_1 receptors, the V_2 receptors

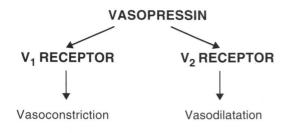

FIGURE 8-15 Vasopressin receptor subtypes. V_1 receptors mediate regulatory vasoconstriction, while counterregulatory vasodilatation is mediated by V_2 receptors. (Modified from Katz, 2000.)

cause water retention, and the V_3 receptors activate aldosterone release. Vasopressin release is normally regulated by increased plasma osmolarity, which stimulates osmoreceptors in the hypothalamus to release this hormone (Fig. 8-16). This physiological response helps in surviving dehydration, when vasopressin released in response to hemoconcentration increases water reabsorption by the kidneys and so reduces plasma osmolarity. The reduced vascular volume often seen in patients with shock also causes vasopressin release.

Unlike the adaptive responses when vasopressin levels are increased by hemoconcentration or volume depletion, where this peptide helps restore blood volume and maintain blood pressure, vasopressin release in chronic heart failure is generally maladaptive. This occurs because vasopressin release in these patients is stimulated by the increased norepinephrine and angiotensin II levels that accompany the hemodynamic defense reaction. Excessive vasopressin secretion can cause a dilutional hyponatremia that may be fatal.

Natriuretic Peptides

One of the more startling recent discoveries in cardiology is that the heart is not only a pump, but also an endocrine organ! This discovery, made when the density of granules in atrial myocardial cells was found to change in response to altered water and electrolyte balance, led to the finding that the atrial granules contain *natriuretic peptides*. These natriuretic peptides allow atrial dilatation to evoke a counterregulatory response that contributes to the body's defense against volume overload by inducing a diuresis and dilating systemic arterioles.

Natriuretic peptides are formed when a propeptide is hydrolyzed by a neutral endopeptidase that is similar to the angiotensin-converting enzyme. There are several different natriuretic peptides: *ANP*, which was originally discovered in the atria; *BNP*, first isolated from the brain and present in small amounts in the adult mammalian ventricles; and *CNP*, which is synthesized in the endothelium. All bind to receptor guanylyl cyclases that stimulate cyclic GMP synthesis.

The amount of BNP produced by the human ventricle is increased when the ventricle becomes hypertrophied as well as when its walls are

PHYSIOLOGICAL

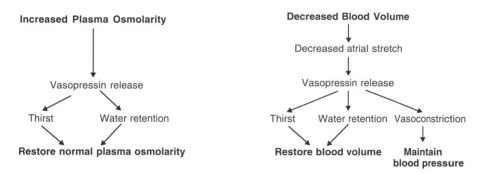

Increased Plasma Osmolarity

Vasopressin release

Thirst   Water retention

Restore normal plasma osmolarity

Decreased Blood Volume

Decreased atrial stretch

Vasopressin release

Thirst   Water retention   Vasoconstriction

Restore blood volume   **Maintain blood pressure**

HEART FAILURE

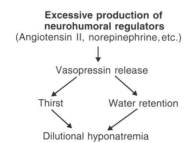

Excessive production of neurohumoral regulators
(Angiotensin II, norepinephrine, etc.)

Vasopressin release

Thirst   Water retention

Dilutional hyponatremia

REGULATION OF VASOPRESSIN RELEASE

FIGURE 8-16   Regulation of vasopressin release. Under physiological conditions, vasopressin secreted in response to increased plasma osmolarity and decreased blood volume increases water retention by the kidneys, increases thirst, and causes vasoconstriction. These adaptive responses, which reduce plasma osmolarity, help restore blood volume and increase blood pressure. In heart failure, where vasopressin release comes under neurohumoral control, inappropriate secretion of this peptide becomes maladaptive when increased thirst and water cause dilutional hyponatremia (Modified from Katz, 2000.)

stretched. For this reason, measurements of blood BNP levels can help identify patients with heart failure and characterize the severity of the hemodynamic abnormality.

Neuropeptide Y; Adrenomedullin; Leptin, Ghrelin, and Related Peptides

Neuropeptide Y, a peptide released by sympathetic nerve endings, can interact with at least five different receptor subtypes, called Y_1 to Y_5. Several are found in the heart and blood vessels, where neuropeptide Y can evoke both functional and proliferative responses. The former include counterregulatory negative inotropic and chronotropic effects on the heart that are mediated by activation of $G_{\alpha i}$, and a vasoconstrictor effect caused when this peptide potentiates the effects of α_1-adrenergic agonists and angiotensin II. Neuropeptide Y also stimulates cardiac hypertrophy, promotes angiogenesis, and increases appetite.

Adrenomedullin is a counterregulatory peptide that is secreted by endothelial cells in response to ischemia and hypoxia, mechanical stress, glucocorticoids, and cytokines. Binding of this peptide to adrenomedullin receptors causes vasodilatation and natriuretic and diuretic responses by the kidneys, and inhibits proliferative responses.

Ghrelin is a peptide produced in the stomach that stimulates appetite and, like neuropeptide Y, decreases sympathetic activity. *Leptin*, a catabolic peptide released from adipose tissue, has opposite effects including inhibition of food intake and increased sympathetic activity; other peptides, including *corticotrophin-releasing factor* and *α-melanocyte–releasing factor*, have effects similar to those of leptin.

Prostaglandins

Prostaglandins are generated when double bonds are inserted into arachidonic acid, a 20-carbon fatty acid, by *cyclooxygenases* (COX). These lipid messengers, which participate in both functional and proliferative signaling, have short half-lives and usually act locally. They can be released from one cell to act on a nearby cell (paracrine effect), or they can bind to a receptor on the cell from which it was released (autocrine effect). Physiologically active prostaglandins bind to G protein–coupled receptors; most important in cardiovascular regulation are *prostacyclin* (PGI$_2$) and *prostaglandin E$_2$* (PGE$_2$), which are vasodilators that inhibit platelet aggregation and adhesion, and *thromboxane* (TxA$_2$), which causes vasoconstriction and has a powerful effect to cause platelet aggregation.

The two major COX isoforms, COX-1 and COX-2, synthesize different prostaglandins. Aspirin, whose benefits in patients with vascular disease are due largely to its ability to acetylate and irreversibly inhibit COX-1, reduces the production of TxA$_2$. Evidence that selective inhibition of COX-2 increases the risk of complications of vascular disease may be due to reduced synthesis of PGI$_2$, a COX-2 product that inhibits endothelial damage and clotting.

Nitric Oxide (NO)

More than 20 years ago, Furchgott and Zawadzki (1980) found that the vasodilator responses to several extracellular messengers are not caused by a direct effect on vascular smooth muscle, but depend instead on a vasodilator synthesized by endothelial cells. This physiological vasodilator, initially called *endothelial-derived relaxing factor* (EDRF), is now known to be *nitric oxide*, a free radical gas whose structural formula is N=O, or more simply, *NO*. Nitric oxide is generated when L-arginine is converted to L-citrulline by a family of enzymes called *nitric oxide synthase* (NOS). Three NOS isoforms are found in the cardiovascular system: two, *eNOS* and *nNOS*, are constitutive

TABLE 8-13 **Major Regulators of Vascular Tone**

Vasoconstrictors	Vasodilators
Catecholamine	*Catecholamine*
Norepinephrine (peripheral, α_1-adrenergic)	Norepinephrine (central α_2-adrenergic)
Peptide	Epinephrine (β_2-adrenergic)
Angiotensin II	Dopamine
Arginine vasopressin	*Peptide*
Endothelin	Natriuretic peptides
Neuropeptide Y	Bradykinin
Lipid	Adrenomedullin
Thromboxane A_2	*Lipid*
	Prostacyclin, prostaglandin E_2
	Gas
	Nitric oxide (NO)

enzymes (*cNOS*) that participate in physiological signaling; the third, *iNOS*, is an inducible enzyme that generates large amounts of NO that act as free radicals during inflammation.

The responses to NO depend on its concentration; smaller amounts of NO generally act as autocrine and paracrine regulators that mediate counterregulatory responses, while high concentrations of this free radical gas are toxic and participate in inflammation. The responses to low NO concentrations include a vasodilator effect caused when NO binds to soluble guanylyl cyclases, a negative chronotropic effect that is probably also mediated by cyclic GMP, and a bimodal effect on contractility that includes a positive inotropic response at lower NO concentrations and as a negative inotropic response at higher concentrations.

Aldosterone

Aldosterone, a steroid hormone produced by the zone glomerulosa of the adrenal cortex, increases sodium reabsorption and promotes potassium loss by the renal tubules. Aldosterone also stimulates fibrosis and in heart failure mediates maladaptive proliferative responses that contribute to the poor prognosis in this syndrome (Chapter 18).

The physiological stimulus for aldosterone release is adrenocorticotrophic hormone (ACTH), a peptide synthesized in the anterior pituitary. Chronic activation of the hemodynamic defense reaction, which occurs in heart failure, causes aldosterone release to be stimulated by regulatory mediators such as norepinephrine, vasopressin, endothelin, and especially angiotensin II.

FUNCTIONAL AND PROLIFERATIVE RESPONSES

The complexity of the hemodynamic defense reaction is apparent in the large number of chemical moieties that regulate vascular tone, several of which interact with different receptors to produce opposing responses (Table 8-13). Proliferative signaling mechanisms (Chapter 9), which from an evolutionary standpoint are more ancient than the neurohumoral responses mediating the hemodynamic defense reaction, are even more complex than those that mediate the functional signals described in this chapter.

BIBLIOGRAPHY

Abassi Z, Karram T, Ellaham S, et al. Implications of the natriuretic peptide system in the pathogenesis of heart failure: diagnostic and therapeutic importance. *Pharmacol Ther* 2004 Jun;102(3):223–241.

Alberts B, Johnson A, Lewis J, et al. *Molecular biology of the cell*, 4th ed. New York: Garland, 2002.

Benigni A, Remuzzi, C. Endothelin antagonists. *Lancet* 1999;353:133–138.

Berk BC. Angiotensin II receptors and angiotensin II–stimulated signal transduction. *Heart Failure Rev* 1998;3:87–99.

Carretero OA, Scicli AG. Kinins as regulators of blood flow and blood pressure. In: Laragh JH, Brenner BM, eds. Hypertension. *Pathophysiology, diagnosis, and management*. New York: Raven Press, 1990:805–817.

Coleman RA, Smith WL, Naruyima S. International Union of Pharmacology Classification of prostanoid receptors: properties, distribution, and structure of the receptors and their subtypes. *Pharmacol Rev* 1994;46:205–229.

Eto T, Kato J, Kitamura K. Regulation of production and secretion of adrenomedullin in the cardiovascular system. *Regul Pept* 2003;112:61–69.

Francis GS. Neuroendocrine activity in congestive heart failure. *Am J Cardiol* 1990;66: 33D–39D.

Francis GS. Vasoactive hormone systems. In: Poole-Wilson PA, Colucci WS, Massie BM, et al., eds. *Heart failure. Scientific principles and clinical practice*. New York: Churchill Livingstone, 1997:215–234.

Hermans E. Biochemical and pharmacological control of the multiplicity of coupling at G-protein-coupled receptors. *Pharmacol Ther* 2003;99:25–44.

Gavras H. Pressor systems in hypertension and congestive heart failure. Role of vasopressin. *Hypertension* 1990;16:587–593.

Hollenberg NK. The role of the kidney in heart failure. In: Cohn JN, ed. *Drug treatment of heart failure*. Secaucus, NJ: ATC, 1988:105–125.

Izumo S, Nadal-Ginard B, Mahdavi V. The thyroid hormone receptor α gene generates functionally different proteins isoforms by alternative splicing. In: Roberts R, Schneider MD, eds. *Molecular biology of the cardiovascular system*. New York: Wiley-Liss, 1990:112–123.

Landry DW, Oliver JA. The pathogenesis of vasodilatory shock. *New Engl J Med* 2001;345: 588–595.

Lefkowitz RJ, Pitcher J, Krueger K, et al. Mechanisms of β-adrenergic receptor desensitization and resensitization. *Adv Pharmacol* 1997;42:416–420.

Levin ER. Endothelins. *New Eng J Med* 1996;333:356–362.

Levin ER, Gardner DG, Samson WK. Natriuretic peptides. *New Eng J Med* 1998;339:321–328.

Massion PB, Feron O, Dessy C, et al. Nitric oxide and cardiac function ten years after, and continuing. *Circ Res* 2003;93:388–398.

Matsumura K, Tsuchihashi T, Fujii K, et al. Neural regulation of blood pressure by leptins and the related peptides. *Reg Peptides* 2003;114:79–86.

Mombouli JV, Vanhoutte PM. Heterogeneity of endothelium-dependent vasodilator effects of angiotensin-converting enzyme inhibitors: role of bradykinin generation during ACE inhibition. *J Cardiovasc Pharmacol* 1992;20[Suppl 9]:S974–S982.

Moncada S, Higgs A. The L-arginine-nitric oxide pathway. *New Eng J Med* 1993;329:2002–2012.

Olson EN. A decade of discoveries in cardiac biology. *Nat Med* 2004;10:467–474.

Protas L, Qu J, Robinson RB. Neuropeptide Y: neurotransmitter or trophic factor in the heart. *News Physiol Sci* 2003;18:181–185.

Raasch W, Schäfer, Chun J, et al. Biological significance of agmatine, an endogenous ligand at imidazoline binding sites. *Br J Pharmacol* 2001;133:755–780.

Raine AEG. Renal abnormalities in congestive heart failure. In: Fozzard H, Haber E, Katz AM, et al., eds. *The heart and cardiovascular system*, 2nd ed. New York: Raven Press, 1992:1379–1391.

Remme WJ. Dopaminergic agents in heart failure: rebirth of an old concept. *Cardiovasc Drugs Therap* 15:107–109.

Tang CM, Insell PA. GPCR expression in the heart. "New" receptors in myocytes and fibroblasts. *Trends Cardiovasc Med* 2004;14:94–99.

Thibonnier M. Vasopressin receptor agonists in heart failure. *Curr Opin Pharm* 2003;3:683–687.

Urata H, Arakawa K. Angiotensin II–forming systems in cardiovascular diseases. *Heart Failure Rev* 1998;3:119–124.

Villarreal F, Zimmermann S, Makhsudova L, et al. Modulation of cardiac remodeling by adenosine: in vitro and in vivo effects. *Mol Cell Biochem* 2003;251:17–26.

Warner TD, Mitchell JA. Cyclooxygenases: new forms, new inhibitors, and lessons from the clinic. *FASEB J* 2004;18:790–804.

Wright DH, Abran D, Bhattacharya M, et al. Prostanoid receptors: ontogeny and implications in vascular physiology. *Am J Physiol Regul Integr Comp Physiol* 2001;281:R1343–R1360.

Xiao RP, Zhu W, Zheng M, et al. Subtype-specific β-adrenoceptor signaling pathways in the heart and their potential clinical implications. *Trends Phamacol Sci* 2004;25:358–365.

REFERENCES

Ahlquist PR. A study of the adrenotropic receptors. *Am J Physiol* 1948;153:586–600.

Clapham DE, Neer EJ. G protein βγ subunits. *Ann Rev Pharmacol* 1997;37:167–203.

Eichhorn EJ. Beta-blocker withdrawal: the song of Orpheus. *Am Heart J* 1999;138:387–389.

Furchgott RF, Zawadzki JV. The obligatory role of endothelial cells in the relaxation of arterial smooth muscle by acetylcholine. *Nature* 1980;288:373–376.

Harris P. Evolution and the cardiac patient. *Cardiovasc Res* 1983;17:313–319, 373–378, 437–445.

Haywood GA, Gullestad L, Katsuya T, et al. AT_1 and AT_2 receptor gene expression in human heart failure. *Circulation* 1997;95:1201–1206.

Herbette LG, Mason RP. Techniques for determining membrane and drug-membrane structures: A reevaluation of the molecular and kinetic basis for the binding of lipid-soluble drugs to their receptors in the heart and brain. In: Fozzard H, Haber E, Katz A, et al., eds. *The heart and circulation*, 2nd ed. New York: Raven Press, New York, 1991:417–462.

Katz AM. *Heart failure: pathophysiology, molecular biology, clinical management.* Philadelphia: Lippincott Williams & Wilkins, 2000.

Laugwitz KL, Allgeier A, Offermanns S, et al. The human thyrotropin receptor: a heptahelical receptor capable of stimulating members of all four G-protein families. *Proc Acad Sci USA* 1996;93:116–120.

Luttrell LM, Ferguson SSG, Daaka Y, et al. β-arrestin-dependent formation of β$_2$ adrenergic receptor-src protein kinase complexes. *Science* 1999;283:655–661.

9

SIGNAL TRANSDUCTION: PROLIFERATIVE SIGNALING

Proliferative signaling, which regulates cell size, shape, and composition, along with cell division, plays an important role in the pathophysiology of cardiac disease. In heart failure, maladaptive proliferative responses worsen prognosis by causing progressive ventricular dilation (*remodeling*) and myocardial cell death. Maladaptive growth responses also cause systemic and pulmonary hypertension by stimulating blood vessel growth, contribute to endothelial damage in atherosclerosis that leads to myocardial infarction and stroke, and increase arrhythmogenic currents across the plasma membrane.

Cardiac myocytes in the adult human heart are terminally differentiated cells with little or no ability to proliferate; they rarely divide, and synthesis of DNA and protein is slow—the half-lives of myofibrillar proteins, for example, can be several days. In contrast, the connective tissue cells that produce the heart's fibrous matrix undergo rapid mitosis. Severely overloaded cardiac myocytes exhibit a limited capacity to divide (Ring, 1950), but this abortive mitotic response does not regenerate significant amounts of functioning heart muscle (Rumyantsev, 1977). It is for this reason that the adult heart cannot adapt to a sustained overload by increasing cell number (hyperplasia); instead, cardiac myocytes can only become larger (hypertrophy). This hypertrophic response is well suited for the heart, which cannot suspend its pumping to generate new myocytes. As noted by Goss (1966): "By giving up the potential for hyperplasia in favor of the necessity for constant function, [the heart . . . has] adapted a strategy that enables [it] to become hypertrophic to a limited extent while doing [its jobs] efficiently." There is, however, a "price": when injured or overloaded, wall stress in the adult heart cannot be normalized by the generation of new myocytes; instead, cardiac myocytes can only hypertrophy by a process that shortens survival in patients with heart failure (Chapter 18).

THE CELL CYCLE

The most obvious characteristic of a terminally differentiated cell is its inability to participate in *mitosis*, the mechanical separation of two daughter cells, each of which contains a set of genes duplicated from the mother cell. Mitosis, which involves more than cell division (*cytokinesis*), depends on a highly regulated process, called the *cell cycle*, in which cell enlargement, DNA replication, and nuclear division (*karyokinesis*) precede cytokinesis. A terminally differentiated cell, by definition, has withdrawn from the cell cycle.

In *prokaryotes* (the name comes from the absence of a formed nucleus), the cell cycle plays a critical role in allowing members of a population to survive an environmental challenge. Because these primitive life forms lack internal membrane structures and therefore have little ability to control their *milieu intèrieur*, prokaryotes survive a change in environment by literally growing their way out of trouble. Rapid cell division is facilitated by the circular structure of prokaryotic DNA, which maintains a continually active cell cycle that allows these cells to replicate without pause; for this reason, prokaryotes can be viewed as growth machines. Because each prokaryote represents an independent entity with its own complement of genes, when a population of these organisms encounters a major environmental change, selection of cells whose phenotype is best able to withstand the new stress helps some of the population to survive. Even when a vast majority of the cells die, their rapid cell cycling can allow a few survivors to multiply and fill the new environment. This is seen in bacteria, which are modern prokaryotes that can divide as rapidly as every 20 minutes, allowing a single cell to generate more than 4 billion descendants—almost the human population of this planet—within 10 hours. The genetic diversification made possible by this rapid proliferation is the basis for the antibiotic resistance commonly seen in bacteria.

The cell cycle in eukaryotes (*eukaryote*, meaning "discrete nucleus") is not continuous, as seen in proliferating prokaryotes, but occurs in spurts. DNA replication, which must be completed before cell division, requires pauses between mitotic events that also allow the newly formed "daughter cells" to rebuild and reorganize their internal structure. The rate of cell cycling varies greatly among eukaryotic cells, with pauses averaging 10 to 20 hours, but often much longer. In terminally differentiated cells, like adult human cardiac myocytes in which effective cell division is not possible, the pause lasts until the cell dies.

Nuclear division and cell division are usually tightly coordinated in eukaryotes so that mitosis gives rise to daughter cells containing a single nucleus. When karyokinesis occurs without cytokinesis, the cell cycle generates a *multinucleate* cell, while DNA replication without either cytokinesis or karyokinesis results in *polyploid* cells, whose nuclei contain more than two sets of chromosomes. In the normal adult human heart, approximately one-fourth of cardiac myocytes are diploid, and more than one-half are tetraploid (Rumyantsev, 1977); the degree of ploidy increases with aging and also when the heart hypertrophies.

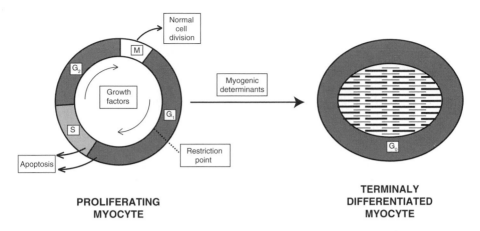

PROLIFERATING
MYOCYTE

TERMINALY
DIFFERENTIATED
MYOCYTE

FIGURE 9-1 Schematic depiction of the cell cycle and the transition to a terminally differentiated cell. **Left**: The cell cycle, such as occurs in proliferating cells of the fetal heart, proceeds in a clockwise direction. Mitosis (M) is followed by a "gap" phase (G_1) during which cells enlarge and carry out their physiological functions; from the standpoint of the cell cycle, however, this phase is quiescent. Cells become "committed" to the cell cycle when they pass a restriction point in G_1, after which the cell cycle proceeds though a phase of DNA synthesis (S), a second gap phase (G_2), and cell division (M). Cells are most susceptible to programmed cell death (apoptosis) late in the G_1 phase and during the S phase. **Right**: Myogenic determinants cause cells to withdraw from the cell cycle and enter a prolonged quiescent phase of terminal differentiation, called G_0.

Phases of the Cell Cycle

The cell cycle can be divided into four phases; in two, the cycle is active, while the other two are relatively quiescent. The two active phases are the *S phase*, characterized by DNA replication, and the *M phase*, in which cell division occurs (Fig. 9-1). These active phases are separated by two phases in which most processes related to cell division are temporarily suspended in order to allow cells to enlarge and carry out their physiological functions; these are the G_1 *phase*, between M and S, and the G_2 *phase*, between S and M. The G_1 *restriction point*, which occurs late in G_1, represents a major pause in cell cycling (Pardee, 1989). Once this restriction point is passed, cell division becomes independent of *external* stimuli, which means that the cell has become committed to dividing; however, even after a cell is committed to proliferation, most steps of the cell cycle remain under the control of *internal* regulatory mechanisms.

In terminally differentiated cells, the G_1 phase is prolonged in a quiescent state that resists stimuli that would otherwise activate cell cycling. This quiescent state, called G_0 in this text, can be viewed as a "detour" out of the cell cycle. In describing this quiescent state in cardiac myocytes, the term G_0 is not strictly correct because it was initially used to describe the cell cycle arrest associated with low metabolic activity in serum-depleted cultured cells. Although a more correct term for terminally differentiated adult cardiac myocytes might be "permanent arrest in the G_1 phase," with apologies to experts, the simpler term G_0 is used in this text.

Even when exposed to activators that stimulate cell division in less differentiated cells, adult cardiac myocytes have virtually no ability to re-enter the cell cycle. When severely stressed, the latter do make abortive attempts to divide, but these efforts to reverse the transition from G_1 to G_0 turn out badly. This is evident in failing hearts, where deleterious features of myocyte hypertrophy contribute to a maladaptive growth response that can accelerate cell death, hasten progression of the hemodynamic disorder, and worsen the prognosis (Chapter 18).

Cyclins, CDK, and Related Proteins

The cell cycle is controlled by *cyclin-dependent protein kinases* (CDK) and *cyclins* (Fig. 9-2), which regulate transitions both within and between the phases shown in Figure 9-1. CDKs are serine–threonine kinases, while cyclins regulate CDK activity. Members of large families of cyclins and CDK isoforms form "matched pairs" in which a given CDK regulates a specific cyclin. Some cyclin–CDK pairs stimulate cell growth in G_1, while others promote DNA replication in S, induce cell division in M, and stimulate transitions from G_2 to M and from G_1 to S. Not all cyclin–CDK pairs regulate the cell cycle; some interact with the myogenic determinants that regulate cell differentiation; others regulate a variety of transcription factors (see below).

CDKs are enzymatically inactive unless bound to an appropriate cyclin, but cyclins generally cause only partial activation of their corresponding CDKs. Complete activation requires the participation of additional

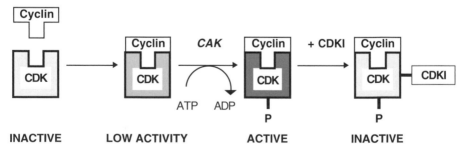

FIGURE 9-2 Cyclin-dependent protein kinases (CDKs) regulate the cell cycle when they interact specifically with regulatory proteins called *cyclins* to form cyclin–CDK pairs. Cyclins cause partial activation of CDK activity; full activation occurs when the cyclin-bound CDKs are phosphorylated by other protein kinases called *CAK* (CDK-activating kinases). Phosphorylated cyclin–CDK pairs are inactivated by CDKIs (cyclin-dependent kinase inhibitors). Additional regulators (*not shown*) include phosphatases that dephosphorylate the CDKs.

protein kinases, called *CDK-activating kinases* (CAK), that phosphorylate cyclin–CDK complexes (Fig. 9-2). *Cyclin-dependent kinase inhibitors* (CDKIs) slow the cell cycle by inhibiting active cyclin–CDK pairs. Other regulatory proteins, not shown in Figure 9-2, include phosphatases that inhibit cell cycling by dephosphorylating CDKs and protein kinases that catalyze inhibitory phosphorylations that inactivate cyclin–CDK pairs.

Tumor Suppressor Proteins

Proliferative signaling is regulated by proteins whose prototype is the *retinoblastoma protein* (pRb); in the heart, the most important member of this family is *p107*. These proteins are substrates for cyclin–CDK-catalyzed phosphorylations that inhibit tumor formation, so they are often called *tumor suppressor proteins*. Retinal cells in children who lack both copies of the retinoblastoma gene undergo malignant transformation and can form metastasizing tumors.

Tumor suppressor proteins are sometimes referred to as *pocket proteins* because their structure includes a pocket that reversibly binds transcription factors (Fig. 9-3); in the inhibitory (hypophosphorylated) state, in which few serine and threonine residues are phosphorylated, these proteins bind and inactivate transcription factors such as E2F (see below). Serine and threonine phosphorylations convert the tumor suppressor proteins to the activated growth-permissive (hyperphosphorylated) state by "kicking" E2F out of the pocket. These proteins provide a "convergence point" at which cyclin–CDK pairs, peptide growth factors, tyrosine kinase receptors, steroid receptors, G protein–coupled receptors, and cytoskeletal proteins regulate proliferative signaling.

E2F and Related Transcription Factors

Transcription factors called *E2F* activate the cell cycle when they are released from hyperphosphorylated tumor suppressor proteins. Conversely, binding of E2F when these proteins are hypophosphorylated arrests the cell cycle early in the G_1 phase, which favors differentiation by allowing cells to enter G_0. E2F, which often functions as a heterodimer with transcription factors called *DP-1*, has additional functions, including induction of apoptosis.

Several mechanisms can inactivate E2F; it can be phosphorylated by a cyclin–CDK pair (cyclin A–CDK2), it can bind directly to this cyclin–CDK pair, and it can form a complex with hypophosphorylated tumor suppressor proteins (Fig. 9-4). This transcription factor also is regulated by changes in the rate at which it is synthesized; for example, its growth-promoting effect can be amplified late in the G_1 phase by increased levels of the mRNA that encodes E2F.

REGULATION OF GENE EXPRESSION

Gene expression is regulated by *transcription factors* that interact with genomic DNA (the DNA found in chromosomes) to activate, inhibit,

A.

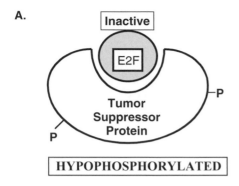

HYPOPHOSPHORYLATED

B.

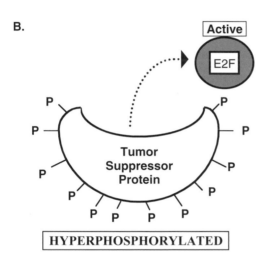

HYPERPHOSPHORYLATED

FIGURE 9-3 Regulation of tumor suppressor proteins. **A:** In the hypophosphorylated state, these proteins bind and inactivate transcription factors such as E2F. **B:** Phosphorylation of serine and threonine residues reduces the affinity for these transcription factors, which are released in an active form that regulates proliferative signaling.

or otherwise modify gene transcription. After it is activated, the gene serves as a template for mRNA that is transported to the cytosol, where it modifies cell growth, protein synthesis, and other proliferative responses.

Promoter, Enhancer, and Repressor DNA Sequences

In addition to coding the amino acid sequence of cellular proteins, genomic DNA contains nucleic acid sequences that turn genes on and off and control the rate at which genes are transcribed. These regulatory sequences include *promoter* regions located at the 5'-end of the gene, "upstream" from the *start site* where DNA transcription begins, and *enhancer* and *repressor* regions that increase and decrease the rate of gene expression, respectively (Fig. 9-5). One of the most important promoter regions is the *TATA box*, so named because its DNA sequence includes thymidine (T) and adenine (A) in the sequence TATA. This sequence represents a weak point in the structure of double-stranded DNA where the helix is most easily unwound to separate the single strands used for copying.

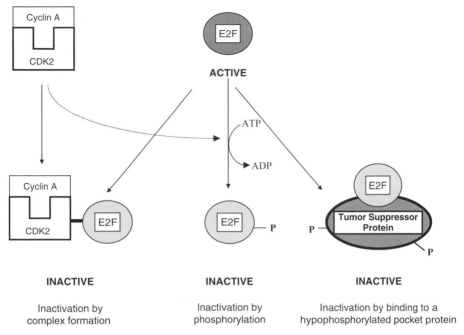

FIGURE 9-4 E2F can be inactivated by several mechanisms: when it forms a complex with cyclin A–CDK2, a cyclin–CDK pair (*left*), by CDK-catalyzed phosphorylation (*center*), and when it binds to a hypophosphorylated tumor suppressor protein (*right*).

Gene transcription is initiated when a promoter forms a multiprotein aggregate with an enzyme called *RNA polymerase*. These complexes, which commonly include additional regulatory proteins, bind to the promoter region of a gene whose base pair sequence becomes a template for the synthesis of a primary RNA transcript containing the information

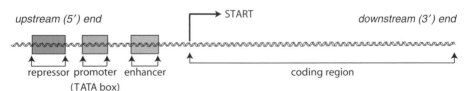

FIGURE 9-5 Gene transcription. Coding regions of genomic DNA that lie downstream (toward the 3' end of the DNA sequence) from a "START" sequence provide templates for the messenger RNA that encodes protein structure. Transcription factors activate gene transcription when they bind to a regulatory sequence located upstream at the 5' end of the gene, called a *promoter*; the *TATA box*, which is made up of thymidine (T) and adenine (A) residues, is among the most important of these promoter regions. Transcription is activated by *enhancers* and inhibited by *repressors*; the latter are found not only upstream from the start site, as shown in the figure, but also downstream and within regulatory sequences in the coding region.

encoded in the gene downstream from the "start site" (Fig. 9-5). The information in this transcript is then encoded in a *messenger RNA* (mRNA) that is transported to the cytosol, where it is used by a ribosome as the template that determines the amino acid sequence of a newly synthesized protein.

Histones

Histones, a family of basic DNA-binding proteins that were initially believed simply to stabilize the acidic DNA within chromosomes, also play an important role in regulating gene expression. Acetylation of histone by *histone acetylases* (HATs) stimulates transcription, while *histone deacetylases* (HDACs) inhibit proliferative responses. Phosphorylation of HDACs increases their deacetylase activity which, by inactivating histones in the heart, inhibits hypertrophic responses.

RNA Processing and Alternative Splicing

Not all of the RNA encoded by genomic DNA serves as a template for protein synthesis. Segments of the primary transcript, called *introns*, are eliminated before the remaining RNA sequences, called *exons*, are assembled into the mRNA that provides the template for protein synthesis (Fig. 9-6).

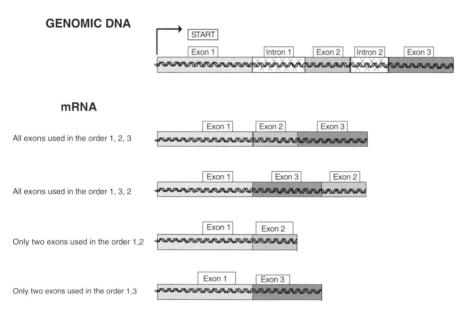

FIGURE 9-6 Alternative splicing. In addition to the *exons* whose sequence is encoded in proteins, primary RNA transcripts often include sequences, called *introns*, that are removed before the synthesis of messenger RNA (mRNA). Selection and rearrangement of exons after elimination of introns allows a single gene to encode several different mRNAs. The four mRNAs derived from a primary transcript containing three exons, shown in this figure, are a few of the possible products of alternative splicing, in which one, two, or all three exons can be combined in various combinations and sequences.

Alternative splicing, which describes the ability of cells to eliminate introns and rearrange selected exons, represents yet another means for regulating proliferative signaling. Examples of this mechanism are illustrated in Figure 9-6, which shows how a gene containing three exons can encode four different mRNAs; this illustration is by no means exhaustive, as the three exons can be used in additional combinations. Some genes contain dozens of exons, so alternative splicing provides an elaborate mechanism for generating many protein isoforms from a single DNA sequence.

Transcription Factors

Key to the regulation of gene expression are transcription factors that recognize and bind to specific DNA sequences. Most transcription factors are proteins and phosphoproteins that turn genes on by binding to a promoter region, accelerate gene expression by binding to an enhancer sequence, or slow gene transcription by binding to a repressor sequence (see Fig. 9-5).

The ability of transcription factors to select a specific gene and then regulate its expression is made possible by structural motifs that provide the tight "fit" needed to identify a specific target DNA sequence. Most transcription factors act as homo- or heterodimers, in which each subunit binds to one of the two strands of genomic DNA. These dimers include *helix-turn-helix*, *helix-loop-helix*, *leucine zipper*, and *zinc finger* structures, in which the subunits are held together by noncovalent linkages that include hydrophobic interactions between leucine residues and divalent zinc atoms (Fig. 9-7). Cooperative interactions between genes and transcription factors permit a single transcription factor to interact sequentially with several functionally related genes to generate a coordinated growth response; these interactions not only allow transcription factors to regulate gene expression, but also allow regulatory regions of some genes to modify the actions of a transcription factor.

Transcription factors can be activated in many ways. Most important is *post-translational modification* of an inactive protein, usually by phosphorylation or dephosphorylation. Transcription factors also can be released from an inactive complex or appear *de novo* when they are synthesized by an activated proliferative signaling cascade. Some genes are regulated by steroid hormones that cross the plasma membrane to bind intracellular *hormone receptor elements* (HREs), which form transcription factors that enter the nucleus.

GROWTH FACTORS

The regulatory mechanisms described above, which operate *within* cells, are generally controlled by factors that originate *outside* cells. The latter include many of the extracellular messengers described in Chapter 8, cell deformation whose effects are mediated by cytoskeletal proteins (see Chapter 5), and extracellular growth factors. The importance of the

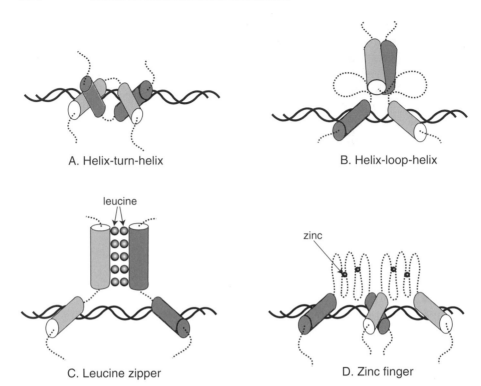

A. Helix-turn-helix   B. Helix-loop-helix

C. Leucine zipper   D. Zinc finger

FIGURE 9-7 Four types of transcription factor. These regulators, which function as dimers, include *helix-turn-helix* and *helix-loop-helix* structures, *leucine zipper* structures in which the two subunits of the dimer are linked by hydrophobic forces between leucine residues, and *zinc finger* structures where zinc atoms stabilize the structure of the transcription factor dimers. Cylinders represent α-helices.

latter became apparent during early efforts to prepare artificial media for culturing mammalian cells, when normal cells were found to lose their ability to grow and divide even after various nutrients, vitamins, and trace elements were included in the culture media. This puzzling observation, which indicated that unknown factors were needed to maintain cell cycling, led to the finding that fetal calf serum could allow these quiescent cells to proliferate; this in turn made it possible to identify the missing ingredients, which were found to be peptides that came to be called *growth factors*.

A large number of *peptide growth factors* are now known to stimulate proliferative responses. Although initially named for the tissues from which they were first isolated, or whose growth they were initially found to stimulate, most growth factors turned out not to be tissue-specific, but instead could mediate proliferative signaling in many cell types throughout the body. These include platelet-derived growth factor (PDGF), epidermal growth factor (EGF), fibroblast growth factor (FGF), insulinlike growth factor (IGF), vascular endothelial growth factor (VEGF), and

TABLE 9-1 **Some Peptide Growth Factors**

Tyrosine kinase ligands
Platelet-derived growth factor (PDGF)
Epidermal growth factor (EGF)
Fibroblast growth factor (FGF)
Insulinlike growth factor (IGF)
Vascular endothelial growth factor (VEGF)
Serine–threonine kinase ligands
Transforming growth factors (e.g., TGF-β)
Cytokines
Tumor necrosis factor-α
Interleukins 2–7, 9–13
Growth hormone
FAS ligand
Erythropoietin
Granulocyte colony-stimulating factor

transforming growth factors (TGF), along with a number of cytokines (Table 9-1). All use paracrine, autocrine, and endocrine pathways to reach receptors on their target cells, most of which include latent tyrosine kinase enzymes. A few, like transforming growth factor-β (TGF-β), bind to receptors with latent serine–threonine kinase activity. Cytokines, which bind to receptors that lack intrinsic protein kinase activity, form aggregates that activate tyrosine kinases in other proteins.

Fibroblast Growth Factor

Fibroblast growth factors (FGF) regulate proliferative signaling in response to mechanical stresses and other changes in the external environment, generally by stimulating growth and proliferation, inhibiting differentiation, and favoring expression of fetal genes (Table 9-2). In blood vessels, FGFs modify growth and responses to endothelial damage, while in the heart, they participate in the healing response to injury and the hypertrophic response to overload. These peptides, which are often divided into acidic and basic FGF, bind to *FGF receptor tyrosine kinases* that contain both a latent tyrosine kinase and a heparin-binding domain (Fig. 9-8).

When bound to FGF, FGF receptor tyrosine kinases form aggregates with *FGF receptor heparan sulfate proteoglycans*; the latter, which are members of a family of connective tissue glycoproteins that link cells to one another, activate the latent receptor tyrosine kinase. This generates a signal that can phosphorylate a variety of intracellular proteins, including

TABLE 9-2 **Some Effects of FGF and TGF-β on the Heart**

FGF

  Stimulates myocyte growth

  Inhibits differentiation and myogenesis

  Causes expression of the fetal gene program

  Inhibits apoptosis

TGF-β

  Stimulates fibrosis

  Stimulates myocyte differentiation and myogenesis

  Causes expression of the fetal gene program

  Promotes apoptosis

mitogen-activated protein (MAP) kinases, phospholipase C, and regulators of other proliferative signal transduction cascades (see below).

FGFs, which are released by mediators of the hemodynamic defense reaction that include angiotensin II and endothelin, activate gene programs that participate in the hypertrophic response to overload. Interactions of FGF receptor heparan sulfate proteoglycans with the extracellular matrix allow cell deformation to initiate proliferative signals that modify cell size, shape, and composition.

Transforming Growth Factor β

Transforming growth factor β (TGF-β) plays a major role in tissue responses to injury by stimulating fibrous tissue growth, cell proliferation, differentiation, embryogenesis, and programmed cell death (Table 9-2). In the heart, these peptides participate in the hypertrophic response of the heart to overload and the reactive fibrosis that accompanies cell damage.

Signaling by TGF-β is mediated by two classes of TGF-β receptors, called *type I* and *type II*; although both contain a latent serine–threonine kinase, only the type II receptors actually bind TGF-β (Fig. 9-9). Signaling begins when a TGF-β homodimer binds two of the type II receptors, which forms a ligand-receptor complex that interacts with two type I receptors. This activates the latent protein kinase of the type II receptors, which phosphorylates and activates the latent protein kinase of the type I receptors. The latter then catalyze serine–threonine phosphorylations that propagate the TGF-β signal down intracellular signaling cascades.

The major substrates for TGF-β–catalyzed phosphorylation are transcription factors called *Smads* (a conflation of the names of the first two members of this family to be described: "Sma" in *C. elegans* and "Mad" in *Drosophila*), The phosphorylated Smads, along with additional members of the Smad family, ubiquitin ligases (called *Smurfs* for "Smad ubiquitination regulator factor"), often interact with scaffolding proteins (see below).

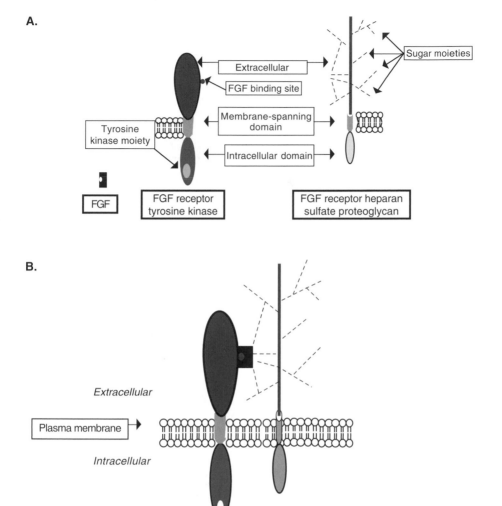

FIGURE 9-8 FGF signaling. **A:** Components include FGF, its plasma membrane receptor (FGF receptor tyrosine kinase), and an FGF receptor heparan sulfate proteoglycan that contains sugar moieties that are linked to the extracellular matrix. **B:** Signaling is initiated when these components form a complex that activates a latent tyrosine kinase in the intracellular domain of the FGF receptor. The latter can then catalyze tyrosine moieties in other "downstream" components of the signal transduction cascade.

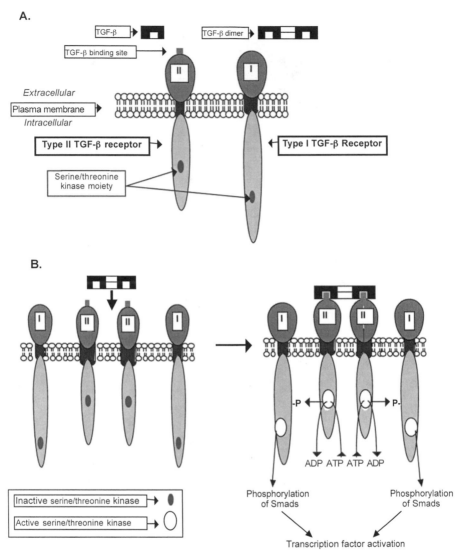

FIGURE 9-9   TGF-β signaling. **A:** Components include TGF-β and type I and type II TGF-β receptors. **B:** These components form a complex made up of the TGF-β homodimer, two type II receptors, and two type I receptors in which a latent serine–threonine kinase in the intracellular domain of the type II receptors is stimulated to phosphorylate the type I receptors. This activates the latter to catalyze tyrosine moieties in other "downstream" components of the signal transduction cascade.

TGF-β, in addition to activating fibroblasts that will cause fibrosis and stimulating a number of proliferative signaling pathways, redirects the pattern of protein synthesis in hypertrophied hearts to favor expression of fetal genes (see Chapter 18). Responses to angiotensin II, which play an important role in causing maladaptive hypertrophy in failing

TABLE 9-3 **Selected Actions of the Cytokines**

Cellular Effects
Inflammation
Cell proliferation
Cell transformation
Apoptosis (programmed cell death)
Signal transduction
Activate tyrosine kinases [e.g., janus kinase (JAK)]
Activate protein kinases-A and C
Activate stress-activated MAP kinases
Activate phospholipases A_2 and C
Increase levels of cyclic AMP and diacylglycerol
Activate signal transducer and activator of transcription (STAT)
Activate NF-κB
Activate immediate-early genes (e.g., *AP-1, c-fos, c-jun*)
Induce Synthesis of:
Inflammatory mediators, including other cytokines
Inducible nitric oxide synthase (iNOS)
Growth factors: PDGF, GM-CSF
Receptors: EGF receptor, IL-2 receptor
Cytoskeletal molecules
Heat shock proteins

hearts (see Chapter 18) are mediated in part when angiotensin II activates TGF-β signaling.

Cytokines

The cytokines are an ancient family of peptides that mediate a variety of biological functions in almost every type of cell (Table 9-3). Cytokines, like peptide growth factors, bind to plasma membrane receptors; however, these receptors do not contain protein kinase moieties, but instead interact with other membrane proteins that contain this enzyme. Some cytokine receptors also contain an amino acid sequence, referred to as a *death domain*, that stimulates apoptosis.

Signal transduction by cytokines begins when the ligand-bound receptors form aggregates that can include an additional coupling protein called *gp130* (Fig. 9-10). The most important mediator of cytokine-mediated signal transduction are intracellular tyrosine kinases called *JAK*. (This acronym, which originally stood for "Just Another Kinase," has been redefined to mean *Janus kinase* because, like Janus—the two-faced

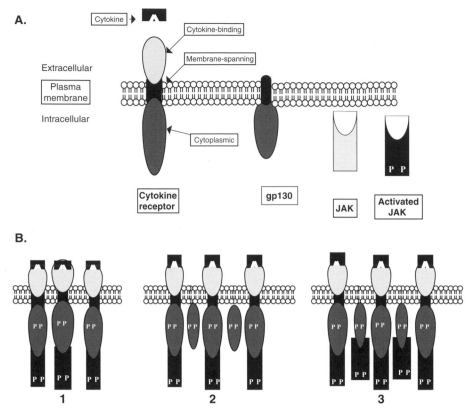

FIGURE 9-10 Cytokine signaling. **A:** Components include the cytokine receptors, which contain cytokine-binding, membrane-spanning, and cytoplasmic domains; the coupling protein gp130; and tyrosine kinases called *JAK*, which in the dephospho form are inactive. **B:** Cytokine binding causes the receptors to form trimeric aggregates (1) that can include gp130 (2 and 3). The aggregated receptors and receptor–gp130 complexes bind to JAK, which activates its latent tyrosine kinase activity. The activated JAKs can phosphorylate themselves (autophosphorylation), the receptors, gp130, and members of the STAT class of transcription factors.

Roman god of doorways who looks both outward and inward—JAKs respond to cytokine binding outside the cell by phosphorylating proteins within the cell.) Although tyrosine phosphorylation is central to most cytokine-mediated cell signaling, serine and threonine phosphorylations participate in some of these regulatory mechanisms.

In addition to their well-known proinflammatory effects, cytokines also regulate other cellular processes, including protein synthesis and apoptosis; in the heart, for example, gp130 plays an important role in the adaptive hypertrophic response to overload (Uozumi et al., 2001). JAKs regulate cytokine signaling by phosphorylating the intracellular domains of cytokine receptors, gp130, and other JAKs (Fig. 9-10). Other substrates for JAK-catalyzed phosphorylations include a transcription factor called *signal transducer and activator of transcription* (STAT) that, when phosphorylated by JAK, moves to the nucleus to regulate gene expression. Proliferative signaling by cytokines also is mediated by stress-activated MAP kinases (see below) and a signaling cascade that phosphorylates a protein called *I*κ*B* that, when phosphorylated, activates NF-κB, a transcription factor that stimulates gene transcription. Cytokine signaling can be "turned off" by inhibition of cytokine-induced phosphorylation pathways, or by specific phosphatases that dephosphorylate the activated signaling proteins.

CROSSOVERS BETWEEN FUNCTIONAL AND PROLIFERATIVE SIGNALING

As recently as the early 1990s, proliferative and functional signaling were viewed as distinct and independently regulated processes (Fig. 9-11). It is now apparent, however, that a single pathway often mediates both types of response. For example, the G protein–linked receptors, which were initially identified as mediating functional signals, modify proliferative responses once believed to be under the "exclusive" control of the enzyme-linked receptors. Conversely, the tyrosine kinase receptors initially thought to regulate only proliferative signals also modify functional

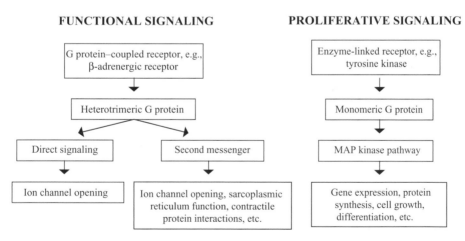

FIGURE 9-11 Early view of cell signaling as two independent systems that generate functional and proliferative responses. Functional signaling (*left*), which is mediated by G protein–coupled receptors and heterotrimeric G proteins, was viewed as regulating functional responses such as myocardial contractility and smooth muscle contraction, whereas proliferative signaling was thought to regulate growth responses when ligands, like peptide growth factors, bind enzyme-linked receptors that activate monomeric GTP-binding proteins. These two pathways also were believed to utilize different signaling mechanisms: functional signaling by membrane-linked or second messenger–mediated mechanisms and cell growth and proliferation by MAP kinase pathways.

responses, such as myocardial contractility. This change in our understanding of signal transduction is described by Bourne (1995) as an advance from "a few discrete clans" of signaling molecules, organized into the two discrete pathways of functional and proliferative signaling, to a series of "wheels within wheels! . . . bustling communication networks within and between clans of signaling proteins. . . ."

Proliferative Signaling by G Proteins

HETEROTRIMERIC G PROTEINS. Most mediators of the functional responses of the hemodynamic defense reaction (see Chapter 8) participate in the hypertrophic response of the heart to overload. These mediators, which include norepinephrine, angiotensin II, vasopressin, and endothelin, stimulate G protein–coupled receptors to activate G_α-GTP and $G_{\beta\gamma}$, both of which can modify proliferative as well as functional responses. Crossovers also are seen in the actions of many downstream mediators of G protein–coupled receptor signaling; for example, cyclic AMP–dependent protein kinases (PK-A) participate in proliferative signaling by phosphorylating transcriptional regulators such as *CREB* (*cyclic AMP receptor element-binding protein*) and *CREM* (*cyclic AMP receptor element modulator*). Angiotensin II, endothelin, vasopressin, and α_1-adrenergic receptor agonists also regulate proliferative signaling pathways by activating $G_{\alpha q}$, which stimulates phospholipase C to release inositol trisphosphate ($InsP_3$) and diacylglycerol (DAG) (see Chapter 8). $InsP_3$ opens intracellular calcium release channels, which provide calcium that mediates proliferative signaling, while DAG activates protein kinase C (PK-C). The latter is a lipid-dependent protein kinase that catalyzes serine–threonine phosphorylation of substrates including the monomeric G protein Ras, which activates mitogen-activated protein kinases (MAP kinases) and other proliferative signaling pathways (see below).

A fascinating example of a crossover between functional and proliferative signaling is the ability of the internalized β-receptor–β-arrestin complex, which although has lost its ability to generate functional responses (see Chapter 8) generates proliferative responses (Luttrell et al., 1999). This crossover occurs when the internalized β-receptor complex forms an aggregate that can activate MAP kinases (see Fig. 9-12). The remarkable ability of the inactivated β-receptor to adopt a new signaling role can be viewed as "informing" a cell that its use of a short-term, cyclic AMP–mediated, functional response has failed to meet a long-term challenge and that a proliferative response is needed instead. Stated simplistically, this mechanism says that the time for a stressed cell to run or fight has ended and that to survive, the cell must grow its way out of trouble!

MONOMERIC G PROTEINS. Proliferative signaling is often coupled by monomeric G proteins, like Ras, that mediate signals generated by activation of enzyme-linked receptors (Fig. 9-13). These small proteins, which like G_α are active when bound to GTP, contain an intrinsic GTPase and

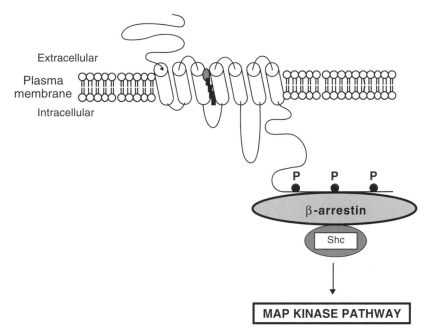

FIGURE 9-12 Stimulation of proliferative responses by internalized β-adrenergic receptors. Aggregates made up of phosphorylated β-arrestin–bound receptors and protein kinases like Shc can provide a scaffold that activates MAP kinase pathways.

are inactivated when the bound GTP is dephosphorylated by an intrinsic GTPase. Unlike the heterotrimeric G proteins, monomeric G proteins do not interact directly with plasma membrane receptors or with proteins analogous to $G_{\beta\gamma}$. Because GTP hydrolysis by the monomeric G proteins is generally slower than that by G_α, the signals that they mediate generally last longer.

Proliferative Signaling by Calcium

Although increased cytosolic calcium is generally linked to such functional responses as contraction and secretion (see Chapter 4), this cation also mediates proliferative responses. The response to calcium depends in part on the rate of rise of cytosolic calcium release; proliferative responses are often initiated by small sustained elevations of cytosolic calcium, whereas functional signals, like those that mediate excitation–contraction coupling, are activated by large, briefer increases (Berridge, 1997). Slow rises in cytosolic calcium occur after the opening of plasma membrane T-type calcium channels, intracellular InsP$_3$-gated intracellular calcium channels, and stretch-operated calcium channels.

Important mediators of proliferative signaling include calcium-calmodulin–dependent protein kinases that phosphorylate a number of regulatory proteins (see Chapter 4). The latter include *histone deacetylases* (*HDACs*) which, in the phosphorylated state, inhibit proliferative signaling,

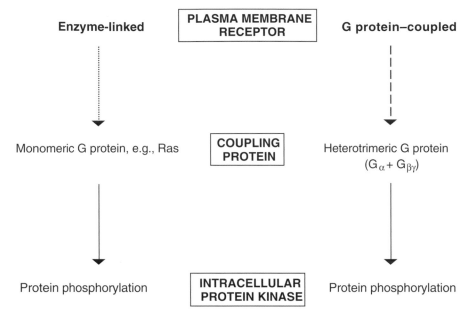

FIGURE 9-13 Parallels between signals generated by enzyme-linked and G protein–coupled plasma membrane receptors. These two classes of receptor utilize different GTP-binding proteins to link receptor activation at the "top" of the cascade to downstream phosphorylations that are catalyzed by protein kinases. G protein–coupled receptors interact directly with heterotrimeric G proteins (*dotted arrow*), whereas enzyme-linked receptors indirectly stimulate monomeric G proteins in reactions that require additional coupling steps (*dashed arrow*).

and transcription factors such as cyclic AMP–response element-binding protein (*CREB*). Calcium also activates a phosphatase called *calcineurin*, which stimulates cardiac hypertrophy by dephosphorylating the inactive form of a transcription factor called *NF-AT3* (*nuclear factor of activated T cells or NFAT*). This allows NFAT to bind to and activate *GATA4* and *MEF2C*, transcription factors that mediate the hypertrophic response of the heart to overload.

MAP KINASE PATHWAYS

Many of the transcription factors that mediate proliferative signaling are activated by MAP kinase pathways that include a sequence of three serine–threonine phosphorylations (Fig. 9-14). MAP kinases were initially identified as regulators of cell growth and proliferation that are activated when peptide growth factors bind to *extracellular receptor kinases* (*ERKs*) (Egan and Weinberg, 1993; Graves et al., 1997). More recently, additional *stress-activated MAP kinase pathways* were found to be activated by inflammatory cytokines and toxic agents, as well as by G protein–coupled receptors and cytoskeletal deformation (Table 9-4). The

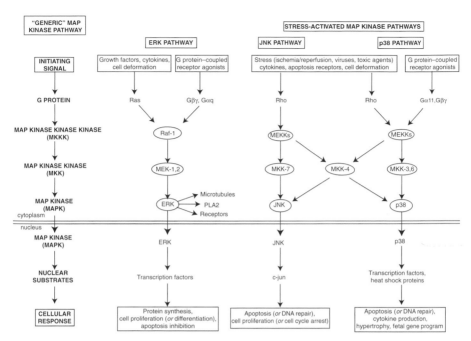

FIGURE 9-14   MAP kinase pathways. The "generic" pathway (*left*) lists key steps that are common to these signaling pathways, all of which utilize a GTP-binding protein to activate a sequence of three serine–threonine kinases: MAP kinase kinase kinase (MKKK), which phosphorylates a MAP kinase kinase (MKK), which phosphorylates a MAP kinase. The latter, when phosphorylated, enters the nucleus, where it can phosphorylate nuclear transcription factors; some MAP kinases also phosphorylate cytosolic proteins. Three MAP kinase pathways are shown: the extracellular receptor–activated kinase (ERK) and two stress-activated pathways (*right*). The ERK pathway can be coupled by Ras when activated by tyrosine kinase receptors, and by the heterotrimeric G proteins, generally $G_{\alpha q}$, when activated by G protein–coupled receptors. The major MKKK in the ERK pathway is Raf-1, the MKKs include MEK-1 and -2, while the most important MAP kinase is ERK. The two stress-activated MAP kinase pathways, which phosphorylate JNK and p38, are generally coupled by monomeric G proteins of the Rho family and, in the case of the p38 pathway, also by $G_{\alpha 11}$ and $G_{\beta \gamma}$. The MKKKs in the stress-activated pathways, called MEKKs, function like Raf-1 to phosphorylate MKKs that phosphorylate JNK and p38. JNK enters the nucleus, where it phosphorylates a transcription factor called *c-jun*, while p38 can phosphorylate nuclear transcription factors and heat shock proteins.

roles of specific MAP kinases in causing adaptive and maladaptive aspects of cardiac hypertrophy are not entirely clear, but there is evidence that concentric and eccentric hypertrophy are mediated by different MAP kinase pathways.

The ERK- and stress-activated MAP kinase pathways are activated by monomeric G proteins: the *Ras* family for the ERK pathway and the *Rho* family for stress-activated pathways. MAP kinases also are activated by heterotrimeric G proteins, both G_α and the $G_{\beta\gamma}$ complex, which provides crossovers between functional and proliferative signaling that allow mediators of the hemodynamic defense reaction, like norepinephrine,

TABLE 9-4   **Some Signals That Regulate Map Kinases in the Heart**

Peptide growth factors (e.g., FGF)
Circulating neurohumoral mediators (e.g., norepinephrine, angiotensin II, endothelin)
Locally released neurohumoral mediators (e.g., angiotensin II)
The cytoskeleton (e.g., integrins, cadherins)
Inflammatory cytokines (e.g., TNF-α)

angiotensin II, and endothelin, to regulate cell growth and composition. Other crossovers that involve MAP kinase pathways include activation of proliferative signaling by the internalized β-receptor–β-arrestin complex (see above), phosphorylations catalyzed by DAG-activated PK-C, and InsP$_3$-induced calcium release.

The "Generic" MAP Kinase Pathway

Signaling by MAP kinase pathways resembles an American square dance in which the signal, like a dancer, moves gracefully along a series of partners. The early steps in this dance often take place on a supporting platform, or "scaffold," that is formed when regulatory proteins aggregate along the inner surface of the plasma membrane; later in the dance, the action moves through the cytosol, crosses the nuclear membrane, and concludes in the nucleus when the activated MAP kinases phosphorylate transcription factors.

Common to all MAP kinase pathways is activation of *MAP kinase kinase kinases* (MKKKs) (Fig. 9-14). These serine–threonine kinases then phosphorylate a second kinase, called *MAP kinase kinase* (MKK), which phosphorylates the *MAP kinase*. Most MAP kinases enter the nucleus, where they phosphorylate transcription factors, but some MAP kinase substrates are cytosolic proteins. Signal diversity is provided by a large number of isoforms of the MKKKs, MKKs, and MAP kinases, and the interactions of these pathways with other signal transduction cascades.

Extracellular Receptor Kinase Pathways

Extracellular receptor kinase (ERK)-mediated signals are generally initiated when ligand binding to a tyrosine kinase receptor causes the latter to form aggregates that simulate the latent tyrosine kinase activity (Fig. 9-15). The latter then autophosphorylates the receptor to form phospho-ester groups that provide "docking sites," which initiate aggregations among signaling proteins, much as the partners in our dance join hands to form a square. Aggregation begins when the activated tyrosine kinase receptors phosphorylate adaptor proteins called *Shc* (from *Src-homology* because of similarities to the gene *src*) and *Grb2* (*growth receptor binding protein*). Scaffolds formed along the inner surface of the plasma membrane

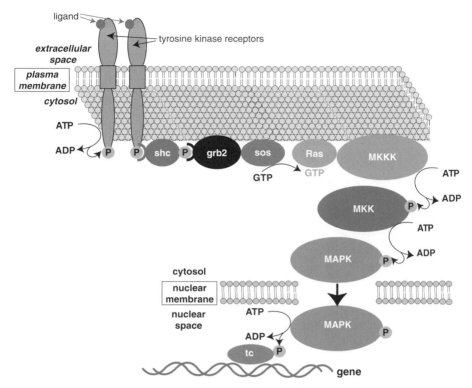

FIGURE 9-15 Proliferative signaling by an enzyme-linked receptor. Binding to the ligand causes the receptor to form an aggregate that activates its latent tyrosine kinase activity. Autophosphorylation of the receptor then creates a "docking site" that binds and then phosphorylates the adaptor protein Shc to create another docking site. This stimulates Shc to add Grb2 to the multiprotein aggregate assembled along the inner surface of the plasma membrane. This aggregate then activates Sos, a guanine nucleotide-exchange factor that exchanges Ras-bound GDP for GTP. The activated Ras-GTP complex stimulates Raf-1, a MAP kinase kinase kinase (MKKK) that phosphorylates and activates the MAP kinase kinase (MKK) MEK-1, which phosphorylates the MAP kinase (MAPK) ERK-2. Translocation of the latter to the nucleus allows the activated ERK to phosphorylate nuclear transcription factors (tc) that interact with specific DNA sequences.

by these multiprotein aggregates interact with a guanine nucleotide-exchange factor called *Sos* (named after the drosophila mutant *son-of-sevenless*), which activates Ras by exchanging its bound GDP for GTP; the latter reaction is analogous to the activation of G_α by ligand-bound G protein–coupled receptors (see Chapter 8). Ras also can be activated by additional signaling cascades, which allows other mediators of proliferative signaling to activate MAP kinase pathways.

The Ras-GTP complex in the ERK pathway activates an MKKK called *Raf-1* (Figs. 9-14 and 9-15) that phosphorylates and activates MKKs called *MEK-1* or *MEK-2* (an abbreviation of *MAP kinase/ERK kinase*). The activated MEKs then phosphorylate ERK, the MAP kinase

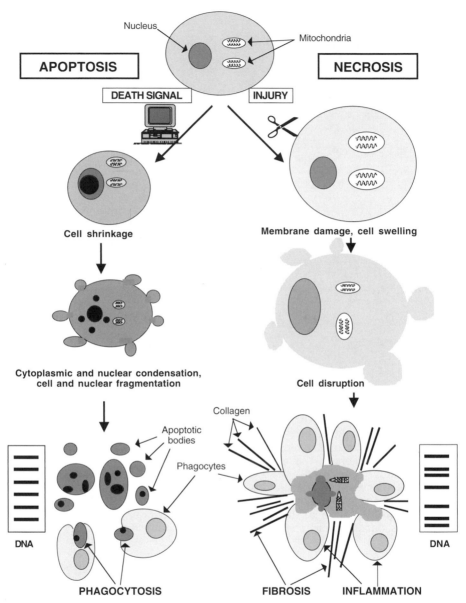

FIGURE 9-16 Apoptosis and necrosis. Apoptosis (*left*) is a highly regulated process of programmed cell death that induces cell shrinkage and condensation of the cytosol and nucleus; this yields cell fragments, called *apoptotic bodies*, that because they are surrounded by plasma membrane can be engulfed and digested by phagocytes without evoking an inflammatory reaction. Apoptosis also is characterized by DNA breakdown into regularly sized fragments that, when fractionated on gels, resemble ladders. Necrosis (*right*) is generally caused when plasma membrane damage impairs its ability to serve as a permeability barrier, which causes cells to swell and eventually to burst. The resulting release of cell contents initiates an inflammatory reaction that leads to fibrosis and scarring. DNA breakdown into random-sized fragments prevents the appearance of the ordered "laddering" seen in apoptosis. (Modified from Katz, 2000.)

that moves to the nucleus to phosphorylate a variety of transcription factors.

Stress-Activated MAP Kinase Pathways

Stress-activated MAP kinase pathways, which are activated by cytokines and cell deformation, play an important role in the hypertrophic response of the heart to overload. The stress-activated MKKKs include several isoforms of both *MEKK* (*MEK kinase*), whose function is analogous to that of Raf-1, and MKKs, whose function is analogous to that of MEK-1. The latter include MKK-7, which mediates JNK signaling; MKK-3 and MKK-6, which operate in the p38 pathway; and MKK-4, which is active in both. The MKKs phosphorylate *c-Jun amino-terminal kinase* (*Jun kinase* or *JNK*), which phosphorylates the transcription factor *c-jun*, and p38, which is itself a transcription factor.

PHOSPHOINOSITIDE 3'-OH KINASE AND AKT

Phosphoinositide 3'-OH kinases (*PI3-kinases*) mediate proliferative signaling by catalyzing the phosphorylation of the 3'-hydroxyl group in phosphatidylinositol trisphosphate (PIP_3), a membrane phospholipid. PI3-kinases can be activated by receptor tyrosine kinases that bind to insulin, insulin growth factor (IGF), and growth hormone; by activated $G_{\beta\gamma}$ subunits of heterotrimeric G proteins; and by cytoskeletal deformation. In the heart, phosphorylation of PIP_3 by a PI3-kinase called *p110a*, activates *Akt*, a serine–threonine kinase named for a related transforming component in the T8 strain of AKR/J mice. Because the structure of Akt is homologous to PK-A and PK-C, this protein kinase is sometimes referred to as *protein kinase-B* (*PK-B*). Akt substrates include transcription factors that participate in the physiological hypertrophy seen in the athlete's heart (see Chapter 18).

APOPTOSIS (PROGRAMMED CELL DEATH)

Cells can die in two fundamentally different ways: they can be killed by extrinsic factors (*necrosis* or accidental cell death), or they can be programmed to die by signal transduction systems that operate within the cell (*apoptosis* or programmed cell death). Apoptosis, in many ways, can be viewed as cell suicide, whereas necrosis represents cell murder.

The hallmark of necrosis, which can be viewed as a "catastrophic failure of cellular homeostasis" (Raffray and Cohen, 1997), is cell rupture that is generally preceded by cell swelling and breakdown of the plasma membrane barrier. Because plasma membrane rupture releases reactive cellular contents that evoke an intense inflammatory response, necrosis usually leads to fibrosis. In the heart, where increased plasma membrane permeability allows calcium to leak into myocytes, exposure of the contractile proteins to high calcium concentrations initiates explosive interactions between the myofilaments that cause *contraction-band necrosis*, which literally tears cells apart (see Chapter 17). In apoptosis, on the other hand, the dead cells vanish. The latter plays an important role in embryogenesis—for example, when the tail of the tadpole is "reabsorbed" without scarring the mature frog, which differs from a third degree burn, where necrosis stimulates a fibrotic response that causes scarring and, sometimes, keloid formation. However, the distinction between these two forms of cell death is not always clear; although the extremes differ markedly, there are gradations between necrosis and apoptosis, and some mechanisms operate in both. In addition, cell death can begin as apoptosis and end as necrosis. For these reasons, necrosis and apoptosis can be viewed as extremes of a continuum (Kroemer et al., 1997).

Before describing *apoptosis*, I cannot refrain from commenting on its pronunciation—and frequent mispronunciation. This term is derived from two Greek words, *apo* (away) and *ptosis* (falling), and there are defensible reasons to pronounce or not to pronounce the second "p" (*apo• ptosis'* or *apo• tosis'*). However, there is no basis for the mispronunciation "*a• pop'• tosis*," which combines parts of the two words to create a third, nonsense, syllable. For this reason, there is no "*pop*" in apoptosis!

Mechanism of Apoptosis

Apoptosis was initially thought to be triggered when cells are injured by viruses, toxins, irradiation, energy starvation, and reactive oxygen species. It is now clear, however, that the highly regulated "programmed cell death" also can be initiated when mediators of the hemodynamic defense reaction activate proliferative signaling pathways. The many similarities between the regulation of apoptosis and proliferation are apparent in rapidly proliferating tissues, like those of the embryo, where programmed cell death is as "natural" as the falling of leaves from a deciduous tree in autumn. In the fetus, apoptosis allows the orderly elimination of cells for which the need has ended; for example, as many as half of the neurons that appear in the developing vertebrate nervous system are eliminated after they form synaptic connections with their target cells (Raff et al., 1993). This is essential for embryonic development, where many cell types appear and then disappear; if cell death in the fetus led to fibrosis, the adult would become a mass of scar tissue. This feature of apoptosis is elegantly described by Savill et al. (1997), who note that it "is beautifully demonstrated in the developing *Drosophila* eye, where to achieve the adult form, thousands of unwanted interommatidal cells undergo programmed death and phagocytosis without disrupting the delicate architecture of the organ." If unneeded cells were not eliminated during early development, we would all have been born blind, with gills and tails, and webs between our fingers and toes!

Apoptosis, which also helps to prevent malignant transformation by eliminating cells with a tendency for unchecked growth (van Noorden et al., 1998), is a highly controlled process—death, after all, is irreversible. In some ways, the control of apoptosis resembles the American legal system, where executions are carried out only after a jury trial, review by the trial judge, and an elaborate appellate process. In apoptosis, the process begins when the "decision" that a cell is to die is initiated either by activation of programs that lead to programmed cell death, or by withdrawal of apoptosis-inhibitory factors that allow a preprogrammed death process to kill the cell.

"Death signals" that initiate apoptosis begin when regulatory programs cause the cell to shrink and eventually to break up into small, membrane-surrounded fragments that often contain bits of condensed chromatin, called *apoptotic bodies* (Fig. 9-16). Maintenance of plasma membrane integrity until late in the apoptotic process prevents release of the reactive cellular contents, instead allowing fragments of the dying cell to be engulfed by macrophages. In this way, apoptosis differs from necrosis, which is characterized by cell swelling and rupture. Another distinction between necrosis and apoptosis is the way that DNA is degraded; in necrosis, the DNA is broken down into randomly sized fragments, whereas DNA breakdown in apoptosis gives rise to regularly sized fragments that when fractionated resemble a ladder.

The ability of phagocytes to ingest cell fragments formed during apoptosis without invoking an inflammatory response by spilling "raw" indigestible cell contents into tissues is like an elegant meal for which the meat is boned, tenderized, and cut into bite-sized pieces; shells are removed from lobsters, shrimp, and clams; and fruits and vegetables are cored and peeled. In necrosis, according to this culinary analogy, the same ingredients are presented in raw form, often still alive, which causes the diner to experience a stomachache that is analogous to the inflammation and scarring that characterize necrosis.

Control of Apoptosis

Factors that initiate apoptosis include plasma membrane receptors called *Fas*, which are activated by peptides called *Fas ligand* (FasL) (Fig. 9-17); the latter are cytokines that occur in both membrane-bound (mFasL) and soluble (sFasL) forms. FasL initiates apoptosis by activating a 70– to 90–amino acid sequence in the Fas receptor, called a *death domain* (Fig. 9-17); similar death domains are found in other cytokine receptors and in caspases (see below). Binding of FasL causes the Fas receptors to form trimers in which the death domains bind to mediator proteins called *adaptors* that contain additional death domains, such as *FADD (Fas-associated death domain protein)*. Apoptosis also is initiated by peptide growth factors, cytoskeletal proteins, and mediators of the hemodynamic defense reaction such as norepinephrine and angiotensin II. Other initiators of apoptosis include gp130, the PI3K–Akt pathway, calcineurin, some CDK–cyclin pairs, NF-κB, and nuclear transcription factors such as *c-fos* and *c-myc*. The fact that many mediators of proliferative

A.

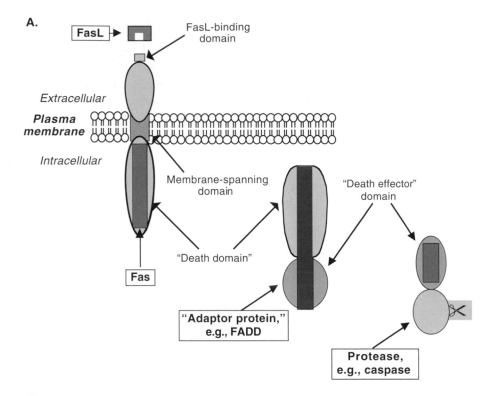

B.

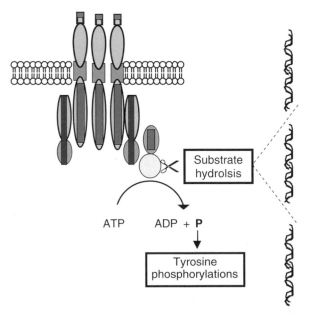

FIGURE 9-17 The Fas/FasL system. A: Components include a cytokine called Fas ligand (FasL); Fas, a plasma membrane receptor that contains a "death domain"; and adaptor proteins, such as FADD. B: Binding of FasL to Fas causes the latter to form a trimeric

signaling also regulate apoptosis has suggested that apoptosis represents a modified form of mitosis (Ucker, 1991).

All of these signaling pathways initiate apoptosis by activating cysteine proteases called *caspases* that, in addition to hydrolyzing proteins, participate in elaborate apoptotic regulatory cascades. Some caspases contain a death effector domain that activates apoptosis when it binds to homologous death effector domains in adaptor proteins; other caspases regulate apoptosis by hydrolyzing tumor suppressors, cytoskeletal and nuclear regulatory proteins, and enzymes that participate in RNA splicing, cell division, and DNA repair and replication.

Mitochondria play an important role in causing apoptosis in energy-starved and calcium-overloaded hearts, where cell death is triggered when *reactive oxygen species* (*ROS*) open pores in the mitochondrial inner membrane. The latter, called *mitochondrial permeability transition pores* (*MPTP*), release an "apoptosis-producing factor," cytochrome C, an endonuclease, and several procaspases into the cytosol from within the mitochondrial matrix. Members of the Bcl family (see below) and calcium-activated signaling pathways also activate apoptosis by opening MPTP. The apoptosis-producing factor, cytochrome C, and a caspase released by the mitochondria form complexes, called *apoptosomes*, that activate other caspase pathways.

Bcl-2 (an acronym for *B-cell lymphoma/leukemia 2 gene*) and related proteins serve many roles in apoptosis: some (e.g., *Bcl-2* and *Bcl-x$_L$*) suppress this process, while others (e.g., *Bak*, *Bax*, and *Bad*) promote cell death by interfering with apoptosis-suppressing proteins. Bcl-2, the proto-type of this family, is a proapoptotic protein that opens MPTP; other proapoptotic Bcl-2 proteins have functions similar to those of adaptor proteins like FADD. Antiapoptotic members of the Bcl-2 family inhibit caspases, protein kinases, and other signaling proteins involved in apoptosis. Because apoptosis can be a calamity for the adult heart, whose myocytes have little capacity to divide, the Bcl-2 proteins that inhibit apoptosis, along with an antiapoptotic cytosolic protein called *FLIP* (*Fas ligand inhibitory protein*), play an important role in preserving cardiac function.

The transcription factor *p53*, a major regulator of cell survival, has been called the *master watchman* of the genome (Saini and Walker, 1998). In normally proliferating cells, p53 contributes to the regulation of normal gene expression, whereas in damaged cells, p53 inhibits proliferative signaling and increases the expression of genes that encode proapoptotic factors. This dual role, which regulates both the cell cycle

---

FIGURE 9-17 (*Continued*) aggregate in which the death domains interact with homologous death domains in the adaptor proteins; this stimulates an active site in the adaptor protein called a death effector domain, which binds homologous death effector domains in caspases and other effectors of apoptosis. Caspases include enzymes that break down cell constituents, tyrosine kinases, and other regulators of programmed cell death.

and apoptosis, allows p53 to carry out a "triage" that helps decide the fate of an injured cell. When DNA damage is mild, p53 provides time for DNA repair by shutting down the cell cycle, but when an injury is so severe that the DNA damage cannot be repaired, its proapoptotic effects kill the cell. In proliferating tissues, the latter effect allows p53 to prevent malignancy by eliminating severely damaged, potentially transformed cells; in terminally differentiated cardiac myocytes, where malignant transformation is very rare, p53 serves mainly to eliminate severely damaged cells.

HEAT SHOCK PROTEINS AND HYPOXIA INDUCIBLE FACTOR

Cell damage in most tissues is minimized by the *heat shock* response, a highly conserved defense mechanism that received its name because it was first observed in tissues exposed to high temperature. This response protects cells from a variety of stresses by activating transcription factors that stimulate the synthesis of *heat shock proteins* (*HSPs*); the latter, which bind to cellular proteins and inhibit their denaturation, are sometimes called *chaperones*. HSP-70, the most important heat shock protein in the heart, also inhibits apoptosis, counteracts some deleterious effects of cytokines, protects against mitochondrial damage, and preserves cytoskeletal structure.

The heart's defenses against energy starvation also are mediated by *hypoxia inducible factor-1α* (*HIF-1α*) that activates genes that encode proteins that help protect key cellular components from hypoxic damage. These include *erythropoietin*, which increases oxygen delivery; *vascular endothelial cell growth factor* (*VEGF*), which promotes blood vessel growth; metabolic enzymes that increase anaerobic ATP production; and signaling molecules that inhibit apoptosis.

PROLIFERATIVE RESPONSES TO STRESS

Gene expression is activated, and in some cases inhibited when cardiac myocytes are subjected to a stress, such as ischemia, stretch, or overload. The first genes to be upregulated, called *immediate-early response genes*, are normally inactive in terminally differentiated cells, but can be activated rapidly after cardiac myocytes are stressed—in some cases, within a few minutes. The speed of this response indicates that the genes are activated by phosphorylations and other post-translational modifications. If the stress is sustained, additional genes, called *late-response genes*, become upregulated in reactions that depend on the synthesis of new proteins. In many cases, late-response genes are activated by transcription factors whose synthesis is stimulated by the immediate-early genes. In the overloaded heart, both immediate-early and late-response genes participate in an adaptive hypertrophic response that initially tends to normalize wall stress; however, these responses come to play a pathogenic role in the maladaptive hypertrophy seen in chronically overloaded failing hearts—for example, by stimulating apoptosis and causing cell elongation ("remodeling," see Chapter 18).

Immediate-Early and Late-Response Genes

Many of the signaling pathways described in this chapter as well as in Chapter 8, activate the immediate-early response when the heart becomes ischemic or is overloaded. This initiates a complex response in which more than 100 different genes are activated and deactivated. Genes whose expression is increased include nuclear transcription factors like *c-myc*, *c-fos*, and *c-jun*; *ras*, which encodes the monomeric GTP-binding protein Ras, and *hsp*-70, which encodes a heat shock protein.

The immediate-early response is followed by the more sustained activation of a different complement of late-response genes, which encode the synthesis of a variety of proteins, including additional transcription factors, cyclins, Cdks, and mitochondrial, cytoskeletal, and myofibrillar proteins. Many of the late-response genes expressed in overloaded hearts encode fetal proteins and protein isoforms normally found in the fetal heart during development (see below).

The appearance and disappearance of the mRNAs encoded in response to stress do not follow a uniform time course. Instead, their synthesis is activated and inactivated at different times during the first minutes and hours after the onset of the stress and then shut off at different rates over the subsequent hours and days. In addition to these temporal heterogeneities, there are spatial heterogeneities in the immediate-early response; for example, overload causes mRNAs encoding specific contractile protein isoforms to be upregulated differently in various regions of the heart (Schiaffino et al., 1989).

REVERSION TO THE FETAL PHENOTYPE

One of the remarkable features of the proliferative response seen in overloaded hearts is the reappearance of the patterns of gene expression normally seen in fetal life. This is due in part to the preferential expression of fetal genes in stressed cardiac myocytes, which can be viewed simplistically as accompanying the "failed" effort of these terminally differentiated cells to proliferate.

The functional consequences of reversion of the heart to the fetal phenotype are complex; for example, increased expression of the low ATPase fetal myosin heavy chain, which replaces the higher ATPase myosin normally found in the adult heart, has both beneficial and detrimental effects. By slowing the turnover of myosin cross-bridges, this isoform shift reduces contractility (see Chapter 4), thereby worsening the

TABLE 9-5 Some Proliferative Signaling Systems That Operate in the Mammalian Cardiovascular System

Extracellular Signal	Receptor	Coupling Proteins	Second Messenger or Mediator System	Intracellular Targets
Mediated by G-protein–coupled receptors				
β-Adrenergic agonists	β-adrenergic receptor	G protein	adenylyl cyclase, cyclic AMP calcium	protein kinase-A calmodulin, calcineurin
α-Adrenergic agonists	α-adrenergic receptor	G protein, ras	phospholipase C, DAG, InsP$_3$	protein kinase-C
Angiotensin II	AT$_1$ receptor	G protein, ras	phospholipase C, DAG, InsP$_3$	protein kinase-C
Endothelin	ET$_A$ receptor	G protein, ras	phospholipase C, DAG, InsP$_3$	protein kinase-C
Mediated by enzyme-linked receptors				
Peptide growth factors	tyrosine kinase receptors	ras		MAP kinases
Inflammatory cytokines	cytokine receptors, gp130	ras		SAPKs
Mediated by the cytoskeleton				
	integrins, titin, etc.	ras		tyrosine kinases, MAP kinases

G protein, heterotrimeric G protein; SAPK, stress-activated protein kinase; MAP kinase, mitogen-activated protein kinase.

hemodynamic abnormalities caused by chronic overloading. At the same time, however, this isoform shift reduces the rate of ATP hydrolysis by the heart's contractile machinery, which has a beneficial energy-sparing effect in the overloaded heart. Another important consequence of the reversion to the fetal phenotype is reduction of the content of sarcoplasmic reticulum which, in addition to reducing contractility, increases the heart's dependence on calcium derived from the extracellular fluid (the "extracellular calcium cycle" described in Chapter 7). Because both calcium entry and calcium efflux across the plasma membrane are accompanied by depolarizing currents, this feature of the reversion to the fetal phenotype contributes to the arrhythmias and sudden death commonly seen in end-stage heart failure (see Chapter 18).

SUMMARY AND CONCLUSIONS

Some of the key reactions that mediate the proliferative response to overload in the failing heart are summarized in Table 9-5. Because control of proliferative signaling is so intricate, this summary is incomplete, which reflects a complexity that will only increase with continued progress in the fast-moving fields reviewed in this chapter. Yet, these new insights can be expected to yield information that will improve therapy for patients with cardiovascular disease.

BIBLIOGRAPHY

Akazawa H, Komuro I. Roles of cardiac transcription factors in cardiac hypertrophy. *Circ Res* 2003;92:1079–1088.

Alberts B, Bray D, Lewis J, et al. *Molecular biology of the cell*, 4th ed. New York: Garland, 2002.

Bartek J, Bartkova J, Lukas J. The retinoblastoma protein pathway in cell cycle control and cancer. *Exp Cell Res* 1997;237:1–6.

Bazzoni F, Beutler B. The tumor necrosis factor ligand and receptor families. *New Engl J Med* 1996;334:1717–1725.

Bernards R. E2F: a nodal point in cell cycle regulation. *Biochim Biophys Acta* 1997;1333:M33–M40.

Brown R. The Bcl-2 family of proteins. *Br Med Bull* 1997;53:466–477.

Bueno OF, Molkentin JD. Involvement of extracellular signal-regulated kinases 1/2 in cardiac hypertrophy and cell death. *Circ Res* 2002;91:776–781.

Bugaisky L, Gupta M, Gupta MG, et al. Cellular and molecular mechanisms of hypertrophy. In: Fozzard H, Haber E, Katz A, et al., eds. *The heart and cardiovascular system*. New York: Raven Press, 1992:1621–1640.

Buja LM, Entman ML. Models of myocardial cell injury and cell death in ischemic heart disease. *Circulation* 1998;98:1355–1357.

Calladine CR, Drew HR. *Understanding DNA*. London: Academic Press, 1992.

Ceci M, Ross J Jr, Condorelli G. Molecular determinants of the physiological adaptation to stress in the cardiomyocyte: a focus on AKT. *J Mol Cell Cardiol* 2004;37:905–912.

Chi NC, Karliner JS. Molecular determinants of responses to myocardial ischemia/reperfusion injury: focus on hypoxia-inducible and heat shock factors. *Cardiovasc Res* 2004;61:437– 447.

Chiarugi V, Magnelli L, Cinelli M. Complex interplay among apoptosis factors: RB, P53, E2F, TGF-β, cell cycle inhibitors and the Bcl-2 gene family. *Pharmacol Res* 1997;35: 257–261.

Clapham DE, Neer EJ. G protein βγ subunits. *Ann Rev Pharmacol* 1997;37:167–203.

Cummins P, ed. *Growth factors and the cardiovascular system*. Boston: Kluwer, 1993.

Detillieux KA, Sheikh F, Kardami E, et al. Biological activities of fibroblast growth factor-2 in the adult myocardium. *Cardiovasc Res* 2003;57:8–19.

ten Dijke P, Hill CS. New insights into TGF-β–Smad signaling. *Trends Biochem Sci* 2004;29:265–273.

Dorn GW II, Force T. Protein kinase cascades in the regulation of cardiac hypertrophy. *J Clin Invest* 2005;115:527–537.

Downward J. (PI 3-kinase, Akt and cell survival. *Sem Cell Develop Biol* 2004;15: 177–182.

Dubois JM, Rouzaire-Dubois B. Role of potassium channels in mitogenesis. *Prog Biophys Mol Biol* 1993;59:1–21.

Dynlacht BD. Regulation of transcription by proteins that control the cell cycle. *Nature* 1997;389:149–152.

English J, Pearson G, Wilsbacher J, et al. New insights into the control of MAP kinase pathways. *Exp Cell Res* 1999;253:255–270.

Field LJ. Modulation of the cardiomyocyte cell cycle in genetically altered animals. *Ann NY Acad Sci* 2004;1015:160–170.

Ford HL, Pardee AB. Cancer and cell cycling. *J Cell Biochem* 1999;75(S32):166–172.

Frey N, Katus HA, Olson EN, et al. Hypertrophy of the heart. A new therapeutic target. *Circulation* 2004;109:1580–1589.

Gustafsson AB, Gottlied RA. Mechanisms of apoptosis in the heart. *J Clin Immunol* 2003;23:447–459.

Haunstetter A, Izumo S. Apoptosis: basic mechanisms and implications for cardiovascular disease. *Circ Res* 1998;82:1111–1129.

Henriksson M, Lüscher B. Proteins of the Myc network: essential regulator of cell growth and differentiation. *Adv Cancer Res* 1996;68:109–182.

Herwig S, Strauss M. The retinoblastoma protein: a master regulator of cell cycle, differentiation, and apoptosis. *Eur J Biochem* 1997;246:581–601.

Hetts SW. To die or not to die: an overview of apoptosis and its role in disease. *JAMA* 1998; 279:300–307.

Hill CS. Signaling to the nucleus by members of the transforming growth factor-β (TGF-β) superfamily. *Cell Signal* 1996;8:533–544.

Hoshijima M, Chien KR. Mixed signals in heart failure: cancer rules. *J Clin Invest* 2002;1098:849–855.

Hu H, Sachs F. Stretch-activated ion channels in the heart. *J Mol Cell Cardiol* 1997;29: 1511–1523.

Ichijo H. From receptors to stress-activated MAP kinases. *Oncogene* 1999;18:6087–6093.

Izumo S. Molecular basis of heart failure. In: Mann DL, ed. *Heart failure*. Philadelphia: Saunders, 2004.

Kardami E, Jiang ZS, Jimenez SK, et al. Fibroblast growth factor 2 isoforms and cardiac hypertrophy. *Cardiovasc Res* 2004;63:458–466.

Kidd VJ. Proteolytic activities that mediate apoptosis. Ann Rev Physiol 60:533-573.

Kudoh S, Akazawa H, Takano H, et al. Stretch-modulation of second messengers: effects on cardiomyocyte ion transport. *Prog Biophys Mol Biol* 2003;82:57–66.

Liang Q, Molkentin JD. Redefining the roles of p38 and JNK signaling in cardiac hypertrophy: dichotomy between cultured myocytes and animal models. *J Mol Cell Cardiol* 2003;35:1385–1394.

Lips DJ, deWindta LJ, van Kraaij DJW, et al. Molecular determinants of myocardial hypertrophy and failure: alternative pathways for beneficial and maladaptive hypertrophy. *Europ Heart J* 2003;24:883–896.

Lodish H, Berk A, Zipursky SL, et al. *Molecular cell biology*, 4th ed. New York: Freeman, 2000.

Manjo G, Joris I. Apoptosis, oncosis, and necrosis. An overview of cell death. *Am J Pathol* 1995;146:3–15.

McFalls EO, Liem D, Schoonerwoerd K, et al. Mitochondrial function: the heart of myocardial preservation. *J Lab Clin Med* 2003;142:141–149.

Molkentin JD, Dorn GW II. Cytoplamic signaling pathways that regulate cardiac hypertrophy. *Annu Rev Physiol* 2001;63:391–426.

Mowat MRA. p53 in tumor progression: life, death and everything. *Adv Cancer Res* 1998; 74:25–48.

Olson EN. A decade of discoveries in cardiac biology. *Nat Med* 2004;10:467–474.

Ono K, Han J. The p38 signal transduction pathway: activation and function. *Cell Signal* 2000;12:1–13.

Peeper DS, Bernards R. Communication between the extracellular environment, cytoplasmic signaling cascades and the nuclear cell-cycle machinery. *FEBS Lett* 1997;410: 11–16.

Petrich BG, Yibin Wang Y. Stress-activated MAP kinases in cardiac remodeling and heart failure new insights from transgenic studies. *Trends CV Med* 2004;14:50–55.

Prasad SVN, Perrino C, Rockman HA. Role of phosphoinositide 3-kinase in cardiac function and heart failure. *Trends Cardiovasc Med* 2003;13:206–212.

Pratt WB, Toft DO. Regulation of signaling protein function and trafficking by the hsp90/hsp70-based chaperone machinery. *Exp Biol Med* 2003;228:111–133.

Ransohoff RM. Cellular responses to interferons and other cytokines: the JAK-STAT paradigm. *New Engl J Med* 1998;338:616–618.

Rao A, Luo C, Hogan PG. Transcription factors of the NFAT family regulation and function. *Annu Rev Immunol* 1997;15:707–747.

Ravitz MJ, Wenner CE. Cyclin-dependent kinase regulation during G1 phase and cell cycle regulation by TGF-β. *Adv Cancer Res* 1997;71:165–207.

Reed JC. Double identity for proteins of the Bcl-2 family. *Nature* 1997;387:773–776.

Rosenkranz S. TGF-β1 and angiotensin networking in cardiac remodeling. *Cardiovasc Res* 2004;63:423–432.

Saini KS, Walker NI. Biochemical and molecular mechanisms regulating apoptosis. *Mol Cell Biochem* 1998;178:9–25.

Sekiguchi K, Li X, Coker M, et al. Cross-regulation between the renin-angiotensin system and inflammatory mediators in cardiac hypertrophy and failure. *Cardiovasc Res* 2004;63:433–442.

Selvetella G, Hirsch E, Notte A, et al. Adaptive and maladaptive hypertrophic pathways: points of convergence and divergence. *Cardiovasc Res* 2004;63:373–380.

Simpson PC. β-protein kinase C and hypertrophic signaling in human heart failure. *Circulation* 1999;93:334–337.

Stroud RM, Wells JA. Mechanistic diversity of cytokine receptor signaling across cell membranes. *Sci STKE* 2004;231:re7.

Sugden PH, Clerk A. "Stress-responsive" mitogen-activated protein kinases (c-jun N-terminal kinases and p38 mitogen-activated protein kinases) in the myocardium. *Circ Res* 1998;83:345–352.

Sussman MA, McCulloch A, Borg TK. Dance band on the Titanic. Biomechanical signaling in cardiac hypertrophy. *Circ Res* 2002;91:888–898.

Thompson EB. The many roles of c-Myc in apoptosis. *Ann Rev Physiol* 1998;60: 575–600.

Thornberry NA. The caspase family of cysteine proteases. *Br Med Bull* 1997;53: 478–490.

van Biesen T, Luttrell LM, Hawes BE, et al. Mitogenic signaling via G protein–coupled receptors. *Endoc Rev* 1996;17:698–714.

van Empel VPM, De Windt LJ. Myocyte hypertrophy and apoptosis: a balancing act *Cardiovasc Res* 2004;63:487–499.

Walsh K, Perlman H. Cell cycle exit upon myogenic differentiation. *Curr Opin Genet Dev* 1997;7:597–602.

Widmann C, Gibson S, Jarpe MP, et al. Mitogen-activated protein kinase: conservation of a three kinase module from yeast to human. *Physiol Rev* 1999;79:143–180.

Wyllie AH. Apoptosis: an overview. *Br Med Bull* 1997;53:451–465.

Zhang T, Brown JH. Role of Ca2 $^+$ /calmodulin-dependent protein kinase II in cardiac hypertrophy and heart failure. *Cardiovasc Res* 2004;63:476–486.

REFERENCES

Berridge M. The AM and FM of calcium signaling. *Nature* 1997;386:759–760.

Bourne HR. Team blue sees red. *Nature* 1995;376:727–729.

Egan SE, Weinberg RA. The pathway to signal achievement. *Nature* 1993;365:781–783.

Goss RJ. Hypertrophy versus hyperplasia. *Science* 1966;153:1615–1620.

Graves LM, Bornfeldt KE, Krebs EG. Historical perspectives and new insights involving the MAP kinase cascades. *Adv Second Messenger Phosphoprotein Res* 1997;31: 49–61.

Katz AM. *Heart failure. Pathophysiology, molecular biology, and clinical management.* Philadelphia: Lippincott Williams & Wilkins, 2000.

Kroemer G, Zamzami N, Susin SA. Mitochondrial control of apoptosis. *Immunol Today* 1997;18:44–51.

Luttrell LM, Ferguson SSG, Daaka Y, et al. β-arrestin-dependent formation of β$_2$ adrenergic receptor-src protein kinase complexes. *Science* 1999;283:655–661.

Pardee AB. G1 events and regulation of cell proliferation. *Science* 1989;246:603–608.

Raff MC, Barres BA, Burne JF, et al. Programmed cell death and the control of cell survival: lessons from the nervous system. *Science* 1993;262:695–700.

Raffray M, Cohen GM. Apoptosis and necrosis in toxicology: a continuum or distinct modes of cell death? *Pharmacol Ther* 1997;75:153–177.

Ring PA. Myocardial regeneration in experimental ischaemic lesions of the heart. *J Path Bact* 1950;62:21–27.

Rumyantsev PP. Interrelations of the proliferation and differentiation of processes during cardiac myogenesis and regeneration. *Int Rev Cytol* 1977;51:187–273.

Saini KS, Walker NI. Biochemical and molecular mechanisms regulating apoptosis. *Mol Cell Biochem* 1998;178:9–25.

Savill J. Recognition and phagocytosis of cells undergoing apoptosis. *BMJ* 1997;53: 491–508.

Schiaffino S, Samuel JL, Sassoon D, et al. Nonsynchronous accumulation of α-skeletal actin and β-myosin heavy chain mRNAs during early stages of pressure-overloaded-induced cardiac hypertrophy demonstrated by in situ hybridization. *Circ Res* 1989;64:937–948.

Ucker DS. Death by suicide: one way to go in mammalian development? *New Biol* 1991;3:103–109.

Uozumi H, Hiroi Y, Zou Y, et al. gp130 plays a critical role in pressure overload-induced cardiac hypertrophy. *J Biol Chem* 2001;276:23115–23119.

van Noorden CFJ, Meade-Tollin LC, Bosman FT. Metastasis. *Am Scientist* 1998;86:130–141.

10

REGULATION OF CARDIAC MUSCLE PERFORMANCE: FUNCTIONAL AND PROLIFERATIVE MECHANISMS

Three different types of mechanism regulate cardiac performance (Katz, 1988); two evoke functional responses, the third depends on proliferative responses (Table 10-1). The most "modern" is regulation by changing *organ physiology*, a functional mechanism that appeared about 600 million years ago with the evolution of large multicellular animals that required a circulatory system. The second functional mechanism, regulation by changes in *cell biochemistry* and *biophysics*, appeared much earlier, about 2,000 million years ago, in single-celled eukaryotes in which internal membrane systems regulated the intracellular environment (*milieu intèrieur*). Regulation by altered *gene expression*, the third, is the most primitive, having appeared at the dawn of life more than 3,500 million years ago. These proliferative mechanisms made it possible for early populations of prokaryotes to survive environmental change by providing a genetic diversity that allowed some individuals to survive in the new surroundings (see Chapter 9). Because proliferative signaling has had the longest time to evolve, it is not surprising that it is the most complex.

Regulation by changing organ physiology adjusts cardiac performance to meet simple hemodynamic challenges like increased venous return (Starling's Law of the Heart). More complex hemodynamic challenges, such as those that occur during exercise, are met by biochemical responses that alter myocardial contractility and relaxation; the most important functional responses are brought about by changes in the calcium fluxes between the cytosol, extracellular fluid, and sarcoplasmic reticulum (see Chapter 7). The third mechanism, which depends on proliferative signaling, allows chronic hemodynamic overloading and other long-term challenges to alter the size, shape, and molecular composition of the heart.

Each of these three types of response follows a different time course. Regulation by changing end-diastolic fiber length (organ physiology) operates most rapidly, on a "beat-to-beat" basis, while changes in contractility

TABLE 10-1 Three Types of Mechanism That Regulate Cardiac Performance

Functional Responses
Organ physiology: changes in end-diastolic fiber length (Starling's Law of the Heart)
Cell biochemistry and biophysics: changes in myocardial contractility and relaxation
Proliferative Responses
"Molecular biology:" changes in the architecture of the heart, its protein and membrane composition, and altered gene expression

and relaxation (cell biochemistry and biophysics) generally require several seconds or minutes to appear and disappear. Most sustained are the responses to proliferative signaling (altered gene expression), such as those that occur in chronically overloaded and damaged hearts, in which long-term changes in cardiac performance result from structural changes that can take days, weeks, and even months to develop.

FUNCTIONAL RESPONSES: REGULATION BY CHANGING END-DIASTOLIC VOLUME AND MYOCARDIAL CONTRACTILITY

Functional control of cardiac performance is usually attributed to two mechanisms: changes in rest length and changes in contractility (see Chapter 6). The former, which allows cardiac performance to respond to changes in end-diastolic volume, is generally referred to as "Starling's Law of the Heart" (Starling, 1918). This physiological mechanism was commonly viewed as the only determinant of myocardial performance until the mid-1950s, when description of the "family of Starling curves" (Sarnoff, 1955) made it possible to distinguish between length-dependent regulation of contractile performance and regulation by changes in contractility.

Regulation by changing end-diastolic fiber length and changing contractility were initially thought to arise from entirely different mechanisms. This interpretation was based largely on the now discarded view that the length–tension relationship in cardiac muscle is caused when changes in the overlap between the thick and thin filaments modify the number of potential interactions between actin and myosin (the "ultrastructural mechanism" described in Chapter 6), whereas contractility is changed when biochemical changes modify the contractile proteins interactions. Even though control by changing end-diastolic volume, like that by changing contractility, is now attributed to variations in excitation–contraction coupling, the traditional distinction remains useful because these regulatory mechanisms serve different physiological functions.

Changes in End-Diastolic Volume

Regulation by changing end-diastolic volume (Starling's Law of the Heart) can be viewed as a "passive" mechanism that equalizes the outputs of the right and left ventricles and allows the heart to respond rapidly to changes such as in preload and afterload.

MATCHING THE OUTPUTS OF THE RIGHT AND LEFT VENTRICLES. The positive feedback that results from the operation of the ventricles on the ascending limbs of their length–tension curves (see Chapter 6) plays an essential role in equalizing the outputs of the two ventricles. For example, when right ventricular output is increased by leg raising, the increased flow of blood through the lungs increases venous return to the left ventricle, which according to Starling's law increases left ventricular ejection. Conversely, reduced ejection by the right ventricle decreases left ventricular filling and therefore reduces left ventricular output.

CHANGING PRELOAD. Increased venous return to the right atrium, as occurs when the legs are raised, causes an elevation in right atrial pressure that is transmitted immediately to the right ventricle, where it increases end-diastolic volume (preload). According to Starling's law, the latter increases the ability of the right ventricle to eject blood, which restores the equilibrium between venous return and right ventricular output. This ability of the heart to increase its output in response to changing venous return represents a positive feedback in which altered blood flow *into* the heart leads to a corresponding change in the flow of blood *out of* the heart.

CHANGING AFTERLOAD. An abrupt increase in aortic pressure (afterload) reduces left ventricular ejection (see Chapter 6), which increases the volume of blood remaining in the ventricle at the end of systole (end-systolic volume). When the venous return during the next diastole is added to this increased end-systolic volume, end-diastolic volume is increased. According to Starling's law, this compensates for the increased afterload by increasing the ability of the ventricle to do work.

The Garden Hose Effect

A peculiar type of length-dependent regulation of cardiac performance was observed many years ago, when coronary perfusion pressure was found to influence the ability of the heart to develop tension even when the ventricle was drained of blood and intraventricular pressure was kept at zero (Salisbury et al., 1960). The unexpected ability of a higher coronary artery pressure to increase cardiac performance is explained because increasing coronary artery pressure elongates the cardiac myocytes by increasing the pressure *within* its walls, much as a garden hose is distended when its internal pressure is increased by occluding its outlet.

Changes in Myocardial Contractility
(Inotropic Properties or Systolic Function)

Although Starling's law plays a major role in beat-to-beat adjustments in cardiac performance, it is of little importance in sustained circulatory changes. This became apparent in the 1930s, when it was found that despite a several-fold increase in cardiac output, the heart could become smaller during exercise. These and other findings made it clear that mechanisms other than end-diastolic fiber length regulate cardiac performance. The most important of these mechanisms are changes in myocardial contractility that occur during the hemodynamic defense reaction as well as those responsible for most responses of the heart to drugs and disease. Because contractility is often referred to as *inotropy*, a *positive inotropic* intervention increases contractility, while a *negative inotropic* intervention reduces contractility.

WHAT IS MYOCARDIAL CONTRACTILITY? Myocardial contractility is a manifestation of *all* of the factors that influence the interactions between the contractile proteins, except for those that depend on preload and afterload. In the heart, the former is end-diastolic volume, which determines sarcomere length, while afterload has a major effect on work performance (see Chapter 6). A simple definition is *the ability of the ventricle to do work that does not depend on preload or afterload*. However, this definition is of limited value because it does not distinguish among the many variables that modify the contractile machinery of the heart. From a practical standpoint, a *change* in myocardial contractility is easier to define; this is simply *any change in cardiac performance that is not caused by a change in initial fiber length (preload) or afterload*. If, for example, a drug increases tension development or shortening in an isolated strip of cardiac muscle contracting at fixed rest length and load, contractility has been increased (Fig. 10-1). Conversely, a drug that reduces the ability of the myocardium to do work at constant length and

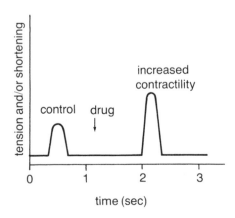

FIGURE 10-1 Increased myocardial contractility enhances the amount of tension developed, the rate of shortening, or both without an increase in rest length.

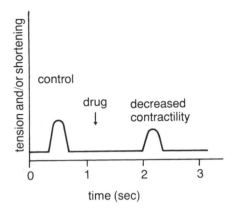

FIGURE 10-2 Decreased myocardial contractility reduces the amount of tension developed, the rate of shortening, or both without a decrease in rest length.

load has decreased contractility (Fig. 10-2). In the intact heart, a change in left ventricular contractility can be defined as a change in the work performed per beat at constant end-diastolic volume and aortic pressure (see Chapter 12).

Although it can be relatively easy to identify a change in myocardial contractility, there remains the more important question as to what, exactly, has been changed. Simple definitions fail because contractility is determined by *all* of the many processes that influence the ability of a muscle to do work. Two commonly used ways to define myocardial contractility are described below; one is based on the principles of muscle mechanics, the other on the interactions between the contractile proteins. While neither has much clinical value, these approaches can be useful in trying to decide what is going on in a patient who experiences an unexpected change in hemodynamics, such as a fall in blood pressure.

CONTRACTILITY DEFINED IN TERMS OF MUSCLE MECHANICS. Muscle mechanics were once believed to be able to quantify myocardial contractility in the face of changing preload and afterload. The latter, which are detailed in Chapter 6, include the ability of a greater preload to increase the ability of muscle to develop tension and shorten, and of increased afterload to slow and reduce the extent of shortening. The value of cardiac mechanics in quantifying the load-independent properties of the contracting heart was thought to lie in its ability to measure the two types of interaction between the myosin cross-bridges and actin: one where the cross-bridges are maintaining tension (see Fig. 3-16), the other in which they are turning over at their maximal intrinsic rate (see Fig. 3-17). Afterload is a major determinant of the distribution of the cross-bridges between these two states. If, for example, a muscle is presented with a heavy load, the developed tension is high and most of the cross-bridges are holding tension, so shortening velocity is low and the load is moved only a short distance. Conversely, in a lightly loaded muscle, where developed tension is low, most of the cross-bridges are free to cycle, so shortening velocity is high and the load is moved a greater distance. These load-dependent changes in tension and shortening velocity do *not* reflect variations in contractility, but instead are different ways that a muscle operating at a given level of contractility is able to do work.

In the 1960s and 1970s, it was believed that the effects of changing the heart's afterload could be eliminated by extrapolating P_o, and V_{max} from force–velocity curves (see Fig. 3-15). These intercepts, which were shown by Hill to be determined by the number and turnover of interactions within the contractile machinery of the frog sartorius, were claimed to distinguish between the effects of changing end-diastolic fiber length and those of changing contractility in the heart. It was stated that changing preload influences P_o, but not V_{max}, because according to the "ultrastructural mechanism" for the length–tension relationship, length-dependent variations in the ability of the heart to do work are caused by changes in the number of active cross-bridges (see Chapter 6). This meant that because changes in length should modify only P_o, a change in contractility would be identified as a change in V_{max}.

However, it is now clear that in cardiac muscle, these measurements can neither define contractility nor distinguish the effects of changing fiber length from those of a change in inotropic state. This is because the portions of the force–velocity curves that can be measured in heart muscle are not hyperbolical, which means that estimates of V_{max} and P_o, the intercepts, depend on imprecise extrapolations. The major underlying problem is that, unlike tetanized skeletal muscle, where active state develops rapidly and remains stable for a reasonable time, active state in cardiac muscle changes throughout systole. This is due to the influence of three time-dependent variables, none of which can be quantified: the rate of onset, duration, and rate of decay of the active state (see Chapter 6). In addition, the spiral arrangement of the fibers in the walls of the heart (see Chapter 1) and high resting tension of cardiac muscle (see Chapter 6) contribute elasticities that, even when the ends of the muscle are fixed, modify developed tension and shortening velocity as active state increases and decreases. These and other limitations mean that P_o and V_{max} cannot be accurately extrapolated in cardiac muscle from measurements of length and tension.

CONTRACTILITY DEFINED IN TERMS OF CONTRACTILE PROTEIN INTERACTIONS. Although accurate measurements of force–velocity curves are not possible in the heart, the underlying concept, that P_o is proportional to the *number* of active cross-bridges and that V_{max} reflects the *maximal rate* of cross-bridge cycling, remains useful. In the heart, most of the major functional mechanisms that modify contractility are brought about by changes in the number of interactions between the myosin cross-bridges and actin. These, in turn, reflect variations in the amount of calcium delivered to the contractile proteins during excitation–contraction coupling and changes in the calcium-affinity of troponin C, both of which should change only

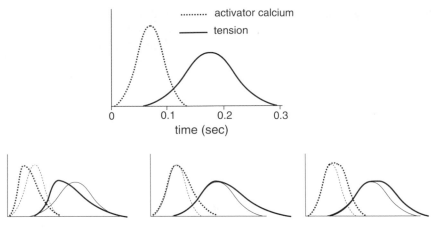

FIGURE 10-3 Three mechanisms by which time-dependent changes in the release of activator calcium in cardiac muscle can increase contractility without changing the maximal release of activator calcium. **Above:** Control, showing the increase in cytosolic calcium (*dotted line*) that precedes tension development (*solid line*). **Below:** Contractility can be increased (*heavy lines*) when the rate of calcium release is increased (a), the rate of calcium removal is reduced (b), or the duration of calcium release is prolonged (c).

P_0. The rate of cross-bridge cycling, which determines V_{max}, the other determinant of myocardial contractility, can be varied by functional signals that initiate post-translational changes, such as phosphorylation of the myofibrillar proteins (see Chapter 4).

Contractility also can be regulated by changes in the time course of calcium release into the cytosol, such as the rate at which calcium is delivered to the contractile proteins, the time that calcium remains bound to troponin C, and the rate at which activator calcium is dissociated from troponins (Fig. 10-3). These changes, which modify the duration of the active state, can be approximated during the development and decay of tension by calcium-sensitive dyes.

"PRACTICAL" VALUE OF THE CONCEPT OF MYOCARDIAL CONTRACTILITY. Even though the complexity of the active state is now known to make it impossible to quantify the level of contractility in the beating heart, the concept is important clinically. This is illustrated by the patient mentioned on p. 286, who experienced an unexplained fall in blood pressure. If the hemodynamic deterioration cannot be attributed to a fall in end-diastolic volume, as might be caused by hemorrhage, vasodilatation, or another disorder that decreases circulating blood volume, a search should immediately be undertaken to identify a pathophysiological process, like myocardial infarction or a drug, that could have reduced myocardial contractility.

Changes in Filling (Lusitropic Properties or Diastolic Function)

The clinical importance of changes in diastolic filling was not recognized until relatively recently. This is largely because the first applications of hemodynamic physiology that followed the introduction of cardiac catheterization in the 1940s focused on pressures, which were readily measured by the equipment available to early workers. Initial efforts to characterize myocardial performance therefore used pressure-based indices, notably the rate of pressure rise during isovolumic contraction (+dP/dt), to quantify myocardial contractility (see Chapter 12). The neglect of relaxation abnormalities reflected the difficulty in interpreting measurements of the rate of pressure fall during isovolumic relaxation (−dP/dt), which is highly dependent on systemic blood pressure and so requires corrections that are both difficult and imprecise. It was not until the 1970s, when echocardiography and nuclear techniques made it possible to measure changes in ventricular volume, that diastolic function could be characterized in terms of the rate and extent of filling (see Chapter 12).

FUNCTIONAL MECHANISMS THAT REGULATE MYOCARDIAL CONTRACTILITY AND RELAXATION

Most functional changes in contractility and relaxation are initiated by post-translational signals that modify the calcium fluxes that control the contractile protein interactions. These physiological mechanisms generally result from phosphorylation of the contractile proteins and the membrane proteins that participate in excitation–contraction coupling and relaxation. The following discussion, which is based on the schematic depiction of the extracellular and intracellular calcium cycles shown in Figure 7-20, highlights a few key regulatory mechanisms, including the staircase phenomena, postextrasystolic potentiation, and the responses of the heart to energy starvation, sympathetic stimulation, cardiac glycosides and calcium sensitizing drugs.

Changes in Calcium Fluxes across the Plasma Membrane

PLASMA MEMBRANE CALCIUM CHANNELS. Calcium entry by way of L-type calcium channels ("dihydropyridine receptors"), which is among the most important determinants of myocardial contractility, serves two functions: It triggers the opening of the intracellular calcium release channels in the sarcoplasmic reticulum and contributes to the filling of internal calcium stores. Only a small amount of the calcium that enters the cytosol through these channels binds to the contractile proteins of the adult heart because most of the activator calcium is provided by the intracellular calcium cycle.

The positive inotropic effects of β-adrenergic agonists and phosphodiesterase inhibitors, both of which increase cyclic AMP levels, are due in part to phosphorylation of these calcium channels by cyclic AMP–dependent protein kinases (PK-A). Because phosphorylation increases the probability of channel opening (see Chapter 13), more calcium enters the cytosol (Fig. 10-4) to cause a positive inotropic response. β-Adrenergic receptor blockers reduce contractility by inhibiting the channel opening caused by basal sympathetic activity; L-type calcium

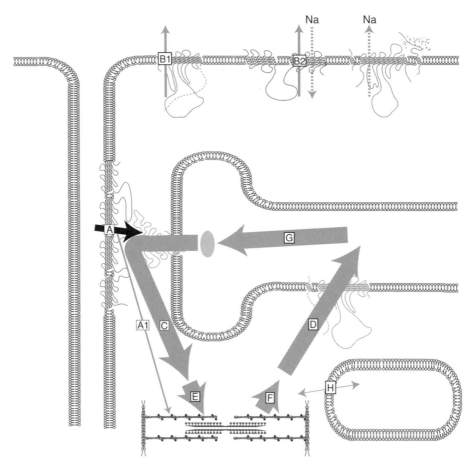

FIGURE 10-4 Increased calcium entry through L-type plasma membrane calcium channels (*larger arrow* A) contributes to several positive inotropic mechanisms, including the positive staircase, postextrasystolic potentiation, and the inotropic response caused by cyclic AMP. In the staircase, increased stimulation frequency causes more calcium channel openings per unit of time, which increases net calcium influx across the plasma membrane. Postextrasystolic potentiation occurs when premature depolarization of the plasma membrane increases the opening of these channels; as virtually all of the additional calcium goes into the sarcoplasmic reticulum, contractility is increased in subsequent beats. The positive inotropic effect of cyclic AMP is due in part to increased calcium channel opening, which increases the amount of calcium that enters the cytosol through these channels.

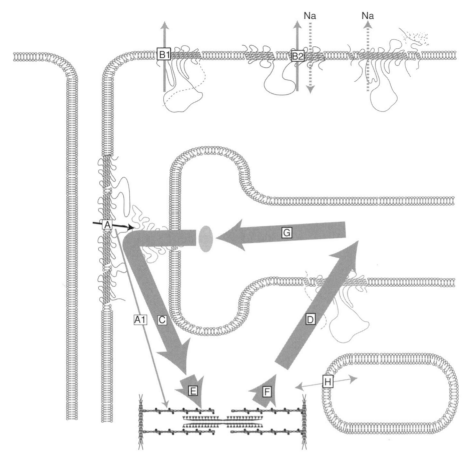

FIGURE 10-5   Drugs that inhibit L-type calcium channel opening (calcium channel blockers) reduce calcium entry across the plasma membrane (*smaller arrow* A).

channel blockers, which directly inhibit channel opening, also have a negative inotropic effect (Fig. 10-5). Calcium entry is reduced in the energy-starved heart when decreased ATP concentration attenuates an allosteric effect that facilitates calcium channel opening (see Chapter 7).

THE POSITIVE (BOWDITCH) STAIRCASE. Bowditch (1871) was the first to observe that the tension developed by cardiac muscle increases when the frequency of stimulation is increased, and that slowed stimulation reduces tension (Fig. 10-6). The stepwise increase in tension seen when heart rate is accelerated, called the *positive staircase* or *treppe* (the latter is the German word for *staircase*), is a manifestation of rate-dependent variations in contractility known collectively as the *force–frequency relationship*. These rate-dependent changes in contractility are caused by altered stimulation *frequency*, not *intensity*, and so do not violate the *all-or-none law* (also first described by Bowditch) stating that the magnitude of a

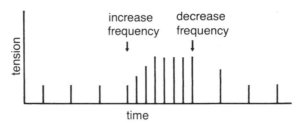

FIGURE 10-6 The positive (Bowditch) staircase. Tension developed by cardiac muscle during a series of isometric contractions (*shown as vertical lines*) increases in a stepwise manner after stimulation frequency is increased and decreases when stimulation frequency is reduced.

response is independent of the intensity of the stimulus. The positive staircase is due simply to the fact that more frequent opening of plasma membrane calcium channels at higher rates of stimulation increases calcium flux from the extracellular space into cytosol (Fig. 10-4).

POSTEXTRASYSTOLIC POTENTIATION. Contractions that follow a premature systole (often referred to as an *extrasystole*) manifest a positive inotropic effect, called *postextrasystolic potentiation*, that is among the most intense seen in cardiac muscle (Fig. 10-7). The magnitude of the increase in contractility is not correlated with the tension developed by the premature systole; in fact, a large postextrasystolic potentiation can occur when the premature beat comes so early as merely to delay relaxation after the preceding normal beat.

Postextrasystolic potentiation occurs because premature depolarizations increase calcium entry through plasma membrane calcium channels, which adds to the calcium stored in the sarcoplasmic reticulum. Unlike the positive staircase, where filling of these stores is increased by more frequent channel openings, postextrasystolic potentiation occurs when premature stimuli increase the extent to which the channels open. This mechanism was elucidated by Wood et al. (1969), who induced small changes in membrane potential during the absolute refractory period by applying currents through an intracellular electrode (Fig. 10-8). Because these currents appeared at a time when heart cannot generate an action potential (see Chapter 14), they did not affect tension development during

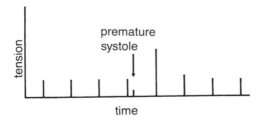

time

FIGURE 10-7 Postextrasystolic potentiation. The tension developed by the contraction immediately following a premature systole (sometimes called an *extrasystole*) is potentiated by a positive inotropic state left behind by the premature systole.

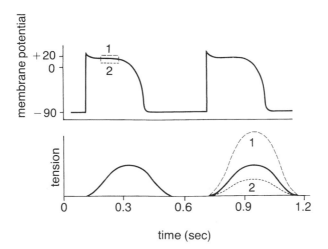

FIGURE 10-8 Effects of altered membrane potential during an action potential plateau (*top*) on contractile performance in the following beat. Depolarizing (1) or hyperpolarizing (2) currents applied during the plateau of the cardiac action potential have no effect on tension developed during the contraction in which the current is applied. However, tension developed in the subsequent contraction (*bottom*) is increased by the current (1) and decreased by a hyperpolarizing current (2).

the beat in which they were applied. Instead, depolarizing currents that caused membrane potential to become more negative increased tension developed in the *following* systole (1, Fig. 10-8); conversely, hyperpolarizing currents that shifted membrane potential toward the resting level reduced tension in the subsequent beat (2, Fig. 10-8). These findings reflect the ability of the small changes in membrane potential to modify the opening of the L-type calcium channels in *subsequent* contractions: Depolarization prolongs calcium channel opening, while reducing membrane potential accelerates their closing.

THE SODIUM–CALCIUM EXCHANGER. The Na–Ca exchanger, which exchanges sodium and calcium in both directions across the plasma membrane (see Chapter 7), has important effects on both myocardial contractility and membrane potential. The latter include afterdepolarizations, which are caused by depolarizing currents generated when divalent calcium ions leave the cytosol in exchange for three univalent sodium ions (see Chapter 14).

Competition between the sodium and calcium fluxes mediated by the Na–Ca exchanger allows changes in the extracellular concentrations of these ions to modify calcium influx; this explains why myocardial contractility is directly proportional to the ratio between extracellular sodium and calcium. Increased calcium influx by way of the Na–Ca exchanger also accounts for the ability of increased extracellular calcium or decreased extracellular sodium to increase contractility (Fig. 10-9), while the negative inotropic effect of decreased extracellular calcium and increased extracellular sodium are caused by reduced calcium influx.

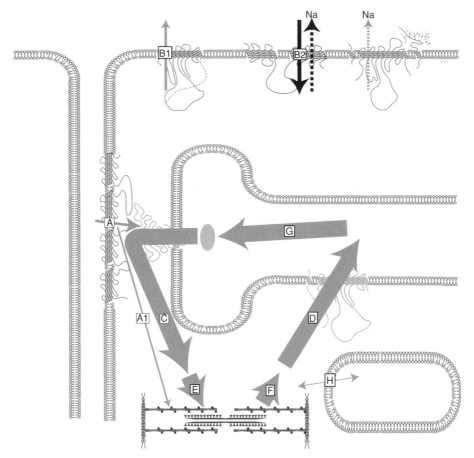

FIGURE 10-9 Increased extracellular calcium and decreased extracellular sodium cause a positive inotropic effect by increasing calcium entry by way of the Na–Ca exchanger (*larger inward arrow* B2).

Inhibition of the sodium pump by cardiac glycosides (see Chapter 7) increases intracellular sodium concentration, which increases intracellular calcium stores by two mechanisms, both of which involve the Na–Ca exchanger. The first is the ability of increased cytosolic sodium to reduce calcium efflux by competing with calcium at the intracellular site of the exchanger (Fig. 10-10). The second occurs when some of the sodium that would have been exchanged for extracellular potassium by the sodium pump is, instead, exchanged for extracellular calcium (Fig. 10-11). Both responses increase intracellular calcium, and so have a positive inotropic effect.

THE SODIUM–HYDROGEN EXCHANGER. Protons generated during anaerobic energy production are transported out of the cytosol in exchange for sodium by a Na–H exchanger (see Chapter 7). The resulting increase in

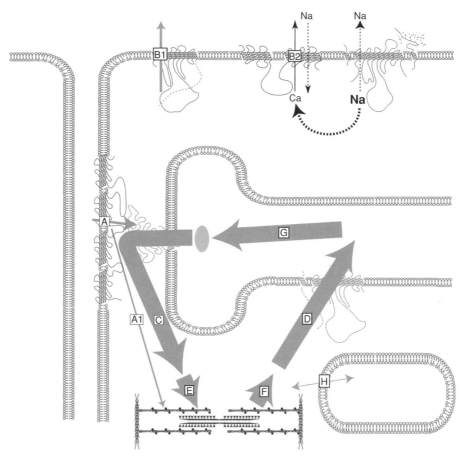

FIGURE 10-10 Cardiac glycosides, by inhibiting the sodium pump, increase cytosolic sodium concentration. The higher intracellular sodium concentration (*curved dotted arrow*) increases calcium stores within the cell by reducing calcium efflux by way of the Na–Ca exchanger (*smaller arrow* B2).

intracellular sodium increases contractility by reducing calcium efflux by way of the Na–Ca exchanger (see above).

THE PLASMA MEMBRANE CALCIUM PUMP. The plasma membrane calcium pump, which like the Na–Ca exchanger transports calcium out of the myocardial cell, is stimulated by calcium–calmodulin-dependent protein kinase (see Chapter 7), By increasing calcium flux out of the cytosol (Fig. 10-12), this response helps to avoid calcium overload, but also has a negative inotropic effect.

Changes in Calcium Fluxes across the Sarcoplasmic Reticulum Membrane

Contraction and relaxation in the adult human heart are controlled mainly by calcium fluxes across the sarcoplasmic reticulum membrane.

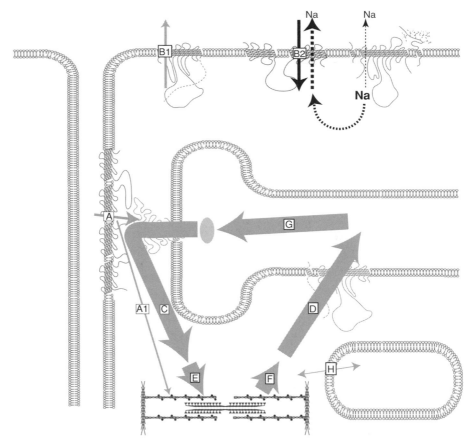

FIGURE 10-11 Cardiac glycosides, by inhibiting the sodium pump, reduce the amount of sodium exchanged for potassium. The higher intracellular sodium concentration (*curved dotted arrow*) increases sodium efflux by way of the Na–Ca exchanger, which increases calcium influx (*larger inward arrow* B2).

The most important determinants of the amount of calcium released are the calcium content of the sarcoplasmic reticulum and the amount of "trigger" calcium that enters the cell by way of L-type plasma membrane calcium channels (see Chapter 7).

CALCIUM RELEASE CHANNELS. Calcium is released from the cardiac sarcoplasmic reticulum through intracellular calcium release channels ("ryanodine receptors"). Decreased intracellular calcium stores and attenuation of the signal initiated by calcium influx through L-type calcium channels reduces this calcium release and therefore have a negative inotropic effect (Fig. 10-13). Conversely, increased calcium stores and calcium influx increase contractility. Because allosteric effects of high ATP concentrations facilitate the opening of the calcium release channels (see Chapter 7), ATP depletion in energy-starved hearts can blunt the response of these channels to calcium-triggered calcium release and so reduce contractility (Fig. 10-13).

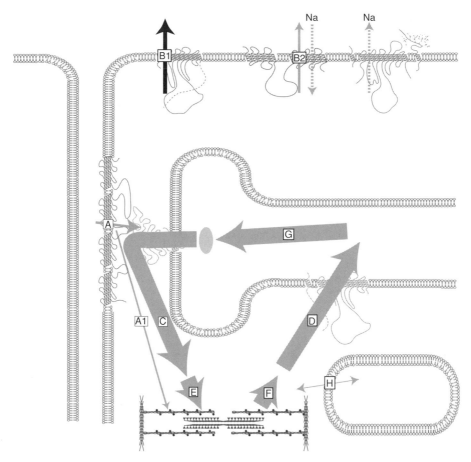

FIGURE 10-12 Acceleration of the plasma membrane calcium pump by calcium-calmodulin–dependent protein kinase increases active transport of calcium out of the cell (*larger arrow* B1).

CALCIUM PUMP ATPASE. Cytosolic calcium concentration, which is the most important physiological regulator of calcium uptake by the sarcoplasmic reticulum calcium pump (SERCA), accelerates calcium removal from the cytosol, thereby playing a key role in matching the amount of calcium taken up during diastole to that released during systole. Agents that increase cyclic AMP levels, either by stimulating the synthesis of this intracellular second messenger (β-adrenergic agonists) or inhibiting its breakdown (phosphodiesterase inhibitors) have important inotropic and lusitropic effects. The latter are caused when PK-A catalyzes the phosphorylation of phospholamban, a regulatory protein that in its dephospho form inhibits the pump. Reversal of this effect by phospholamban phosphorylation increases the calcium sensitivity of the pump, which stimulates calcium uptake into the sarcoplasmic reticulum (Fig. 10-14). This accelerates relaxation directly and, by increasing the amount of calcium retained in this intracellular membrane system, also has a positive inotropic effect.

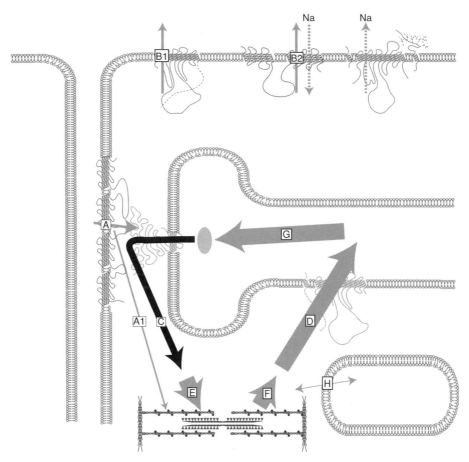

FIGURE 10-13 Calcium efflux through calcium release channels in the sarcoplasmic reticulum (*smaller arrow* C) is reduced when less "trigger" calcium enters by way of the plasma membrane calcium channels, when intracellular calcium stores are depleted, and when ATP is depleted in an energy-starved heart.

The allosteric effect of ATP stimulates calcium uptake by the sarcoplasmic reticulum (see Chapter 7) so that energy starvation impairs relaxation (Fig. 10-15). A fall in ATP concentration also inhibits the calcium pump by decreasing the free energy released during ATP hydrolysis, an effect that is amplified by an accompanying rise in ADP levels (see Chapter 7).

Changes in Calcium Fluxes within the Sarcoplasmic Reticulum

Transfer of calcium from the sarcotubular network, where this activator is taken up by the calcium pump ATPase, to the subsarcolemmal cisternae from which this ion is released through calcium release channels is mediated by passive diffusion. This process may become rate limiting at

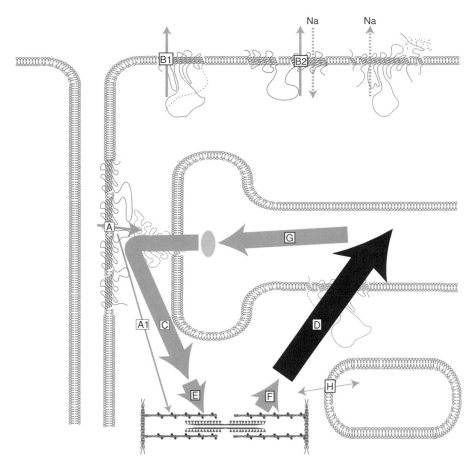

FIGURE 10-14 Increased calcium uptake into the sarcoplasmic reticulum caused by phosphorylation of phospholamban (*larger arrow* D) favors relaxation by increasing the rate and extent of calcium removal from the cytosol.

rapid heart rates because of the small cross-sectional area of the lumen within these membranes.

THE NEGATIVE (WOODWORTH) STAIRCASE. Woodworth (1902), a few decades after Bowditch described the positive staircase, observed another staircase phenomenon in which tension decreases as heart rate is accelerated (Fig. 10-16). This feature of the force–frequency relationship, which is opposite to the Bowditch staircase, is often called the *negative* or *Woodworth staircase*. The negative staircase is most prominent at higher stimulation frequencies, where a decrease in stimulation frequency can cause a transient increase in tension. An increase in the tension developed by the first beat following a pause, sometimes called the *recuperative effect of a pause*, also is a manifestation of the negative staircase.

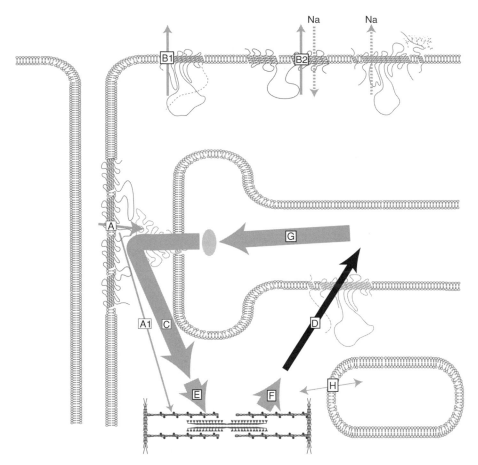

FIGURE 10-15 Calcium uptake into the sarcoplasmic reticulum can be slowed by a fall in ATP concentration, acidosis, and a reduced number of calcium pump ATPase molecules (*smaller arrow* D). All of these effects impair relaxation.

Both the negative (Woodworth) and positive (Bowditch) staircases can appear when stimulation frequency is changed (Fig. 10-17). The negative staircase, which evolves more rapidly, causes an initial fall in tension when stimulation frequency is increased (1, Fig. 10-17) and a transient rise in tension when heart rate is decreased (3, Fig. 10-17); the latter also explains the recuperative effect of a pause. Any fall in tension caused by the negative staircase is quickly overwhelmed in subsequent contractions by the more slowly developing positive staircase (2, Fig. 10-17); conversely, the initial increase in tension seen when stimulation frequency is decreased is followed by a fall in tension as the more slowly evolving positive staircase wears off (4, Fig. 10-17). These force–frequency relationships are altered in failing hearts, where the positive staircase is attenuated and may disappear completely.

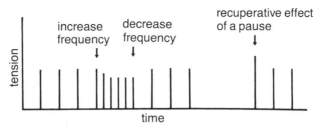

FIGURE 10-16 The negative (Woodworth) staircase. The tension developed during a series of contractions by cardiac muscle decreases in the first few beats after stimulation rate is increased and augmented when stimulation is slowed. Another manifestation of the negative staircase is the recuperative effect of a pause, which increases tension in the first beat after stimulation is interrupted.

The rapid changes in contractility associated with the negative staircase may reflect a redistribution of calcium within the cell; according to this hypothesis, the rapid fall of tension that follows an increase in stimulation frequency occurs when slow diffusion of this activator to the calcium release channels in the subsarcolemmal cisternae causes calcium to accumulate within the sarcotubular network (Fig. 10-18). This mechanism also could explain the recuperative effect of a pause, as the latter would allow calcium that had accumulated in the sarcotubular network to diffuse to the subsarcolemmal cisternae, where its release would augment tension developed in the subsequent contraction (Fig. 10-19). Alternative mechanisms include slow reactivation of the calcium release channels following a short cycle, which would cause short cycles to reduce calcium release by not permitting enough time for the calcium release channels to recover fully from a refractory state left behind after the preceding beat.

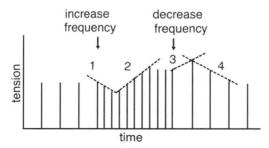

FIGURE 10-17 Simultaneous appearance of the positive and negative staircases. The initial response to an increase in stimulation frequency is a transient fall in tension (1, *the negative staircase*), which is then overcome by a rise in tension caused by the more slowly evolving positive staircase (2). Conversely, the initial response to a decrease in stimulation frequency is a transient rise in tension (3, *the negative staircase*), followed by a fall in tension as the positive inotropic effect of the positive staircase wears off (4).

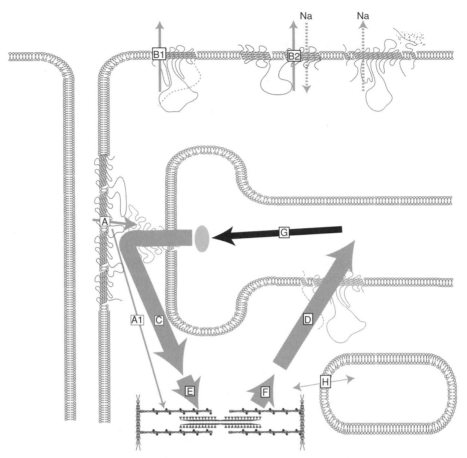

FIGURE 10-18 Possible mechanism for the negative staircase. Diffusion of calcium from the sarcotubular network to the calcium release site in the subsarcolemmal cisternae may, at rapid heart rates, fail to allow all of the calcium to move from the former to the latter (*smaller arrow* G). Another explanation for the negative staircase (*not shown*) is the refractory state of the sarcoplasmic reticulum calcium release channels.

Regulation by Changes in the Contractile Proteins

Modifications of the myofibrillar proteins that can alter myocardial contractility include changes in the interactions between the myosin cross-bridges and actin, which can modify cross-bridge cycling, and changes in the calcium sensitivity of the troponin complex.

Cyclic AMP-dependent protein kinases (PK-A), in addition to stimulating calcium uptake into the cardiac sarcoplasmic reticulum (see above), catalyze myosin light chain phosphorylations that increase contractility by accelerating cross-bridge cycling. PK-A also phosphorylates troponin I, which by decreasing the calcium affinity of the contractile proteins has a negative inotropic effect; however, the most important consequence is to facilitate relaxation (Fig. 10-20).

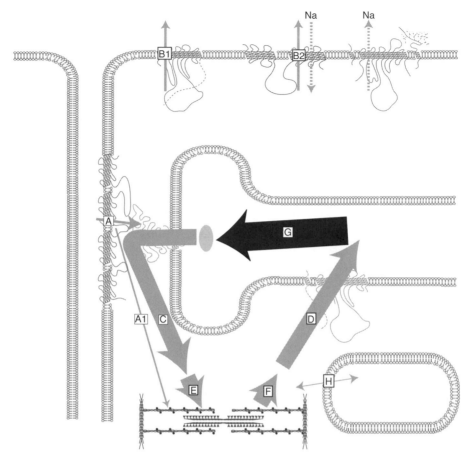

FIGURE 10-19 Possible mechanism for the recuperative effect of a pause. Rapid heart rates can cause calcium to accumulate in the sarcotubular network, and a pause allows this calcium to diffuse to the calcium release site in the subsarcolemmal cisternae (*larger arrow* G) and increase tension developed in contractions after the pause.

Angiotensin II, α_1-adrenergic stimulation, and endothelin cause a weak positive inotropic response by activating signaling pathways that release diacylglycerol (DAG) and inositol trisphosphate (InsP$_3$) (see Chapter 8). The latter increases cytosolic calcium by opening InsP$_3$-gated intracellular calcium release channels (see Chapter 9), while DAG activates protein kinase C-catalyzed phosphorylations that increase the calcium affinity of troponin (Fig. 10-21). The latter effect does not depend on an increase in cytosolic calcium, and so avoids the arrhythmogenic consequences of increased electrogenic calcium efflux via the sodium-calcium exchanger (see Chapter 7). The theoretical advantages of this positive inotropic mechanism stimulated the development of "calcium sensitizers", such as levosimendan, that increase the number of active acting-myosin interactions at any level of cytosolic calcium (Sorsa et al, 2002). Although

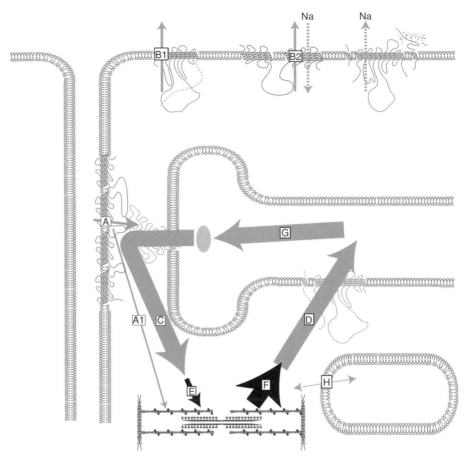

FIGURE 10-20 Decreased calcium affinity of the troponin complex, shown as a smaller association arrow (E) and larger dissociation arrow (F), favor dissociation of this ion from its binding site on the contractile proteins. The result would decrease contractility but facilitate relaxation.

these drugs can increase myocardial contractility without the adverse consequences of cytosolic calcium overload, they have the theoretical disadvantage of impairing relaxation.

Extracellular Potassium, ATP, and Acidosis

At the time that the first edition of this text was written, elevated extracellular potassium was believed to play a role in regulating cardiac performance by depressing myocardial contractility. It is now apparent, however, that the negative inotropic effect of high extracellular potassium is indirect and due largely to decreased resting potential across the plasma membrane (see Chapter 14).

The role of ATP in providing energy for contraction process (see Chapter 2) led early workers to suggest that a fall in ATP level depressed

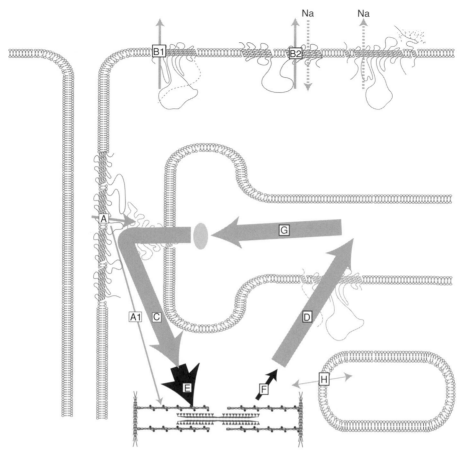

FIGURE 10-21   Increased calcium affinity of the troponin complex, shown as a larger association arrow (E) and smaller dissociation arrow (F), increases contractility by increasing
the binding of activator calcium to troponin; this change also would impair relaxation.

myocardial contractility in the energy-starved heart. This response, however, is not due to lack of ATP for binding to the substrate sites on the contractile proteins because the latter are saturated at very low ATP concentrations, below 1 μM, while cytosolic ATP levels are normally greater than
1 mM. Lack of ATP for binding to these substrate sites therefore does not
alter contractility, except in the dying heart, where complete hydrolysis of
ATP causes rigor (see Chapter 4).

The profound negative inotropic effects of acidosis are due in part to
a competition between protons and calcium for the high-affinity calcium-
binding sites on troponin. This allows a fall in pH to shift the calcium sensitivity of tension development to higher calcium concentrations. In addition, acidosis inhibits excitation–contraction coupling and relaxation
because protons inhibit most of the pumps, channels, and exchangers that
mediate calcium fluxes into and out of the cytosol (see Chapter 7).

TABLE 10-2 **Major Responses of Heart Muscle to β-Adrenergic Stimulation**

Response	Cellular Effect	Physiological Role
Functional Responses		
Increased energy production		
Accelerated glycogenolysis	Increased ATP regeneration	Energy provision for increased work
Phosphorylation of plasma membrane Ca channels		
Atria and ventricles	Increased Ca entry, increased contractility	Increased ejection ($\downarrow$ ESV)
Sinoatrial node	Accelerated heart rate	Increased cardiac output
Atrioventricular node	Accelerated conduction velocity	Maintained AV conduction
Phosphorylation of the Na pump		
Increased Na efflux	Increased Ca efflux by way of Na–Ca exchange	Increased filling ($\uparrow$ EDV)
Phosphorylation of phospholamban		
Increased Ca pump turnover	Increased Ca uptake into the SR	Increased filling ($\uparrow$ EDV)
	Increased Ca stores in the SR	Increased ejection ($\downarrow$ ESV)
Increased Ca-sensitivity of Ca pump	Increased Ca uptake into the SR	Increased filling ($\uparrow$ EDV)
	Increased Ca stores in the SR	Increased ejection ($\downarrow$ ESV)
Phosphorylation of troponin I	Decreased Ca affinity of troponin C	Increased filling ($\uparrow$ EDV)
Phosphorylation of myosin	Accelerated cross-bridge cycling	Increased ejection ($\downarrow$ ESV)
Proliferative Responses		
Hypertrophy	More sarcomeres	Increased ejection ($\downarrow$ ESV)

ESV, end-systolic volume; EDV, end-diastolic volume; SR, sarcoplasmic reticulum.

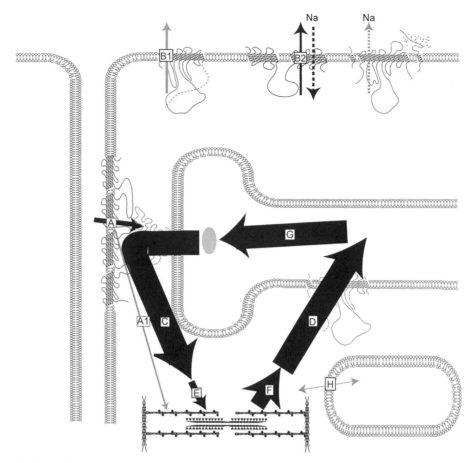

FIGURE 10-22 Effects of β-adrenergic stimulation. Increased calcium entry through plasma membrane calcium channels (*larger arrow* A) and increased calcium release from the calcium release channels in the sarcoplasmic reticulum (*larger arrow* B) increase contractility. At the same time, relaxation is accelerated by a decrease in the calcium affinity of the troponin complex (*smaller arrow* E and *larger arrow* F) and by increased calcium uptake into the sarcoplasmic reticulum (*larger arrow* D).

Regulation of Myocardial Contractility by β-Adrenergic Stimulation: An Integrated Functional Response

Sympathetic stimulation, the most important mediator of the hemodynamic defense reaction, has many effects on the cardiovascular system (Table 10-2). The most important functional responses of the heart result from cyclic AMP–stimulated phosphorylations (Fig. 10-22), some of which favor contraction (e.g., increased calcium entry through plasma membrane calcium channels), while others favor relaxation (e.g., accelerated calcium uptake into the sarcoplasmic reticulum and decreased calcium affinity of troponin). These responses, which at first glance appear to oppose one another, are parts of an integrated response that allows the heart both to

A. Control

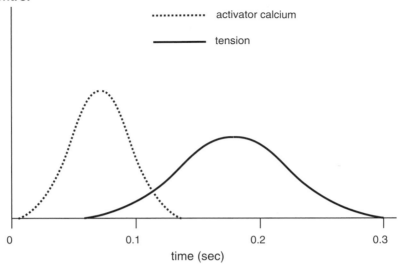

B. Cyclic AMP–activated

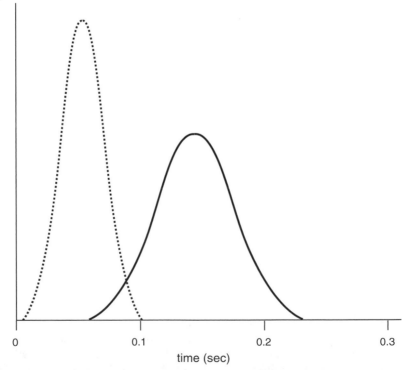

FIGURE 10-23 Increased cellular cyclic AMP levels caused by β-adrenergic stimulation and phosphodiesterase inhibition increase the amount of calcium that enters and leaves the cytosol during each cardiac cycle (*dotted lines*). These effects increase maximum tension development and shorten the duration of systole response (*solid line*).

increase its contractility and relax completely when sympathetic stimulation accelerates heart rate.

Although β-adrenergic stimulation increases the rate of rise of cytosolic calcium and tension, both follow abbreviated time courses (Fig. 10-23). The inotropic response is caused by increased calcium influx across the plasma membrane, which is due mainly to phosphorylation of the L-type calcium channels, and by an increase in the amount of calcium stored in the sarcoplasmic reticulum, which occurs when phospholamban phosphorylation stimulates calcium uptake into this internal membrane system. Troponin I phosphorylation facilitates calcium dissociation from the troponin complex, which along with the increased rate of calcium uptake into the sarcoplasmic reticulum accelerates relaxation. A positive lusitropic effect also is brought about by phosphorylation of phospholamban, which accelerates calcium uptake into the sarcoplasmic reticulum. On balance, the positive inotropic effect of the increased calcium fluxes into the cytosol overcomes the tendency of the increased calcium removal from troponin to reduce contractility. However, relaxation also must be accelerated during sympathetic stimulation because β-adrenergic agonists increase heart rate (see Chapter 14), which shortens diastole. The lusitropic effects of cyclic AMP are therefore necessary to allow the larger amount of activator calcium that enters the myocardial cell to be pumped out of the cytosol during a shorter diastolic interval.

PROLIFERATIVE RESPONSES THAT REGULATE MYOCARDIAL CONTRACTILITY AND RELAXATION

The functional responses described above, which allow the heart to meet short-term challenges like exercise and hemorrhage (see Chapter 8), rarely persist for more than a few hours or days. In chronic disease, where the challenges last much longer, an entirely different group of *proliferative* responses are evoked (see Fig. 8-1). The examples described below, which are part of the "reversion to the fetal phenotype" seen in hypertrophied and failing hearts, illustrate two of the many mechanisms by which proliferative responses modify contractility and relaxation.

ISOFORM SHIFTS INVOLVING THE CONTRACTILE PROTEINS. One of the first observations suggesting a role for abnormal proliferative signaling in diseased hearts was published by Alpert and Gordon (1962), who reported a reduction in the ATPase activity of myofibrils isolated from failing human hearts. This abnormality was immediately recognized as a possible explanation for the depressed myocardial contractility generally seen in these patients and led to studies demonstrating that chronic overloading causes isoform shifts that are now known to involve a variety of myofibrillar proteins (see Chapter 18).

The most extensively studied of these isoform shifts occurs in the myosin heavy chains, where overload causes the high ATPase α isoform normally found in adult hearts to be replaced by the slower β isoform. Because the latter predominates in the embryonic heart, this isoform shift is an example of reversion to the fetal phenotype (see Chapter 9). The opposite response, replacement of slow with fast myosin heavy chains, accompanies the physiological hypertrophy of the "athlete's heart" (Scheuer and Buttrick, 1985). Overloading also causes isoform shifts in the myosin light chains and replacement of cardiac α-actin with skeletal α-actin, the gene product found in the fetal heart. Other isoform shifts occur in the regulatory proteins, including troponin T and troponin I, both of which cause allosteric effects that modify calcium binding by troponin C. However, the latter, which along with tropomyosin is the most highly conserved of the myofibrillar proteins, does not itself participate in these isoform shifts.

Overload-induced changes in the cardiac contractile proteins are not caused simply by an overall stimulation of myocyte growth because not all of the myofibrillar proteins participate in this proliferative response; isoform shifts involving the myosin heavy chains and actin can follow different time courses (Izumo et al., 1988); and the fetal myosin and actin isoforms initially appear in different locations (Schiaffino et al., 1989). Furthermore, pressure overload and volume overload, like physiological and pathological hypertrophy (see above), do not lead to identical molecular changes (Calderone et al., 1995). This demonstrates that different loading conditions activate different proliferative signaling pathways.

Proliferative responses similar to those seen in overloaded hearts also are seen in chronic endocrinopathies; for example, hyperthyroidism increases the content of the high-ATPase myosin heavy chain isoform, which aids in the adaptation to the rapid heart rate and low peripheral resistance also caused by excessive thyroid hormone release.

Preferential expression of the gene that encodes the slow β-myosin heavy chain isoform has a negative inotropic effect because it reduces the maximal velocity of contraction; however, this isoform switch also improves the efficiency of the overloaded heart because muscles containing the slow β-myosin heavy chains generate tension more efficiently than those with the faster α isoform (Table 10-3). For this reason, replacement of the fast myosin heavy chain with the slow isoform is not entirely maladaptive; although it does reduce myocardial contractility by slowing the cross-bridge cycle, this

TABLE 10-3 Physiological Effects of Myosin Heavy Chain Isoform Switches

Ratio of Fast (α) to Slow (β) Myosin Heavy Chain Isoforms	Rate of Cross-Bridge Cycling	Tension–Time Integral during a Single Contraction	Efficiency of Tension Development
Increased	Increased	Decreased	Decreased
Decreased	Decreased	Increased	Increased

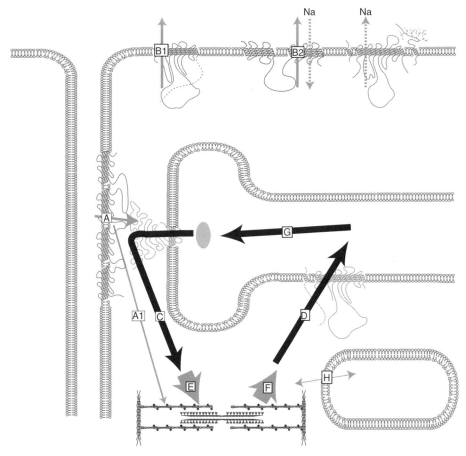

FIGURE 10-24 Reduction of the intracellular calcium cycle, which occurs when reversion to the fetal phenotype in chronically overloaded and failing hearts reduces the densities of the calcium release channels (*smaller arrow* C) and the calcium pump ATPase (*smaller arrow* D).

isoform shift has an energy-sparing effect that can be beneficial in severely pressure-overloaded and failing hearts, which are usually energy starved.

CHANGES IN THE SARCOPLASMIC RETICULUM PROTEINS. The number of calcium release channels, calcium pump ATPase molecules, and phospholamban molecules have all been reported to decrease in chronic heart failure (see Chapter 18). These changes, which slow the intracellular calcium cycle (Fig. 10-24), contribute to the depressed contractility and impaired relaxation generally seen in this syndrome. They also are part of the reversion to the fetal phenotype that accompanies the hypertrophic response to overload; this reflects the fact that more primitive cardiac myocytes rely mainly on the extracellular calcium cycle for excitation–contraction coupling and relaxation and therefore contain smaller amounts of the components that contribute to the intracellular

TABLE 10-4 **Mechanisms Regulating the Contractile Performance of Skeletal and Cardiac Muscle**

Mechanism	Role in Skeletal Muscle	Role in Cardiac Muscle
Summation of individual contractile events (partial and complete tetanus)	Minor	None
Variations in number of active motor units	Major	None
Length-dependent changes (length–tension relationship, Starling's Law of the Heart	Usually minor	Major in beat-to-beat regulation, minor in sustained responses
Ability to vary intrinsic contractile properties	Minor	Major in sustained responses, minor in beat-to-beat regulation

calcium cycle (see Chapter 7). The opposite response is seen in the physiological hypertrophy of the athlete's heart, where the content of structures that participate in the intracellular calcium cycle is increased (Scheuer and Buttrick, 1985).

REGULATION OF PERFORMANCE IN SKELETAL MUSCLE AND THE HEART

The interplay between the regulatory mechanisms discussed above can be appreciated by comparing the regulation of cardiac performance with that of skeletal muscle (Table 10-4).

Summation of Contractions

The tension developed by a skeletal muscle can be increased when rapid stimulation causes summation or a tetanic contraction (see Chapter 6). This response is possible because of the short duration of the skeletal muscle action potential, which ends before the active state begins to decay. However, summation is of little physiological importance in skeletal muscle because most contractions are brief tetani; although extraocular muscle contractions are twitches, these brief contractile responses—which resemble the knee jerk reflex—would not be useful for most movements.

Summation can play no role in the heart because action potentials normally last almost to the end of the active state. For this reason, cardiac muscle cannot respond to electrical stimuli until relaxation is well under way, which makes it impossible for tetanic contraction and summation to be used for physiological regulation.

Variations in the Number of Active Motor Units

Skeletal muscles are composed of groups of myocytes, called *motor units*, which are innervated by single motor neurons that operate independently of one another. This allows performance to be regulated by variations in the number of active motor units, a control mechanism that is integrated within the central nervous system. For example, only a small fraction of the motor units are activated in a muscle that lifts a light load, whereas a much greater proportion of the motor units are activated by way of their motor neurons when the same muscle lifts a heavy load. This mechanism is the major determinant of skeletal muscle performance.

In the heart, the number of active muscle fibers cannot be varied because the many gap junctions in the intercalated discs provide low electrical resistance pathways that link the interiors of adjacent cardiac myocytes (see Chapter 13). For this reason, the heart is a functional syncytium, so when any region of the normal heart is depolarized, the entire heart is activated.

Changes in Sarcomere Length

The length–tension relationship allows preload to influence the performance of both skeletal and cardiac muscle. In most skeletal muscles, however, rest length is determined largely by the angles at the joints; as these are generally chosen to optimize leverage, rather than to set muscle length along a length–tension curve, variations in rest length are of little regulatory importance.

Changes in rest length are more important in walls of the heart, where chamber volume determines fiber length. However, the fact that the heart is a hollow viscus constrains the role of changing sarcomere length because, according to the Law of Laplace (see Chapter 12), when volume increases, more wall stress is required to generate a given pressure. This means that the heart's sarcomeres must function on the ascending limb of their length–tension curves to maintain the steady state needed to match ejection to filling (see Chapter 12). For this reason, the major regulatory function of length-dependent changes in the heart is to "fine tune" performance so as to match venous return and cardiac output.

Changes in Contractility

Changes in contractility play little role in skeletal muscle, where the high content of sarcoplasmic reticulum allows excitation–contraction coupling to deliver enough calcium to saturate virtually all of the binding sites on troponin C; as a result, even under resting conditions, skeletal muscle tension is at or near the maximum that the muscle can generate. The situation in the heart, however, is quite different because under basal conditions, excitation–contraction coupling does not provide enough activator calcium to saturate all of the troponin C in normal myocardial cells. This allows a variety of stimuli to regulate myocardial contractility by modifying the calcium cycles described in Chapter 7. Therefore, the heart relies on changing contractility to vary the strength of cardiac contraction to respond to such challenges as the neurohumoral response and the administration of cardiac drugs.

CONCLUSION

The regulatory mechanisms described in this chapter operate in the intact heart to allow this muscular pump to adapt its performance to the changing demands of the circulation.

REFERENCES

Alpert NR, Gordon MS. Myofibrillar adenosine triphosphatase activity in congestive heart failure. *Am J Physiol* 1962;202:940–946.

Bowditch HP. Über die Eigenthümlichkeiten der Reizbarkeit, welche die Musklefasern des Herzens zeigen. Berichte der Kön Sächs Gesellschaft der Wissenschaften Mathematisch-Physische Classe 1871;23:652–689.

Calderone A, Takahashi N, Izzo NJ Jr, et al. Pressure- and volume-induced left ventricular hypertrophies are associated with distinct myocyte phenotypes and differential induction of peptide growth factor mRNAs. *Circulation* 1995;92:2385–2390.

Izumo S, Nadal-Ginard B, Mahdavi V. Protooncogene induction and reprogramming of cardiac gene expression produced by pressure overload. *Proc Nat Acad Sci USA* 1988;85:339–343.

Katz AM. Molecular biology in cardiology, a paradigmatic shift. *J Mol Cell Cardiol* 1988;20:355–366.

Salisbury PF, Cross CA, Rieben PA. Influence of coronary artery pressure upon myocardial elasticity. *Circ Res* 1960;8:794–800.

Sarnoff SJ. Myocardial contractility as described by ventricular function curves: observations on Starling's law of the heart. *Physiol Rev* 1955;35:107–122.

Scheuer J, Buttrick P. The cardiac hypertrophic response to pathologic and physiologic loads. *Circulation* 1985;75[Suppl I, Pt 2]:I-63–I-68.

Schiaffino S, Samuel JL, Sassoon D, et al. Nonsynchronous accumulation of α-skeletal actin and β-myosin heavy chain mRNAs during early stages of pressure-overloaded-induced cardiac hypertrophy demonstrated by in situ hybridization. *Circ Res* 1989;64:937–948.

Sorsa T, Pollesello P, Solaro RJ. The contractile apparatus as a target for drugs against heart failure: Interaction of levosimendan, a calcium sensitiser, with cardiac troponin c. Mol Cell Biochem 2004:266:87–107.

Starling EH. *The Linacre lecture on the law of the heart*. London: Longmans, Green and Co., 1918.

Wood EH, Hepner RL, Weidmann S. Inotropic effects of electrical currents. *Circ Res* 1969;24:409–445.

Woodworth RS. Maximal contraction, "staircase" contraction, refractory period, and compensatory pause of the heart. *Am J Physiol* 1902;8:213–249.

Normal Physiology

11

THE HEART AS A MUSCULAR PUMP

Unlike the contractions of a skeletal muscle or a strip of cardiac muscle, which are characterized by changes in tension and length, the heart generates *pressure* and ejects a *volume* of blood. For this reason, when describing the work of this hollow muscular structure, changes in tension and length must be redefined as changes in pressure and volume (Fig. 11-1).

CAVITY VOLUME AND FIBER LENGTH: A GEOMETRIC RELATIONSHIP

The relationship between length and volume is determined by the laws of geometry. In a sphere, for example, volume is defined by the equation:

$$V = \tfrac{4}{3}\pi R^3 \qquad\qquad [11\text{-}1]$$

where V = volume and R = radius. Because circumference is equal to $2\pi R$, volume also is related to the third power of circumference, which means that a 50% reduction of circumference reduces volume to one-eighth $(\tfrac{1}{2}^3)$ of its original value. Although the left ventricle is not a sphere, its shape can be approximated as an ellipsoid with three axes: anterior-posterior diameter (DA), lateral diameter (DL), and maximal length (LM) (Fig. 11-2). These can be used to estimate left ventricular volume according to an equation that describes the volume of an ellipse:

$$V = \tfrac{4}{3}\pi \; (DA/2) \times (DL/2) \times (LM/2) \qquad\qquad [11\text{-}2]$$

CAVITY PRESSURE AND WALL STRESS: THE LAW OF LAPLACE

The forces exerted around the circumference of a thick-walled ventricle represent a *stress*; although *tension* is sometimes used, this is not

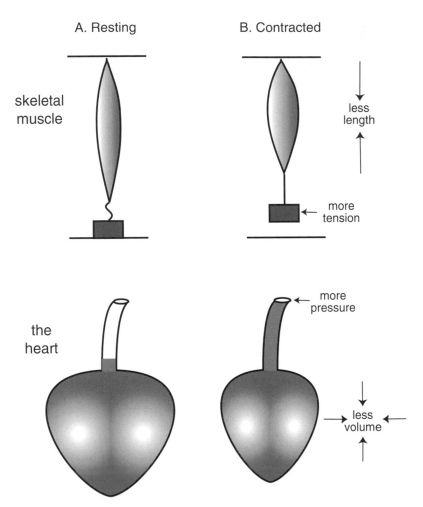

FIGURE 11-1 Comparison of a skeletal muscle, which shortens and develops tension (*above*), and the heart, whose contraction reduces cavity volume and increases pressure (*below*).

correct because tension is a force exerted along a line (e.g., dynes/cm), whereas stress is a force exerted across an area (e.g., dynes/cm^2). Even though individual cardiac myocytes develop tension, it is a stress that appears in the ventricular walls.

Wall stress generates a *pressure* within the ventricular cavity; this pressure, like stress, is a force exerted across an area, and both have the same units (dynes/cm^2). However, pressure is a distending force exerted at right angles to the ventricular walls, whereas wall stress describes the force directed around the circumference of the ventricle. Pressures in the cardiovascular system are usually described in millimeters of mercury or centimeters of water; these represent the height of a column of mercury or

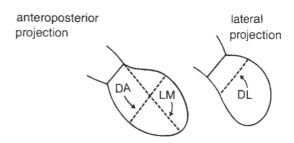

FIGURE 11-2 Outline of the cavity of the left ventricle viewed in anteroposterior and lateral projections. Volume can be estimated by assuming the cavity to be an ellipse whose long axis is LM and whose short axes are DA and DL.

water that exerts the corresponding force per unit of surface area. The commonly used pressure units mm Hg and cm H_2O are converted to gram-centimeter-second (cgs) units in Table 11-1.

The relationship between wall stress and interventricular pressure, like that between length and volume, is influenced by cavity size and shape. These relationships are quantified by the Law of Laplace, which relates wall stress and cavity pressure to wall thickness and the curvature of the ventricular walls. In its simplest form, as applied to a cylinder having an infinitely thin wall (Fig. 11-3), the Law of Laplace states that wall tension is equal to the pressure within the cylinder times its radius:

$$T = P \times R \qquad\qquad [11\text{-}3]$$

where T is wall tension (dynes/cm), P is pressure (dynes/cm^2), and R is radius (cm). The Law of Laplace therefore states that *when the pressure within a cylinder is held constant, the tension on its walls increases with increasing radius, and vice versa.* The reason that a greater wall stress is needed to achieve a given cavity pressure when radius increases is that a smaller fraction of the wall stress is directed toward the center of the cavity (Fig. 11-4). A familiar application of the Law of Laplace is seen in the trucks used to transport fluids and gases in which, to minimize the hazard of bursting, tanks that carry compressed gasses at high internal pressures are constructed with smaller radii than tanks that carry liquids at low pressures (Fig. 11-5).

The tendency of a tank to burst also can be reduced by increasing the thickness of its walls simply because the greater wall thickness reduces the

TABLE 11-1 **Units of Pressure**

Unit	Dynes/cm^2
1 mm Hg	1,330
1 cm H_2O	980

A

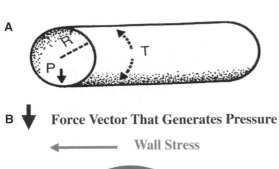

B ⬇ **Force Vector That Generates Pressure**

⬅——— **Wall Stress**

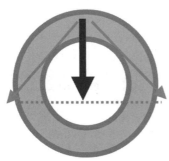

FIGURE 11-3 The Law of Laplace. **A:** In a thin-walled cylinder, the Law of Laplace relates wall tension (T) to the pressure within the cylinder (P) and the radius of curvature (R). **B:** In the heart's cavities, pressure is determined by that portion of the force vectors generated in the walls that are directed toward the center of the cavity.

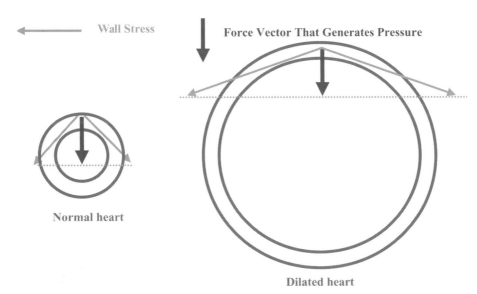

Normal heart

Dilated heart

FIGURE 11-4 Mechanism by which dilatation increases the wall stress needed to achieve a given pressure. In the dilated heart, a smaller proportion of the wall stress is directed toward the center of the cavity than in the normal heart, which means that more wall stress must be developed to achieve a given cavity pressure.

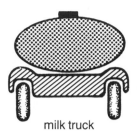
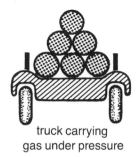

milk truck

truck carrying
gas under pressure

FIGURE 11-5   A practical application of the Law of Laplace. Trucks used to transport gas under high pressure contain several cylindrical tanks, each with a short radius of curvature (*right*). A single tank with a large radius of curvature is used in a milk truck, where the pressure in the tank is low (*left*).

stress on each element in the wall. The Law of Laplace as applied to a thick-walled cylinder is therefore:

$$T \alpha \frac{P \times R}{h} \qquad \text{[11-4]}$$

where h is wall thickness. For this reason, when hypertrophy increases wall thickness, it reduces the stress on the individual muscle fibers by distributing the load among a greater number of sarcomeres.

Even though the complex geometry of the ventricles makes it impossible to calculate wall stress with precision, two fundamental facts should not be obscured: *dilation increases the tension that must be developed by the muscle fibers in the walls of the heart to generate a given cavity pressure*, and *at any given cavity pressure, increased wall thickness (hypertrophy) reduces the amount of tension on each muscle fiber*.

Distribution of Stress across the Walls of the Heart

Stress is not distributed uniformly in all layers of the walls of the heart. This can be modeled as a series of concentric elastic spheres enclosing a pressurized cavity, where increasing the pressure in the cavity causes the greatest increase in wall stress on the innermost layer (Wong and Rautaharju, 1968; Fenton et al., 1978). Although this might appear to contradict the Law of Laplace, which states that wall stress increases as diameter increases (equation 11-3), there is no contradiction because the *distribution* of stress among the layers of a thick-walled ventricle differs from the *average amount* of stress in the walls of ventricles that have different radii of curvature.

Differences in the stresses developed by various layers of the ventricle are especially marked in hearts that undergo concentric hypertrophy. In these hearts, the high stress in the endocardial layers increases energy expenditure. This contributes to the vulnerability of the endocardium to energy starvation, an effect that is exacerbated because high wall stress also increases the compression of the muscular branches of the coronary arteries that traverse the ventricular walls before reaching the endocardium (see Fig. 1-9). Together, the higher wall stress and lower coronary flow make the subendocardium especially vulnerable to energy starvation when energy demand is increased or energy supply is decreased.

CYCLES OF CONTRACTION AND RELAXATION: PRESSURE–VOLUME LOOPS

Ventricular pressure and volume undergo a sequence of changes during each cardiac cycle that can be displayed as "pressure–volume loop," where changing pressure is plotted as a function of volume (see below). These diagrams, which are useful in appreciating how physiological and pathophysiological interventions influence cardiac function, can be understood by first examining a preloaded skeletal muscle that lifts a heavy afterload (Fig. 11-6). The *preload* is a small weight placed on the resting muscle before it is stimulated to contract, while the *afterload* is a heavier weight that rests on a support and therefore is lifted by

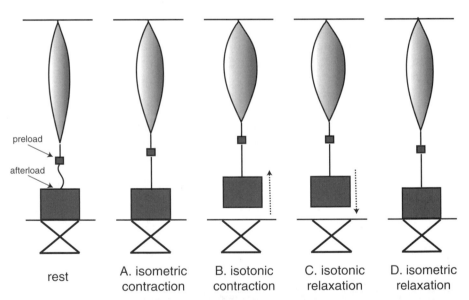

preload

afterload

| rest | A. isometric contraction | B. isotonic contraction | C. isotonic relaxation | D. isometric relaxation |

FIGURE 11-6 Cycle of contraction and relaxation in an afterloaded skeletal muscle. A small preload stretches the resting muscle, while the heavier afterload rests on a support until after the muscle has started to contract. The first phase in the cycle is isometric contraction (A), during which tension developed by the muscle increases until it equals the afterload. In the second phase, isotonic contraction (B), the muscle shortens while lifting the afterload. Relaxation is initially isotonic when the afterload is lowered to the support (C). Isometric relaxation (D) begins when the afterload reaches the support and continues until muscle tension returns to zero.

the contracting muscle only after it develops a tension equal to the weight of the afterload (see Chapter 3).

Skeletal Muscle

The cycle of contraction and relaxation depicted in Figure 11-6 can be divided into four phases; two of contraction and two of relaxation. The first phase, *isometric contraction* (A, Fig. 11-6), begins when the activated muscle starts to develop tension; however, as long as muscle tension is less than the afterload, shortening cannot occur. The second phase, *isotonic contraction* (B, Fig. 11-6), begins when active tension equals the afterload, at which time the muscle begins to lift the load. Shortening then continues at a constant tension, which is equal to the weight of the afterload (the small preload is ignored). The third phase, *isotonic relaxation* (C, Fig. 11-6), begins when the (relaxing) muscle starts to lengthen while still bearing the afterload. Lengthening continues at the constant tension of the afterload until the latter returns to the support and so is removed from the muscle. This marks the beginning of the fourth phase, *isometric relaxation* (D, Fig. 11-6), during which tension is dissipated in the unloaded muscle. These four phases can be plotted as a "work diagram" (Fig. 11-7), which shows how tension and length change during the contraction shown in Figure 11-6. Because the muscle shortens and lengthens with the same afterload, the curves for isotonic contraction and isotonic relaxation in Figure 11-7 are superimposed.

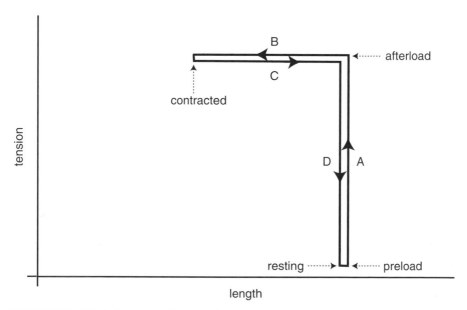

FIGURE 11-7 Work diagram of the contraction–relaxation cycle depicted in Figure 11-6. **A:** isometric contraction; **B:** isotonic contraction; **C:** isotonic relaxation; **D:** isometric relaxation. The two isometric curves (**A** and **D**) and two isotonic curves (**B** and **C**) should be superimposed but are separated for clarity.

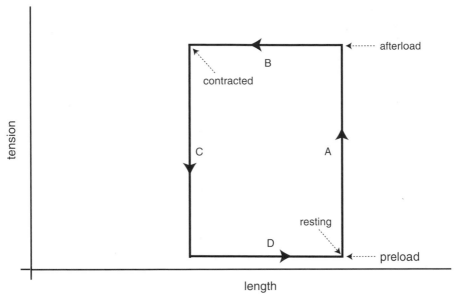

FIGURE 11-8 Work diagram of a muscle from which the afterload is disengaged when relaxation begins. Isometric contraction (**A**) and isotonic contraction (**B**) occur as in the contraction depicted in Figures 11-6 and 11-7. However, because the afterload is removed before the muscle begins to relax, tension during isotonic relaxation (**C**) is equal to the weight small preload, which stretches the muscle during isometric relaxation (**D**).

If instead of relaxing under the same loading conditions that were present during contraction the afterload is removed at the end of isometric contraction (B, Fig. 11-6), isometric relaxation will occur with the muscle bearing only the small preload. This contraction can be described by the work diagram shown in Figure 11-8.

The Left Ventricular Pressure–Volume Loop

The work diagram in Figure 11-8 resembles the pressure–volume loop generated by the left ventricle (Fig. 11-9) because the ventricle, like the skeletal muscle, carries a small preload—in this case, the diastolic pressure generated by the venous return and atrial systole. Ventricular afterload, which is related to aortic pressure, does not influence the pressure in the left ventricular cavity during diastole because the closed aortic valve has "disconnected" the ventricle from the blood in the aorta.

Each cycle of contraction and relaxation in the left ventricle can be depicted as a pressure-volume loop that begins at end-diastole and is inscribed in a counterclockwise direction (Fig. 11-9). Like the skeletal muscle contraction shown in Figure 11-8, the pressure-volume loop proceeds through four phases. *Isovolumic contraction*, the first phase of systole, begins when tension is developed by the ventricular myocardium. Increasing intraventricular pressure first closes the mitral valve, after

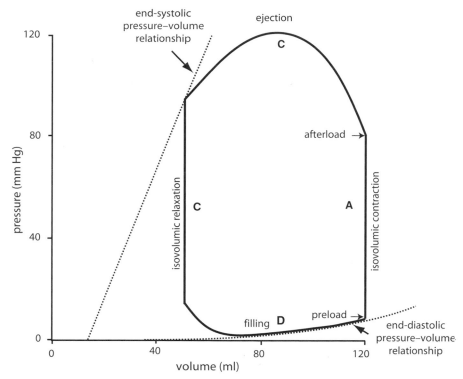

FIGURE 11-9   Pressure–volume loop (work diagram) of the left ventricle. The preload, which is generated during diastole by the venous return and atrial systole, determines the point along the end-diastolic pressure–volume relationship (the lusitropic state) at which systole begins. After the onset of systole, the mitral valve closes, and pressure increases sharply. Because both the aortic and mitral valves are closed, contraction is isovolumic (A). Ejection begins when the aortic valve opens and the ventricle meets its afterload, the aortic pressure. Systole ends when ventricular pressure and volume reach the end-systolic pressure–volume relationship, which describes the inotropic state of the ventricle. After aortic valve closure removes the afterload (aortic pressure) from the ventricular cavity, blood can neither enter nor leave the ventricle; as a result, relaxation begins under isovolumic conditions (C). When left ventricular pressure falls below that in the left atrium, the mitral valve opens, and blood flows from the atrium into the ventricle during the phase of filling (D). The cycle ends when ventricular pressure and volume reach the end-diastolic pressure–volume relationship, and the next cycle begins.

which intraventricular pressure rises until it exceeds that in the aorta, which causes the aortic valve to open. Until this happens, blood can neither enter nor leave the ventricle, so pressure increases at a constant volume to inscribe an upward, vertical deflection (A, Fig. 11-9). The second phase, *ejection*, begins after the heart meets its afterload, when blood is ejected into the aorta (B, Fig. 11-9). The reduction in ventricular volume during ejection causes the pressure-volume loop to turn to the left. Aortic pressure first rises during ejection because blood is flowing into the aorta faster than it is running out into the tissues, and then falls as slowing of ejection allows blood to flow out of the aorta more rapidly than it enters from the ventricle. Even though aortic pressure rises and falls during ejection, wall stress falls steadily throughout this phase of the cardiac cycle because of the decreasing cavity volume and thickening of the ventricular walls. Systole ends at a point along the *end-systolic pressure-volume relationship* that describes the inotropic state of the ventricle.

The third phase, *isovolumic relaxation* (C, Fig. 11-9), marks the start of diastole. During this phase, which begins after aortic valve closure "disconnects" the ventricle from the afterload, both the aortic and mitral valves are closed so that ventricular volume remains constant. The ventricle continues to relax with no change in volume until left ventricular pressure falls below that in the left atrium, which allows the mitral valve to open. This initiates the final phase of *filling* (D, Fig. 11-9), during which blood flows across the mitral valve from the atrium into the relaxing ventricle. Left ventricular pressure and volume rise gradually during this phase as blood returning from the lungs generates the preload for the next contraction. Diastole ends at a point on the *end-diastolic pressure-volume relationship*.

Two pressure-volume relationships (abbreviated as *PV relationships* in this text) constrain the pressure-volume loop: the *end-systolic PV relationship*, which defines the inotropic properties of the contracting ventricle, and the *end-diastolic PV relationship*, which reflects the lusitropic properties of the relaxed heart. *End-diastolic volume* is determined by end-systolic volume (the "residual" volume left behind after the previous cardiac cycle), venous return, and the lusitropic properties of the ventricle (Table 11-2). *End-systolic volume* is determined by end-diastolic volume, aortic pressure, and the inotropic state. Changing pressures in the circulation modify cardiac performance by shifting the end-diastolic and end-systolic points along the two PV relationships, but the limits imposed by the latter cannot be exceeded. Changes in inotropic and lusitropic state, on

TABLE 11-2 Determinants of the Work of the Heart

Filling

Venous return: flow of blood in the veins toward the heart

End-systolic volume: blood left behind from the pervious systole

Lusitropy: ability of the heart to fill, the end-diastolic pressure–volume relationship

Ejection

Aortic diastolic pressure: ability of the aorta to receive blood from the heart

End-diastolic volume: amount of blood at the start of systole

Inotropy: ability of the heart to eject, the end-systolic pressure–volume relationship the other hand, alter these limits by shifting the end-diastolic and end-systolic PV relationships.

The end-systolic PV relationship, which is a measure of contractility, is determined by the many variables that regulate the number and turnover rate of the interactions between the myosin cross-bridges and actin (see Chapters 4, 7, and 10). The end-diastolic PV relationship, which measures lusitropy, is influenced by the rate and extent of calcium uptake into the sarcoplasmic reticulum, the ease with which calcium dissociates from troponin (i.e., the calcium affinity of troponin), and the extent to which the contractile proteins are dissociated after the activator calcium has been removed from the troponin complex (see Chapters 7 and 10). Compliance also is influenced by the cytoskeleton, the extracellular matrix, the pericardium, and the geometry and thickness of the ventricular walls.

THE CARDIAC CYCLE

Each time the heart contracts, the spread of a wave of electrical depolarization initiates a series of mechanical events that cause blood to flow into and out of the ventricles and the valves to open and close. Together, these electrical and mechanical events constitute the *cardiac cycle* or *"Wiggers' Diagram,"* which is the foundation of modern cardiology. The following description of the cardiac cycle and Figure 11-10 are modified from the 1949 edition of Carl J. Wiggers' classic text *Physiology in Health and Disease.*

> The series of superimposed curves that are reproduced in Figure 11-10 unfold at a glance the story of cardiodynamic events in the left side of the heart, which may be briefly summarized as follows:
>
> At the onset of ventricular systole the pressures are approximately equal in the atrium and ventricle, and the atrioventricular (AV) valves are in the act of floating into apposition. After the pressure has risen slightly within the ventricle, the AV valves close completely giving rise to the first heart sound [S_1]. Since the aortic valve is still closed, the ventricle contracts isovolumically, and the intraventricular pressure rises rapidly. The aortic valve opens when left ventricular pressure exceeds that in the aorta. As a result, aorta and ventricle become a common cavity, and the two pressure curves follow one another closely.
>
> With the rapid expulsion of blood during the early moments of ejection—indicated by volume changes of the ventricles—the pressures in the left ventricle and aorta rise to a summit because the rate at which blood is expelled into the aorta exceeds that at which it flows from its branches through the arterioles. The rise is rounded chiefly because, with rather constant ejection rate, the runoff increases gradually with the progressive rise of aortic pressure. The rounded summit is reached when ejection and runoff become equal. Since the rate of ejection diminishes during the latter part of systole while flow out of the aortic branches continue to be high, aortic and ventricular pressures

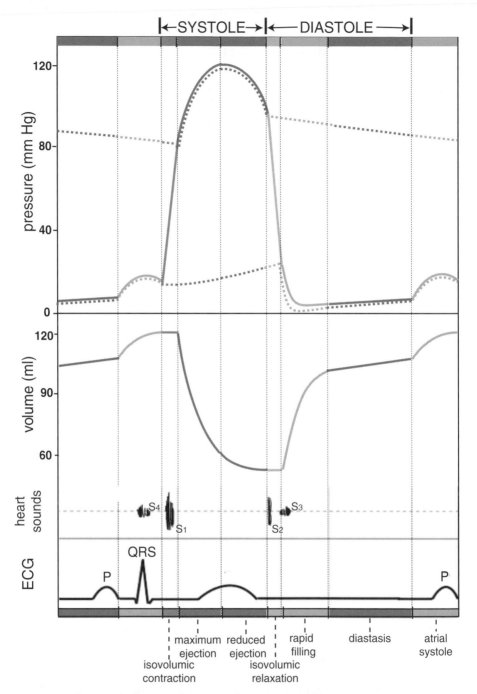

FIGURE 11-10 The cardiac cycle (Wiggers diagram) showing seven phases of left ventricular systole. By convention, the cycle begins with contraction of the ventricle so that atrial systole is placed at the end of ventricular diastole. The *top three curves* represent aortic pressure (*upper dashed line*), left ventricular pressure (*solid line*), and left atrial pressure (*lower dashed line*). The *solid line* below these pressure curves is left ventricular volume, below which are the heart sounds: S_4, atrial (or fourth) sound; S_1, first heart sound; S_2, second heart sound; S_3, third heart sound. The *bottom line* shows the timing of the electrocardiogram (ECG), which records the electrical events during the cardiac cycle.

gradually decline. On the basis of pressure curves it is possible to separate the period of ejection into two phases, viz., maximum ejection and reduced ejection. Summarizing, the rise and fall of aortic and ventricular pressures always represent a balance between the rate at which blood is ejected into the aorta and the rate at which it leaves by its branches. However, the changes in rate of ventricular ejection normally dominate the shape of the curves during ejection.

At the onset of ventricular diastole, aorta and ventricle are still in communication. The first effect of relaxation consists in a sharp drop in pressure in the ventricle and aorta, the latter being quickly terminated by the closure of the semilunar valves, after which the aortic curve declines very gradually for the remainder of diastole. The closure of the semilunar valves is associated with the second heart sound [S_2].

Within the ventricle, pressure declines rapidly until the AV valves open, and the phase of isovolumic relaxation terminates. During this phase of ventricular relaxation the atrial pressure continues to rise slowly. As soon as intraventricular pressure has declined to a level lower than that in the atrium, the AV valves are opened again by the difference of pressure and a rapid inflow of blood into the ventricle begins. While this continues, pressures in the atrium and ventricle decline together, but the atrial pressure remains a trifle higher than the ventricular. In long cycles this is followed by a phase of slowed filling, or diastasis, during which ventricular inflow is exceedingly slow, and the pressure rises very gradually both in the atrium and ventricle. In young normal individuals, and in some pathological states, the rapid inflow of blood into the ventricle is associated with an audible sound, the third heart sound [S_3]. Occasionally, atrial systole also produces a sound sometimes called the fourth heart sound [S_4].

The Phases of the Cardiac Cycle: The succession of atrial and ventricular events constitutes the cardiac cycle. Since ventricular contraction is dynamically the most important it is fitting to start the cycle with this event. Accordingly, the cardiac cycle can be divided advantageously into ventricular systole and diastole, but each of these periods must be further subdivided. For the sake of clarity these subdivisions are designated as phases of systole and diastole. The vertical lines of [Figure 11-10] serve to demarcate the successive periods and phases of systole and diastole. The first phase of systole is called isovolumic contraction, for the ventricle contracts essentially in this manner with all valves closed. The second phase is best referred to as ejection; it can be further subdivided by reference to the aortic pressure curve alone or with the aid of the ventricular volume curve into the phase of maximum ejection, and the phase of reduced ejection.

Diastole begins with closure of the semilunar valves. It is followed by isovolumic relaxation, which ends as soon as atrial pressure exceeds that in the ventricle. With opening of the AV valves, rapid filling supervenes, and this is followed by a phase of slowed filling or diastasis, whose length depends on the heart rate. Finally, atrial systole terminates the period of ventricular diastole and the cycle begins again.

The durations of these successive phases have been repeatedly studied but with varying degrees of accuracy. The average values in seconds

TABLE 11-3 **Durations (in Seconds) of the Phases
of the Cardiac Cycle***

Isovolumic contraction	0.05
Maximum ejection	0.09
Reduced ejection	0.17
Total systole	**0.31**
Isovolumic relaxation	0.08
Rapid inflow	0.11
Diastasis	0.19
Atrial systole	0.11
Total systole	**0.49**

*Values are for the human left ventricle at a heart rate of
75/min. (Modified from Wiggers, 1949.)

[Table 11-3] derived from an analysis of many pressure pulses, are sufficient to give an idea as to the relative duration in man of the most commonly used phases.

A schematic drawing of the electrocardiogram showing its relationship to the cardiac cycle is included in Figure 11-10. The P wave is inscribed during atrial depolarization, while the QRS complex originates from ventricular depolarization; both of these electrical events *precede* the corresponding mechanical events. The T wave is due to ventricular repolarization.

The first and second heart sounds, although related to valve closure, do not arise in the valves; instead, they are caused by vibrations in the walls of the ventricles, and to a lesser extent the great vessels, that are initiated by rapid acceleration and deceleration of the moving stream of blood. This resembles a drum, where sound is initiated by the drumstick (analogous to valve closure or rapid filling of a venticle) but is actually generated by the head of the drum (analogous to vibrations in the walls of the ventricle).

END-DIASTOLIC VOLUME AS A DETERMINANT
OF VENTRICULAR FUNCTION: STARLING'S LAW
OF THE HEART (THE FRANK–STARLING RELATIONSHIP)

The relationship between the volume of blood in ventricles at the moment they begin to contract (end-diastolic volume or EDV) and the systolic pressure that can be developed by the heart is a manifestation of the length–tension relationship (see Chapter 6). Although this relationship was well known to physiologists in the latter half of the 19th century, it is commonly referred to as Starling's Law of the Heart or the Frank–Starling relationship because of studies of the working mammalian heart by Ernest Starling in 1914 and of the isolated frog heart by Otto Frank in 1895.

The operation of this physiological law is seen when a balloon placed within the relaxed left ventricle is filled with increasing volumes of an incompressible fluid (Fig. 11-11). When the volume in the balloon is increased, end-diastolic pressure increases; the curve relating the changing pressures and volumes at the end of the diastole is, of course, the end-diastolic PV relationship (Fig. 11-9). The pressure that can be developed during systole is modified by the volume of fluid contained in the balloon. Over the normal range of end-diastolic volume, the heart's ability to generate pressure increases linearly as the balloon fills. Arrows drawn to connect each end-diastolic pressure with the corresponding pressure at the end of systole are vertical in Figure 11-11 because the volume in the balloon cannot change, which means that the heart is contracting under isovolumic conditions. When the lengths of these arrows, which represent the pressures developed during systole (systolic pressure minus diastolic pressure), are plotted as a function of the end-diastolic

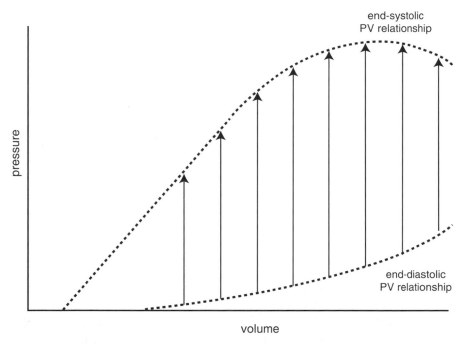

FIGURE 11-11 Starling's Law of the Heart. Systolic pressures (*vertical arrows*) that develop in a series of isovolumic contractions increase with increasing end-diastolic volume. At very high end-diastolic volumes, systolic pressure can decline with increasing volume. The *lower dashed line* is the end-diastolic pressure–volume (PV) relationship; the *upper dashed line* is the the end-systolic PV relationship.

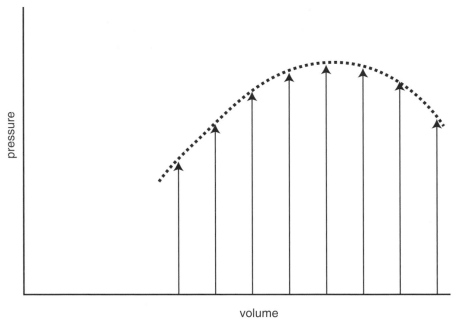

volume

FIGURE 11-12 Ascending and descending limbs of the Starling curve, plotted as the vertical arrows in Figure 11-11. The increase in developed pressure that accompanies an increase in end-diastolic volume is the ascending limb of the Starling curve; the fall in developed pressure as the ventricle dilates at very high volumes is the descending limb.

volume (Fig. 11-12), the resulting curve (often called a *Starling curve*) is analogous to the length–tension relationship of a skeletal muscle (see Chapter 6).

The Descending Limb of the Starling Curve

The heart normally operates on the left-hand portion of the Starling curve, which like the left-hand part of the length–tension curve is called the *ascending limb* (see Chapter 6). This means that increasing preload enhances the ability of the heart to empty, which allows the heart to respond to increased end-diastolic volume by increasing ejection pressure, stroke volume, or both. Only at very high, nonphysiological filling pressures can the heart move onto the descending limb; however, the low compliance of cardiac muscle, along with the stiff pericardium, normally prevent this from occurring. This is very important because the heart determines the "leverage" of its contraction and because, even for a short time, the heart *must* eject during systole what it receives during diastole. However, the ventricle cannot achieve a steady state when it operates on the descending limb (Katz, 1965). Although this was noted briefly by Starling in 1918, the view that failing hearts operate on the descending limb of the Starling curve was taught until the 1970s.

A ventricle operating on the descending limb of the Starling curve would respond to even a small increase in venous return by dilating to the maximum volume allowed by the low compliance of the myocardium and pericardium. "Runaway dilatation" would then occur because additional filling reduces the ability of the ventricle to eject, which would increase end-systolic volume, which would cause more dilatation, which would decrease ejection further, and so initiate a vicious cycle where increased filling decreases the ability to eject and decreased ejection increases filling. The heart has no way to recover from this cycle, so were it not for its low compliance, a heart that enters the descending limb of the Starling curve would burst like an overfilled balloon. Instead of causing the heart to rupture, however, overdilatation causes *acute pulmonary edema*, which in the 19th century was called *acute dilatation*. Faced with a patient in whom this disaster is unfolding, the physician must try to reduce ventricular volume. This was once done using rotating tourniquets and even phlebotomy to lower preload, and morphine (which has a vasodilator effect) along with reassurance to reduce afterload—which decreases end-diastolic volume by facilitating ejection. Therapy for acute pulmonary edema now uses diuretics to reduce preload and vasodilators to reduce afterload. When successful, these measures can return the heart to the steady state that occurs on the ascending limb of the Starling curve.

The challenge to a heart operating on the descending limb of the Starling curve is quite different from that in an overstretched skeletal muscle, where opposing muscles can reverse any tendency for an excessive increase in rest length. Because skeletal muscles do not determine their preload, they can operate on the descending limb of their length–tension curves without increasing the load at the start of the next contraction.

THE PERICARDIUM

The pericardium, along with the low compliance of the ventricular walls, plays an important role in limiting ventricular filling and preventing high diastolic pressures from causing the heart to enter the descending limb of the Starling curve. If the pericardium shrinks, as can occur following chronic inflammation (constrictive pericarditis), or if the pericardial cavity fills with fluid (pericardial effusion), the heart becomes unable to fill. The major consequence of these conditions is impaired filling of the thin-walled right ventricle, so these patients suffer mainly from low cardiac output and complications of increased systemic venous pressure. If a pericardial effusion develops rapidly, or if blood leaks into the pericardial cavity from a ruptured ventricle or aortic dissection, the condition (called *pericardial tamponade*) can be rapidly fatal.

Although the pericardium limits acute dilatation of the heart, the pericardial sac generally enlarges slowly when stretched chronically. For this reason, the pericardium plays little role in limiting the progressive dilatation (remodeling) of the failing heart.

THE ATRIUM AS A PRIMER PUMP

Atrial systole plays an important role in determining ventricular end-diastolic volume. The timing of atrial systole immediately before ventricular systole allows its small contraction to add to the volume of blood in the ventricles at that instant (end-diastole) when ventricular volume determines ventricular performance, which avoids the need for atrial pressure to remain high throughout diastole.

Loss of the atrial "kick," which occurs most commonly when effective atrial contraction ceases in patients with atrial fibrillation, has two hemodynamic consequences, both bad (Fig. 11-13). The first is a fall in ventricular *end-diastolic* pressure and volume that reduces ejection and decreases cardiac output, while the second, a rise in *mean* atrial pressure, impedes the return of blood to the heart and as a result increases venous pressures. These effects are sometimes well tolerated in individuals who have a normal heart, but when cardiac function is compromised, as in patients with heart failure, atrial fibrillation seriously worsens the clinical disorder. Another dangerous complication is increased risk of emboli caused by the tendency of clots to form in the fibrillating atria. Because emboli formed in the left atria often travel to the cerebral circulation, where they can cause a cerebrovascular accident ("stroke"), the clinical significance of this arrhythmia can be devastating, even when the hemodynamic abnormality is mild.

The importance of the atrial primer pump can be understood by viewing atrial systole as a mechanism that increases diastolic volume at the instant (end-diastole) when diastolic volume determines ventricular performance. In this way, atrial systole provides the ventricle with a high end-diastolic volume without the need to maintain a high atrial pressure throughout diastole. Loss of atrial systole cancels both; ventricular end-diastolic volume decreases, which reduces cardiac output, while the higher mean atrial pressure increases venous pressure, which can cause—or worsen—the manifestations of "backward failure" (see Chapter 18).

CONCLUSIONS

Two laws govern the relationship between ventricular volume and cardiac pump performance. The first, the Law of Laplace, is a physical law stating that when the ventricle dilates, the wall stress needed to achieve a given intraventricular pressure is increased. The second, Starling's Law of the Heart, is a physiological law stating that when a ventricle dilates, its ability to perform work increases. In a normal heart operating within the normal range of ventricular volumes, the physiological law predominates: When the ventricle dilates, the increased capacity to generate pressure is much more important than the increased wall stress. However, in the failing heart, the increased wall stress caused by ventricular dilation adds to the energy cost of cardiac contraction, so that the detrimental effects of ventricular dilatation can outweigh the beneficial effects.

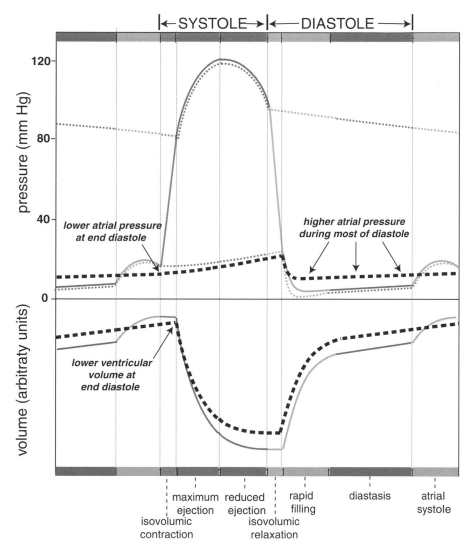

FIGURE 11-13 Effects of loss of atrial systole. In the normal cardiac cycle, atrial contraction (*lower dotted line*) increases left ventricular pressure at the end of diastole so that loss of atrial systole (*heavy dashed line*) causes end-diastolic pressure to fall. Because atrial systole is no longer present to cause an additional rise of pressure at the end of diastole, maintenance of ventricular end-diastolic volume requires an increase in *mean* left atrial pressure. Despite this rise, which impedes venous return, end-diastolic pressure remains low, and ejection is reduced.

BIBLIOGRAPHY

Baim DS, Grossman W. *Grossman's cardiac catheterization, angiography, and intervention,* 6th ed. Philadelphia: Lippincott Williams & Wilkins, 2000.

Burton AC. Physical principles of circulatory phenomena: the physical equilibria of the heart and blood vessels. In: Hamilton WF, Dow P, eds. *Handbook of physiology.* Section 2: Circulation, Vol. 1. Washington, DC: American Physiological Society, 1962:85–106.

Covell JW, Ross J Jr. Systolic and diastolic function (mechanics) of the intact heart. In: Page E, Fozzard HA, Solaro RJ, eds. *Handbook of physiology*. Section 2: The cardiovascular system, Vol. 1, The heart. Oxford: University Press, 2002:741–785.

Luisada AA, Portaluppi F. The main heart sounds as vibrations of the cardiohemic system: old controversy and new facts. *Am J Cardiol* 1983;52:1133–1136.

Suga N. Ventricular energetics. *Physiol Rev* 1990;70:247–277

REFERENCES

Fenton TR, Cherry JM, Klassen GA. Transmural myocardial deformation in the canine left ventricular wall. *Am J Physiol* 1978;235:H523–H530.

Katz AM. The descending limb of the Starling curve and the failing heart. *Circulation* 1965;32:871–875.

Wiggers CJ. *Physiology in health and disease*. Philadelphia: Lea & Febiger, 1949:651–654.

Wong AYK, Rautaharju PM. Stress distribution within the left ventricular wall approximated as a thick ellipsoidal shell. *Am Heart J* 1968;75:649–662.

12

THE WORKING HEART

The heart performs two very different types of work: *external work* that propels blood from the left ventricle into the aorta and from the right ventricle into the pulmonary artery, and *internal work* that is expended to stretch elasticities and lengthen viscous elements in the walls of the contracting ventricles. Much of the energy expended to do internal work is degraded to heat when the heart relaxes and so contributes inefficiency to the performance of the heart.

EXTERNAL WORK

Stroke Work

Most of the external work of the heart is used to eject blood under pressure into the aorta and pulmonary artery (Table 12-1). This is the *stroke work* (sometimes called *pressure-volume work*), which can be estimated by multiplying the volume of blood ejected during each stroke (the stroke volume, abbreviated SV) and the pressure at which the blood is ejected (P):

$$\text{Stroke work} = P \times SV \qquad [12\text{-}1]$$

The product of *pressure* (dynes/cm^2) and *volume* (cm^3) has the correct cgs units for work (dynes cm). In the left ventricle, when mean ejection pressure is 105 mm Hg and stroke volume is 70 mL, stroke work is 7,350 mm Hg mL, which in cgs units is $\sim 9.3 \times 10^6$ dynes cm.

Because aortic and pulmonary artery pressures rise and fall during ejection (see Chapter 11), stroke work is more accurately calculated as the integral of pressure and the volume change:

$$\text{Stroke work} = \int P dV \qquad [12\text{-}2]$$

where P is the pressure at which each increment (dV) of the stroke volume is ejected. For most purposes, however, the stroke work of the left ventricle pressure can be calculated simply by multiplying stroke volume by either peak or mean aortic pressure.

TABLE 12-1 **Determinants of the External Work of the Left Heart**

Cardiac Output (stroke volume × heart rate)
Stroke volume: end-diastolic volume−end-systolic volume
End-diastolic volume: filling
End-systolic volume: ejection
Heart rate (chronotropy): firing rate of the sinoatrial node pacemaker
Aortic Systolic Pressure (pressure within the aorta as blood leaves the ejecting ventricle)

Stroke volume is the difference between end-diastolic volume (EDV), the amount of blood within the ventricle at the end of filling, and end-systolic volume (ESV), the amount that remains when ejection has ended (Table 12-1). This allows equation 12-1 to be expanded as:

$$\text{Stroke work} = P \times (EDV - ESV). \qquad [12\text{-}3]$$

Each determinant of stroke work is controlled differently. End-diastolic volume is determined by three variables; two, which together define the *preload*, are venous return and end-systolic volume, the third is the lusitropic state of the ventricle. End-systolic volume is determined by end-diastolic volume and stroke volume; the latter being determined by the inotropic state of the ventricle and the *afterload*. At steady state, the stroke volumes of the two ventricles are the same, but because pulmonary artery pressure is approximately one-fifth that of aortic pressure, the stroke work of the right ventricle is less than that of the left ventricle.

RESISTANCE AND IMPEDANCE. Aortic pressure, which is closely related to but not the same as left ventricular afterload, is determined by the amount of blood ejected into the aorta and aortic *impedance*. Although aortic *impedance* is often equated to *peripheral resistance*, there is a difference. Resistance, in electricity, is the ratio between a potential difference and the flow of *direct current*; similarly, peripheral resistance describes the relationship between cardiac output and the pressure difference between the arteries and veins:

$$\text{Resistance} = \frac{\Delta \text{pressure}}{\text{Flow}} \qquad [12\text{-}4]$$

Electrical impedance, on the other hand, describes the relationship between current flow and the changing potential differences of an *alternating current*. Aortic impedance therefore takes into account the changes in pressure and flow velocity that occur throughout the cardiac cycle; because this calculation is complex, resistance is almost always used for clinical measurements.

The distinction between resistance and impedance has important implications; consider, for example, two patients in whom cardiac output and venous pressure are the same, but in whom aortic pressures are 110/80 and 170/50 mm Hg (the latter is often called "systolic hypertension"). Because mean aortic pressure (which can be estimated as aortic diastolic pressure +1/3 pulse pressure) is approximately 90 mm Hg in both patients, their peripheral resistances also are the same. However, because of the higher systolic pressure, the left ventricle ejects against a higher afterload in the patient with systolic hypertension because aortic impedance is greater.

Kinetic Work

In addition to stroke work, a small amount of *kinetic work* is performed to impart velocity to the blood as it leaves the ventricles to enter the aorta and pulmonary artery. The kinetic energy of this moving stream of blood, according to the laws of physics, is proportional to the square of the velocity at which blood leaves the ventricle:

$$\text{Kinetic work} = 1/2mv^2 \tag{12-5}$$

where m is the mass of blood moving out of the left ventricle into the aorta or from the right ventricle to the pulmonary artery, and v is the velocity at which this blood crosses the semilunar valves. The kinetic work of the left ventricle is normally less than 5% of the stroke work, but in the right ventricle, where systolic pressure is low, kinetic work represents a greater proportion of the smaller amount of total work performed.

Stroke volume contributes to both m (cm^3) and v^2 [$(cm^3/sec)^2$] in equation 12-5, so the kinetic work is proportional to the cube of the stroke volume (SV^3). For this reason, when stroke volume is abnormally high (as occurs in aortic insufficiency or severe anemia), kinetic work can represent a significant portion of the work of the left ventricle (although rarely more than 10%).

Kinetic energy is converted to pressure as velocity slows when blood moves through the circulatory system. Therefore, kinetic work—like stroke work—contributes to the "useful" work that pumps blood through the body.

Atrial Work

The work done when the atria pump blood into the ventricles makes only a negligible contribution to the energy expended by the heart because atrial systole moves only part of the stroke volume at a low pressure. Even though it adds little to overall energy expenditure, atrial systole is an important determinant of ventricular end-diastolic volume because of its timing (see Chapter 11).

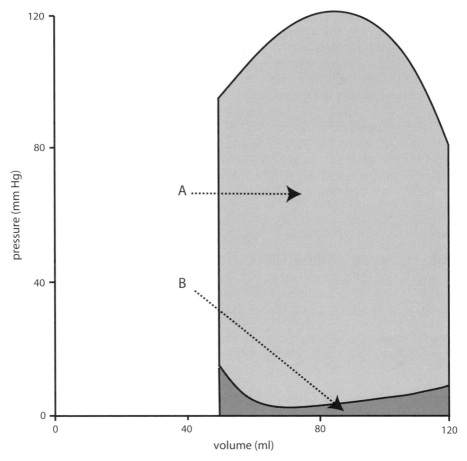

FIGURE 12-1 Work of the left ventricle. Useful work is the work done by the ventricle **(A)** plus the work contributed by atrial systole and the inertia of the venous return **(B)**.

Work Done to Fill the Ventricle

Calculations of the work of the heart often subtract the energy expended to fill the ventricles (Fig. 12-1), but this is usually a small fraction of total stroke work. The energy that fills each ventricle during diastole is provided by the momentum of the venous return and so is generated by opposite ventricle; blood pumped out of the right ventricle helps fill the left ventricle, and blood that leaves the left ventricle helps fill the right ventricle. Atrial systole, although important because of its timing, normally makes only a small contribution to ventricular filling.

INTERNAL WORK

In addition to the external work that circulates blood under pressure through the vascular system, the heart uses a large amount of energy to perform internal work. Much of this internal work stretches elasticities and elongates viscous elements in the myosin cross-bridges, the cytoskeleton (see Chapter 5), and the connective tissue that supports the heart (see Fig. 1-10). Energy also is used to rearrange the spiral bundles that make up the muscular architecture of the ventricle (see Fig. 1-4) and to effect the substantial shape changes that occur during isovolumic contraction, when the normally elongated left ventricle becomes more spherical as the apex is pulled toward the base (Hawthorne, 1961). Another form of internal work is the downward movement of the entire heart during ejection, sometimes referred to as the *"descent of the base"*; the latter, which is a consequence of Newton's Third Law ("to every action there is an equal and opposite reaction"), reflects the fact that when blood ejected into the aorta moves toward the head, the heart must move in the opposite direction, toward the feet. The descent of the base is the major cause of the *x descent* in the jugular venous pulse, a downward pulsation seen immediately after the upward *a wave* caused by atrial systole. This movement also explains the bouncing of the needle seen when one stands quietly on a scale, and provided the rationale for *ballistocardiography*, a now discarded method to estimate stroke volume.

Much of the energy expended as internal work is degraded to heat and contributes to the inefficiency of the heart. Internal work is directly proportional to wall stress, so the resulting loss of efficiency is greater when the heart becomes dilated (a consequence of the law of Laplace) or ejects against a high afterload. Not all of the energy used to stretch the elasticities within the heart and its supporting structures is wasted because wall stress decreases during ejection, when radius decreases and wall thickness increases; this allows some of the potential energy stored in the stretched elasticities to perform external (useful) work. Conversion of this potential energy to useful work accounts for the energy-sparing effect of interventions that reduce afterload; conversely, decreased utilization of this potential energy to perform useful work is among the adverse consequences of a high afterload. The latter is especially deleterious in the energy-starved hearts of patients with coronary occlusions or heart failure.

VENTRICULAR ARCHITECTURE

The law of Laplace was first applied to the heart in 1892, when Woods noted that "the thickness of the heart at any place bears a direct proportion to the relative tension at that place." Using measurements of wall thickness and radii of curvature, and assuming that wall stress is uniform throughout the heart, Woods not only predicted that left ventricular pressure is higher than that in the right ventricle, but that the difference is less in the neonatal heart where, as we now know, pulmonary pressure is the same as that in the aorta. The law of Laplace also explains how cardiac architecture is adapted to intraventricular pressure (Fig. 12-2). For example, in the giraffe left ventricle, where systolic pressure often exceeds 300 mm Hg, wall stress is kept low by thick walls and a narrow cavity,

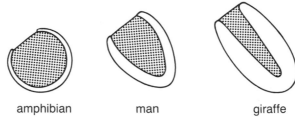

amphibian   man   giraffe

FIGURE 12-2 Relationship between ventricular cavity shape and systole pressure. The thin-walled ventricle of the amphibian heart, which develops a low pressure, is almost spherical, while that of the thicker human left ventricle, which develops a much higher pressure, is more elongated. In the giraffe, where left ventricular systolic pressure is extremely high, the cavity of the thick-walled ventricle is almost tubular.

whereas the amphibian ventricle, which generates low pressures, is thin walled and almost spherical. The law of Laplace also explains the different shapes of the right and left ventricles, where the radius of curvature of the walls of the more conical left ventricle is less than in the right ventricle, which has a crescentic cross-sectional shape (Fig. 12-3) (see also Fig. 1-3). This architecture allows the left ventricle to generate high intraventricular pressures with the same wall stress as the right ventricle.

The interventricular septum is thick because it normally functions as part of the left ventricle (Weber et al., 1991). However, when right ventricular pressure is elevated—for example, in pulmonary hypertension—the septum contracts "paradoxically" and moves away from the left ventricular cavity to assist in right ventricular ejection.

MINUTE WORK

Clinical descriptions of the work of the heart generally refer to the external work performed per minute, or *minute work*. Minute work, which is really a *power* (work per time), is calculated by multiplying the work per beat (stroke work) by the number of beats per minute (HR = heart rate):

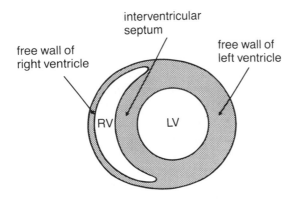

interventricular septum

free wall of right ventricle

free wall of left ventricle

RV   LV

FIGURE 12-3 Cross section of the human heart showing the thin-walled, crescentic right ventricle (RV), where systolic pressure is approximately 1/5 that of the thick-walled, narrower left ventricle (LV). The thick interventricular septum normally functions as part of the left ventricle.

$$\text{Minute work} = \text{HR} \times \text{SV} \times \text{P} \qquad [12\text{-}6]$$

Because the product of HR $\times$ SV in equation 12-6 is *cardiac output* (CO), minute work also is the product of pressure $\times$ cardiac output:

$$\text{Minute work} = \text{P} \times \text{CO} \qquad [12\text{-}7]$$

Cardiac output in humans is normally about 5 liters per minute.

Determinants of Minute Work

Each of the variables in equation 12-6 makes an independent contribution to the minute work, which can be increased by increasing ejection pressure, heart rate, stroke volume, or any combination of these variables. Because stroke volume = EDV – ESV, there are actually four determinants of minute work:

$$\text{Minute work} = \text{P} \times \text{HR} \times (\text{EDV} - \text{ESV}) \qquad [12\text{-}8]$$

Each of these four variables has a different impact on cardiac energetics, so total minute work provides only a rough index of the energy demands of the heart (see below).

WORK OF THE ISOLATED HEART

The variables that determine minute work are most readily analyzed in isolated heart preparations, where each can be varied independently. The preparation illustrated in Figure 12-4, which is similar to a working turtle heart that the author studied as a medical student in 1953, considers the work of a single ventricle—this is not a problem in the turtle heart, which has only one ventricle. Filling pressure (preload) can be varied by adjusting the height of the venous reservoir and ejection pressure (afterload) by raising or lowering the outlet of a flexible tube connected to the aorta; heart rate is controlled by electrical stimulation. The following discussion examines the effects of changing stroke volume, ejection pressure, and heart rate, while the other determinants of minute work are kept constant.

Varying Stroke Volume

Changing the height of the venous reservoir directly modifies ventricular end-diastolic pressure and end-diastolic volume (preload). The effects on cardiac performance are predicted by Starling's Law of the

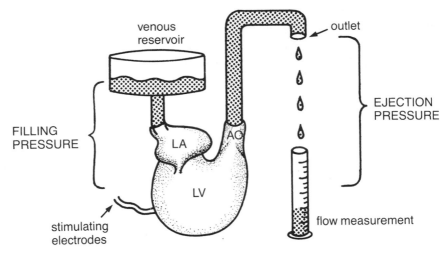

FIGURE 12-4 Isolated turtle heart preparation. Blood flows from the venous reservoir into the left atrium (LA) at a pressure determined by the height of the reservoir. When the ventricle (LV) contracts, blood is pumped across the aortic valve (AO) into a tube in which the height of the outlet, relative to the center of the ventricle, is the ejection pressure. Stroke volume is the amount of blood ejected during each beat.

Heart; as long as the heart functions on the ascending limb, stroke volume will increase with increasing filling pressure (Fig. 12-5). Because stroke work equals stroke volume times ejection pressure, which is held constant, stroke work can be substituted for stroke volume on the ordinate in Figure 12-5; as heart rate also is kept constant, minute work can be placed on the ordinate of Figure 12-5.

Varying Ejection Pressure

Raising or lowering the outlet of the tube connected to the aorta directly affects ejection pressure (afterload). However, stroke volume also will change because afterload is a major determinant of the ability of a muscle to shorten (see Chapter 3); for this reason, increased afterload will reduce stroke volume, and decreased afterload will increase ejection. To satisfy the requirement that only one variable be changed at any time, the level of the

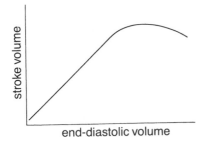

FIGURE 12-5 Operation of Starling's law of the heart under conditions where heart rate and ejection pressure are constant and only filling pressure is allowed to vary. Under these conditions, stroke volume rises as filling pressure increases. The descending limb shown at high end-diastolic volumes in this and the next figure is not seen in the normal mammalian heart.

FIGURE 12-6 Operation of Starling's law of the heart under conditions where heart rate and stroke volume are constant, therefore only ejection pressure can vary. When ejection pressure is increased, end-diastolic pressure also must be increased to meet the requirement that stroke volume remain constant, and vice versa.

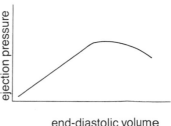

end-diastolic volume

venous reservoir must be adjusted to maintain a constant stroke volume. This means that when afterload is increased, the venous reservoir must be raised to maintain stroke volume; conversely, when reduced ejection pressure allows stroke volume to increase, the venous reservoir must be lowered. Varying the height of the venous reservoir also alters end-diastolic volume, which allows Starling's law to maintain a constant output in the face of the changing afterload (Fig. 12-6). As heart rate is kept constant, stroke work and minute work can replace ejection pressure on the ordinate in Figure 12-6.

Varying Heart Rate

When heart rate is varied at constant ejection pressure and venous pressure, stroke volume will be independent of heart rate as long as diastole lasts long enough to allow the ventricle to relax completely. Under these conditions, cardiac output and minute work will vary directly with heart rate. However, these effects are not the same in the intact animal, where cardiac output is generally independent of heart rate. This is because the major determinant of blood flow through each organ is the caliber of the arterioles that control tissue perfusion. This mechanism, called *autoregulation*, adjusts blood flow to match the needs of the tissue, which means that cardiac output is normally determined by the needs of the body, rather than the ability of the heart to pump blood. Except at very low and very high heart rates, therefore, cardiac output will be independent of heart rate (Warner and Toronto, 1960) (Fig. 12-7). However, cardiac output falls at very rapid heart rates because diastole does not last long enough to allow the ventricle to fill completely; this is due both to the limited flow velocity across the mitral valve and lack of time for the myocardium to relax completely. In humans, cardiac output begins to fall at heart rates greater than about 160 beats per minute, and less when there is heart failure. Cardiac output also falls when heart rate reaches extremely slow rates, as in patients with complete heart block, where rates can be as low as 20 beats per minute. Under these conditions, even though there is ample time for filling, increases in end-diastolic volume are limited by the low diastolic compliance of the heart (see Chapter 6). The adverse clinical effects of these very slow heart rates include profound weakness and clinical evidence of heart failure, both of which can be relieved by pacing the heart with an electronic pacemaker.

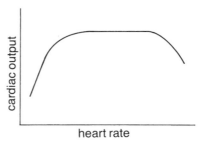

FIGURE 12-7 Effects of heart rate on cardiac output in the intact animal. Because blood flow through the tissues is normally determined largely by local metabolic needs, cardiac output remains constant when heart rate changes, which means that stroke volume varies inversely with heart rate. Cardiac output becomes dependent on heart rate only at rates so high that the brief duration of diastole does not allow the heart to relax fully, or at rates so low that increasing the duration of diastole cannot allow additional filling of the ventricle.

ENERGY COST OF THE WORK OF THE HEART

Energy utilization by the heart can be estimated by measuring cardiac oxygen consumption because cardiac muscle meets its energy needs by oxidizing fat, carbohydrates, and to a minor extent, protein (see Chapter 2). Because aerobic energy production is virtually independent of the substrate oxidized, calculation of the energy made available from the consumption of a given amount of oxygen is easy; even though oxidation of each gram of fat yields approximately 9 calories, while that of carbohydrate and proteins yields only about 4 calories/g, more oxygen is consumed by the oxidation of fat. For this reason, when energy release is expressed per liter of oxygen consumed, the value for all three substrates is approximately 4.8 calories/gm.

Cardiac Efficiency

The efficiency of cardiac contraction can be estimated by dividing the external work of the heart by the energy equivalent of the oxygen consumed:

$$\text{Cardiac efficiency} = \frac{\text{external work}}{\text{energy equivalent of oxygen consumption}} \qquad [12\text{-}9]$$

Although equation 12-9 does not describe a thermodynamic efficiency, the simpler variable provides a useful index of the overall economy of the heart. When calculated in this manner, the efficiency of the working heart ranges between 5% and 20%, the exact value depending on the nature and amount of work performed (see below).

The heart's low efficiency is due in large part to the energy expended during isovolumic contraction because, even when ventricular pressure fails to open the aortic and pulmonic valves and no external work is performed, energy is expended to perform internal work. When even a small amount of blood is ejected, external work is performed and a numerator appears in the equation for cardiac efficiency (equation 12-9). Although extra energy is required to eject this blood, efficiency generally increases with decreasing afterload because the energy expended to perform internal work becomes a smaller proportion of the total energy expenditure.

PRESSURE WORK AND FLOW WORK. The importance of afterload in cardiac energetics was first shown by Evans and Matsuoka (1915), who found that oxygen consumption increases when the heart does more work (Fig. 12-8); as noted in Chapter 5, this is a manifestation of the Fenn effect. Evans and Matsuoka also found that oxygen consumption and efficiency depend not only on the *amount* of work performed, but *how* it is performed (Fig. 12-9). Although increases in pressure and flow both require extra oxygen consumption, the extra expenditure of energy is greater when the heart contracts against a higher afterload than when it ejects a larger volume of blood. As a result, a*n increase in pressure generated by the heart is energetically more costly than a similar increase in ejection.* These differences are due mainly to the effects of afterload on the energy expended in performing internal work, which as noted above is directly proportional to wall stress. In addition, when the left ventricle ejects, its radius of curvature becomes smaller and wall thickness increases, both of which reduce wall stress. Reduced afterload therefore increases efficiency by allowing a greater amount of the energy stored in stretched elasticities to perform useful work.

The extra expenditure of energy at high wall stress is greater in cardiac muscle than in the frog sartorius, where heat liberation during

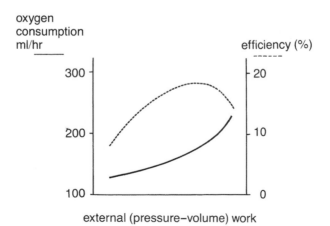

FIGURE 12-8 Relationship between external work and the energetics of ventricular contraction. Oxygen consumption (*solid line*) increases when more work is done, while efficiency (*dashed line*) first rises and then falls. Based on Evans and Matsuoka (1915).

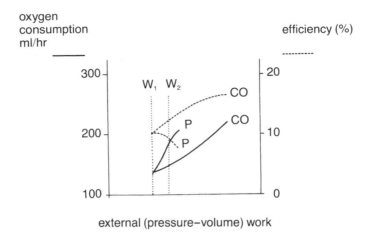

FIGURE 12-9 Influence of the type of external work on oxygen consumption (*solid lines*) and efficiency (*dashed lines*). Increasing cardiac work from W_1 to W_2 by increasing ejection pressure (P) causes a greater increase in oxygen consumption than when work is increased to a similar extent by increasing cardiac output (CO). For this reason, efficiency is greater when cardiac output is increased than when ejection pressure is increased. Based on Evans and Matsuoka (1915).

contraction is essentially independent of load (Fig. 12-10). This difference was explained many years ago by Fenn, who found that not all skeletal muscles contract efficiently at high loads; in the frog gastrocnemius, for example, total energy expenditure does not decline appreciably with increasing load as it does in the sartorius (Martin, 1928). These differences

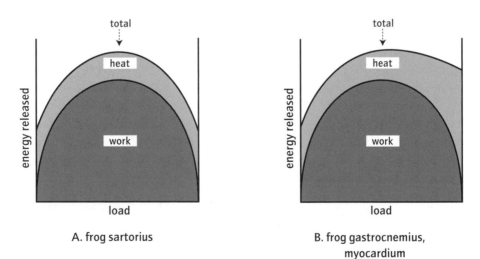

FIGURE 12-10 Relationship between load, work, and total energy liberation in two types of skeletal muscle. **A:** In the frog sartorius, heat production is independent of load, so work and total energy expenditure are maximal at intermediate loads **B:** In the frog gastrocnemius, as in the myocardium, total energy expenditure and heat production increase disproportionately at high loads.

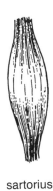

sartorius

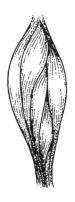

gastrocnemius

FIGURE 12-11 Arrangement of muscle fibers in the frog sartorius muscle, where the fibers are parallel and oriented longitudinally, and the gastrocnemius, where the non-parallel organization of fiber bundles increases internal work at higher tensions.

are the result of differences in the internal work expended to rearrange the fiber bundles when the muscles develop tension. Unlike the sartorius, where the fiber bundles run parallel to one another from one end of the muscle to the other, the gastrocnemius has an asymmetrical bipennate arrangement (Fig. 12-11) that allows significant shape changes to occur even when the ends of the muscle are fixed in an isometric contraction. Although the extent of sarcomere shortening is small, the tension developed during isometric contraction of the gastrocnemius allows small shape changes to generate high levels of internal work that, when degraded to heat, increase energy expenditure (Fig. 12-10B). In the sartorius muscle, where the parallel arrangement of the fiber bundles allows much less shape change during contraction (Fig. 12-10A), the internal work and energy wastage associated with tension development are less; this is one reason that A. V. Hill chose the frog sartorius as the standard preparation for his classical studies of muscle energetics (see Chapter 5). The complex architecture of the heart, which resembles the gastrocnemius much more than the sartorius, is the major reason for the higher energy cost of increasing pressure than increasing cardial output (Fig. 12-9).

Effect of Dilatation on Efficiency

Dilatation adds to the inefficiency of the heart because increased cavity size reduces the fall in wall stress that normally occurs during ejection; this is due simply to the geometry of a dilated heart, where ejection of a given volume is associated with a smaller change in dimensions than in a normal heart. These relationships are apparent in a simple spherical model in which dilatation has doubled wall stress at the same cavity pressure (Fig. 12-12, Table 12-2). In this example, ejection of 70 cm^3 by the normal ventricle reduces wall tension by almost 40% (from 3.72×10^5 to 2.26×10^5 dynes/cm), whereas ejection of the same volume by the dilated

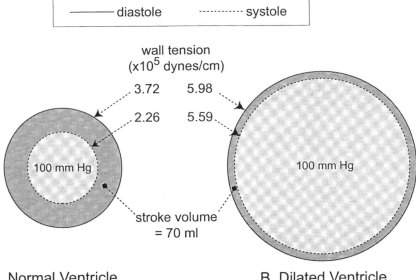

A. Normal Ventricle   B. Dilated Ventricle

FIGURE 12-12 Effects of cavity volume on the relationships between pressure, wall tension, and the change in circumference during ejection by a normal ventricle (A) and a
dilated ventricle (B). Cavity outlines are shown at end-diastole (*solid circles*) and at end-
systole (*dashed circles*); the shaded areas between each pair of circles, which are the
same, represent the stroke volume. The dilated ventricle ejects its stroke volume with a
smaller decrease in circumference than the normal ventricle, so wall tension falls less
during ejection. (The data used in this figure are found in Table 12-2.)

ventricle decreases wall tension less than 10% (from 5.98×10^5 to 5.59×10^5 dynes/cm).

These architectural consequences of dilatation explain the lower
efficiency of the larger heart because in ejecting the same volume of blood
at the same pressure, not only is wall stress higher, but there is less wall
shortening than in the smaller heart. The latter reduces the extent to
which wall stress falls during ejection by the dilated heart, and so allows
less of the internal work expended in stretching elasticities to be used for
ejection.

Changing Heart Rate

The high energy cost of internal work helps explain the inefficiency
associated with increased heart rate. Because internal work must be done
each time that pressure develops during isometric contraction, and
because much of this work is converted to heat during relaxation, more
energy is wasted to perform internal work when more isovolumic contractions are performed per unit time. Another reason that increasing
heart rate is a costly way to increase the minute work of the heart is that
energy must be expended during each cardiac cycle to restore ion gradients

TABLE 12-2 **Effects of Dilatation on Ventricular Energetics+**

Variable	Normal Ventricle	Dilated Ventricle
At start of ejection		
Pressure (mm Hg*)	100	100
Volume (cm³)	92	380
Radius (cm)	2.8	4.5
Circumference (cm)	17.5	28
Wall tension (dynes/cm)	3.72×10^5	5.98×10^5
Stroke volume (cm³)	70	70
At end of ejection		
Pressure (mm Hg*)	100	100
Volume (cm³)	22	310
Radius (cm)	1.7	4.2
Circumference (cm)	11	26.5
Wall tension (dynes/cm)	2.26×10^5	5.59×10^5
External stroke work (dynes/cm)	9.3×10^6	9.3×10^6
Conditions of external work		
Average wall tension (dynes/cm)	2.99×10^5	5.79×10^5
Change in circumference (cm)	6.5	1.5
As % end-diastolic circumference	~40	~5
Ejection fraction	70%	18%

+Volumes, radii, circumferences, and wall tensions are calculated by assuming that the ventricle is a thin-walled sphere that ejects at a constant pressure.
*One mm Hg = 1.33×10^3 dynes/cm².

across the plasma membrane and to pump calcium into the sarcoplasmic reticulum.

Clinical Estimates of the Energy Cost of Cardiac Work

The product of heart rate and aortic pressure correlates closely with cardiac oxygen consumption and can be used to estimate the energy expenditure of the intact heart (Gerola et al. 1956; Katz and Feinberg, 1958):

Energy expenditure α HR $\times$ P   [12-10]

This product, HR $\times$ P, is generally referred to as the *double-product*. A somewhat more elaborate index of myocardial oxygen consumption, *the*

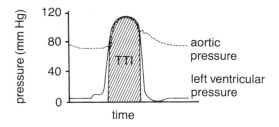

FIGURE 12-13 Cardiac oxygen consumption can be estimated as the tension–time index (TTI), which is the area under the ejection phase of the left ventricular pressure–volume loop.

tension-time index (Sarnoff et al., 1958), multiplies average ejection pressure by the duration of ejection (Fig. 12-13); however, this more cumbersome index has not been shown to be more useful clinically than the double-product.

Even though the double product (equation 12-10) includes only two of the three terms of the equation for minute work (equation 12-6), as it omits stroke volume, the latter is the least important determinant of the energy costs of cardiac work. A more important limitation of this index is that it does not take into account the effects of chamber size in determining wall stress. Despite these limitations, the double-product is widely used to measure cardiac energy consumption—for example, during clinical stress testing.

CHANGES IN MYOCARDIAL CONTRACTILITY (INOTROPY): THE FAMILY OF STARLING CURVES

Each Starling curve defines the effect of changing rest length on myocardial performance at any level of contractility, whereas a change in contractility generates a new Starling curve. This allows contractile performance to be described by a "family of Starling curves," each of which reflects the effects of changing end-diastolic volume at a different inotropic state. This interplay is shown in Figure 12-14, where points C, A, and B lie along a control Starling curve, therefore defining a level of contractility. Changes in end-diastolic volume can cause stroke work to increase (A → B) or decrease (A → C). A positive inotropic intervention, which by definition increases the ability of the heart to do work at any given end-diastolic volume, shifts the heart to a higher Starling curve (curve containing D); conversely, a negative inotropic intervention causes a shift to a lower Starling curve (curve containing E). Thus, Figure 12-14 illustrates two mechanisms that change stroke work: vary end-diastolic volume or vary contractility.

The energy cost of these two mechanisms is not the same because when cardiac performance is increased by a greater end-diastolic volume (Starling's Law of the Heart), the response requires cavity dilatation, which increases wall stress and reduces efficiency. When contractility is increased, on the other hand, wall stress does not increase because increased ejection reduces cavity volume.

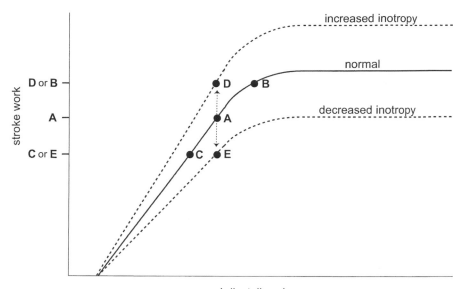

FIGURE 12-14 Family of Starling curves. The *solid line* (**CAB**) is an end-systolic pressure–volume relationship (Starling curve) that describes myocardial contractility; point A along this line represents the basal state. The two *dashed lines* represent additional Starling curves recorded after contractility has changed. Changes in end-diastolic volume at a constant level of contractility shift the end-systolic point along a given Starling curve; an increase in venous return increases stroke work from **A** to **B**, and a decrease in venous return decreases stroke work from **A** to **C**. The work of the heart also can be changed by interventions that modify myocardial contractility, which increase or decrease stroke work at any end-diastolic volume; for this reason, positive and negative inotropic interventions cause a shift to a new Starling curve. Starting from the basal state (*point A*), a positive inotropic intervention increases stroke work (**A** to **D**) and a negative inotropic intervention decreases work from (**A** to **E**).

CHANGES IN MYOCARDIAL RELAXATION (LUSITROPY): THE FAMILY OF FILLING CURVES

Changes in the lusitropic (relaxation) properties of the heart, which represent an additional mechanism that regulates cardiac performance, generate a family of *filling curves* (Fig. 12-15). Points V, X, and W, which lie along one such filling curve, show the effects of changing preload on ventricular pressure and volume at a constant lusitropic state. A change in diastolic properties that causes a shift to a new filling curve changes end-diastolic volume at any filling pressure (preload) (X → Y or Z in Fig. 12-15), which means that the lusitropic state has changed.

INTERPLAY BETWEEN CHANGING INOTROPY AND LUSITROPY

The curves depicted in Figure 12-15 are the same as the PV relationships that enclose the pressure volume loop (see Fig. 11-9), which allows

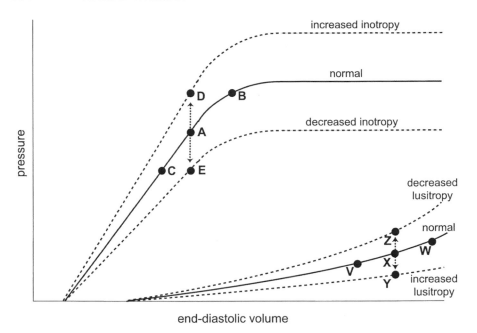

FIGURE 12-15 Family of filling curves. Three end-diastolic PV relationships have been added to the end-systolic pressure–volume relationships shown in Figure 12-14. The basal end-diastolic pressure–volume relationship contains point **X**. A positive lusitropic intervention, which improves the ability of the ventricle to fill, shifts the end-diastolic PV relationship to the right and downward (*curve containing point* **Y**), while a negative lusitropic intervention, which impairs ventricular filling, shifts this relationship to the left and upward (*curve containing point* **Z**).

pressure-volume loops to be used to illustrate the interplay between changing inotropic and lusitropic states. In the following discussion, four interventions are described: two alter contractility (inotropic properties) and two modify relaxation (lusitropic properties). For simplicity, only the first beat after an abrupt change is shown.

Effects of a Negative Inotropic Intervention

A decrease in contractility shifts the end-systolic PV relationship (the Starling curve) to the right and downward (Fig. 12-16). If the first beat after the negative inotropic intervention encounters the same aortic pressure, the initial effect is to reduce stroke volume.

Because the decreased ejection leaves behind a greater end-systolic (residual) volume, end-diastolic volume increases in subsequent beats. This will shift the loop to the right along the end-diastolic PV relationship and allow the operation of Starling's law to return stroke volume toward normal. An additional compensatory response is provided by the hemodynamic defense response (see Chapter 8), which responds to a fall in cardiac output by causing both vasoconstriction and cardiac stimulation.

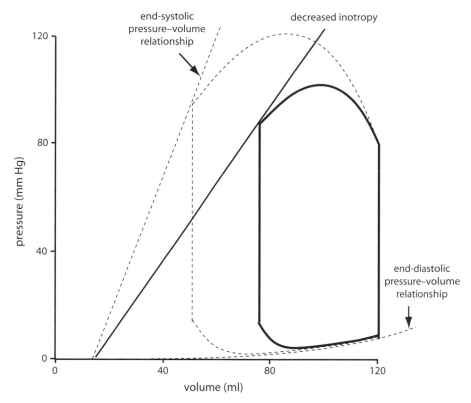

FIGURE 12-16 A negative inotropic intervention (*solid lines*) shifts the end-systolic pressure–volume (PV) relationship to the right and downward; if aortic pressure remains constant, stroke volume will be reduced. The control loop and control end-systolic and end-diastolic pressure–volume relationships are shown as *dashed lines* in this and the following three figures.

Effects of a Positive Inotropic Intervention

When contractility is increased, the end-systolic PV relationship shifts to the left and upward (Fig. 12-17). If aortic pressure remains the same in the first beat after the inotropic intervention, the greater ability of the ventricle to eject increases stroke volume.

Because increased ejection reduces end-systolic volume, subsequent beats will be shifted to lower volumes along the unchanged end-diastolic PV relationship. This will decrease end-diastolic volume, which according to Starling's law reduces ejection and so returns stroke volume toward the control level.

Effects of a Negative Lusitropic Intervention

An intervention that impairs ventricular filling by altering lusitropic properties shifts the end-diastolic PV relationship to the left and upward, which raises the pressure needed to achieve a given increment in diastolic

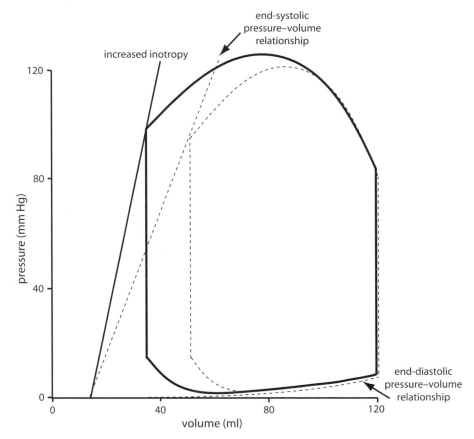

FIGURE 12-17 A positive inotropic intervention (*solid lines*) shifts the end-systolic PV relationship to the left and upward (*solid curves*); if aortic pressure remains constant, stroke volume will increase.

volume (Fig. 12-18). If the first beat after the change begins at an unchanged end-diastolic pressure and encounters the same aortic pressure, stroke volume will be reduced.

The fall in stroke volume, like that which follows the negative inotropic intervention described above, will increase preload in subsequent beats, resulting in a rightward shift along the new end-diastolic PV relationship. By increasing end-diastolic volume, this shift allows Starling's law to return stroke volume toward normal.

Effects of a Positive Lusitropic Intervention

A positive lusitropic intervention shifts the end-diastolic PV relationship to the right and downward (Fig. 12-19). If filling pressure and aortic pressure do not change, the increased end-diastolic volume increases stroke volume. The latter, by decreasing end-systolic volume, would allow Starling's law to return stroke volume toward normal.

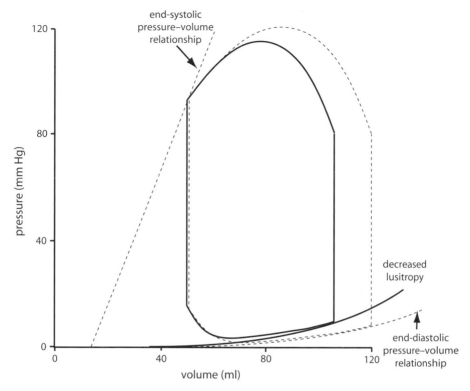

FIGURE 12-18 A negative lusitropic intervention (*solid lines*) shifts the end-diastolic PV relationship to the left and upward; if aortic pressure remains constant, stroke volume will be reduced.

Effects of Changing Preload and Afterload

Interactions of the heart with the circulation allow changes in venous return and aortic pressure to alter the pressure–volume loop. A change in preload moves the end-diastolic point along the end-diastolic PV relationship, while changing afterload moves the point at which the aortic valve opens upward or downward along the curve inscribed during isovolumic contraction.

INTERPLAY BETWEEN VENOUS RETURN AND CARDIAC OUTPUT

In the intact circulation, where blood flows in a circle, venous return must equal cardiac output. This means that to maintain a steady state, cardiac output must be matched to venous return, and venous return to cardiac output. In terms of *cardiac output*, this steady state is maintained by Starling's Law of the Heart, which increases stroke volume when more blood returns to the heart and decreases stroke volume when venous

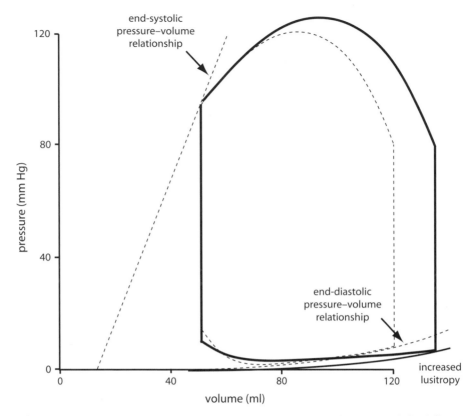

FIGURE 12-19 A positive lusitropic intervention (*solid lines*) shifts the end-diastolic PV relationship to the right and downward; if aortic pressure remains constant, stroke volume will increase.

return is reduced. In terms of *venous return*, the steady state is maintained because decreased stroke volume increases atrial pressure, which reduces venous return, and increased stroke volume decreases atrial pressure, which increases venous return. The interplay between stroke volume and venous return is not due to a physiological law but instead results from the simple interplay between atrial pressure and blood flow from the veins into the heart.

The mechanism by which atrial pressure matches venous return to cardiac output is shown in Figure 12-20, which illustrates how changing the height of a hose leading out of a reservoir affects flow. Raising the outlet of the hose, which represents atrial pressure, slows the rate of flow out of the reservoir; flow stops altogether when the pressure at the outlet of the hose is the same as that in the reservoir (D). This interplay is shown graphically in Figure 12-21 (often described as a "Guyton diagram" after Arthur Guyton, who devised this diagram), which depicts the relationship between right atrial pressure and venous return (blood flow into the heart), and between atrial pressure and cardiac output (blood flow out of the heart).

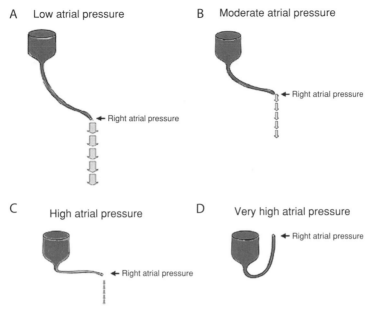

FIGURE 12-20 Effect of raising and lowering the outlet of a hose connected to a reservoir. Flow out of the reservoir depends on the pressure gradient between the outlet of the hose, which in the heart represents atrial pressure, and the pressure exerted by the fluid in the reservoir. When the outlet of the hose is at a low level (A), flow out of the reservoir is rapid. Flow is reduced by raising the outlet of the hose (B and C) and stops altogether when the pressure at the outlet of the hose is the same as that in the reservoir (D). The fluid level in the reservoir is equivalent to the mean circulatory filling pressure.

When viewed *from the circulation*, increased atrial pressure reduces blood flow *toward* the heart, whereas when viewed *from the heart*, increased atrial pressure increases the ejection of blood *from* the heart (Starling's Law of the Heart). The effects of atrial pressure on flow described by these two relationships are therefore opposite to one another; venous return falls with increasing atrial pressure, while cardiac output rises when atrial pressure increases (Fig. 12-21). At any steady state, the unique intersection of the two curves defines the atrial pressure where venous return and cardiac output are equal to one another. The maximal level to which right atrial pressure can rise in the intact circulation, which can be measured when the heart is stopped and all pressures in the cardiovascular system come to equilibrium, is the *mean circulatory filling pressure*; this is the pressure at which venous return (and cardiac output) fall to zero.

The Guyton diagram helps to clarify the interplay between atrial pressure, venous return, and cardiac output (Figs. 12-22 and 12-23). A fall in venous return, by shifting the end-diastolic point along the Starling curve down and to the left, reduces cardiac output (Fig. 12-22, N → D), while increased venous return shifts this end-diastolic point up and to the right, which increases cardiac output (Fig. 12-22, N → I). A positive inotropic intervention increases ejection and therefore lowers atrial pressure

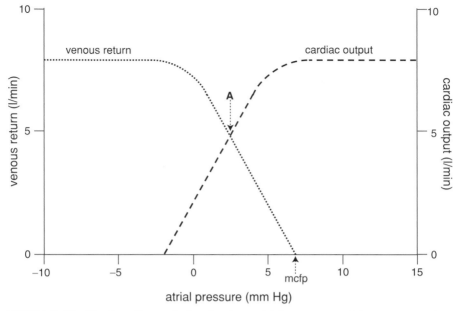

FIGURE 12-21 "Guyton diagram" showing how atrial pressure matches venous return (*dotted line*) and cardiac output (*dashed line*). Elevating atrial pressure increases cardiac output (Starling's law of the heart) but decreases venous return, whereas decreasing atrial pressure has the opposite effect. At any steady state, the two curves intersect at the atrial pressure at which flow into and out of the heart are the same (**A**). The pressure recorded when the heart is stopped is the mean circulatory filling pressure (mcfp).

(Fig. 12-23, N → I); the resulting fall in the resistance to blood flow into the heart increases venous return, which shifts the intersection of the two curves up and to the left. Conversely, a negative inotropic intervention reduces ejection, increasing atrial pressure (Fig. 12-23, N → D). The latter, by reducing venous return, shifts the intersection down and to the right. Thus, changes in the interplay between the amount of blood returning from the periphery and the amount leaving the heart establish new steady states that can be characterized by the points at which venous return and cardiac output are equal.

CLINICAL INDICES OF MYOCARDIAL CONTRACTILITY (INOTROPY)

Efforts to identify clinical indices of myocardial contractility were stimulated in the 1960s by the need to identify the optimal time for surgical repair of valvular heart disease. Correct timing remains a challenge because if valve replacement is performed too soon, exposure to such hazards as embolism, infection, and deterioration of the prosthetic valve is unnecessarily prolonged, whereas if surgery is delayed too long, even a technically perfect operation cannot help the patient because prolonged

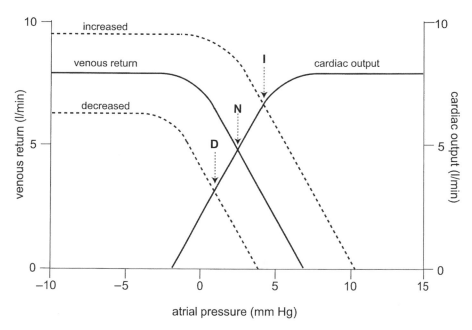

FIGURE 12-22 Curves relating venous return and cardiac output showing effects of changing atrial pressure. Increased atrial pressure reduces venous return, whereas decreased atrial pressure allows venous return to increase. **N**, normal; **I**, increased atrial pressure; **D**, decreased atrial pressure.

overload irreversibly damages the myocardium (see Chapter 18). The clinical use of these indices has decreased recently because modern imaging modalities give a clearer picture of the pathological anatomy of diseased hearts, and because depressed contractility is now recognized to be only one of several determinants of outcome in these patients. The following discussion highlights a few clinical indices to illustrate the practical use of the physiological principles described in this text.

The most direct measurement of ventricular function might seem to be the clinical state of the patient. However, the hemodynamic defense reaction has a major influence on the severity of the signs and symptoms of heart failure (see Chapter 18), so clinical evaluation provides little information regarding the state of the myocardium.

Systolic Time Intervals

External carotid pulse recording, phonocardiography, and electrocardiography allow the phases of the cardiac cycle to be timed and related to the mechanical events occurring in the left ventricle (Fig. 12-24, Table 12-3). The duration of left ventricular systole can be estimated as the $Q-S_2$ interval, which begins with the QRS complex on the electrocardiogram and ends with S_2, the second heart sound caused by aortic valve closure. Left ventricular systole can be subdivided into three phases: *the $Q-S_1$ interval*, measured from the beginning of the QRS complex to mitral valve

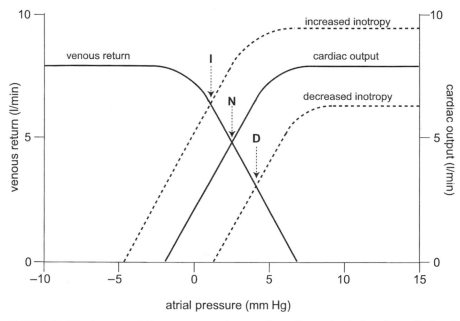

FIGURE 12-23 Curves relating venous return and cardiac output showing effects of changing inotropic state. Increased contractility decreases right atrial pressure, which allows venous return to increase. Conversely, decreased contractility raises atrial pressure and therefore lowers venous return. **N**, normal; **I**, increased contractility; **D**, decreased contractility.

closure, which generates S_1 (the first heart sound); *isovolumic contraction time*, between S_1 and aortic valve opening; and *left ventricular ejection time* (LVET), measured from the upstroke of the carotid pulse (the beginning of left ventricular ejection) to the dicrotic notch (aortic valve closure). Because there is a delay in the transmission of the pulse wave from the aortic root to the carotid artery, isovolumic contraction time is estimated by subtracting the interval between S_2 and the dicrotic notch from the interval between S_1 and the carotid upstroke. The *pre-ejection period* (PEP), obtained by subtracting LVET from the Q–S_2 interval, measures the interval between the onset of ventricular depolarization and the beginning of ejection. When contractility is depressed, PEP is prolonged and LVET is shortened, so the ratio PEP/LVET can be used to identify patients with depressed myocardial contractility. The systolic time intervals, which must be corrected for heart rate, provide only rough estimates of contractility because they are influenced by preload and afterload as well as abnormalities in left ventricular depolarization.

Hemodynamic Indices

Left ventricular filling pressures can be estimated by "wedging" an end-hole catheter passed from a systemic vein into a small pulmonary artery; this records pulmonary wedge pressure, which is generally close to

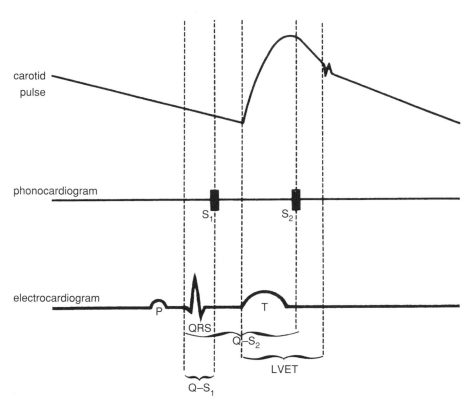

FIGURE 12-24 Systolic time intervals can be calculated from the carotid pulse (*upper*), phonocardiogram (*middle*), and electrocardiogram (*lower*). Delayed transmission of the arterial pulse from the aortic root to the carotid artery causes S_2 to precede the dicrotic notch in the aortic pulse tracing. LVET (left ventricular ejection time) is the interval between the carotid upstroke and the dicrotic notch. The Q–S_2 interval represents the total duration of electromechanical systole. Subtraction of LVET from the Q–S_2 interval yields the pre-ejection period (PEP).

left atrial pressure. The catheters used to measure wedge pressure also can be used to measure cardiac output and can help clarify the state of the left ventricle in patients with severely abnormal hemodynamics.

Isovolumic Indices

Several indices of myocardial contractility are based on analyses of pressure measurements obtained during isovolumic contraction. A major advantage is that data are collected before the aortic valve opens, so these indices are independent of afterload. The simplest isovolumic index of left ventricular contractility is dP/dt_{max}, the maximum rate of pressure rise. However, dP/dt_{max} is only a crude index of contractility because it is influenced by the size and thickness of the left ventricle, regional abnormalities in left ventricular function, a leaky mitral valve, loss of the normal synchronicity of contraction, and end-diastolic volume (preload). The quotient $(dP/dt)/P$, obtained by dividing dP/dt continuously by instantaneous left

TABLE 12-3 **Systolic Time Intervals**

Interval	Measurement	Physiological correlation
$Q–S_2$	From beginning of QRS to first frequency vibration of S_2	Total electromechanical systole
$Q–S_1$	From beginning of QRS to beginning of S_2	Excitation–contraction coupling
Isovolumic contraction	From S_1 to onset of rise in aortic pressure	Excitation contraction-coupling
Left ventricular ejection time (LVET)	From onset of carotid upstroke to the dicrotic notch	Total ejection
Pre-ejection period (PEP)	$Q–S_2$ *minus* LVET	Isovolumic contraction plus $Q–S_1$ interval

ventricular pressure, is influenced less by preload than dP/dt_{max} but is not very sensitive to changes in contractility.

The velocity of fiber shortening during isovolumic contraction (V_{CE}) uses pressure measurements to estimate shortening velocities in the walls of the ventricle. This requires the selection of a stiffness constant (K) to convert changing wall stress to changes in the length of the contractile elements. In the equation for V_{CE},

$$V_{CE} = \frac{dT/dt}{KT} + C \qquad [12\text{-}11]$$

T is the tension developed by the contractile elements, dT/dt is the rate of rise of wall tension calculated according to the law of Laplace, and K is the stiffness constant of the series elasticity (C, a small stiffness extrapolated for zero load, is generally ignored in calculating V_{CE}). Because K has the units dT/dl, V_{CE} can be expressed as a change in muscle length. Estimates of V_{CE}, like other pressure-derived indices, are subject to the limitations described for dP/dt_{max}.

Indices Based on Measurements of Volume and Dimensions

Measurements of ventricular volume and wall motion, while they cannot define the contractile state of the left ventricle, provide indispensable characterizations of ventricular architecture and allow serial determinations to be made during the natural history of the disease in an individual patient. These noninvasive measurements are useful in ischemic heart disease, where regional wall motion abnormalities can identify patients in whom occlusion of one or more coronary arteries has caused a localized contractile abnormality. Methods to quantify regional wall motion are difficult and are used mainly in research. In clinical practice, wall motion is usually described visually. Mild impairment causes *asyneresis* (reduced inward movement) or *asynchrony* (disturbed temporal sequence of contraction). More severe impairment of function causes *akinesis* (failure of a damaged segment to participate in ejection), while the most severe is *dyskinesis*, where the damaged segment bulges outward during systole. A large dyskinetic region is commonly referred to as an *aneurysm*.

EJECTION FRACTION. *Ejection fraction* (EF), which has become the most commonly used index of left ventricular function, is the fraction of the end-diastolic volume that is ejected as the stroke volume:

$$EF = \frac{SV}{EDV} \qquad [12\text{-}12]$$

Because EF is inversely related to end-diastolic volume, it is reduced in patients with dilated hearts. The extent to which EF is depressed is a very good predictor of long-term prognosis, but EF correlates poorly with the severity of symptoms because the major cause of the low EF is not a decrease in stroke volume, the numerator in equation 12-12, but dilatation, which increases EDV, the denominator. EF is of little value as an index of myocardial contractility because it is determined largely by changes in EDV; furthermore, EF is influenced by preload and heart rate, and especially by afterload.

EF, which is normally >55%, can fall below 20% in patients with heart failure; however, many patients with heart failure do not have a dilated ventricle and therefore EF is normal. The abnormality in these patients is often called "diastolic heart failure" in contrast to "systolic heart failure," where EF is low.

Fractional wall shortening, which is analogous to EF except that it is calculated using dimensions measured by echocardiography instead of cavity volumes, has the same limitations as a measure of contractility.

INDICES OF FILLING (LUSITROPY)

Much less attention has been paid to abnormalities of relaxation because, until noninvasive methods to measure volumes became available, it was quite difficult to estimate lusitropic properties. (The fact that ejection by a hydraulic pump is generally more impressive than its filling undoubtedly contributed to the general neglect of diastole by all but a few 20th-century cardiologists!)

Lusitropic abnormalities can modify three features of ventricular relaxation (Fig. 12-25). Two depend on relaxation rate: the rate of pressure

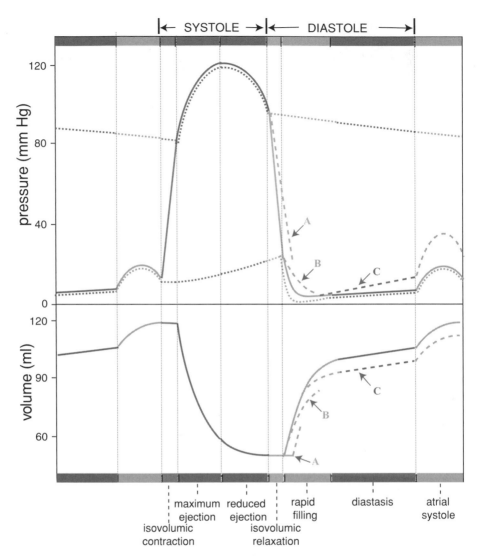

FIGURE 12-25 Pathophysiological mechanisms that can impair diastolic function. **(A)** Slowed rate of pressure fall during isovolumic relaxation (−dP/dt); **(B)** slowed filling during early diastole; and **(C)** slowed filling throughout diastole. A decrease in slope of the curve relating the increase in volume to the increase in pressure throughout diastole defines a decrease in compliance (or an increase in stiffness).

fall during isovolumic relaxation (−dP/dt) and the rate of filling during early diastole (dV/dt). The other is the slope of the curve relating the increase in ventricular volume to the pressure rise in late diastole, which can be viewed either as compliance (dV/dP, the slope of the curve relating the change in volume for each increment of pressure) or stiffness, its reciprocal (dP/dV, the slope of the curve relating the change in pressure to that of volume) (Fig. 12-26).

A. Decreased compliance   B. Increased stiffness

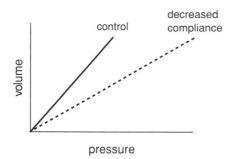
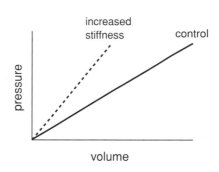

FIGURE 12-26   Graphic representations of decreased compliance (**A**) and increased stiffness (**B**). These differ simply in the way that the relationship between changing pressure and changing volume are plotted.

There are many causes of impaired diastolic function (Table 12-4), but it is usually impossible to relate the hemodynamic abnormalities shown in Figure 12-25 to any of these causative mechanisms, which tend to occur together. The rate of pressure fall during isovolumic relaxation ($-dP/dt$) and the rate of filling during early diastole (dV/dt) are influenced by the number, turnover rate, and calcium-sensitivity of the calcium pump of the sarcoplasmic reticulum and the calcium affinity of the troponin complex. Diastolic compliance and the rate of filling during early diastole are influenced by persistence of bonds linking the thick and

TABLE 12-4   Mechanisms That Can Modify Filling of the Heart

1. Structural abnormalities
   Valvular disorders—e.g., mitral stenosis
   Pericardial effusion
   Architectural abnormalities—e.g., concentric hypertrophy
2. Physiological abnormalities
   Abbreviation of systole (tachycardia)
   Increased end-systolic (residual) volume
3. Nonmyocyte abnormalities
   Increased connective tissue, fibrosis
   Constrictive pericarditis
4. Cardiac myocyte abnormalities
   Decreased rate of calcium uptake by the sarcoplasmic reticulum
   Decreased extent of calcium uptake by the sarcoplasmic reticulum
   Increased calcium affinity of the contractile proteins

thin filaments, cytoskeletal abnormalities, changes in the extracellular matrix such as fibrosis, and infiltrative diseases like amyloidosis. Cytosolic calcium overload, which can be caused by excessive calcium influx or impaired calcium removal from the cytosol, impairs all of these lusitropic indices.

Diastolic function can be evaluated clinically by such simple methods as auscultation, where an audible third or fourth heart sound implies that the ventricle has become stiff. Doppler measurements of the flow across the mitral valve provide useful noninvasive indices of diastolic function. These include the E/A ratio, which measures the ratio between early and late maxima of flow velocity; the former (E) is related to rapid filling, while the latter (A) is due to atrial systole. More elaborate indices of diastolic function include the percentage of end-diastolic filling that occurs during the first third of diastole, average rapid filling rate, peak filling rate, and the time to peak filling rate. Like the indices used to estimate contractility, these are generally rather imprecise.

A traditional index of diastolic function is the maximum rate of left ventricular pressure fall during isovolumic relaxation, $-dP/dt_{max}$, but because this is highly dependent on aortic pressure, corrections must be made to obtain a pressure-independent index. If the decline in left ventricular pressure is assumed to be exponential with time, $-dP/dt$ can be expressed as an exponential function. This makes it possible to calculate a time constant, τ, based on the time required for ventricular pressure to decline to either 1/2 or 1/e of its value at the time of aortic valve closure. As the fall of left ventricular pressure during isovolumic relaxation is not usually exponential, more elaborate equations are often used to calculate τ. The complexity of these determinations, however, generally limits these measurements to the research laboratory.

CONCLUSIONS

The hemodynamic principles described in this chapter represent the foundation of modern cardiology and must be understood by all who care for patients with heart disease. Although conceptual and technological advances are providing new and useful tools to evaluate cardiac performance, definition of pathophysiology and formulation of a therapeutic plan still require a trained clinician who can organize and synthesize the growing array of data. It can be argued that, as we learn more about pathophysiology and how it causes disease, even greater skill is needed to integrate the flood of data obtained from an individual patient. Of course, this is not always possible. This was noted many years ago by a colleague who said: "If you can't put everything together, the first thing to do is to throw out the high technology." This view is also stated in an old aphorism: "Listen to the patient."

BIBLIOGRAPHY

Hugenholtz PG, Rutishauser W, eds. Symposium: assessment of left ventricular function. *Eur J Cardiol* 1974;1:229–334 .

Krayenbuehl HP, Hess OM, Turina J. Assessment of left ventricular function. *Cardiovasc Med* 1978;2:883–910.

Mirsky I. Assessment of diastolic function: suggested methods and future considerations. *Circulation* 1984;69:834–841.

Pasipoularidies A. Clinical assessment of ventricular ejection dynamics with and without outflow obstruction. *J Am Coll Cardiol* 1990;15:859–892.

Pouleur H, Rousseau MF, van Eyll C, et al. Assessment of left ventricular contractility from late systolic stress-volume relations. *Circulation* 1982;65:1204–1212.

Sagawa K. Editorial: the end-systolic pressure-volume relation of the left ventricle: definition, modifications and clinical use. *Circulation* 1981;63:1223–1227.

Weissler AM, Garrard CL Jr. Systolic time intervals in cardiac disease. *Mod Concepts Cardiovasc Dis* 1971;40:1–8.

See also the bibliography for Chapter 11.

REFERENCES

Evans CL, Matsuoka Y. The effect of various mechanical conditions on the gaseous metabolism and efficiency of the mammalian heart. *J Physiol (Lond)* 1915;49:378–405.

Gerola A, Feinberg H, Katz LN. The oxygen cost of cardiac hemodynamic activity. *The Physiologist* 1956;1:31.

Hawthorne EW. Instantaneous dimensional changes in the left ventricle of dogs. *Circ Res* 1961;9:110–119.

Katz LN, Feinberg H. The relation of cardiac effort to myocardial oxygen consumption and coronary flow. *Circ Res* 1958;6:656–669.

Martin DS. The relation between work performed and heat liberated by the isolated gastrocnemius, semitendinosus and tibialis anticus muscles of the frog. *Am J Physiol* 1928;33:543–547.

Sarnoff SJ, Braunwald E, Welch GH Jr, et al. Hemodynamic determinants of oxygen consumption of the heart with special reference to the tension-time index. *Am J Physiol* 1958;192:148–156.

Warner HR, Toronto AF. Regulation of cardiac output through stroke volume. *Circ Res* 1960;8:549–552.

Weber KT, Janicki JS, Shroff SV, et al. Contractile mechanics and interaction of the right and left ventricles. *Am J Cardiol* 1981;47:686–695.

Woods RH. A few applications of a physical theorem to membranes in a state of tension in the human body. *J Anat Physiol* 1892;26:362–370.

13

CARDIAC ION CHANNELS

Cardiac myocytes are activated by an electrical signal, the *action potential*, in which changes in electrical potential across the plasma membrane (E_m) result from an elaborate sequence of openings and closings of ion channels. These action potentials, which differ in various regions of the heart, organize the mechanical events of the cardiac cycle and help provide the homogeneity of activation that optimizes the efficiency of cardiac contraction (see Chapter 6).

MEMBRANE POTENTIAL

A microelectrode inserted through the plasma membrane of a resting cardiac myocyte records an intracellular potential that is more negative than that outside of the cell (Fig. 13-1). How this potential difference is described is determined by convention. When expressed in terms of the potential recorded within the cell, with the surrounding medium viewed as zero, resting potential is negative. If, on the other hand, resting potential is described in terms of the potential outside the cell, and intracellular potential is viewed as zero, resting potential is positive. No small confusion arises because different conventions are used in cardiac electrophysiology and electrocardiography!

The convention employed by membrane electrophysiologists, who place electrodes inside the cell and measure the potential of the cell interior relative to that in the surrounding medium, is to describe resting potential as negative. Clinical electrocardiographers, on the other hand, place electrodes on the body surface and so view the myocardium from the outside, which at rest is positively charged. This and the next chapter, which describe cellular events, view resting potential as negative, whereas the two subsequent chapters, which describe electrocardiograms, consider resting potential to be positive.

A change in membrane potential that decreases the electronegativity inside a resting myocyte is called *depolarization* (Fig. 13-2). The return of membrane potential toward its resting level in a depolarized myocyte is *repolarization*, whereas an increase in the resting potential of an unexcited cell is *hyperpolarization*. *Action potentials* therefore include at least two phases: one of depolarization and the other of repolarization.

370

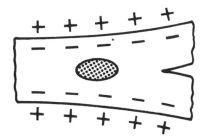

FIGURE 13-1 Resting cardiac muscle cell. The normal resting potential is negative inside the cell and positive at the cell surface.

Action potential *amplitude*, which is usually expressed in millivolts (mV), defines the extent to which cellular electronegativity changes from its resting level, including any reversal to electropositivity.

MEMBRANE CURRENTS

The most important physiological currents in the heart, carried by ions that cross the plasma membrane, known as *ionic currents*. By convention, ionic currents are described as if they were carried by positively charged ions—this is easily remembered because cations are the most important charge carriers in the heart.

Inward and Outward Currents

An *inward current*, according to electrophysiological convention, represents the flux of charge that would result if a positive ion moved into the cell. Because the interior of the resting cell is negatively charged, inward currents cause depolarization. Most inward currents in the heart are generated when positively charged sodium and calcium ions enter the cell. Because the outward movement of a negative ion has the same effect on membrane potential as the inward movement of a positive ion, the efflux of an anion like chloride also generates an inward current (Table 13-1).

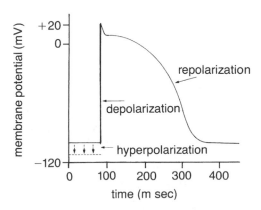

FIGURE 13-2 Some conventions of cardiac electrophysiology. The resting cell is viewed from within and is negatively charged. Hyperpolarization increases resting potential. Depolarization occurs when resting potential is decreased, while repolarization occurs when membrane potential returns to its resting level at the end of an action potential. The amplitude of the action potential is the extent to which cellular electronegativity has changed from its resting level, including any reversal to electropositivity.

TABLE 13-1 Ions As Charge Carriers across Cell Membranes

Ion Potential	Charge	Direction of Passive Flux	Current Generated	Effect on Membrane
Calcium	Positive	Inward	Inward	Depolarization
Sodium	Positive	Inward	Inward	Depolarization
Potassium	Positive	Outward	Outward	Repolarization
Chloride	Negative	Inward	Outward	Repolarization

An *outward current* can result either from the movement of a positively charged ion out of the cell interior, or from the flux of a negatively charged ion into the cell. Both increase electronegativity within the cell. In the resting cell, outward currents cause hyperpolarization, while outward currents that follow depolarization, therefore returning membrane potential toward the resting negativity, cause repolarization (Fig. 13-2).

Ionic and Capacitive Currents

Capacitive currents occur in biological tissues because the phospholipid bilayer, like a capacitor, includes an insulator (the hydrophobic core) surrounded by two layers of polar molecules (the phospholipid head groups) (see Chapter 1). In a resting cell, where the extracellular surface of the plasma membrane is positively charged, a cathode placed outside the cell draws positive charge from its external surface and causes negative charge to move away from the internal surface (Fig. 13-3A). These charge movements, which are carried by electrons, discharge the capacitance and cause the membrane to depolarize. A similar response is generated when a cation enters the cell (Fig. 13-3B); the major difference between capacitive and ionic currents is that in the latter, currents occur when ions cross the

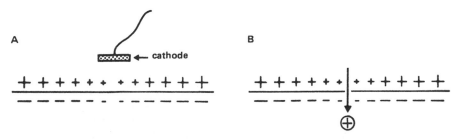

FIGURE 13-3 Differences between capacitive and ionic currents. **A:** A capacitive current is generated when a cathode is placed outside a resting cell. Movement of electrons from the cathode toward the extracellular surface of the plasma membrane discharges the positive potential outside the cell and causes electrons to move away from the inner surface. **B:** An inward ion current is generated when cations move across the membrane from outside to inside the cell.

lipid barrier in the center of the bilayer, whereas capacitive currents are generated by the movements of electrons relative to the membrane surface.

Action potentials in the heart are normally initiated by capacitive currents that are generated when a wave of depolarization approaches a region of the resting heart. These currents occur when the depolarized region causes the outside of the plasma membrane to become negative and the inside to become positive, which depolarizes the resting membrane (Fig. 13-3). This process becomes regenerative when depolarization opens channels that carry inward current (see Chapter 14).

MEMBRANE RESISTANCE, PERMEABILITY, AND CONDUCTANCE

The ratio between membrane potential and current flow is *membrane resistance*, which can be described according to Ohm's law:

$$R = \frac{E}{I} \qquad\qquad [13\text{-}1]$$

where R is resistance, E is potential, and I is current flow. *Membrane conductance*, designated g, is the reciprocal of membrane resistance, so

$$g = \frac{I}{E} \qquad\qquad [13\text{-}2]$$

Permeability and conductance, both of which define the ability of a substance to cross a membrane, are not the same. *Permeability* (P) measures the ability of a membrane to allow the movement (flux) of molecules in both directions, from one side of the membrane to the other, while *conductance* describes charge movements in only one direction across the membrane. Permeability most commonly describes systems at or near equilibrium, while conductance characterizes the currents generated by the flux of an ion down a pre-existing electrochemical gradient.

Permeability, which characterizes the ability of an uncharged molecule to cross a membrane, is defined by the relationship:

$$\text{Flux} = -P_{molecule} \times \Delta c_{molecule}, \qquad\qquad [13\text{-}3]$$

which states that net flux is equal to the permeability coefficient for the molecule ($-P_{molecule}$) times the difference in the concentration of the molecule at the two sides of the membrane ($\Delta c_{molecule}$).

Conductance describes the current flow when an ion moves across a membrane. Ionic currents are determined by the conductance for that ion and the potential difference (driving force) across the membrane. The latter is the difference between the actual transmembrane potential (E_m) and the potential at which there is no net ion flux (E_{ion}, the equilibrium potential, see Chapter 14). For example, the current carried by potassium ions (i_K) is:

$$i_K = g_K \times (E_m - E_K),\ \ \ \ \ \ \ \ \ \ \ \ [13\text{-}4]$$

where g_K is the potassium conductance. Depending on the difference between E_K and E_m, current can flow in either direction across the membrane, although not in both directions at any given time. Biological currents are expressed in *Siemens*, a unit that is similar to the mho, the reciprocal of the ohm that measures resistance.

GENERATION OF THE ACTION POTENTIAL

In 1902, J. Bernstein, who was aware that mammalian cells contain a high concentration of potassium, proposed that the plasma membrane is selectively permeable to potassium ions, and that the fixed negative charge of the cytosolic proteins establishes a Donnan equilibrium that concentrates potassium ions in an electronegative cytosol. Intracellular potentials were first measured shortly before the outbreak of World War II, when A. L. Hodgkin and A. F. Huxley in England, and K. S. Cole and H. J. Curtis in the United States, inserted microelectrodes into squid giant axons. Initial measurements confirmed Bernstein's prediction of electronegativity within resting cells and showed that this negativity decreased during excitation. However, intracellular recordings carried out after World War II, when more advanced equipment had become available, yielded a surprise. This was that membrane potential did not simply decrease to zero during excitation, as would be expected if changing potassium permeability alone was responsible for activation. Instead, membrane potential was found to reverse during excitation, when the cell interior became positive. This meant that action potentials are generated by processes more complex than dissipation of the potassium gradient.

The Voltage Clamp

In the 1950s, Hodgkin, Huxley, and Bernard Katz published a series of classical experiments that characterized the ionic basis for the action potential in squid giant axons. Conceptually, their approach was simple: Instead of measuring potential changes during an action potential, when ionic currents depolarized and repolarized the membrane, they measured the currents needed to hold voltage constant. This was done by placing an electrode inside the axon, exciting the membrane, and then applying currents across the membrane to keep membrane potential from changing. The applied currents, which exactly matched the currents that would have otherwise caused membrane potential to change, represent the "voltage clamp." By measuring these applied currents, Hodgkin, Huxley, and Katz were able to quantify both the magnitude and timing of physiological ionic currents that, by flowing in the opposite direction, generated the squid axon action potential. Interventions such as changing sodium and potassium concentrations inside and outside the axon demonstrated that depolarization occurs when sodium ions enter the cell, that repolarization is caused by potassium efflux, and that reversal of membrane potential at the peak of the action potential is due to a large inward sodium current.

GENERAL PROPERTIES OF PLASMA MEMBRANE IONIC CURRENTS

Most of the ion fluxes responsible for plasma membrane depolarization and repolarization are passive and do not require the expenditure of energy because the ions move downhill along their electrochemical gradients. These ion fluxes are now known to be mediated by members of an extended family of membrane proteins that contain ion-selective pores which, when open, favor the passage of a single ion species. In most cardiac channel proteins, changes in membrane potential open and close these pores, so they are generally referred to as *voltage-gated* ion channels. The exceptions are ion channels that respond to chemical signals and are called *receptor-operated* channels.

Most voltage-gated ion channels, once opened, do not remain in the open state but instead cycle through at least two closed states (Fig. 13-4). In the case of the heart's sodium and calcium channels, the physiological transition from the closed (resting) to the open state, called *activation*, occurs when depolarization increases the probability of channel opening (see below). At the same time, however, depolarization also increases the probability that these channels will assume the closed (inactive) state, a process that is called *inactivation*. This means that the same depolarizing signal that opens the resting channel causes it to close. Once the channel has closed, it assumes a closed (inactive) state; this is called a *refractory* state because the channel cannot be reopened by additional depolarizing stimuli.

Depolarization causes sodium and calcium channels to open transiently because activation is faster than inactivation. The dual response to membrane depolarization is an example of a general principle in biological regulation, discussed in Chapter 8, that to prevent runaway signaling, mechanisms that initiate a response also set into motion slower processes that end the response. In this way, ion channels resemble the water taps commonly found in public washrooms, where flooding is prevented when the same signal that starts the flow of water also shuts off the tap, albeit more slowly.

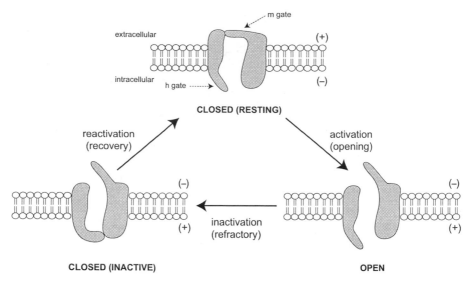

FIGURE 13-4 Three states of a voltage-gated ion channel. Depicted are the two closed and one open state. Transitions between these states (*arrows*) open the channel (activation), close the channel in a refractory state where it cannot be reopened (inactivation), and reactivate the channel by ending this refractoriness (recovery).

Reactivation (recovery), the transition from the closed (inactive) state to the closed (resting) state where the channel can again be opened by depolarization, requires an additional signal. In the heart, sodium and calcium channels are reactivated when repolarizing (outward) currents carried by potassium channels return membrane potential to its resting level. Once sodium and calcium channels are reactivated and their refractoriness ends, they can again be opened by depolarizing stimuli.

ION CHANNEL GATING

The mechanisms that control the states of an ion channel are often called *gating mechanisms*. Initially presented as mathematical concepts, channel gating can now be related to conformational changes in specific regions of the ion channel molecules.

Sodium Channels

Hodgkin and Huxley (1952) developed equations that characterize the behavior of the sodium current that depolarizes the squid axon in terms of maximal channel conductance and two coefficients, m and h. Because m is a coefficient of channel *opening* while h is a coefficient of channel *closing*, sodium current increases when m increases and h decreases. Sodium current is maximal when m is 1 (100% probability of being open) and h is 0 (0% probability of being closed). This relationship is described by the following equation:

TABLE 13-2 **Sodium Channel Gating**

Channel State	State of the m Gate	State of the h Gate
Closed (resting)	Closed	Open
Open (active)	Open	Open
Closed (inactive)	Open	Closed

$$i_{Na} = m^3 h g_{Na} (E_m - E_{Na})$$ [13-5]

Equation 13-5 states that the inward sodium current (i_{Na}) is determined by the maximal sodium conductance (g_{Na}), the difference between actual membrane potential (E_m) and the sodium equilibrium potential (E_{Na}), and the two coefficients, m and h. E_{Na}, which is the potential that would be recorded if the membrane were permeable only to sodium ions, is generally about $+20$ mV (see Chapter 14). The two coefficients, m and h, are now known to describe two regions of the sodium channel (see below). Measurements of these coefficients predict that depolarization rapidly opens the m gate while, at the same time, causes the h gates to close more slowly. The different time-dependent properties of m and h explain why the first effect of depolarization is to open the m gate, which activates the channel; why the slower increase in h inactivates the channel; and why the open state is brief. The Hodgkin–Huxley equations therefore define three channel states: an open state in which both gates are open, and *two* closed states (Table 13-2). In one of the latter, the m gate is closed and the h gate open (closed, resting); in the other, the m gate is open and the h gate closed (closed, inactive). The difference between the two closed states is that in the closed, resting state, the m gate is readily opened by membrane depolarization, while in the closed, inactive state, the h gate can be opened only by repolarization, which occurs when outward potassium currents return membrane potential to its resting level (see below). Because repolarization causes the m gates to close more rapidly than the h gates open, the sodium channel does not reopen during recovery.

One of the more remarkable facts about the Hodgkin–Huxley model is that it anticipated key features of the structure of voltage-gated ion channels; as described below, an α-helical transmembrane segment rich in positively charged amino acids corresponds to the activation (m) gate, while the inactivation (h) gate is an intracellular peptide chain that responds to depolarization by occluding the inner mouth of the channel pore.

Potassium and Calcium Channels

Hodgkin and Huxley developed additional equations to describe the potassium channel, whose activation gate is designated n. The opening of potassium channels was found to depend on the fourth power of the coefficient n:

$$i_K = n^4 g_K (E_m - E_K)$$ [13-6]

More than a decade after Hodgkin and Huxley published their classical studies, a third class of plasma membrane channel, the L-type calcium channel, was found to play a major role in maintaining the plateau phase of the cardiac action potential.

ION CHANNEL PROTEINS

Ion channels are members of a family of tetrameric proteins whose primitive ancestor was probably a monomer whose gene underwent duplication and divergence to give rise to the modern channels. Around the time that eukaryotes evolved from prokaryotes, the ancestral monomeric channel protein appears to have given rise to cyclic nucleotide–gated channels, whose opening is controlled by cAMP and cGMP, and potassium channels, whose four domains are not linked covalently. The most primitive channels whose four subunits are covalently linked are the calcium channels; later, when multicellular metazoan phyla evolved at the beginning of the Cambrian period, the gene encoding the calcium channels seems to have diverged to give rise to sodium channels, whose large action potentials conduct much more rapidly than calcium-dependent action potentials. The rapid conduction of sodium currents probably explains why these channels are found in multicellular organisms whose survival depends on the coordination among different regions of their bodies.

Pores and Gates

One of the fundamental properties of plasma membrane channels is their ion selectivity, which means that sodium channels conduct sodium ions, calcium channels conduct calcium ions, and the like. While this selectivity is not absolute, the preferences of different channels for one or another ion can be quite stringent; for example, calcium channels under physiological conditions conduct mainly calcium in spite of the almost 100-fold greater concentration of sodium ions in the extracellular fluid. Ion size cannot account for this selectivity because if size was the major determinant, all channels would be expected to select for the smallest ions. Instead, the preferred ions interact with specific sites within the channel in a manner that allows only the "correct" ion to enter the channel. Detailed structural analysis of potassium channels has shown an arrangement of anionic groups within the pore that recognizes potassium (Fig. 13-5). Because other ion species bind with lower affinity to these anionic sites, they are excluded from the selectivity filter by the preferred

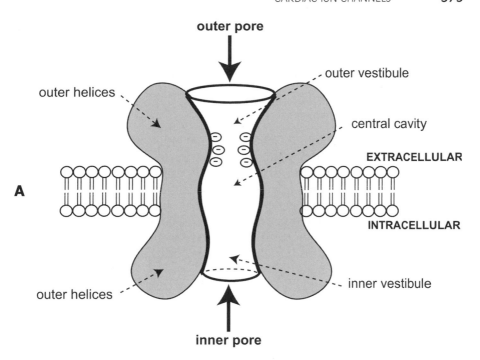

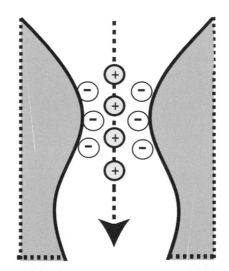

FIGURE 13-5 Structure of an ion channel pore showing two "vestibules," a central cavity, and portions of the outer helices that interact with the membrane bilayer (A). The selectivity filter, which lies between the outer vestibule and the central cavity of the pore, is lined with anionic groups that recognize the cation that is allowed to pass through the open channel. An enlarged view of the selectivity filter shows the cations moving in single file through the channel as they interact with anionic binding sites on the two sides of this narrow region of the pore (B).

ion. The direction of the ion flux is determined by the concentration gradient across the bilayer; ions enter the channel from the side of the membrane containing the higher ion concentration because these ions are most likely to displace ions already bound within the channel.

Gating Currents, Inactivation Gates, and Inactivation Particles

To explain the effects of changing membrane potential on channel gating, Hodgkin and Huxley predicted that parts of the sodium channel contain charged regions that generate small "gating currents" when they move in response to changing membrane potential. Careful measurements carried out in the 1960s, using conditions that eliminated or corrected for changing membrane capacitance and ion fluxes, identified these gating currents, which are now known to be caused by movements of positively charged regions of the sodium channel that correspond to the activation (m) gates (see below).

Closure of the h gates occurs when depolarization causes an inactivating "particle" within the cytosol to block the inner mouth of the open channel. This mechanism, called a *ball and chain*, inactivates the channel when a cytoplasmic portion of the channel binds to the intracellular side of the pore (Fig. 13-6).

Channel Subunits and Domains

Voltage-dependent ion channels generally contain several subunits, called α_1, α_2, β, γ, and δ. Although considerable progress has been made in defining structure–function relationships of the major, pore-containing α-subunits, the roles of the smaller β, γ, and δ subunits are less well understood. Not all ion channels contain small subunits; for example, functional sodium channels may contain zero, one, or two β-subunits.

Most channels contain four pore regions derived from three types of *domain* (Fig. 13-7). The larger domains (Fig. 13-7A), which are found in sodium, calcium, and outward-rectifying potassium channels, contains six

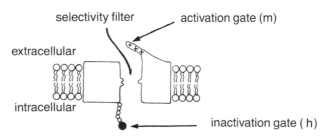

FIGURE 13-6 Simplified cartoon of an ion channel showing a positively charged activation (m) gate at the extracellular surface of the bilayer and an inactivation (h) gate that is represented by a "ball and chain." A "selectivity filter" within the channel determines the ion species that the channel allows to cross the membrane.

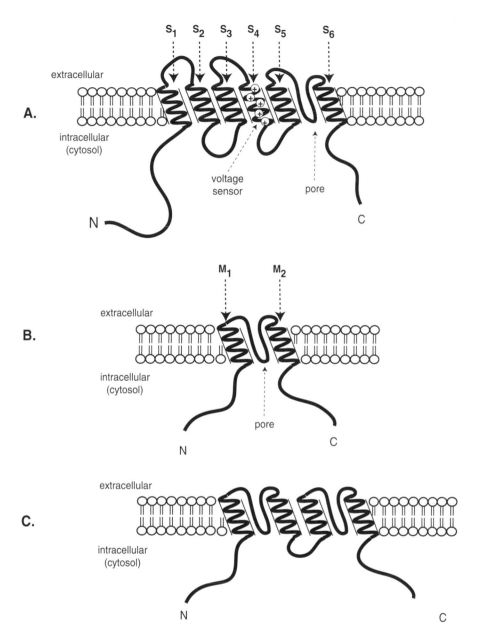

FIGURE 13-7 Schematic representation of three types of ion channel domain. **A:** The domains in sodium and calcium channels, and outward rectifier potassium channels, contain six transmembrane α-helices. The positively charged S_4 transmembrane segment in each of these domains provides the voltage sensor that responds to membrane depolarization by opening the channel. In sodium channels, this is the "m gate" described by the Hodgkin–Huxley equations. The "pore region" of the channel is made up of the S_5 and S_6 transmembrane segments and the intervening loop that "dips" into the membrane bilayer. **B and C:** Inward rectifier potassium channels are made of smaller domains that are homologous to the S_5 and S_6 transmembrane segments of the larger domain shown in **A**. Single-pore domains are largely the pore, made up of the M_1 and M_2 transmembrane segments along with the intervening loop (**B**). Two-pore domains are made up of two of the pore regions (**C**). The absence of a charged transmembrane segment homologous to S_4 explains why the response of inward rectifying channels to membrane depolarization differs from that of channels made up of the larger domains depicted in **A**.

α-helical transmembrane segments, designated S_1–S_6, while the smaller domains in the inward-rectifying potassium channels contain either one (Fig. 13-7B) or two (Fig. 13-7C) pores.

In sodium and calcium channels, the four large channel domains are connected covalently by relatively short linking segments (Fig. 13-8A). The potassium channels that carry transient outward and outward rectifying currents (see Chapter 14) also contain four of the larger domains, but these are not linked covalently (Fig. 13-8B). Assembly of different functional channels from these domains is limited because the latter contain "identity tags" that favor interactions between some and limit those between others. Inward rectifying potassium channels contain four smaller noncovalently-linked pore regions derived either from four single pore structures (Fig. 13-8Ca) or two two-pore structures (Fig. 13-8Cb).

The 6 α-helical transmembrane segments in the larger channel domains are organized in the membrane so that the S_5 and S_6 α-helices, along with an intervening peptide loop, line the pore through which a given ion species can selectively penetrate the open channel. The S_1, S_2,

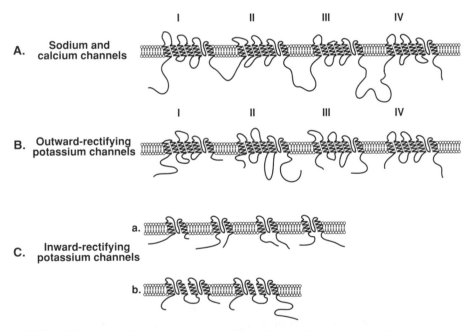

FIGURE 13-8 Schematic representation of three types of voltage-gated ion channel. **A:** Sodium and calcium channels are covalently linked tetramers made up of four of the larger domains shown in Figure 13-7 (numbered I–IV), each of which contains six α-helical transmembrane segments. **B:** Outward rectifying potassium channels also are made up of the larger domains shown in Figure 13-7, but the domains are not linked covalently. **C:** Inward rectifier potassium channels include either four of the smaller one-pore domains (a) or two of the two-pore domains (b) shown in Figure 13-7.

and S_3 α-helical segments are present on the surface of the channel that interacts with the surrounding membrane lipids. The *m gate* or "voltage sensor" is the S_4 α-helix, which contains positively charged arginine and lysine residues; movement of this charged peptide, which is responsible for the gating currents described above, allow membrane depolarization to open the channel (Figs. 13-9 and 13-10). Channels are inactivated by intracellular peptide loops, called *inactivation particles*, that can occlude the inner surface of the pore. In sodium channels, the inactivation particle is the cytoplasmic loop connecting the S_6 transmembrane segment of domain III to the S_1 segment of domain IV, which therefore represents the *h gate* (Fig. 13-9). Similar mechanisms in potassium channels allow portions of other intracellular peptide chains to plug and thus inactivate these channels. Like a ball swinging at the end of a chain, inactivation particles bind to and block the inner mouth of the pore in response to changing membrane potential. The high degree of recognition between the channel pore and the inactivation particles can be documented when the "ball and chain" region is synthesized as a small peptide that, even though it is not linked to the channel protein, can inactivate the channel.

The most important physiological regulator of the opening and closing of the voltage-gated channels is, of course, membrane voltage;

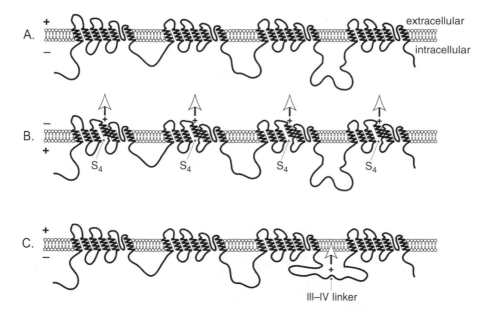

FIGURE 13-9 Three states of a sodium channel. **A:** Closed (resting) state, in which the extracellular surface of the membrane is positively charged and the interior is negatively charged. **B:** The transition to the activated (open) state occurs when membrane depolarization shifts the positions of the S_4 transmembrane segments (the m gates or voltage sensors). **C:** The transition to the closed (inactive) state is brought about when the intracellular peptide chain that connects the III and IV domains (the h gate or inactivation particle) swings toward the membrane to block the inner mouth of the pore.

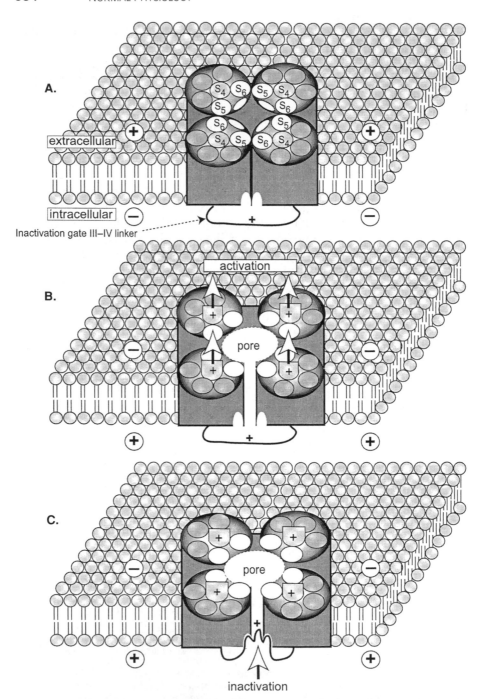

FIGURE 13-10 Three-dimensional representation of the three major states of the sodium channel. The S_5 and S_6 α-helical transmembrane segments along with the intervening peptide chains of the four domains surround the pore, while the S_1, S_2, and S_3 α-helical transmembrane segments (not labeled) allow the channel to interact with the

FIGURE 13-11 Response of a single calcium channel to membrane depolarization. When the membrane is depolarized from −20 to +50 mV (*upper tracing*), the channel begins to alternate between its closed and open states (*middle tracing*). Later, when depolarization is continued, the channel tends to open less frequently so that membrane current (*lower tracing*), after initial increasing (*downward deflection*), begins to decrease.

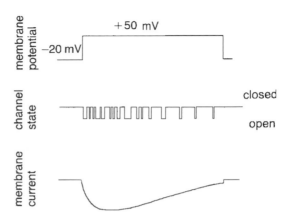

additional control is effected when a number of neurotransmitters, intracellular messengers, and other signaling mechanisms cause post-translational changes in these membrane proteins. The latter generally result from phosphorylations that modify channel gating by altering the charge on various regions of the channel. Many drugs that modify channel function bind to the S_5 and S_6 α-helices and intervening peptide loop that surround the pore. Several heritable disorders that result from mutations in the major channel subunits and smaller regulatory subunits can cause lethal arrhythmias (see Chapter 14).

SINGLE CHANNEL RECORDINGS

Characterization of single channel opening and closing has revolutionized our understanding of ion fluxes across biological membranes. Recordings from single calcium channels show that shortly after the application of a current that depolarizes the membrane from −20 mV to +50 mV, the channel begins to flicker into its open state (Fig. 13-11). Each channel opening and closing is extremely rapid, so the slower changes in membrane currents recorded from whole cells—which represent the sum of all channel openings and closings—tell us little about the rate of the molecular transitions in a single channel.

Most functional changes in the magnitude and time course of cardiac ion currents are determined by changes in the probability that the channel will be in its open state, rather than by changes in the magnitude or speed of channel openings. For example, phosphorylation of L-type calcium

bilayer. **A:** In the resting state, the pore is closed. **B:** The channel is opened when the four charged S_4 transmembrane segments (the m gates or voltage sensors) shift their positions in response to membrane depolarization. **C:** The channel closes and becomes refractory when the intracellular peptide chain that connects the III and IV domains (the h gate or inactivation particle) occludes the inner mouth of the pore.

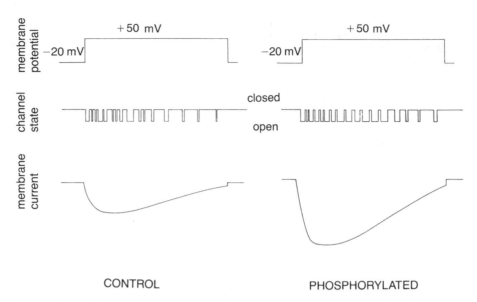

FIGURE 13-12 Response of a single calcium channel to phosphorylation by a cyclic AMP–dependent protein kinase. In response to the same depolarization (*upper tracing*), the phosphorylated channel spends more time in its open state (*middle tracing*) so that membrane current (*lower tracing*) is increased.

channels in response to β-adrenergic stimulation promotes calcium entry by increasing the probability of finding the channel in the open state after the membrane is depolarized (Fig. 13-12).

Ion Channel Sub-States

The view that voltage-gated ion channels exist in only three functional states—open, closed (resting), and closed (inactivated) (see above)—has had to be modified on the basis of analyses of single channel recordings, which have demonstrated many additional sub-states. The existence of these sub-states explains such puzzling phenomena as the ability of some calcium channel blocking drugs to both activate and inhibit calcium channel opening and, even more remarkably, to do so at the same time! These apparently paradoxical responses reflect the ability of these drugs to modify transitions among several states of the calcium channel (Hess et al., 1984). In addition to the closed state (Mode 0), described earlier as closed (resting), L-type calcium channels can open in two states: brief openings (Mode 1) and long-lasting openings (Mode 2), both of which are natural states of the channels (Fig. 13-13). Phosphorylation of these channels in response to sympathetic stimulation favors the appearance of long-lasting openings (Mode 2). The importance of these sub-states is highlighted by evidence that some of the more than 80 sodium channel mutations that cause the heritable "Long QT" and "Brugada" syndromes (see Chapter 14) favor abnormal sub-states of this channel.

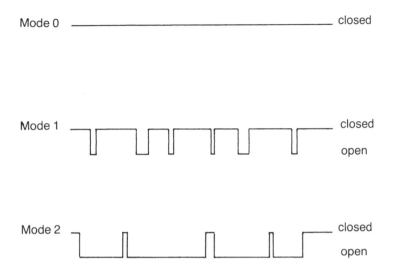

FIGURE 13-13 Different open substates of a calcium channel. Mode 0, closed; Mode 1, brief openings; Mode 2, long-lasting openings.

ION CHANNELS OF THE INTERCALATED DISC: THE GAP JUNCTION AND CONNEXINS

Action potential propagation in biological tissues depends on electrical circuits that resemble those in an undersea cable, where longitudinal currents flow in both the sea water outside the cable and within its copper core (see Chapter 16). Similarly, impulse conduction in the heart depends on current flow through the extracellular space and between the interiors of adjacent cells (Fig. 13-14). These longitudinal currents depend

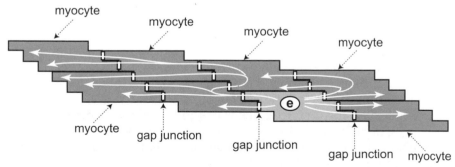

FIGURE 13-14 Current flow in the myocardium. Cardiac myocytes are separated by intercalated discs that contain gap junctions. *Dark lines* represent the plasma membrane, which has a high electrical resistance. The flow of current (*white arrows*) from a depolarized cell (*lighter myocyte labeled e*) is transmitted primarily in a longitudinal direction through the gap junctions in the intercalated discs; very little current flows transversely across the plasma membranes.

on channels that are entirely different from the voltage-gated channels that allow the transverse flow of currents across the plasma membrane.

Intracellular longitudinal currents are carried by a special class of nonselective channels found in the gap junction, or nexus, of the intercalated disc (see Fig. 1-22). These gap junction channels are permeable to large charged molecules; for example, radioactive potassium injected at one end of a bundle of myocardial cells diffuses across the intercalated discs from cell to cell almost as rapidly as this ion would diffuse in an aqueous medium. They provide the low electrical resistance pathway between adjacent cells that is essential for longitudinal conduction.

Gap junction channels are made up of *connexon* (Fig. 13-15), an ancient protein that is found today in simple organisms like coelenterates and ctenophores as well as in higher animals. Each channel is made up of two connexon molecules, one in the plasma membrane of each adjacent cell. Connexon molecules contain six *connexin* subunits that include four transmembrane α-helices. Several connexin isoforms are found in the mammalian myocardium (their names are based on their molecular weight in kD); most abundant is connexin 43 (Cx43). Connexin 45 (Cx45), which forms lower conductance channels than Cx43, is the most abundant connexin in the SA and AV nodes and the His–Purkinje system and appears to be a substrate for regulatory phosphorylations. Connexin 40 (Cx40), a high conductance isoform, also is expressed in the rapidly conducting cells of the His–Purkinje system. Isoform shifts involving the connexins alter conduction velocity in diseased hearts. Interactions between connexins and cytoskeletal proteins also appear to participate in proliferative signaling.

Acidosis and high cytosolic calcium close the gap junction channels. The former operates by a "ball and chain" mechanism, where movement of a "gating particle" in the C-terminal end of the molecule blocks the channel in a manner similar to the inactivation of voltage-gated sodium and potassium channels (see above). In addition to limiting the spread of acidosis through the heart, this response slows impulse propagation by causing the electrical uncoupling of adjacent cells. Closure of the gap junctions by calcium is essential in limiting cell death when portions of the heart become irreversibly damaged, as occurs after a myocardial infarction, where plasma membrane damage allows uncontrolled calcium entry into the cytosol. In order for these damaged hearts to survive, the interiors of dead cells must be uncoupled from those of its viable neighbors; like the closing of bulkhead doors when a ship takes on water, closure of connexin channels by calcium prevents a situation that is as dangerous to the heart as flooding in an ocean liner.

STRETCH-ACTIVATED CHANNELS

Cell deformation has long been known to evoke, or to modify, electrical signals in the heart. The property, called *mechano-electrical feedback,*

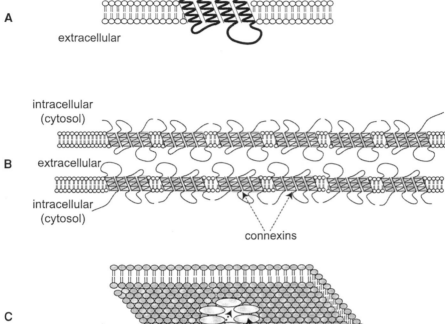

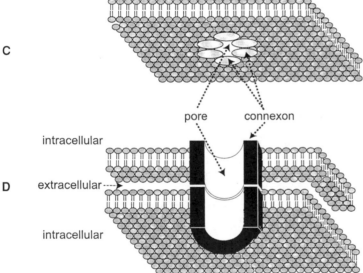

FIGURE 13-15   Structure of the connexin, connexon, and gap junction channels. A: A single connexin molecule showing the four transmembrane α-helices. B: Two connexon channels, each made up of six connexin subunits, are found in the membranes of adjacent cells in the nexus structures of the intercalated disc. C: Three-dimensional view of a gap junction channel in one membrane bilayer showing the pore surrounded by six connexon molecules. D: Three-dimensional view of a gap junction highlighting the pore that links the interiors of the adjoining cells.

is mediated by a variety of ion channels in both cardiac myocytes and nonmyocytes. Stretch-activated currents can be carried by potassium, chloride, and nonselective cation channels, many of which are linked to other signal transduction systems. The latter include second messenger–mediated signals as well as molecular signals that are mediated by cytoskeletal proteins (see Chapter 5).

CONCLUSIONS

The relationships between channel structure and channel function described in this chapter are central to understanding normal and abnormal cardiac electrophysiology. This is apparent in the following chapter, when we see how different ion channels generate the currents that give rise to the cardiac action potential.

BIBLIOGRAPHY

Antzelevitch C, Brugada P, Borggrefe M, et al. Brugada syndrome report of the second consensus conference. *Circulation* 2005;111:659–670.

Armstrong CM. Sodium channels and gating currents. *Physiol Rev* 1981;61:644–683.

Bers DM. Excitation-contraction coupling and cardiac contractile force, 2nd ed. Dordrecht: Kluwer, 2001.

Hille B. Ionic channels of excitable membranes, 3rd ed. Sunderland, MA: Sinauaer, 2001.

Jalife J, Morley GE, Vaidya D. Connexins and impulse propagation in the mouse heart. *J Cardiovasc Electrophysiol* 1999;10:1649–1663.

Jan LY, Jan YN. Tracing the roots of ion channels. *Cell* 1992;69:715–718.

Kohl P, Ravens U. Cardiac mechano-electric feedback: past, present, and prospect. *Prog Biophys Mol Biol* 2003;82:3–9.

Nerbonne JM. Molecular basis of functional voltage-gated K^+ channel diversity in the mammalian myocardium. *J Physiol (Lond)* 2000;525:285–298.

Priori AG. Inherited arrhythmogenic disorders. The complexity beyond monogenic disorders. *Circ Res* 2004;94:140–145.

Snyders DJ. Structure and function of cardiac potassium channels. *Cardiovasc Res* 1999;42:377–390.

Strong M, Chandy KG, Gutman GA. Molecular evolution of voltage-sensitive ion channel genes: on the origins of electrical excitability. *Mol Biol Evol* 1993;10:221–242.

Yeager M. Structure of cardiac gap junction intercellular channels. *J Struct Biol* 1998;121:231–245.

REFERENCES

Bernstein J. Untersuchungen zur Thermodynamik der bioelektrischen Ströme. PflügersArch ges Physiol 1902;92:521–562.

Hess P, Lansman JB, Tsien RW. Different modes of Ca channel gating behaviour favoured by dihydropyridine calcium agonists and antagonists. *Nature* 1984;311:538–544.

Hodgkin AL, Huxley AF. A quantitative description of membrane current and its application to conduction and excitation in nerve. *J Physiol (Lond)* 1952;117:500–544.

14

THE CARDIAC ACTION POTENTIAL

The cardiac action potential, which results from the orchestrated opening and closing of the ion channels described in Chapter 13, is more complex than the action potentials in skeletal muscle and nerve, where depolarization lasts only a few milliseconds (Fig. 14-1). In the heart, action potentials last several hundred milliseconds, consist of several phases, and vary in characteristics from region to region. Purkinje fiber action potentials, for example, are large, rapidly rising, last over 300 msec, and include at least five distinct phases (Fig. 14-2). These include a large rapid upstroke (phase 0), which is followed by transient repolarization (phase 1) and a plateau (phase 2) that do not have clear counterparts in nerve and skeletal muscle. Purkinje fiber action potentials end when repolarization (phase 3) brings membrane potential back to its resting level after which, during diastole (phase 4), these myocytes often exhibit spontaneous depolarization (pacemaker activity). Action potentials in the working cells of the ventricles are similar to those of Purkinje cells, except that they are somewhat smaller and lack pacemaker activity; atrial action potentials resemble those of the ventricles except that they are briefer, while action potentials in the sinoatrial (SA) and atrioventricular (AV) nodes are even smaller and lack a plateau.

RESTING POTENTIAL

Resting potential in myocardial cells is related to the electrochemical gradient for potassium across the plasma membrane, which is permeable to potassium but impermeable to the large anionic proteins and organic phosphates found in the cytosol; this establishes a *Donnan equilibrium*, where $[K^+]_i$ is higher than $[K^+]_o$ and the cytosol is negatively charged (see Chapter 13). In this Donnan equilibrium, the tendency for potassium to move down its concentration gradient out of the cell is balanced by a negative intracellular resting potential that favors potassium influx; in other words, the ability of the potassium concentration gradient to cause potassium efflux is countered by an electrical gradient that causes potassium influx.

The Nernst and Goldman-Hodgkin-Katz Equations

The plasma membrane in resting cardiac myocytes is not perfectly selective for potassium. There is, for example, a small permeability to sodium which, because of the higher sodium concentration outside the

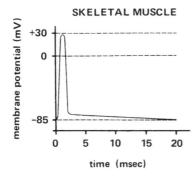

SKELETAL MUSCLE

FIGURE 14-1 The skeletal muscle action potential is a brief biphasic event in which rapid depolarization (*upward deflection*) is quickly followed by repolarization (*downward deflection*). A small positive after potential causes an approximately 10 msec delay prior to return of the membrane potential to its resting level.

cell (Table 14-1), favors a membrane potential opposite in polarity to that associated with the potassium gradient. The membrane potential that results from the distributions of these and other ions is described by the Nernst and Goldman-Hodgkin-Katz equations, which define the *equilibrium potential* (where there is no net flux of ions) established by ion concentration gradients across the plasma membrane. The Nernst equation describes the equilibrium potential for a single ion, while the Goldman-Hodgkin-Katz equation describes the potential across a membrane that is permeable to several ions.

THE NERNST EQUATION. The membrane potential established by a concentration difference for a single ion across a semipermeable membrane is described by the Nernst equation:

$$E_m = \frac{RT}{zF} \ln \frac{Pa_o}{Pa_i} \qquad [14\text{-}1]$$

where E_m is the membrane potential, R the gas constant, T the absolute temperature, z the valence of the ion, F the Faraday constant, P the

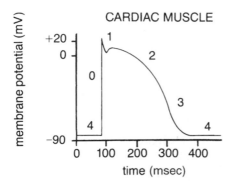

CARDIAC MUSCLE

FIGURE 14-2 The Purkinje fiber action potential lasts over 300 msec and consists of five phases. Phase 0 (*the upstroke*) corresponds to depolarization and phase 3 (*repolarization*) to repolarization in skeletal muscle. Phases 1 (*early repolarization*) and 2 (*plateau*) have no clear counterpart in skeletal muscle, while phase 4 (*diastole*) corresponds to the resting potential.

TABLE 14-1   Ion Activities Inside and Outside Mammalian Myocytes

Ion	Intracellular Concentration	Intracellular Activity	Extracellular Concentration	Extracellular Activity
Sodium	5–34*	8	140	110
Potassium	104–180*	100	5.4	4
Chloride	4.2+	45	117	88
Calcium		0.0002‡	3	1

Values are in mM. Activities are "averages" weighted arbitrarily by the author for use in
   various equations.
*Based on data from Walker, (1986).
+Based on data from Hille, 2001.
‡Based on data for resting cells from Blinks, (1986).

permeability to the ion, and a_o and a_i the activities of the ion outside and
inside the membrane. In the case of an alkali metal ion like sodium or
potassium, $z = 1$, so for a freely permeable membrane ($P = 1$) at 37° C, the
Nernst equation can be written for ordinary (base 10) logarithms as:

$$E_m = 61.5 \log \frac{a_o}{a_i} \qquad [14\text{-}2]$$

Equation 14-2 states that a 10-fold difference in the activity of a
monovalent cation, where $a_o/a_i = 10$, generates a potential difference of
+61.5 mV. If the concentration gradient is reversed and $a_o/a_i = 0.1$, Em is
−61.5 mV.

In resting cardiac muscle, where $[K^+]_o$ is about 5.4 mM and $[K^+]_i$ is
about 120 mM, the corresponding potassium ion activities are approximately 4 and 100 mM (Table 14-1). If the resting myocardium were freely
permeable to potassium and impermeable to all other ions for which a
concentration gradient exists between the inside and outside of the cell,
E_m would equal E_K:

$$E_m = 61.5 \times \log \frac{4}{100} = -86 \text{ mV} \qquad [14\text{-}3]$$

Measured resting potentials in most regions of the heart are close to
that predicted by the Nernst equation for potassium.

Variations in extracellular potassium have an important effect on
resting potential; increased extracellular potassium causes depolarization,
while reduction in extracellular potassium hyperpolarizes the membrane

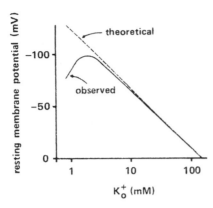

FIGURE 14-3 Relationship between extracellular potassium concentration (K^+_o) and resting membrane potential. Changing extracellular potassium at normal and high K^+_o levels causes membrane potential (*solid line*) to respond in a manner that closely approximates the predictions of the Nernst equation for potassium (*dashed line*). However, at low levels of extracellular potassium, membrane potential decreases unexpectedly because potassium permeability falls.

(Fig. 14-3). At very low extracellular potassium (<3 mM), however, resting potential does not follow the Nernst equation for potassium because hypokalemia reduces potassium permeability (P_K) (Fig. 14-3). This increases the influence of the smaller permeability to other ions, which shifts membrane potential away from that predicted by the Nernst equation for potassium.

THE GOLDMAN-HODGKIN-KATZ EQUATION. More accurate estimates of membrane potential are calculated by the Goldman-Hodgkin-Katz equation, which takes into account the permeabilities and activities of all ion species for which there is a gradient across the membrane. For a membrane permeable to sodium and chloride as well as to potassium, this equation is:

$$E_m = \frac{RT}{zF} \ln \left(P_K \frac{aK_o}{aK_i} + P_{Na} \frac{aNa_o}{aNa_i} + P_{Cl} \frac{aCl_i}{aCl_o} \right) \qquad [14\text{-}4]$$

Equation 14-4 highlights the fact that the contribution of any ion to membrane potential is determined both by the activity gradient across the membrane and the permeability of the membrane to that ion. The contribution of any ion to E_m disappears if there is no activity gradient or if permeability to the ion becomes zero.

THE CARDIAC ACTION POTENTIAL

Threshold

In order for an electrical stimulus to initiate an action potential, depolarization must reach a *threshold*. Smaller (subthreshold) depolarizations cause only local responses because they do not open enough depolarizing channels to initiate a regenerative action potential (Fig. 14-4 A and B). The potential at which an action potential first appears is the threshold, where

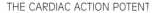

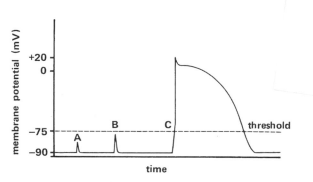

FIGURE 14-4 Threshold for initiation of a propagated action potential. Small depolariz-ing stimuli (A and B) that fail to reach threshold (*dashed line*) are unable to initiate an action potential. When depolarization reaches threshold (C), a regenerative action potential is generated in which subsequent depolarization becomes independent of the initial stimulus.

opening of enough sodium channels—or calcium channels in nodal cells—imitates the sequence of channel openings that generates the action poten-tial. The latter is often called *regenerative* because once threshold is reached, subsequent depolarization is independent of the initial depolar-izing stimulus (Fig. 14-4C). Although small depolarizations that fail to reach threshold do not initiate action potentials, they can have important effects on excitability; for example, subthreshold depolarizations can cause sodium channels to inactivate by closing h gates.

Amplitude and Rate of Rise of the Action Potential

The rate of depolarization (dV/dt) during an action potential upstroke is determined by the rate at which sodium—or in nodal cells, calcium—enters the cytosol. In cells whose action potentials depend on sodium influx, initial depolarizing currents develop rapidly, are very large, and last only a short time; for this reason, sodium currents are often referred to as *fast inward currents*. The action potentials in the SA and AV nodes have a lower amplitude and slower rate of rise because depolarization depends on the slower opening of smaller (lower conductance) calcium channels.

Membrane potential immediately prior to stimulation is an impor-tant determinant of sodium channel opening and thus determines the amplitude and rate of rise of the action potential. In Purkinje fibers at the normal resting potential of between -80 and -90 mV, depolarizing stimuli that exceed threshold generate large action potentials with a rapid upstroke (Fig. 14-5a). However, if the cell is partially depolarized prior to stimulation, the same depolarizing stimulus produces a smaller, more slowly rising action potential (Fig. 14-5b) because the prior sub-threshold depolarization inactivates some of the sodium channels by closing their h gates. Sodium channels also are inactivated when thresh-old is approached at a slow rate. If threshold is reached quickly, sodium conductance increases rapidly so that action potential upstroke is rapid

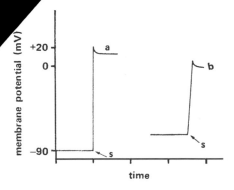

FIGURE 14-5 The rate and extent of depolarization depend on the resting membrane potential prior to stimulation. A large, rapidly rising action potential is produced by a stimulus (s) when the resting potential is high (a), whereas partial depolarization prior to stimulation (b) causes the same stimulus to produce a small, slowly rising action potential. These changes in the action potential upstroke reflect the voltage-dependent closing of the inactivation (h) gates of the sodium channels.

and the amplitude high (Fig. 14-6a), whereas if threshold is approached more slowly, some of the h gates close and the channel is inactivated. By reducing the number of available sodium channels, therefore, slow depolarization generates a small action potential with a slow upstroke (Fig. 14-6b). These manifestations of the voltage-dependent inactivation of sodium channel opening are important clinically because conditions like ischemia reduce resting potential and so inactivate sodium channels, which slows impulse propagation and provides a substrate for arrhythmias (Chapter 17).

Refractory Periods

Attempts to activate the heart before it has recovered from a preceding depolarization also produce small, slowly rising action potentials. The mechanism, inactivation of the channels normally responsible for depolarization, reflects the slow rate of channel reactivation. In the case of the sodium channels, delay in reactivation is due to the slow recovery of h gates, which can require more than 100 msec to reopen after membrane potential has returned to its resting level.

The period of depressed excitability that begins when depolarization closes the h gates of sodium channels is called the *refractory period* and is generally divided into two phases (Fig. 14-7). The first is the *absolute*

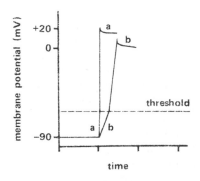

FIGURE 14-6 The rate and extent of depolarization depend in part on the rate at which membrane potential approaches threshold. A large, rapidly rising action potential is produced when the stimulus reaches threshold rapidly (a), whereas a stimulus that slowly reaches threshold produces a small, slowly rising action potential (b).

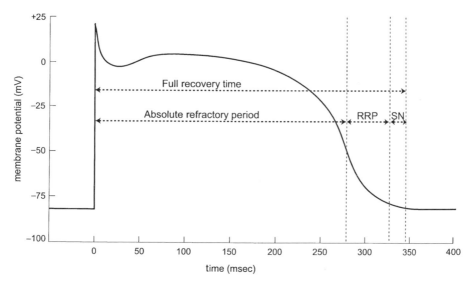

FIGURE 14-7 Refractory periods. Closing of the h gates immediately after membrane depolarization causes the absolute refractory period, during which no stimulus regardless of its strength is able to initiate a propagated action potential. This is followed by a relative refractory period (RRP) during which only stimuli that exceed the normal threshold can cause a propagated action potential. The functional refractory period, which includes the absolute and relative refractory periods, is followed by a supernormal period (SN), during which subthreshold stimuli slightly less than those that reach the normal threshold can generate a propagated action potential. Action potentials generated during the relative refractory and supernormal periods are small and slowly rising because of incomplete recovery of the sodium channels. The full recovery time begins with depolarization and ends after the supernormal period, when normal stimuli produce normally propagated action potentials.

refractory period, when no stimulus, whatever its magnitude, can evoke a propagated response. This is followed by the *relative refractory period*, when only stimuli that exceed the normal threshold can initiate a propagated response. The interval between the onset of depolarization and the return of normal excitability, sometimes called the *full-recovery time*, encompasses the effective and relative refractory periods as well as the supernormal period described below. The long refractory period of myocardial cells is due both to the prolonged plateau of the action potential, which delays the return of membrane potential to the resting level at which the sodium channels reactivate, and the slow rate of channel recovery after the membrane has repolarized.

Action potentials evoked during the heart's relative refractory period depolarize slowly and are of low amplitude, and therefore conduct slowly (see above). Because slow conduction is an important substrate for reentrant arrhythmias (see Chapter 16), small action potentials that are generated during the refractory periods are an important cause of sudden cardiac death.

Supernormality

A *supernormal period*, sometimes seen at the end of the relative refractory period (Fig. 14-7), is characterized by the ability of stimuli smaller than those needed to reach the normal threshold to produce propagated action potentials. Although threshold is reduced during supernormality, the action potentials generated during this period are of low amplitude. This apparent discrepancy reflects the fact that although threshold is low, not all sodium channels have recovered. The supernormal phase occurs at approximately the same time as the "vulnerable period" (see Chapter 16), but vulnerability and supernormality are different phenomena: Supernormality is a *lowered threshold*, whereas vulnerability describes *increased susceptibility to ventricular fibrillation*.

Supernormality is well documented in isolated His–Purkinje cells but is probably absent in the AV node, atria, and ventricles (Spear and Moore, 1980). Evidence for this mechanism can occasionally be identified on the clinical electrocardiogram (see Chapter 16).

RECTIFICATION

Ion channels often exhibit a property called *rectification*, which means that the ability of the channel to carry a current is influenced by membrane potential. One example of a rectifier is a device that converts alternating current to direct current by allowing current to flow in only one direction. When changes in membrane voltage modify channel opening, the currents carried by these channels are said to be rectified (Fig. 14-8). Rectified currents differ from unrectified (Ohmic) currents, where channel opening is independent of the potential difference (E). In an unrectified potassium current, where resistance (R) is constant, the current (I) is an inverse linear function of voltage:

$$I = \frac{E}{R} \qquad [14\text{-}5]$$

In describing potassium currents across biological membranes, *outward rectification* is said to occur when depolarization *increases* the flow of repolarizing current. Because outward rectifier currents in a depolarized cell return membrane potential toward the resting level, outward rectification is viewed as "true" rectification that "puts things right" by ending the action potential. *Inward rectification* is exactly the opposite, as inward rectifier potassium currents tend to maintain the membrane in a depolarized state; in the heart, this occurs when depolarization *decreases* a repolarizing potassium current. Inward rectification was once considered to be an anomaly and was sometimes called *anomalous* rectification.

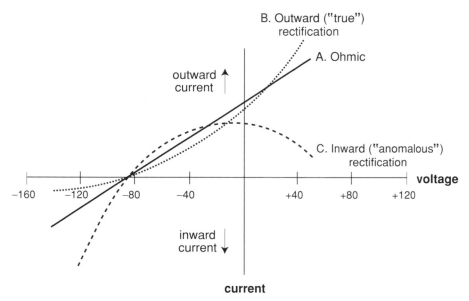

FIGURE 14-8 Rectification of potassium currents. The effects of changing membrane potential (*abscissa*) on ionic currents (*ordinate*) are shown for three different types of potassium channel; inward currents are *downward*, outward currents are *upward*. All potassium currents are zero at −86 mV, the equilibrium potential for potassium. An unrectified (Ohmic) current (*solid line A*) is a linear function of membrane voltage because channel opening is independent of membrane potential. Outward ("true") rectification (*dotted line B*) occurs when depolarization increases potassium channel opening, which tends to bring membrane potential back to the resting level. Inward ("anomalous") rectification (C) occurs when depolarization decreases potassium channel opening, which favors further or sustained depolarization.

As noted below, different classes of potassium channels are responsible for outward and inward rectification.

SODIUM CURRENTS

A high sodium permeability favors a membrane potential opposite in polarity to that caused by the potassium gradient because extracellular sodium concentration is higher than that in the cell interior (Table 14-1). This is apparent in a simplified Goldman-Hodgkin-Katz equation that describes the dependence of membrane potential on both potassium and sodium:

$$E_m \sim P_K \frac{aK_o}{aK_i} + P_{Na} \frac{aNa_o}{aNa_i} \qquad [14\text{-}6]$$

As extracellular sodium concentration is about 140 mM, which corresponds to an activity of about 110 mM, while intracellular sodium activity is about 8 mM (Table 14-1), the Nernst equation for sodium predicts a membrane potential of +70 mV:

$$E_m = 61.5 \times \log \frac{110}{8} = +70 \, mV \qquad [14\text{-}7]$$

Cardiac action potentials do not reach the high positivity predicted by equation 14-7 because of a residual permeability to potassium ($P_K > 0$) and failure of sodium conductance to reach its maximum ($P_{Na} < 1$).

Only one type of sodium channel is normally found in the human heart; this channel, called *hH1*, is encoded by SCN5A. A large number of mutations in this channel have been identified as causes of both "gain-in-function" and "loss-of-function" abnormalities. The abnormal inward currents caused by gain-in-function mutations delay repolarization and cause a long QT syndrome called *LQT3*, while loss-of-function mutations cause an electrocardiographic abnormality called the *Brugada syndrome*; both are substrates for lethal arrhythmias (see Chapters 15 and 16). Sodium channels can be regulated by both PK-A, which increases the inward sodium current, and PK-C, which reduces sodium conductance.

CALCIUM CURRENTS

The calcium gradient across the plasma membrane, like that for sodium, favors an inward (depolarizing) current because extracellular ionized calcium activity is approximately 1 mM, whereas cytosolic calcium during diastole is approximately 0.2 μM (0.0002 mM) (Table 14-1). This 5,000-fold activity gradient for calcium, according to the Nernst equation, establishes a positive calcium equilibrium potential:

$$E_m = \frac{61.5}{2} \log \frac{1}{0.0002} = +114 \, mV \qquad [14\text{-}8]$$

During systole, when intracellular calcium concentration increases, this equilibrium potential falls.

The major calcium current in working cardiac myocytes and Purkinje fibers, which appears after the sodium current has generated phase 0, was initially referred to as a *secondary* or *slow inward current*. The threshold for opening of the heart's calcium channels is higher than that for the sodium channels so that an approaching wave of depolarization does not open the calcium channels until after sodium channel opening.

L-Type and T-Type Calcium Channels

Several types of plasma membrane calcium channels are found in mammalian tissues (Table 14-2). The most important in the cardiovascular system are the L- and T-type calcium channels (Table 14-3), whose names reflect the slower inactivation of L-type calcium channels than T-type channels (L, long-lasting; T, transient).

L-type calcium currents contribute to the action potential plateau (phase 2) in the working cells of the atria and ventricles as well as in Purkinje fibers. When this plateau was first observed, it was not clear whether membrane potential had stabilized because current flow had ceased, or because current flow into and out of the cell had become equal. The answer was provided by Sylvio Weidmann, who measured a high membrane conductance during the early portion of the plateau, which meant that the membrane was carrying *both* inward and outward currents. L-type calcium channels are now known to be responsible for the inward current, while the outward current is carried by delayed rectifier potassium channels (see

TABLE 14-2 Plasma Membrane Calcium Channels

Channel Subtype	Major Function
Voltage-gated calcium channels	
L-type calcium channels	Skeletal excitation–contraction coupling
	Cardiac excitation–contraction coupling
	Cardiac pacemaker activity
	Cardiac atrioventricular conduction
	Smooth muscle excitation–contraction coupling
	Transmitter release (endocrine cells)
T-type calcium channels	Growth regulation
	Cardiac pacemaker activity
N-type calcium channels	Transmitter release (neurons)
P-type calcium channels	Transmitter release (neurons and endocrine cells)
Q-type calcium channels	Transmitter release (neuronal cells)
R-type calcium channels	Transmitter release (neuronal cells)
Receptor-operated calcium channels	Smooth muscle excitation–contraction coupling
	Responses to chemical stimuli (nonmotile cells)
Second messenger–operated calcium channels	Responses to cAMP, cGMP, etc.

TABLE 14-3 **Major Calcium Channels in the Heart**

Property	L-type Calcium Channel	T-type Calcium Channel
Threshold	low (-40 mV)	high (-70 mV)
Inactivation	slow (L, long-lasting)	fast (T, transient)
Size (channel conductance)	large (15–25 picosiemens)	small (7–9 picosiemens)
Major function in heart	sinoatrial node pacemaker	sinoatrial node pacemaker
	atrioventricular conduction	proliferative signaling
	excitation–contraction coupling	? resting tension
Major function in smooth muscle	contraction	contraction

below). The initial depolarizing currents in the SA and AV nodes, unlike those of most working cardiac myocytes and His–Purkinje cells that depend on large inward sodium currents, are carried by the L-type channels.

The α_1-subunits of L-type calcium channels play a central role in cardiac and skeletal muscle excitation–contraction coupling, but they do so in different ways. The cardiac channel carries the inward calcium current that opens the sarcoplasmic reticulum calcium release channels ("calcium-triggered calcium release"), while a different L-type calcium channel isoform provides a plug that occludes the sarcoplasmic reticulum channels in resting skeletal muscle (see Chapter 7). The cardiac α_1-subunit is activated by PK-A–catalyzed phosphorylations, which contribute to the inotropic response to sympathetic stimulation (see Chapters 8 and 10). These channels also bind to the three major classes of calcium channel blocking drugs (dihydropyridine, benzodiazepine, and phenylalkylamine).

The small inward currents generated by the transient openings of T-type calcium channels do not play an important role in depolarization of the atria, ventricles, and His–Purkinje system because these currents occur at the same time as the much larger sodium currents. However, T-type calcium channels participate in SA node pacemaker activity, where their small depolarizations generate an inward current that contributes to the oscillatory potentials that characterize pacemaker cells (see below). T-type calcium channels do not participate in excitation–contraction coupling because they admit only a small amount of calcium at a slow rate; furthermore, these channels are not located in close proximity to the calcium release channels of the sarcoplasmic reticulum. The small calcium signals generated by the T-type calcium channels appear to participate in proliferative signaling and may contribute to resting tension.

POTASSIUM CURRENTS

Potassium currents serve several roles in the heart. Inward rectifier channels are open in resting cells, where they determine the level of the resting potential (phase 4). Outward rectifier channels, which open after the cells are depolarized, generate two different types of current. One is a brief transient current that causes rapid repolarization after the action potential upstroke (phase 1); the other causes the more sustained delayed rectifier currents that initiate phase 3.

The nomenclature of the potassium currents and channels responsible is quite arcane (Tables 14-4–14-6); some names are historical (e.g., i_{K1}), others describe the duration of the open state (e.g., i_{to1}), the timing of

TABLE 14-4 **Some Potassium Currents in the Heart**

Current	Functional Role
Outward Rectifier	
Transient outward current (i_{to1})	Opens briefly immediately after depolarization, regulates action potential duration
Rapid outward (delayed) rectifier (i_{Kr})	Opens early during the plateau, initiates repolarization
Slow outward (delayed) rectifier (i_{Ks})	Opens late during the plateau, initiates repolarization
Ultra-rapid outward (delayed) rectifier (i_{Kur})	Opens very early during the plateau (atrial myocytes), initiates repolarization
Calcium-activated potassium current ($i_{K.Ca}$)	Activated by high cytosolic calcium, accelerates repolarization in calcium-overload
Lipid-activated potassium current ($i_{K.AA}$)	Activated by arachidonic acid and other fatty acids, especially at acid pH
Inward Rectifier	
Inward (anomalous) rectifier (i_{K1})	Maintains resting potential, closes with depolarization to prolong the plateau
ATP-sensitive potassium current ($i_{K.ATP}$)	Normally inhibited by ATP, opens in energy-starved hearts
Acetylcholine-activated potassium current ($i_{K.Ach}$)	Activated by $G_{\alpha i}$ in response to vagal stimulation and adenosine; hyperpolarizes resting cells, slows SA node pacemaker, shortens the atrial action potential

TABLE 14-5 **Potassium Channel α-Subunits in the Heart**

Number of Transmembrane α Helices	α-Subunit	Gene	Current(s)
Six			
*Kv** Shaker family			
	Kv1.4	KCNA4	Transient outward (i_{to1})
	Kv4.1	KCND3	Transient outward (i_{to1})
	Kv4.2	KCND2	Transient outward (i_{to1})
	Kv4.3	KCND3	Transient outward (i_{to1})
	Kv1.5 (HK2)	KCNA5	Delayed rectifier (i_{Kur})
	KvLQT1 (Kv7.1)	KCNQ1	Delayed rectifier (i_{Ks})
eag family			
	HERG (Kv11.1)	KCNH2	Delayed rectifier (i_{Kr})
Two			
Kir‡			
	Kir2.1 (IRK1)	KCNJ2	Inward rectifier (i_{K1})
	Kir2.2 (IRK2)	KCNJ12	Inward rectifier (i_{K1})
	Kir3.1 (GIRK1)	KCNJ3	Acetylcholine-regulated ($i_{K.Ach}$)
	Kir3.4 (GIRK4)	KCNJ5	Acetylcholine-regulated ($i_{K.Ach}$)
	Kir6.2 (BIR)	KCNJ11	ATP-regulated ($i_{K.ATP}$) (with SUR2A†)
Four ("2 pore")			Background ("leak") currents
	$K_{2p}1.1^+$ (TWIK 1)	KCNK-1	
	$K_{2p}2.1$ (TREK-1)	KCNK-6	
	$K_{2p}10.1$ (TREK-2)	KCNK-10	
	$K_{2p}3.1$ (TASK-1)	KCNK-3	
	$K_{2p}5.1$ (TASK-2)	KCNK-5	
	$K_{2p}9.1$ (TASK-3)	KCNK-9	
	$K_{2p}17.1$ (TASK-4)	KCNK-17	
	$K_{2p}13.1$ (THIK)	KCNK-13	

*Kv: voltage gated potassium channel.
‡Kir: inward rectifier potassium channel.
+ K_{2p}: two-pore channel.
†SUR: sulfonylurea receptor.

TABLE 14-6 Potassium Channel β-Subunits in the Heart

Subunit	Gene	Associated Channel	Current	Function
MinK	KCNE1	KvLQT1	i_{Ks}	Channel regulator
MiRP1	KCNE2	HERG	i_{Kr}	Channel regulator
Kvβ1 (Kvβ3)	KCNAB1	Kv1.5 (HK2)	i_{Kur}	Channel regulator
Kvβ2	KCNAB2	Kv1.5 (HK2)	i_{Kur}	Channel regulator
SUR2A	ABCC9	Kir6.2 (BIR)	$i_{K.ATP}$	Channel regulator
KChIP1	KCNIP1	Kv4.1	i_{to1}	Channel regulator
KChIP2	KCNIP2	Kv4.2	i_{to1}	Channel regulator
KChAP		Several		Channel regulator ? regulation of transcription and apoptosis

channel opening (i_{Kr} and i_{Ks}), and substances that open (e.g., $i_{K.Ca}$, $i_{K.Ach}$) or close (e.g., $i_{K.ATP}$) the channel. Cloning of these channels has added to this complexity by providing additional names and numbers (and combinations) that identify both channel proteins and the genes that encode them. Mutations in several of these channels cause human disease, and there is reason to believe that channel protein polymorphisms will identify individuals at risk for sudden cardiac death. For this reason, the lists in Tables 14-4 to 14-6 are provided to help nonexperts keep abreast of this fast-moving field.

Potassium channels fall into two broad classes based on their structures and how they rectify (Table 14-4). Outward rectifier channels include *Shaker* channels, a name based on the behavior of *Drosophila* mutants whose appendages shake when fruit flies that express this gene are anesthetized; these channels, which are referred to by the prefix *Kv* (voltage-regulated K channels), are tetramers made up of the noncovalently linked channel domains that contain six transmembrane α-helices (see Fig. 13-7A and Fig. 13-8B). Additional Shaker channels are responsible for i_{to1}, a small but important transient outward current that helps to determine action potential duration and the time course at which other channels open and close. Another outward rectifier potassium channel, whose domains also contain six transmembrane α-helices but with a longer C-terminal peptide than the Kv channels, resembles a *Drosophila* potassium channel called *eag* (for *ether-a-go-go* because expression of a homologous gene product in the fruit fly causes ether-induced leg shaking); the human counterpart of eag is called *HERG* (*human ether-a-go-go*). Outward rectifier potassium channels, like sodium and calcium channels, open when depolarization shifts the position of a charged S_4 transmembrane helix. They are inactivated by a "ball and chain" structure similar to that which closes sodium channels; the "balls" can be derived from the N-terminal region, where they bind to the intracellular side of the pore ("N-type inactivation"), or a portion of the C-terminal region that occludes the extracellular mouth of the pore ("C-type inactivation").

Inward rectifiers are the second major type of potassium channel. Most important are the *Kir* (inward rectifier K) channels that are made up of four "pore" domains, each of which contains two transmembrane α-helical segments (Fig. 13-8Ca). The most recently discovered inward rectifiers are the K_{2P} channels, which contain two tandem repeat domains (Fig. 13-8Cb). Both types of inward rectifier channels regulate resting potential; their lack of an S_4 transmembrane segment explains their unusual rectification.

Outward Rectifier Potassium Currents

The atria, ventricles, and Purkinje fibers, which have large sodium-dependent action potentials, generate two types of outward rectifier potassium current. Transient repolarization (phase 1) is caused in part by a transient outward current called i_{to1}, while delayed rectifier currents (i_{Kr}, i_{Ks}, and i_{Kur}) contribute to phase 3.

TRANSIENT OUTWARD CURRENT (i_{to1}). Phase 1 (early repolarization) is caused by two repolarizing currents. One, i_{to1}, is a potassium current, while the other, i_{to2}, is a chloride current (see below). These brief repolarizing currents shorten action potential duration by accelerating the cycling of channels that open later during the action potential. In diseased hearts, stress-induced changes in the expression of the genes that encode the i_{to1} channels modify action potential duration. For example, a decrease in channel density and isoform shifts prolong cardiac action potentials in the hearts of elderly individuals and patients with heart failure. Stress-induced changes in i_{to1} channels are a major cause for T-wave "evolution" following myocardial infarction, post-tachycardia T-wave abnormalities, and other long-lasting repolarization abnormalities sometimes called *cardiac memory* (see Chapter 17). Activation of i_{to1} channels by PK-A–catalyzed phosphorylations helps shorten the action potential during sympathetic stimulation.

OUTWARD (DELAYED) RECTIFIER POTASSIUM CURRENTS (i_{Kr}, i_{Ks}, AND i_{Kur}). The major repolarizing currents in the heart are carried by outward rectifier potassium channels that, because they open after the initial depolarizing event, are called *delayed rectifiers*. The major delayed rectifier currents in Purkinje fibers and the ventricles are i_{Kr} and i_{Ks}; the subscripts *r* and *s* refer to the rate at which these channels open (r, rapid; s, slow). The short action potentials that characterize atrial myocardium (see below) are caused by "ultra-rapid" delayed rectifier channels called i_{Kur}.

The major subunit of the i_{Ks} channel, KvLQT1 (Kv7.1) is a member of the Kv (Shaker) class, while that of i_{Kr} is the eag channel called *HERG*

(Kv11.1) (see Table 14-5). Activation of i_{Ks} begins shortly after depolarization and, after this current reaches its peak toward the end of the plateau, these channels close as the cell begins to repolarize. In contrast, i_{Kr} follows an unusual time course because the HERG channels open rapidly, but only partially at the beginning of the action potential plateau, whereas at the end of the plateau, they open more fully.

Mutations in the channel proteins responsible for i_{Kr} and i_{Ks} account for several classes of long QT syndrome, which are important substrates for sudden death. Loss of function mutations in HERG (responsible for i_{Kr}) cause the long QT syndrome called *LQT2*, while LQT6 is caused by loss of function mutations in the regulatory protein MiRP1. Similarly, loss of function mutations in KvLQT1 (responsible for i_{Ks}) cause LQT1, while LQT5 is caused by mutations in the regulatory protein MinK. As knowledge of these heritable syndromes increases, so does their complexity—it is now clear, for example, that *gain* of function mutations in HERG cause equally dangerous short QT syndromes. The greater sensitivity of I_{Ks} than i_{Kr} to activation by β-adrenergic agonists is an important reason why patients with KvLQT1 mutations are prone to sudden death following sympathetic stimulation.

LIPID-ACTIVATED POTASSIUM CURRENTS ($i_{K.AA}$). Lipid-activated delayed rectifier potassium channels shorten the cardiac action potential in acidotic hearts and when concentrations of fatty acids and their derivatives are increased. This response may provide an energy-sparing mechanism that abbreviates systole when fatty acids and protons accumulate in ischemic hearts.

CALCIUM-ACTIVATED REPOLARIZING CURRENTS: $i_{K.Ca}$ AND i_{to2}. Two repolarizing currents can be activated by a rise in cytosolic calcium concentration. One, $i_{K.Ca}$, appears to be a Kv potassium channel, while the other is i_{to2}, the calcium-activated chloride channel described below. Both respond to increased cytosolic calcium by generating repolarizing currents that shorten the action potential plateau, thereby providing a negative feedback that limits calcium entry into calcium-overloaded hearts. Activation of these repolarizing currents explains why the QT interval (an index of action potential duration, see Chapter 15) is shortened by hypercalcemia and cardiac glycosides, which increase cellular calcium, and why hypocalcemia prolongs the QT interval.

Inward Rectifier Potassium Currents

The cardiac plasma membrane contains several inward rectifier channels that regulate resting potential and, in the SA node, influence the rate of pacemaker discharge. The inward rectifier channels responsible for the high potassium permeability of the resting heart are members of the Kir family called i_{K1}. Other Kir channels participate in the responses to parasympathetic stimuli ($i_{K.Ach}$) and changing ATP levels ($i_{K.ATP}$).

VOLTAGE-REGULATED INWARD RECTIFIER POTASSIUM CURRENTS (i_{K1}). The i_{K1} channels which open in resting cells are the major determinants of resting potential. Because these channels close in response to depolarization (inward rectification), loss of their outward current makes an important contribution to the long duration of the normal cardiac action potential.

ATP-INHIBITED INWARD RECTIFIER POTASSIUM CURRENTS ($i_{K.ATP}$). The $i_{K.ATP}$ channels are heterotetrameric inward rectifier channels made up of two Kir channels and two molecules of a sulfonylurea receptor called *SUR1*. (The value of sulfonylureas in diabetic patients reflects a role for these channels in regulating insulin release by the pancreas). These ligand-gated inward rectifier channels are opened by ADP and inhibited by physiological levels of ATP so that like a contented house cat asleep before the hearth, $i_{K.ATP}$ channels spend most of their life in a dormant state. Their opening in energy-depleted hearts reduces contractility and so is energy-sparing.

ACETYLCHOLINE-ACTIVATED INWARD RECTIFIER POTASSIUM CURRENTS ($i_{K.Ach}$). Another class of ligand-gated inward rectifier channels, called $i_{K.Ach}$, mediates hyperpolarizing responses to vagal stimulation. The $I_{K.Ach}$ channels are heterotetramers that contain two different Kir channels called *GIRK* (*G protein inward rectifier K channel*). Opening of $i_{K.Ach}$ channels in the atria, which shortens the action potential, is largely responsible for the negative inotropic response to vagal stimulation, while the hyperpolarizing response caused by opening of $i_{K.Ach}$ channels in the SA node slows the sinus pacemaker (see below). These effects occur when acetylcholine binding to cardiac muscarinic receptors activates heterotrimeric G proteins that are coupled directly to these channels within the plasma membrane (see Chapter 8). Binding of adenosine and other purines to purinergic receptors also activates these inward rectifier channels.

CHLORIDE CURRENTS

The Donnan equilibrium responsible for the potassium gradient across the plasma membrane (see above) also establishes a chloride gradient in which intracellular chloride activity is about 4 mM, nearly 5% that outside the cell (~80 mM) (Table 14-1). According to the Nernst equation, the chloride equilibrium potential is about −80 mV:

$$E_{Cl} = 61.5 \times \log \frac{Cl_i}{Cl_o} = \frac{4}{80} = -80 \text{ mV} \qquad [14\text{-}9]$$

Most chloride currents, which are repolarizing, are small and contribute mainly to volume regulation. Other chloride channels in the heart include CFTR (cystic fibrosis transmembrane conductance regulator), a γ-amino butyric acid–regulated channel, and members of an extended family of voltage-gated chloride channels (ClC). The latter, which are outward rectifiers, contain 12 or 13 transmembrane α-helices and differ structurally from the other voltage-gated ion channels described in this chapter. Chloride channels that carry the transient inward current i_{to2} are activated by PK-A, which helps to shorten the action potential during sympathetic activation, and by calcium, which allows calcium overload to reduce action potential duration.

MEMBRANE CURRENTS GENERATED BY THE SODIUM PUMP AND THE SODIUM–CALCIUM EXCHANGER

The sodium pump generates an outward ionic current because it transports three sodium ions out of the cell in exchange for two potassium ions (see Chapter 9). While the effect on membrane potential is normally small, increases in this "background" repolarizing current can become significant in sodium-overloaded cells, as occurs, for example, when the heart rate is accelerated.

A more important membrane current is generated by the Na–Ca exchanger, which because it exchanges one calcium ion for three sodium ions, contributes a small outward current when cytosolic sodium increases after the action potential upstroke in working cardiac myocytes and His–Purkinje cells, and an inward current when calcium leaves these cells during diastole (see Chapter 7). The latter, which tends to occur at the time when the ventricles are most "vulnerable" to fibrillation (see Chapter 16) is especially important in calcium-overloaded cells, where inward currents generated by the Na–Ca exchanger can lead to afterdepolarizations and potentially lethal arrhythmias (see below).

REGENERATIVE ASPECTS OF REPOLARIZATION

Repolarization is governed largely by local factors, the most important of which is the opening of delayed rectifier potassium channels. Although repolarization is not propagated in the same way as depolarization, it is, in a minor way, regenerative because regions that have already repolarized generate capacitive currents that tend to return membrane potential toward the resting level in adjacent depolarized regions of the heart.

THE INTERVAL–DURATION RELATIONSHIP

The *interval–duration relationship* is an essential physiological mechanism that adjusts cardiac action potential duration to the length of the cardiac cycle; the response is especially important at high heart rates, where cycle length must be shortened to allow sufficient time for the rapidly beating ventricles to fill. This is apparent from a simple calculation. The normal ventricular action potential duration is about 0.35 seconds

Heart rate

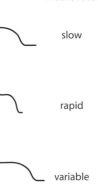

A   slow

B   rapid

C   variable

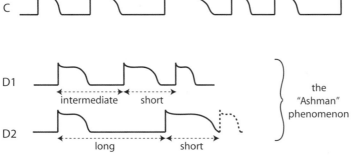

D1

intermediate   short

D2

long   short

the "Ashman" phenomenon

FIGURE 14-9 Interval–duration relationship. At slow heart rates, where diastolic intervals are long, action potential duration is long (A). Where the diastolic interval is short, action potential duration is also short (B). When cycle length varies, action potential duration is determined by the preceding diastolic interval (C). Because the length of the refractory period is correlated with action potential duration, a wave of depolarization that arrives after a short cycle is less likely to encounter refractoriness left behind by a preceding cycle if the short cycle occurred after a previous short cycle than a previous long cycle (D1). For this reason, a wave of depolarization that arrives after a short cycle preceded by a long cycle is more likely to encounter the refractory period of the preceding cycle and will fail to generate an action potential (dashed D2).

when the heart rate is 75 beats per minute (total cycle length = 0.80 sec), yet trained athletes can achieve heart rates in excess of 180 beats per minute, where total cycle length is only 0.33 seconds. Obviously, the heart could not beat at the more rapid rate unless action potentials became shorter. The normal inverse relationship between heart rate and cycle length (Fig. 14-9A and B), which is called the interval–duration relationship, also allows a long diastolic interval to prolong the duration of the following action potential and shortens the action potential when the preceding diastolic interval is abbreviated. This relationship explains the normal inverse relationship between heart rate and the QT interval (see Chapter 15).

    The interval–duration relationship also explains the influence of preceding cycle length on action potential duration when cardiac rhythm is irregular, as in patients with atrial fibrillation (Fig. 14-9C), and accounts for an electrocardiographic phenomenon called the *Ashman phenomenon*. In the latter, action potential prolongation after a long cycle can cause the next wave of depolarization that follows a short cycle to fall during the refractory period (Fig. 14-9D2), whereas the same wave of depolarization at the same short cycle length arriving after a shorter preceding cycle may not encounter refractoriness (Fig. 14-9D1). This is the mechanism for a phenomenon called *aberrant conduction* (see Chapter 16).

Several mechanisms explain the interval–duration relationship. Abbreviation of the action potential at rapid heart rates is due in part to increases in cytosolic calcium and sodium caused by the more frequent action potentials: The increased calcium accelerates repolarization by opening $i_{K.Ca}$ and i_{to2} channels, while elevated cytosolic sodium shortens the action potential by increasing the repolarizing current generated by the sodium pump. Incomplete decay of the delayed rectifier currents i_{Kr} and i_{Ks} at rapid heart rates also contributes outward currents that reduce action potential duration. An additional mechanism, which shortens the action potential when the heart rate is increased by sympathetic stimulation, occurs when PK-A catalyzes phosphorylation of i_{to1} and i_{to2}.

AFTERDEPOLARIZATIONS AND TRIGGERED RESPONSES

Afterdepolarizations are spontaneous depolarizations that appear during repolarization (phase 3) or shortly after the cell has repolarized (phase 4). Neither depends on external stimuli, but both are seen when the heart becomes calcium overloaded. When afterdepolarizations are small, they cause only small oscillations of membrane potential; however, large afterdepolarizations can initiate *triggered responses*, which are important causes of lethal arrhythmias. The increased likelihood of this dangerous arrhythmogenic mechanism caused by calcium overload is a major reason why inotropic drugs and energy starvation often cause sudden death in cardiac patients.

There are two general types of afterdepolarizations: *early afterdepolarizations* and *delayed afterdepolarizations* (Fig. 14-10). The former appear before the end of the action potential, when membrane potential is in the range between -10 and -30 mV; the latter appear after membrane potential has returned to its resting level. Unlike most arrhythmias, which are suppressed when the heart is paced rapidly (a phenomenon called *overdrive suppression*, see Chapter 17), delayed afterdepolarizations are made worse by increasing the heart rate, probably because of a gain in cytosolic calcium (see Chapter 10).

Early Afterdepolarizations

Early afterdepolarizations appear toward the end of the plateau of the cardiac action potential, especially when the latter is prolonged by bradycardia, disease, or drugs. They can be caused by both i_{CaL} and the inward current carried by the Na–Ca exchanger when it removes calcium

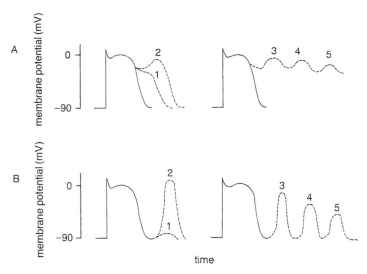

FIGURE 14-10 Afterdepolarizations. **A:** Early afterdepolarizations showing a subthreshold afterdepolarization (1), and larger afterdepolarizations that cause a single (2) and repetitive (3-4-5) triggered responses. **B:** Late afterdepolarizations showing a subthreshold afterdepolarization (1) and afterdepolarizations that reach threshold so as to produce one (2) or a series (3-4-5) of triggered responses. (Modified from Wit and Rosen, 1981.)

from the cell. The underlying mechanisms are not fully understood but may include oscillatory calcium release by the sarcoplasmic reticulum calcium pump (see Chapter 7). The ability of cyclic AMP to increase i_{CaL} is one reason why β-adrenergic agonists and phosphodiesterase inhibitors provoke triggered responses.

Delayed Afterdepolarizations

Delayed afterdepolarizations occur after the cell has repolarized, during phase 4 of the action potential, and are commonly seen in calcium-overloaded hearts; for this reason, their appearance is another unwanted side effect of inotropic therapy with drugs that increase cyclic AMP. The major cause of delayed afterdepolarizations is the inward current generated when calcium is removed from the cytosol by the Na–Ca exchanger.

CHANGES IN IONIC COMPOSITION DURING ACTION POTENTIAL

Each action potential brings small amounts of sodium, calcium, and chloride into working cardiac myocytes and the cells of the His–Purkinje system, while potassium is lost (Table 14-7). To restore the original conditions, sodium, calcium, and chloride must be pumped out of the cytosol, and the cell must regain potassium. It is a common misconception that the concentration gradients for sodium and potassium across the plasma membrane are dissipated during each action potential. However,

TABLE 14-7 Major Ion Fluxes during the Purkinje Fiber Action Potential

Current	Ion	Flux	Current	Phase of Action Potential	Physiological Role
i_{Na}	Na^+	Inward	Inward	0	Depolarization
i_{to1}	K^+	Outward	Outward	1	Early repolarization
i_{to2}	Cl^-	Inward	Outward	1	Early repolarization
i_{CaL}	Ca^{2+}	Inward	Inward	2	Plateau
i_{Kr}	K^+	Outward	Outward	3	Repolarization
i_{Ks}	K^+	Outward	Outward	3	Repolarization
i_{K1}	K^+	Outward	Outward	4	Resting potential
i_f	Na^+	Inward	Inward	4	Pacemaker depolarization

a single depolarization causes only a very small change in the chemical composition of the cardiac cell, as evidenced by the large number of action potentials that can be generated after the Na-K ATPase is poisoned. Although rapid stimulation causes a measurable gain in cytosolic sodium, the increase is small; for example, stimulation of a sheep Purkinje fiber at 2 Hz increases intracellular sodium content by only about 10% (Cohen et al., 1982).

ACTION POTENTIALS IN SPECIFIC REGIONS OF THE HEART

The action potentials in the cardiac myocytes found in different regions of the heart reflect their specialized electrophysiological functions (Fig. 14-11).

Purkinje Fibers

The cells of the His–Purkinje system have very large, rapidly rising action potentials; resting potentials are about -90 mV, and the overshoot can reach $+30$ mV, so action potential amplitude can be greater than $+120$ mV (Fig. 14-11). These features, along with a low internal resistance, favor rapid conduction. The long duration of these action potentials helps to prevent impulses transmitted from the His–Purkinje system to the ventricular myocardium from reactivating the former, and so provides an important safeguard against re-entrant arrhythmias (see Chapter 16). The currents responsible for the Purkinje fiber action potential are depicted in Figures 14-12 and 14-13. Figure 14-12 shows the changes in total current flow during a free-running action potential, while major individual currents are shown in Figure 14-13.

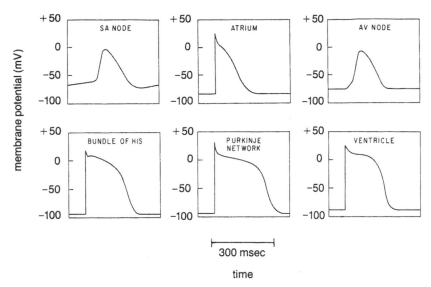

FIGURE 14-11 Action potential configurations in different regions of the mammalian heart.

Sinoatrial Node

The SA node, which serves as the normal *cardiac pacemaker*, is a band of spontaneously depolarizing cells located in the right atrium near its junction with the superior vena cava (Chapter 1). Coordinated interactions among these cells determine the timing of SA node discharge, and shifts in the pacemaker site within this band of nodal cells explain a benign arrhythmia called *wandering pacemaker*. Spontaneous depolarization of the SA node, also called *phase 4 depolarization* or the *pacemaker potential*, normally initiates the wave of depolarization that usually activates all regions of the heart (Chapter 15).

Resting potential in the SA node is low, about 70 mV; the action potentials are small and have a slow upstroke that reflects the absence of fast sodium channels (Fig. 14-11). At least six currents are now believed to participate in pacemaker activity, the hallmark of the SA node (Fig. 14-14); four are inward currents, and the other two are outward potassium currents.

INWARD CURRENTS. Spontaneous pacemaker depolarization begins with the opening of nonspecific cation channels that carry an inward current called i_f because of the unusual characteristics of this current (f stands for "funny"). As membrane potential decreases, the thresholds for two additional channels are reached: T- and L-type calcium channels. The T-type channels, which have the lower threshold, are first to open, which adds a second small depolarizing current to that carried by i_f. When membrane potential reaches the threshold for the L-type calcium channels, the latter generate the major depolarizing current. The fourth inward current, which is

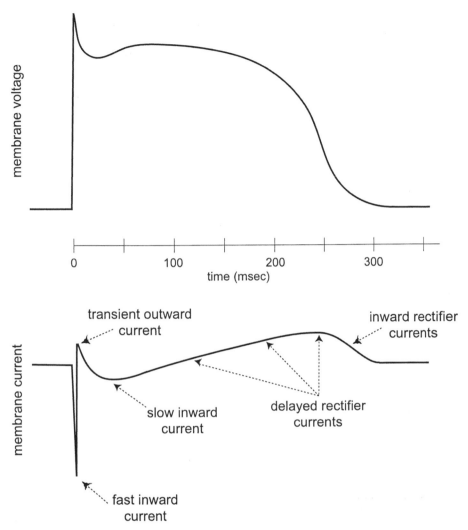

FIGURE 14-12 Purkinje fiber action potential (*upper tracing*) and membrane currents (*lower tracing*); inward currents are *downward*, outward currents are *upward*. The approximate timing of five different types of ionic current are shown.

generated by the electrogenic sodium–calcium exchanger, occurs when each calcium ion that has entered the cytosol through the T- and L-type calcium channels is extruded in exchange for three sodium ions (see Chapter 7).

OUTWARD CURRENTS. Decreases in two outward potassium currents operate synergistically with the increasing inward currents described above. The most important is a delayed rectifier current, called i_K, that restores the resting membrane potential; acceleration of this repolarizing current shortens the pacemaker cycle and therefore increases the heart rate by allowing the i_f channels to depolarize the SA node at an earlier

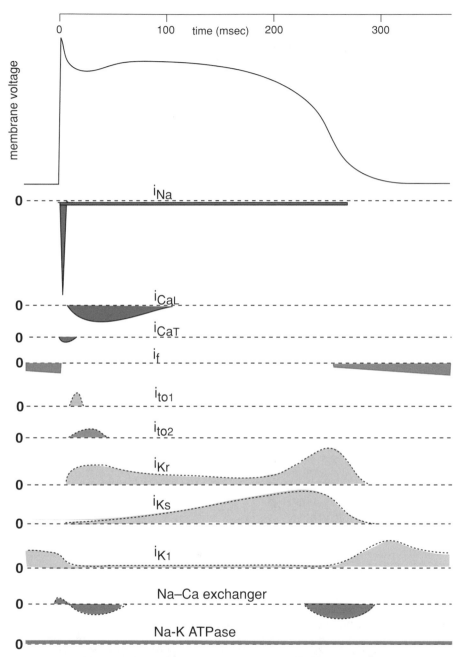

FIGURE 14-13 Individual currents responsible for the Purkinje fiber action potential. *Upper tracing* shows voltage changes. *Lower tracings* show 11 different currents; inward currents are *downward*, outward currents are *upward*. Depolarizing ionic currents include i_{Na}, i_{CaL}, i_{CaT}, and i_f, while repolarizing ionic currents include three outward potassium currents (i_{to1}, i_{Kr}, and i_{Ks}), the transient outward chloride current (i_{to2}). Resting potential is maintained by the inward rectifier i_{K1}. Currents generated by the Na–Ca exchanger and Na-K ATPase are shown at the bottom of the figure.

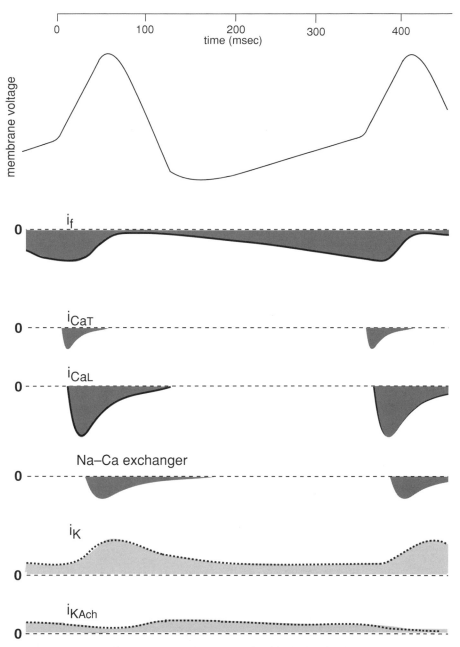

FIGURE 14-14 Individual currents responsible for depolarization of a pacemaker cell in the SA node. *Upper tracing* shows voltage changes. Diastolic depolarization is caused by increases in three inward ionic currents (i_f, i_{CaT}, and i_{CaL}) and an inward current generated when calcium leaves the cell by the Na–Ca exchanger. Increases in the outward rectifier current i_K ends the pacemaker cycle. Pacemaker activity is slowed by $i_{K.Ach}$, which stabilizes resting potential.

time. Opening of the inward rectifier $i_{K.Ach}$ slows the heart rate by maintaining membrane potential at its resting level.

AUTONOMIC CONTROL OF THE SA NODE PACEMAKER. The heart rate is normally under both sympathetic and parasympathetic control. In resting myocardial cells, the most important is a high level of parasympathetic tone that slows spontaneous depolarization of the SA node. This can be demonstrated in a normal person with a resting (basal) heart rate of 60 beats per minute, where administration of atropine, a muscarinic receptor blocker, increases the heart rate to about 120 beats per minute (Fig. 14-15). A lower level of resting sympathetic tone is evidenced by a smaller fall in the heart rate, to about 50 beats per minute, following administration of the β-adrenergic receptor blocker propranolol. Blockade of both sympathetic and parasympathetic activity increases the heart rate to about 100 beats per minute, which represents the "true" resting heart rate. Sympathetic stimulation becomes dominant during exercise, when the heart rate can exceed 180 beats per minute in a trained athlete.

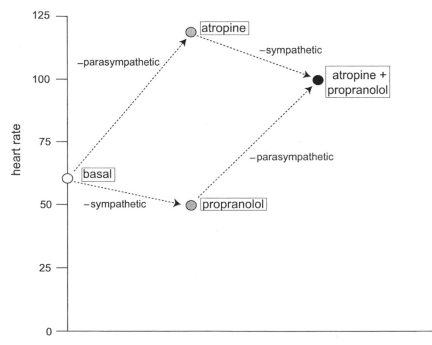

FIGURE 14-15 Effects of autonomic blockade on sinus pacemaker rate. In an individual with a basal heart rate of 60 beats per minute (*open circle*), the muscarinic receptor blocker atropine increases rate to 120 beats per minute, while the β-adrenergic receptor blocker propranolol slows the rate to 50 beats per minute. The decrease in rate from 60 to 50 beats per minute represents the effect of abolishing sympathetic tone, while the increase from 60 to 120 beats per minute results from abolishing parasympathetic tone (*shaded circles*). Block of both autonomic influences by atropine plus propranolol reveals a "true" intrinsic pacemaker rate of 100 beats per minute (*closed circle*).

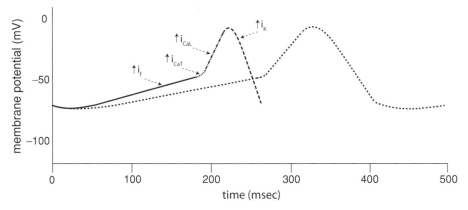

FIGURE 14-16 Acceleration of the SA node pacemaker by sympathetic stimulation. Cyclic AMP increases i_f by interacting directly with these cyclic nucleotide–gated channels to accelerate diastolic depolarization. Cyclic AMP also increases the depolarizing currents carried by i_{CaT} and i_{CaL} by activating PK-A to phosphorylate these channels. Cycle length also is shortened when PK-A phosphorylation of i_K accelerates repolarization.

Autonomic control of the SA node is mediated largely by $G_{\alpha i}$ and $G_{\alpha s}$. The increase in the heart rate caused by sympathetic stimulation occurs when $G_{\alpha s}$ stimulates adenylyl cyclase to increase cyclic AMP production. One effect of this intracellular second messenger is a direct action on i_f that increases the opening of these depolarizing channels. Cyclic AMP also activates PK-A, which phosphorylates i_{CaT}, i_{CaL}, and i_K channels. Phosphorylation of the two types of calcium channel accelerates the heart rate by increasing their depolarizing currents, while phosphorylation of i_K shortens cycle length by accelerating repolarization (Fig. 14-16). Parasympathetic slowing occurs when $G_{\alpha i}$ activates the inward rectifier current $i_{K.Ach}$ which, by increasing outward resting current, inhibits SA node depolarization. $G_{\alpha i}$ also slows the heart rate by inhibiting cyclic AMP production.

Atria

Atrial action potentials are of shorter duration than those of the Purkinje fibers (Fig. 14-11) and usually lack pacemaker activity. Depolarization (phase 0), which is effected by sodium channel opening, is rapid and is followed by a phase of rapid repolarization (phase 1) and a brief plateau (phase 2). The latter merges into the phase of repolarization (phase 3), so separate phases 2 and 3 often cannot be identified. The relatively brief duration of the atrial action potential is due to the "ultrarapid" delayed rectifier current called i_{Kur} (see above). Vagal stimulation shortens both the action potential and refractory period in the atria by activating outward potassium currents. This effect, by reducing calcium channel opening during the plateau, contributes to the negative inotropic response of the atria to vagal stimulation.

Atrioventricular Node

The AV node is a region of slow conduction, which explains the normal delay in impulse transmission from the atria to the ventricles. As the AV node provides the only electrical connection between these regions of the heart, the delay between atrial and ventricular contraction allows atrial systole to determine ventricular end-diastolic volume (see Chapter 11). Resting potential in the AV node is approximately −80 mV, and membrane potential during depolarization usually does not exceed +5 to +10 mV. Action potential duration in the AV node is longer than in the atrium, but much shorter than in the Purkinje fibers.

The AV node can be divided functionally into three regions (Fig. 14-17): the AN region (upper or atrionodal portion), the N region (middle or nodal portion), and the NH region (lower or nodal–His bundle portion). Resting potential is lowest in the N region, while action potentials are shortest in the AN region, increasing progressively in duration through the N region to the NH region. Spontaneous pacemaker activity, which is found in all regions of the AV node, is most rapid in the lower (H and NH) regions and slowest in the N region.

Atrioventricular conduction is slow for several reasons. One is the low amplitude, slowly rising action potential (Fig. 14-11), which depends on small calcium currents. Slow conduction in the AV node is also due to a high internal resistance, which is caused both by the small diameter of the AV nodal cells, especially in the N region, and relatively small number of gap junctions. The rate of depolarization and the amplitude of the AV node action potentials are under autonomic control; sympathetic stimulation accelerates AV conduction by increasing the calcium inward current, while vagal stimulation slows conduction through this structure by inhibiting these depolarizing currents.

Conduction through the AV node is normally precarious because the currents generated during depolarization are barely sufficient to propagate the action potential; for this reason, the AV node is said to have a low *safety factor*. This property limits the frequency with which impulses can be transmitted from the atria to the ventricles and so protects against excessive rates of ventricular beating during atrial flutter and fibrillation. Failure of conduction through the AV node is an important cause of atrioventricular block (see Chapter 16).

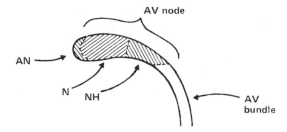

FIGURE 14-17 Atrioventricular conduction system. The AV node can be divided functionally into three regions: AN (upper, or atrionodal), N (middle, or nodal), and NH (lower, or nodal–His bundle).

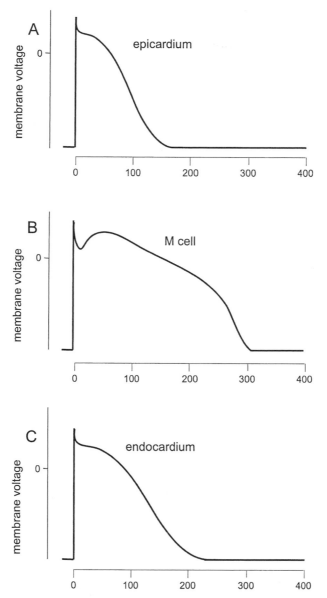

FIGURE 14-18   Action potential configurations in different layers of the ventricular wall. **A:** epicardium; **B:** M cells of the midmyocardium; **C:** endocardium. (Based on data from Liu and Antzelevitch, 1995.)

Ventricles

Ventricular action potentials are smaller than those of the Purkinje fibers (Fig. 14-11), which accounts for the slower conduction velocity in the ventricles. The duration of the plateau is longer than in the atria, and shorter than that of the His–Purkinje system. Spontaneous diastolic depolarization is not normally seen in the ventricular myocardium.

Action potential durations differ in the different layers of the ventricular wall. These heterogeneities, which are due largely to uneven distribution of repolarizing i_{to1} and i_{Ks} channels, explain a puzzling finding described in Chapter 15; that the polarities of the waves inscribed during depolarization and repolarization in the electrocardiogram are the same. This finding, which occurs because the first areas of the ventricle to be depolarized are the last to be repolarized, is due in part to a longer action potential duration in the endocardium than in the epicardium (Fig. 14-18). The long action potentials in the midmyocardial cells (called *m cells*) are due to smaller numbers of both i_{to1} and i_{Ks} channels.

CONCLUSIONS

The practical importance of the ionic currents described in this chapter, which can be recorded from the body surface as the electrocardiogram, is highlighted by a growing number of abnormalities in channel function now recognized to cause cardiac arrhythmias. The material covered in this and the preceding chapter therefore serves as the foundation for understanding clinical electrocardiography, for managing clinical arrhythmias, and for preventing sudden cardiac death.

BIBLIOGRAPHY

Baumgarten CM, Clemo HF. Swelling-activated chloride channels in cardiac physiology and pathophysiology. *Prog Biophys Mol Biol* 2003;82:25–42.

Clancy CE, Kass RS. Inherited and acquired vulnerability to ventricular arrhythmias: cardiac Na^+ and K^+ channels. *Physiol Rev* 2005;85:33–47.

Deal KK, England SK, Tamkun MM. Molecular physiology of cardiac potassium channels. *Physiol Rev* 1996;76:49–67.

Hille B. *Ionic channels of excitable membranes*, 3rd ed. Sunderland, MA: Sinauer, 2001.

Hoffman BF, Cranefield P. *Electrophysiology of the heart.* New York: McGraw Hill, 1960.

Kane GC, Liu X-K, Yamada S, Olson TM, Terzic A. Cardiac K_{ATP} channels in health and disease. J Mol Cell Cardiol 2005;38:937–943. (Note: The June and July 2005 issues of J Mol Cell Cardiol contain additional excellent reviews of K_{ATP} channels.

Katz B. *Nerve, muscle and synapse.* New York: McGraw-Hill, 1966.

Noble D. *The initiation of the heartbeat*, 2nd ed. Oxford: Clarendon Press, 1979.

O'Connell AD, Morton MJ, Hunter M. Two-pore domain K^+ channels—molecular sensors. *Biochim Biophys Acta* 2002;1566:152–161.

Pogwizd SM, Bers DM. Cellular basis of triggered arrhythmias in heart failure. *Trends CV Med* 2004;14:61–66.

Pogwizd SM, Schlotthauer K, Li L, et al. Arrhythmogenesis and contractile dysfunction in heart failure: roles of sodium-calcium exchange, inward rectifier potassium current, and residual beta-adrenergic responsiveness. *Circ Res* 2001;88:1095–1096.

Pourrier M, Schram G, Nattel S. Properties, expression and potential roles of cardiac K^+ channel accessory subunits: MinK, MiRPs, KChIP, and KChAP. *J Membrane Biol* 2003;194:141–152.

Pusch M, Jentsch TJ. Molecular physiology of voltage-gated chloride channels. *Physiol Rev* 1994;74:813–827.

Seino S. ATP-sensitive potassium channels: a model of heteromultimeric potassium channel/receptor assemblies. *Annu Rev Physiol* 1999;61:337–362.

Snyders DJ. Structure and function of cardiac potassium channels. *Cardiovasc Res* 1999; 42:377–390.

Sorota S. Insights into the structure, distribution and function of the cardiac chloride channels. *Cardiovasc Res* 1999;42:361–376.

Tamargo J, Caballero R, Gómez R, et al. Pharmacology of cardiac potassium channels. *Cardiovasc Res* 2004;62:9–33.

Tsien RW. Key clockwork component cloned. *Nature* 1998;391:839–841.

Tsien RW, Tsien RY. Calcium channels, stores, and oscillations. *Ann Rev Cell Biol* 1990; 6:715–760

Wit AL, Rosen MR. Afterdepolarizations and triggered activity. Distinction from automaticity as an arrhythmogenic mechanism. In: Fozzard H, Haber E, Jennings R, et al., eds. *The heart and cardiovascular system*, 2nd ed. New York: Raven Press, 1992:2113–2165.

Wong KR, Trezise AE, Bryant S, et al. Molecular and functional distributions of chloride conductances in rabbit ventricle. *Am J Physiol* 1999;277:H1403–H1409.

Yamada M, Inanobe A, Kurachi Y. G protein regulation of potassium ion channels. *Pharmacol Rev* 1998;50:723–757.

Yu H, McKinnon D, Dixon JE, et al. Transient outward current, i_{to1}, is altered in cardiac memory. *Circulation* 1999;99:1898–1905.

Zipes D, Jalife F. *Cardiac electrophysiology. From cell to bedside*, 3rd ed. Philadelphia: WB Saunders, 1995.

REFERENCES

Blinks JR. Intracellular Ca^{2+} measurements. In: Fozzard H, Haber E, Katz A, et al., eds. *The heart and cardiovascular system*. New York: Raven Press, 1986:671–701.

Cohen CJ, Fozzard HA, Sheu SS. Increase in intracellular sodium ion activity during stimulation in mammalian cardiac muscle. *Circ Res* 1982;50:651–662.

Liu DW, Antzelevitch C. Characteristics of delayed rectifier current (I_{Kr} and I_{Ks}) in canine ventricular epicardial, midmyocardial, and endocardial myocytes. A weaker I_{Ks} contributes to the longer action potential of the M cell. *Circ Res* 1995;76:351–365.

Spear JF, Moore EN. Supernormal conduction in the canine bundle of His and proximal bundle branches. *Am J Physiol* 1980;238:H300–H306.

Walker J. Intracellular inorganic ions in cardiac tissue. In: Fozzard H, Haber E, Katz A, et al. *The heart and cardiovascular system*. New York: Raven Press, 1986:561–572.

Wit AL, Rosen MR. Cellular electrophysiology of cardiac arrhythmias. Part I. Arrhythmias caused by abnormal impulse generation. *Mod Conc Cardiovasc Dis* 1981;50(1):1–8.

Clinical Physiology

15

THE ELECTROCARDIOGRAM

Three of the five major properties of cardiac muscle can be evaluated by the electrocardiogram, which records the electrical activity of the heart from electrodes placed on the body surface. These are automaticity (*chronotropy* or pacemaker activity, the ability to initiate an electrical impulse), conductivity (*dromotropy*, the ability to conduct an electrical impulse), and irritability (*bathmotropy*, the ability to respond to direct stimulation). All of these electrical properties, along with contractility (*inotropy*) and the ability to relax (*lusitropy*), are found in primitive myocardial cells, but as the heart matures and specialized structures appear, many cardiac myocytes lose some of these properties. All adult cardiac myocytes retain conductivity and irritability, but contractility and relaxation are prominent only in the working cells of the atria and ventricles, which generally lack automaticity. Rapidly firing pacemaker cells are found in the sinoatrial (SA) node, while more slowly depolarizing pacemaker cells are found in the atrioventricular (AV) node and His–Purkinje system. Because the latter are activated by impulses conducted from the SA node, their pacemaker activity is normally dormant. Conduction is very slow in the cells of the SA and AV nodes, whereas rapid conduction by the His–Purkinje system synchronizes ventricular contraction.

CHRONOTROPY: PACEMAKERS AND IMPULSE FORMATION

The primary pacemaker of the heart is the SA node, which is derived from the sinus venosus, the most rapidly beating portion of the tubular embryonic heart. These embryonic hearts, like those of primitive animals, can be divided into four regions: the sinus venosus, atria, ventricles, and truncus arteriosus (Fig. 15-1). Although the atria and ventricles often contain pacemaker cells, their spontaneous depolarizations are suppressed by faster sinus venosus pacemaker; this reflects the fact that the intrinsic rate of pacemaker depolarization decreases as one proceeds from the "higher" venous to the "lower" arterial end of the embryonic heart. Unless the lower pacemaker cells are isolated from the more rapidly firing sinus venosus, they do not have time to initiate a propagated wave of depolarization.

A similar hierarchy of pacemaker activity exists in the adult human heart. Impulses conducted from the SA node pacemaker normally suppress

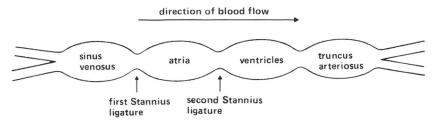

FIGURE 15-1 Embryonic or primitive heart. Blood flow in this tubular heart is from left to right. The intrinsic rates of the intrinsic pacemaker activity of each chamber decreases as one moves downstream; this was demonstrated by Stannius, who in 1852 placed tight ligatures at the sinoatrial junction (first Stannius ligature) and AV junction (second Stannius ligature). Elimination of the influence of the more rapid higher ("upstream") pacemakers revealed the previously suppressed activity of pacemaker cells in the lower ("downstream") regions.

the intrinsic activity of lower pacemakers, whose diastolic depolarization is too slow to reach threshold before these cells are discharged by the wave of depolarization propagated from the SA node. The activity of lower pacemakers can become apparent only when their firing is accelerated, when the SA node pacemaker is slowed, or when impulse conduction is blocked (see Chapter 16).

The SA node in the human heart normally fires 60 to 100 times each minute, whereas the most rapid of the lower pacemakers, generally found in the lower nodal–His (NH) region of the AV node, have an intrinsic rate of approximately 40 to 55 beats per minute. Pacemaker cells in the His–Purkinje system fire at rates of approximately 25 to 40 beats per minute (Table 15-1). Despite their large number, however, lower pacemaker cells often fail to initiate a propagated wave of depolarization when they become isolated electrically from the SA node pacemaker. The resulting cessation of ventricular contraction is an important cause of cardiac arrest.

DROMOTROPY: IMPULSE PROPAGATION THROUGH THE HEART

All conduction in the heart is by way of cardiac muscle; nerves serve only to regulate impulse generation and conduction. The normal activation sequence, shown in Table 15-1, reflects the heart's anatomy and embryology. The impulse that originates in the SA node first activates the atria and then the ventricles; in the latter, the last regions to be activated are the outflow tracts, parts of which are derived from the truncus arteriosus.

Conduction velocities differ in various regions of the heart (Table 15-1). The wave of depolarization is propagated most rapidly in the AV bundle, bundle branches, and Purkinje network; conduction is less rapid in atrial and ventricular myocardium and very slow in the SA and AV nodes.

TABLE 15-1 **Normal Activation Sequence**

Structure	Conduction Velocity (m/sec)	Rate of Pacemaker Discharge (min^{-1})
SA node ⇓	<0.01	60–100
Atrial myocardium ⇓	1.0–1.2	None
AV node ⇓	0.02–0.05	40–55
AV bundle ⇓	1.2–2.0	40–55
Bundle branches ⇓	2.0–4.0	25–40
Purkinje network ⇓	2.0–4.0	25–40
Ventricular myocardium	0.3–1.0	None

Although the latter is a small structure, slow conduction through the AV node causes a delay that plays an important role in timing atrial and ventricular systole (see Chapter 11).

Atrial Depolarization

The wave of depolarization that originates in the SA node spreads first into contiguous areas of the right atrium, and then through atrial myocardium to the left atrium and AV node. Propagation follows a complex path that can vary, which explains changes in morphology of the P waves of the normal electrocardiogram called *wandering pacemaker* (see Chapter 16).

INTERNODAL TRACTS. Rapidly conducting pathways in the atria, called *internodal tracts*, have been described as preferred conduction pathways linking the SA and AV nodes. Three such tracts are generally identified (Fig. 15-2). The *anterior* tract has two branches; one links the SA and AV nodes, the other, called *Bachmann's bundle*, crosses the atrial septum to transmit impulses from the right atrium to the left atrium. The other two, the *middle* and *posterior* internodal tracts (named after *Wenckebach* and *Thorel*, respectively), represent preferential conduction pathways between the SA and AV nodes.

Despite electrophysiological evidence for these conduction pathways, most histological studies fail to demonstrate clearly demarcated bundles of specialized cells that can explain the rapid conduction observed physiologically. For this reason, the internodal tracts are functional rather than

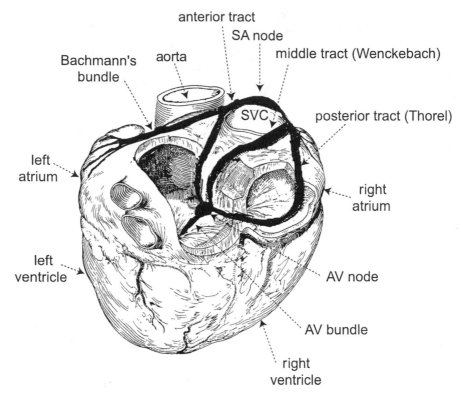

FIGURE 15-2 Internodal tracts as seen in a posterior view of the heart. The anterior, middle, and posterior internodal tracts provide preferential conduction pathways between the SA and AV nodes. A branch of the anterior internodal tract, sometimes called *Bachmann's bundle*, provides a conduction pathway that links the right and left atria. (Redrawn from James, 1967.)

anatomical pathways. The anatomical basis for rapid impulse conduction in the atria may include bundles of pectinate muscles or regions enriched in rapidly conducting Purkinje-like cells.

Atrioventricular Conduction

The role of the fibrous skeleton of the heart as an electrical insulator separating the atria and ventricles (see Chapter 1) is key to understanding AV conduction. Normally, the wave of depolarization that originates in the SA node crosses this connective tissue barrier only through a strand of specialized muscle tissue called the *AV bundle, bundle of His, His bundle,* or *common bundle*. Electrical access to the AV bundle is controlled by the *AV node*, a strand of small nodal cells located near the coronary sinus on the posterior wall of the right atrium. In the normal heart, the AV node provides the only electrical connection between the atria and AV bundle and so regulates all electrical communication between the atria and ventricles (Fig. 15-3).

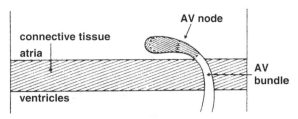

FIGURE 15-3 The AV node and AV bundle provide the only conduction pathway that normally transmits impulses across the central fibrous body. The latter can be viewed as a connective tissue insulator that lies between the atria (*above*) and ventricles (*below*).

Abnormal electrical connections sometimes link the atria and ventricles in human hearts (Fig. 15-4). These include *accessory pathways*, sometimes called the *bundle of Kent*, which are strands of atrial myocardium that cross the central fibrous body at various locations. Although generally dormant, these abnormal conduction pathways can become active and cause arrhythmias. Because accessory pathways conduct more rapidly than the AV node, these structures can provide a "short circuit" that bypasses the normal delay caused by slow AV nodal conduction. Inappropriate impulse transmission between the atria and ventricles through an accessory pathway provides the anatomical substrate for a condition called *pre-excitation* or the *Wolff-Parkinson-White syndrome* (WPW, see Chapter 16). Additional abnormal conduction pathways, called *bypass fibers of James*, can link the atria to the upper portion of the AV bundle; like accessory pathways, they bypass the normal conduction delay in the AV node. *Mahaim fibers* provide another abnormal pathway that can transmit impulses from the upper part of the AV bundle to the

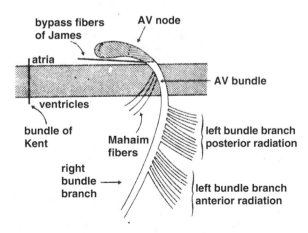

FIGURE 15-4 Abnormal conduction pathways that can link the atria and ventricles. These include accessory pathways (bundle of Kent), whose locations vary; bypass fibers of James, which connect the atrial myocardium to the upper portion of the AV bundle; and Mahaim fibers, which connect the AV bundle to abnormal sites in the ventricles.

ventricles. Accessory pathways, James fibers, and Mahaim fibers can all create arrhythmogenic re-entrant circuits.

Activation of the Ventricles: Bundle Branches, Fascicles, and Purkinje Network

The specialized conduction system of the heart includes the AV bundle, bundle branches, fascicles, and Purkinje network, all of which are made up of rapidly conducting Purkinje fibers. The AV bundle divides at the top of the interventricular septum into the *right* and *left bundle branches* (see Chapter 1). The right bundle branch (Fig. 15-5) is generally a discrete strand of conducting tissue that reaches the right ventricular free wall within a structure called the *moderator band*, whereas the left bundle branch usually fans out over the left ventricle.

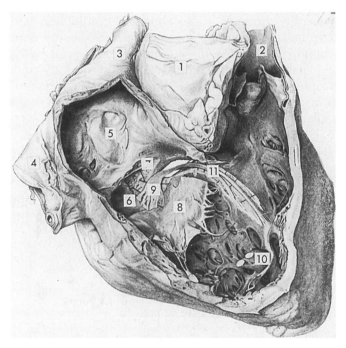

FIGURE 15-5 Conduction system of the human right ventricle viewed from the right after removal of a portion of the right atrial and ventricular walls. Note the aorta (1); pulmonary artery (2); superior vena cava (3); inferior vena cava (4); fossa ovale of the interatrial septum (5); Thebesian valve overlying the coronary sinus (6); false tendon (7); and medial leaflet of the tricuspid valve, which has been separated from its point of insertion (8). The AV node (9), which lies in the right atrium above the tricuspid valve, receives fingerlike branches from the atria and continues toward the ventricles where it merges into the AV bundle at the top of the membranous septum (which has been partially opened in this preparation). The latter divides into the right and left bundle branches; the right bundle branch (11) runs along the right side of the interventricular septum and continues within the moderator band, usually without branching, to reach the anterior papillary muscle of the right ventricle (10). (Modified from Wenckebach and Winterberg, 1927.)

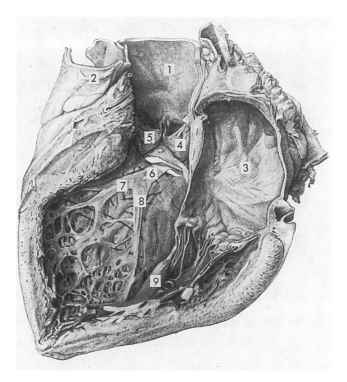

FIGURE 15-6 The same heart as shown in Figure 15-5, viewed from the left after removal of a portion of the left atrial and left ventricular walls. Note the aorta (1); pulmonary artery (2); left atrium (3); and two cusps of the aortic valve (4,5). The left bundle branch, which emerges through an opening made by removal of a portion of the membranous septum, originates as a wide, flat band (6). The left bundle branch then fans out into anterior (7) and posterior (8) fascicles, which run toward the anterior (*not shown*) and posterior (9) papillary muscles of the left ventricle. (Modified from Wenckebach and Winterberg, 1927.)

The left bundle branch is viewed by electrocardiographers as dividing into two branches, called *anterior* and *posterior fascicles* (Fig. 15-6). This terminology was introduced to characterize the electrocardiographic abnormalities that are seen when conduction in these fascicles is interrupted (see below); block in the anterior fascicle produces *left anterior fascicular block* (or *left anterior hemiblock*), while conduction block in the posterior fascicle causes *left posterior fascicular block* (or *left posterior hemiblock*). Even though the fascicular blocks are well-defined electrocardiographic entities, their anatomic basis is tenuous because division of the left bundle branch is highly variable, and discrete anterior and posterior fascicles are uncommon (Fig. 15-7).

The working myocardial cells of the ventricles are depolarized by the *Purkinje network*, a system of rapidly conducting fibers that arise from the bundle branches and course within the inner third of the ventricular walls. Rapid conduction by these fibers coordinates electrical activation of

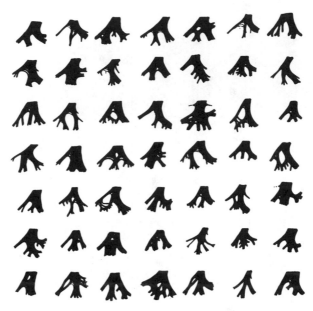

FIGURE 15-7 Sketches of the division of the left bundle branch in 49 human hearts showing that simple bifurcation into anterior and posterior fascicles is uncommon. (From Demoulin JC, Thesis.)

the ventricles and therefore provides the synchrony needed for efficient ventricular ejection.

THE ELECTROCARDIOGRAM

The *electrocardiogram* (abbreviated *ECG* or *EKG*) is a record of potential differences arising within the heart that are measured by electrodes placed on the body surface (Fig. 15-8). The conventional speed of these recordings is 25 mm/sec, so each large horizontal division (time) represents 0.20 sec, and each small division is 0.04 sec. In the normally standardized ECG, each large vertical division (voltage) equals 0.5 mV, and the small divisions are 0.1 mV. The waves recorded by the ECG were named at the beginning of the 20th century by Willem Einthoven, who invented the string galvanometer that made possible the first high fidelity recording of the ECG. To avoid controversies engendered by earlier nomenclature, Einthoven started in the middle of the alphabet and named his deflections PQRST (Fig. 15-9).

It is sometimes forgotten that the ECG records only electrical activity and is *not* a measure of the mechanical behavior of the heart. Although there is a very rough correlation between the amplitude of the deflections inscribed during atrial or ventricular depolarization and the force of contraction, these correlations are tenuous and of limited diagnostic value.

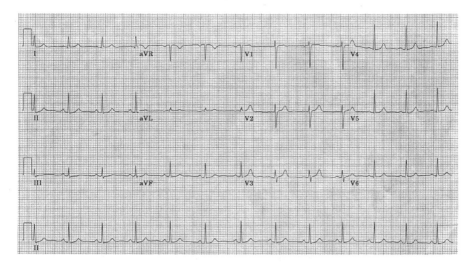

FIGURE 15-8 Normal twelve-lead ECG. The leads recorded in the *upper three tracings* are changed and labeled automatically; the *lower tracing* is a continuous lead II. The vertical "box" at the left is a standardization artifact caused by a 1 mV pulse; when standardization is normal, this causes a 1.0 mm upward shift in the baseline. Paper speed is 25 mm/sec, so each heavy division is 0.2 sec, and each of the smaller, lighter, divisions is 0.04 sec.

The P Wave: Atrial Depolarization

The first deflection recorded by the ECG, named the *P wave* by Einthoven, is caused by atrial depolarization. Although depolarization of the SA node precedes atrial depolarization (Table 15-1; Fig. 15-10), these pacemaker potentials are very small and cannot be recorded from the body surface.

The width (duration) of the P wave, which reflects the time taken for the wave of depolarization to spread over the atria, can be prolonged by atrial enlargement or an intra-atrial conduction delay. Potential differences

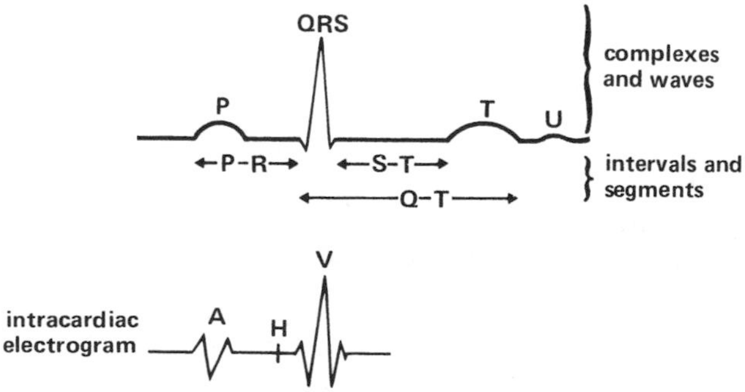

FIGURE 15-9 Body surface and intracardiac electrograms. **Above:** Normal waves, complexes, and intervals measured at the body surface. **Below:** The initial electrical events as recorded by an electrode catheter placed within the heart (Fig. 15-11).

generated during atrial repolarization can be recorded as the T_P *wave* (the "T" of the P), but these are rarely seen because they are small and usually "buried" in the much larger QRS complex. T_P waves are most often seen when P waves are not followed by QRS complexes, as in AV block (see Chapter 16).

The PR Interval: Atrioventricular Conduction

The ECG returns to its baseline between the end of atrial depolarization and the onset of ventricular depolarization; however, a great deal is going on during this "silent" period (Fig. 15-10). The interval between atrial and ventricular activation, called the *PR interval*, begins with the first deflection of the P wave and ends with the first deflection of the QRS complex (whether the latter is a Q wave or an R wave as defined below). During the PR interval, the wave of depolarization that originated in the SA node is propagated through the AV node, AV bundle, bundle branches, fascicles of the left bundle branch, and Purkinje network (Fig. 15-10). Activation of these structures, although extremely important, does not influence the body surface ECG because of their small size.

Electrode catheters passed into the right heart can be placed over the AV bundle (Fig. 15-11) where they record a *His bundle (intracardiac) electrogram* that can be used to time the passage of the wave of depolarization through this structure (Fig. 15-9).

The QRS Complex: Ventricular Depolarization

The *QRS complex* is generated by potential differences that originate from the upstrokes of the ventricular action potentials as the wave of

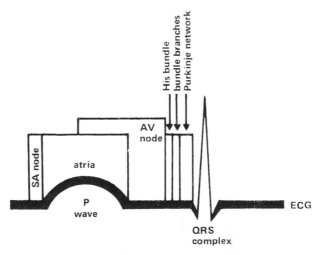

FIGURE 15-10 Tissues depolarized by a wave of activation commencing in the SA node are shown as a series of blocks superimposed on the deflections of the ECG. Depolarization of many important structures during the PR interval does not generate potential differences sufficiently large to be recorded at the body surface.

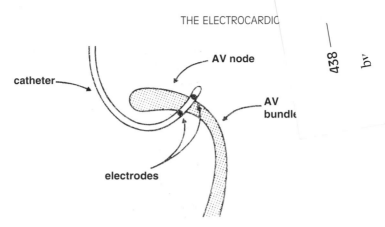

FIGURE 15-11 Depolarization of the AV bundle (see Fig. 15-10) can be recorded by an electrode catheter introduced into the right atrium and placed over this structure.

depolarization passes through the ventricular myocardium (Fig. 15-12). The amplitude of the QRS complex is greater than that of the P wave because the ventricular mass is much larger than that of the atria. The short duration of the QRS complex, which is about the same as that of the P wave, reflects the synchronous activation of the right and left ventricles by rapid conduction through the bundle branches and the His–Purkinje system (Table 15-1).

The "waves" (deflections) of the QRS complex are named according to the following convention: Q, any initial downward deflection followed

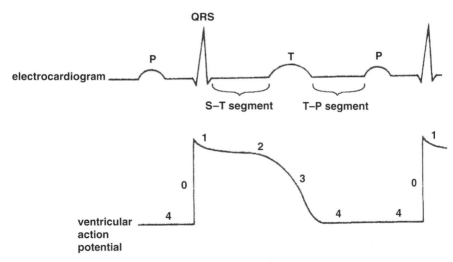

FIGURE 15-12 Temporal relationships between the ECG (*top*) and a representative cardiac action potential (*bottom*). The QRS complex is produced by the upstrokes (phase 0) of all of the action potentials in the ventricles; the isoelectric S–T segment corresponds to the plateau (phase 2), while the T wave is inscribed during repolarization (phase 3) of the ventricular mass. The isoelectric segment that follows the T wave, called the *T–P segment*, is inscribed during ventricular diastole (phase 4).

ɹn upward deflection (if there is only a downward deflection, this is ·alled a *QS*); R, any upward deflection whether or not it is preceded by a Q wave; and S, any downward deflection preceded by an R wave. Additional upward deflections after S waves are called R', R", etc. and additional downward deflections after R waves are S', S", etc.

The QRS complex is prolonged when the normal synchrony of right and left ventricular depolarization is lost; this can occur when conduction is blocked in one of the bundle branches (bundle branch block), or when the ventricles are depolarized by an ectopic focus that activates one ventricle before the other (ventricular premature depolarizations). Slowed conduction in the distal His–Purkinje system also can prolong the QRS complex in patients with severe cardiac disease, notably end-stage heart failure; this is sometimes called *arborization block.*

The S–T Segment: Plateau of the Ventricular Action Potential

Following inscription of the QRS complex, the ECG normally returns to, or very nearly to, its baseline, where it remains until the beginning of repolarization, which inscribes the T wave. This isoelectric phase, called the *S–T segment*, corresponds to the plateau (phase 2) of the ventricular action potentials (Fig. 15-12), when there are no potential differences at the body surface because *all regions of the ventricle are depolarized.*

The reason why the ECG does not record a potential difference during either the S–T segment or the T–P segment (which is inscribed before the QRS complex) can be confusing; after all, the S–T segment is recorded when the ventricles are depolarized, while the T–P segment occurs when the ventricles are fully repolarized and at their resting potential. The reason that the record is at the baseline at both times is because there are no potential differences when *all* regions of the ventricles are depolarized or when *all* regions are at resting potential. The ECG therefore provides no information regarding the absolute level of membrane potential because it cannot measure *"zero"* potential; instead, these tracings record only potential *differences.* For this reason, when the S–T segment appears to be displaced upward or downward relative to the T–P segment, it is not possible to determine whether the abnormality is due to an abnormal potential difference in the resting ventricles (during the T–P segment), or an abnormal potential difference during depolarization (the S–T segment); because the T–P segment is assumed *by convention* to represent the baseline ("zero" potential), both are described as S–T segment shifts. This convention must be understood in evaluating injury currents generated in the ischemic heart (see Chapter 17).

The T Wave: Ventricular Repolarization

Repolarization of the ventricles generates the T wave (Fig. 15-12). Unlike the rapidly changing potential differences that give rise to the sharp deflections of the QRS complex, which reflect the high speed at which the wave of depolarization is propagated over the ventricles, the broader T wave reflects the fact that repolarization proceeds more slowly because it is not due to a propagated wave. The influence of local factors on repolarization (see Chapter 14) explains why the sequence of ventricular repolarization differs from that of depolarization (see below).

The U Wave

Small deflections, called *U waves*, sometimes occur after the end of the T wave. (The small undulations after the T waves in lead V_2–V_5 in Fig. 15-8 are normal U waves.) U waves may be generated by M cells, ventricular myocytes with long action potentials that are located in the midmyocardium (see Chapter 14), although there remains some doubt as to this explanation (Wu et al, 2002).

The QT Interval

The time between the onset of the QRS complex and the end of the T wave, called the *QT interval*, provides a useful index of ventricular action potential duration (Fig. 15-9). Measurements of this interval can be used to evaluate the effects of drugs and diseases on the time-dependent properties of the ion channels responsible for ventricular depolarization and repolarization. QT prolongation is very important clinically because delayed repolarization is a substrate for arrhythmias and sudden death.

A number of drugs can prolong the QT interval, as can electrolyte disorders and several heritable disorders. The latter include mutations in the sodium and delayed rectifier potassium channels (see Chapter 14), the inward rectifier i_{K1} (Lange et al., 2003), and the cytoskeletal protein ankyrin (Table 15-2). The importance of these and other ion channel mutations, which are a leading cause of death in young individuals, is highlighted by a greatly increased risk of sudden death in asymptomatic individuals who are given one of the many drugs that modify the QT interval.

Relationship between the ECG and the Ventricular Action Potential

As a first approximation, the QRS complex corresponds to the upstroke of the ventricular action potentials (phase 0), the S–T segment to the plateau (phase 2), and the T wave to repolarization (phase 3) (Fig. 15-12). The relationship between electrical events in the ventricles and the potential differences at the body surface, however, is more complex than shown in Figure 15-12 because the ECG is influenced by *all* of the action potentials in the millions of cells that are depolarized and repolarized during each cardiac cycle.

NORMAL INTERVALS AND DURATIONS IN THE ECG

Approximate values for the durations of some key waves and intervals of the normal adult ECG are listed in Table 15-3. Most are age-dependent,

TABLE 15-2 **Some Heritable Causes of QT Abnormalities in the Human Heart**

Clinical Syndrome	Mutated Protein/Gene
LQT1: long QT, ventricular arrhythmias	KVLQT1 (Kv7.1)/KCNQ1
LQT2: long QT, ventricular arrhythmias (Some HERG mutations cause short QT syndromes.)	HERG (Kv11.1)/KCNH2
LQT3: long QT, ventricular arrhythmias (SCN5A mutations also cause Brugada syndrome, progressive cardiac conduction system disease, and progressive cardiac dilatation.)	hH1/SCN5A
LQT4: long QT, ventricular arrhythmias	Ankyrin B
LQT5: long QT, ventricular arrhythmias	MinK/KCNE1
LQT6: long QT, ventricular arrhythmias	MirP1/KCNE2
Andersen-Tawil syndrome: long QT, ventricular arrhythmias	Kir2.1/KCNJ2

some vary with heart rate, and the QT interval is slightly longer in women than in men. Formulae have been devised to quantify the relationship between the QT interval and heart rate, but the calculations are complex. Reference to a table of normal QT intervals at various heart rates in men and women is probably the best way to determine whether the QT interval is abnormal in a given patient.

THE HEART AS A DIPOLE IN A VOLUME CONDUCTOR

The electrical activity of the heart is measured by the *twelve-lead electrocardiogram* that records potential differences between electrodes placed at standard positions on the body surface (see below). The pioneers in electrocardiography, in an effort to make their interpretations more scientific, evaluated the magnitude and direction of the electrical vectors responsible for these potential differences by using a simple model that viewed the heart as a *dipole* in a *volume conductor* (Fig. 15-13).

TABLE 15-3 **Some Normal Values in the Normal Adult Human ECG**

	Duration (sec)
PR interval	0.12–0.20 sec
QT interval	0.35–0.40 sec (depends on heart rate)
QRS duration	<0.12 sec (values of 0.10 and 0.11 sec can be abnormal)

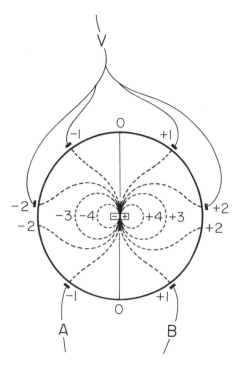

FIGURE 15-13 The partially depolarized ventricles can be depicted as an electrical dipole in a volume conductor. The dipole is the rectangle in the center of the figure, which is positively charged to the right and negatively charged to the left. The volume conductor is shown as a circle (*solid line*) within which are drawn isopotential lines (*dashed lines*). Potentials (*indicated in milli-volts*) can be recorded from the surface of the volume conductor using electrodes such as A and B, where potentials are −1 and +1 mV, respectively. Also shown is an indifferent electrode (V), which is con-nected to four electrodes placed on the surface of the volume conductor so that the sum of the potentials is zero.

A *dipole* is an electrical source, such as an asymmetrically distrib-uted electrical charge. At any instant during depolarization, the heart can be viewed as a dipole because cells in the excited regions are negatively charged, while those in the unexcited regions are electropositive. These polarities reflect the fact that the outside of a depolarized cell is negatively charged relative to the cytosol, whereas the outside of a resting cell is pos-itively charged (Chapter 14). The dipole in Figure 15-13, which is analo-gous to a single frame in a motion picture, depicts the ventricles at one instant during depolarization, when an electrical dipole is created by a resting (positive) region on the right and a depolarized (negative) region on the left.

Recording of the potentials generated by the cardiac dipole depends in part on the conducting medium, or *volume conductor*, that lies between the heart and the recording electrodes. In the model shown in Figure 15-13, the volume conductor is a dish of salt water; in electrocar-diography, the body tissues provide the volume conductor that transmits potentials generated by the heart to electrodes placed on the body sur-face. The isopotential lines in Figure 15-13 show that the potentials in the one-half of the volume conductor occupied by the negative pole are neg-ative, while those in the other one-half are positive. Projection of the isopotential lines to the surface of the volume conductor illustrates that the major determinant of the magnitude of the potentials recorded on the ECG is *the angle between the cardiac dipole and the leads on the body surface.* Potential also falls in proportion to the square of the distance between an electrode and the dipole; however, distance is much less important than the vector angle in clinical electrocardiography and is usually ignored.

The model of the heart as a dipole in the center of a homogenous volume conductor shown in Figure 15-13 is greatly simplified. In the first place, during depolarization, the heart is not a single dipole because the complex pathways of impulse conduction create multiple simultaneous dipoles. A more serious simplification is that the body is not a homogeneous volume conductor; for example, the lungs represent a region of high electrical resistance, which explains why emphysema or pneumothorax can reduce the amplitude and distort the ECG.

ELECTROCARDIOGRAPHIC LEAD SYSTEMS

Two types of lead system can be used to measure the potential difference generated by a dipole in a volume conductor. The simplest is a *bipolar lead*, which records the potential difference between two electrodes, both of which are influenced by the dipole. In the example shown in Figure 15-13, the potential difference between leads A and B is 2 mV. Whether the recorded potential is +2 mV or −2 mV depends on convention: If electrode A is defined as "zero," then B records +2 mV; if B is chosen as "zero," then A is −2 mV. Because of their simplicity, bipolar lead systems were the first to be used in clinical electrocardiography.

Attempts to make electrocardiography more scientific led to the introduction of *unipolar leads* in which one electrode (the *exploring* electrode) measures the potential generated by the dipole, while the other (the *indifferent* electrode) is assumed not to be influenced by the dipole and thus records "zero" potential. Indifferent electrodes can be created by one of two means. One is to place the electrode far away from the dipole, which takes advantage of the decrease in potential as the distance from the dipole increases. One can, for example, place a patient in one corner of a salt water swimming pool and record from the opposite corner. This method, which records only small potential differences because of distance, is obviously impractical. A second type of indifferent electrode is made by connecting a number of electrodes, all of which are influenced by the dipole, to one another. Such leads are assumed to record "zero" potential because the potentials at the many electrodes tend to cancel one another. If the indifferent electrode (V) in Figure 15-13 is assigned a value of "zero," the potential difference recorded between electrode A and the V lead is −1 mV, while electrode B records a potential of +1 mV relative to the V lead.

The second type of indifferent electrode is used in clinical electrocardiography. This is the *V lead*, devised by Frank Wilson, which is constructed by connecting electrodes placed on the two arms and left leg to a central terminal.

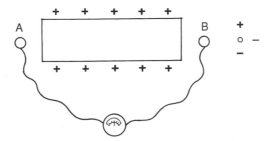

FIGURE 15-14 Resting myocardium. The entire surface is positively charged, relative to the interior of the cells, so that no potential difference is recorded between electrodes A and B. A strip chart recording of the bipolar lead AB (*right*) shows no potential difference and so remains at its baseline.

THE DIPOLE GENERATED DURING VENTRICULAR DEPOLARIZATION

The potential differences (dipoles) generated by the heart change from moment to moment during the cardiac cycle. The deflections generated by these changing potential differences can be understood by using the simple model of a bipolar lead that records the electrical potentials generated by a rectangular strip of cardiac muscle (Figs. 15-14 to 15-18).

Resting

In the resting strip (Fig. 15-14), where the cell surface has a uniform positive charge, no potential differences are recorded. The recording

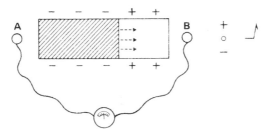

FIGURE 15-15 During depolarization. The strip of myocardium depicted in Figure 15-14 has been stimulated at its left side and is slightly more than one-half depolarized (*shaded area*). The surface of the depolarized area is negatively charged (relative to the interior of the cells of the fiber) so that electrode B faces a region of greater positivity than electrode A. The chart recorder at the right, which has been wired so that an upward deflection is written when electrode B is more positive than A, thus inscribes an upward deflection. The deflection of this bipolar lead reaches its maximum when exactly one-half of the myocardial strip is depolarized. Note that the partially depolarized strip of myocardium is similar to the dipole shown in Figure 15-13.

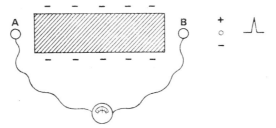

FIGURE 15-16 Fully depolarized. The strip of myocardium depicted in Figures 15-14 and 15-15 is fully depolarized (action potentials of all cells are in phase 2), so their external surfaces are negative relative to their interiors. Because no potential differences exist between the external surfaces of the cells in the strip of myocardium, electrodes A and B both face a similar degree of negativity. The deflection recorded in lead AB (*right*) therefore returns to the baseline.

generated by the bipolar lead AB therefore remains at baseline ("zero" potential).

During Depolarization

Stimulation of the left end of the strip of myocardium initiates a wave of depolarization that is propagated from left to right. As this wave of depolarization moves along the strip, a potential difference appears between electrodes A and B (Fig. 15-15). If electrode A is chosen to represent "zero" potential, electrode B records a positive potential which, according to electrocardiographic convention, causes the recording to move upward. This is because, when a lead faces a region of electropositivity, the recording device is set up to inscribe an upright deflection. As the wave of depolarization moves along the strip, the potential difference first increases, reaching a peak when one-half of the strip is depolarized and then decreases to zero when the entire strip becomes depolarized.

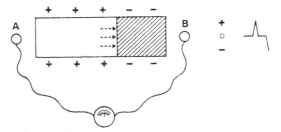

FIGURE 15-17 Repolarization. The strip of myocardium depicted in Figures 15-14 to 15-16 after repolarization has begun in the same region that was first to be depolarized—in this instance, at the left. Because the cell exteriors in the repolarized region have returned to their normal, resting positivity, electrode B faces a region of greater negativity than does electrode A. The chart recorder (*right*) therefore inscribes a downward deflection.

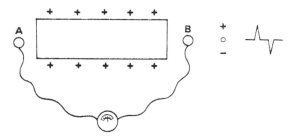

FIGURE 15-18   Fully repolarized. The strip of myocardium depicted in Figures 15-14 to 15-17 in its fully repolarized state is the same as shown in Figure 15-14; the chart recorder (*right*) returns to its baseline.

Fully Depolarized

The potential difference between electrodes A and B returns to zero when the entire strip is depolarized because both electrodes are in a region of electronegativity (Fig. 15-16); for this reason, the record returns to baseline. This highlights the fact that the absence of a potential difference between A and B cannot distinguish between fully depolarized and fully repolarized tissue; as long as there are no potential *differences*, the recording is at zero.

During Repolarization

If repolarization begins at the same point on the strip of myocardium at which the propagated wave of depolarization began, a potential difference opposite in polarity to that seen during depolarization is created (Fig. 15-17). Because electrode B faces an area of electronegativity (relative to A) during repolarization, the conventions described earlier cause a downward deflection to be recorded in the ECG.

Repolarized (Resting)

At the end of the repolarization, when the entire strip is again fully repolarized (Fig. 15-18), no potential differences are recorded. As in Figure 15-14, the record returns to baseline.

A cardinal consequence of the conventions used in electrocardiography is that an *electrode (lead) facing an approaching wave of depolarization records a positive potential and inscribes an upright deflection.* Conversely, a downward deflection is inscribed when a wave of depolarization recedes from a recording electrode, as would have occurred if the strip in Figures 15-14 to 15-18 had been stimulated at the right side or if B rather than A had been chosen to represent zero.

ELECTRICAL VECTORS

In clinical electrocardiography, the potential differences arising in the heart (cardiac dipoles) are represented by electrical vectors whose length and orientation reflect the magnitude and position of the dipole.

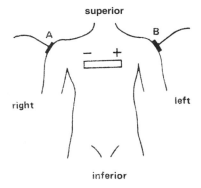

FIGURE 15-19 Cardiac dipole in the human body. The partially depolarized ventricles, which are analogous to the strip of myocardial tissue shown in Figure 15-15, establishes a dipole similar to that shown in Figure 15-13. The potential difference can be recorded between electrodes on the right (A) and left (B) arms.

The dipole shown in Figure 15-19 is oriented transversely in the chest so that an electrode on the right arm (A) records a negative potential and an electrode on the left arm (B) records a positive potential. Whether this is recorded as an upright or inverted deflection depends on which electrode, A or B, is assigned as the "zero" electrode.

Vector arrows that depict cardiac dipoles, by convention, point to the positive pole, while the length of the vector arrow indicates the magnitude of the potential difference (Fig. 15-20). This convention causes the vector arrows to point toward the lead that inscribes an upright deflection, which makes it easy to remember that *electrocardiographic vector arrows point in the direction followed by the wave of depolarization as it passes through the heart.*

QRS Vectors

Because of the complex geometry of the ventricular mass and the fact that the wave of electrical depolarization normally is transmitted synchronously to both ventricles by the right and left bundle branches (see above), many regions of the ventricles are activated simultaneously during inscription of the QRS complex. Furthermore, a different electrical vector is generated at each instant as the wave of depolarization spreads over the ventricles. The sum of *all* of the vectors generated at any moment during depolarization is the *mean instantaneous QRS vector*, while the sum of

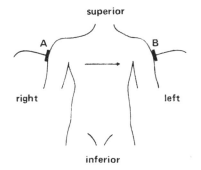

FIGURE 15-20 The dipole shown in Figure 15-19 can be represented by a vector arrow oriented along the dipole axis. By convention, the head of the arrow points to the positive pole of the dipole, and so points in the direction of the propagated wave of depolarization.

FIGURE 15-21 Instantaneous QRS vectors: septal activation. The initial portion of the QRS complex is produced by depolarization of the interventricular septum, which begins at the left ventricular surface of the septum to produce an initial QRS vector that is directed superiorly and to the right.

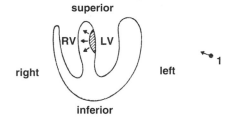

all of the instantaneous vectors generated during ventricular depolarization is the *mean QRS vector*. Whether these vectors cause upright or inverted deflections depends on where the recording electrodes are placed on the body surface and the lead that is selected to represent "zero."

In the following discussion, ventricular activation is divided *arbitrarily* into three phases: septal activation, activation of the apex, and activation of the base, each of which generates a mean instantaneous QRS vector. However, these are not discrete events, but merge from one to the next.

SEPTAL ACTIVATION. The interventricular septum and anterior portion of the base are the first regions to be depolarized during normal ventricular activation. Septal activation begins in the endocardium of the left ventricle, which generates a small electrical vector that is directed to the right (Fig. 15-21). In leads facing the left ventricle, this septal vector gives rise to a small initial downward deflection, called the *septal Q wave.*

ACTIVATION OF THE APEX. Ventricular activation continues as the wave of depolarization is transmitted toward the apex through the Purkinje network, which runs in the endocardium. The much larger mass of the left ventricle causes leftward electrical forces to predominate over those directed to the right so that the second arbitrarily defined vector is directed inferiorly and to the left (Fig. 15-22).

ACTIVATION OF THE BASE. The last regions of the ventricles to be depolarized are the bases of the left and right ventricles. Again, activation proceeds from endocardium to epicardium, and left ventricular forces dominate so that this vector is directed superiorly and to the left (Fig. 15-23).

FIGURE 15-22 Instantaneous QRS vectors: activation of the apex. The midportions of the QRS complex are produced by depolarization of the apex of the heart, which begins at the endocardial surfaces of the ventricles. Because left ventricular forces are dominant, this generates a vector that is directed inferiorly and to the left.

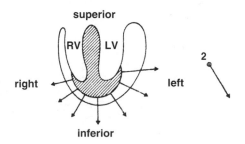

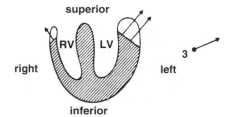

FIGURE 15-23 Instantaneous QRS vectors: activation of the base. The terminal portions of the QRS complex are produced by depolarization of the base of the heart, which begins at the endocardial surfaces. Because left ventricular forces are dominant, this generates a vector that is directed superiorly and to the left.

THE VECTOR LOOP. All three of the mean instantaneous QRS vectors in Figures 15-21 to 15-23 share a common "zero" potential so that the tails of the three vector arrows can be superimposed (Fig. 15-24). If *all* of the other instantaneous vector arrows recorded during the QRS complex are included, their heads inscribe a "vector loop," shown in Figure 15-25A, that starts at zero when the QRS complex begins and returns to zero when the QRS has ended.

THE MEAN QRS VECTOR. *All* of the mean instantaneous QRS vectors inscribed during ventricular activation can be added together to generate the *mean QRS vector*, which represents the average electrical vector generated during depolarization of the ventricles (Fig. 15-25B).

The clinical information provided by the mean QRS vector is limited by the fact that the ECG normally records less than 10% of the total electrical activity generated during ventricular depolarization. This is due largely to mutual cancellation of vectors oriented in opposite directions, which occurs because different regions of the heart are activated at the same time; for example, the left and right ventricles are depolarized in opposite directions. Mutual cancellation also occurs because the Purkinje fibers that penetrate the inner third of the ventricular wall cause ventricular activation to begin within the myocardium (Fig. 15-26A). As long as the wave of depolarization remains beneath the surface of the ventricles, potential differences are not recorded by the ECG; only after depolarization reaches the surface of the ventricles can a potential difference be recorded at the body surface (Fig. 15-26B).

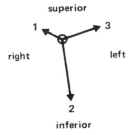

FIGURE 15-24 Because the tails of the three QRS vector arrows shown in Figs. 15-21 to 15-23 all represent "zero" potential, they have been superimposed. This allows the vectors produced by septal activation (1), activation of the apex (2), and activation of the base (3) to be projected in a single figure.

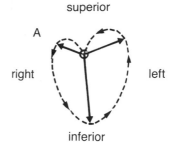

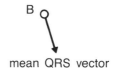

mean QRS vector

FIGURE 15-25 QRS vector loop and mean QRS vector. The vector arrows in Figure 15-24, which are reproduced in A, represent only three of the many instantaneous QRS vectors generated during ventricular depolarization. When the heads of all of these instantaneous vectors are connected (*dashed line*), a loop is formed (A). The mean QRS vector (B) is the sum of all instantaneous vectors generated at all times and in all regions of the ventricles during their depolarization.

BIPOLAR LIMB LEADS AND THE EINTHOVEN TRIANGLE

The first systematic approach to evaluating the potential differences recorded by the ECG was devised by Einthoven, who utilized electrodes placed on the left arm, right arm, and left leg to construct three bipolar limb leads that he called *leads I, II* and *III*. (The electrode usually placed on the right leg in recording the clinical ECG serves as a ground.) Lead I records the potential difference between the right arm and left arm, lead II records that between the right arm and left leg, and lead III records the potential difference between the left arm and left leg. Einthoven chose to define the potential at the right arm electrode as "zero" in leads I and II, while the left arm electrode was chosen as "zero" in lead III (Table 15-4); this assignment of zero electrodes was based on his desire to obtain

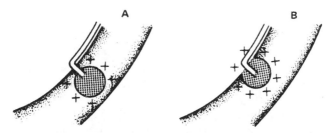

FIGURE 15-26 A wave of depolarization that begins at the end of a Purkinje fiber within the ventricular wall (A) does not generate a potential difference that can be recorded by electrodes outside the heart. Potential differences can be recorded at the body surface only after the depolarized area has expanded to include at least one surface of the ventricular wall (B).

TABLE 15-4 **Standard Limb Leads**

Lead	Potential Difference Between	"Zero" Electrode
Bipolar (Einthoven) Leads		
I	Right arm and left arm	Right arm
II	Right arm and left leg	Right arm
III	Left arm and left leg	Left arm
Unipolar Limb Leads (Augmented)		
aVR	Right arm and a "V" lead made by connecting the left arm and left leg electrodes	The "V" lead
aVL	Left arm and a "V" lead made by connecting the right arm and left leg electrodes	The "V" lead
aVF	Left leg and a "V" lead made by connecting the left arm and right arm electrodes	The "V" lead

upright QRS complexes in these three leads, rather than any mathematical consideration. According to Einthoven's conventions, an upright deflection lead I is recorded when the left arm is positive relative to the right arm; in lead II is recorded when the left leg is positive to the right arm; and in lead III recorded when the left leg is positive to the left arm. An upright QRS is therefore recorded in lead I when the wave of depolarization that activates the ventricles approaches the left arm and in leads II and III when the wave of depolarization approaches the left leg.

THE EINTHOVEN TRIANGLE

Einthoven used his three bipolar leads to calculate electrical vectors by assuming that the right arm, left arm, and left leg electrodes were at the corners of an equilateral triangle, called the *Einthoven triangle*, and that the heart was at the center of this triangle (Fig. 15-27). The net potential recorded in each of the bipolar leads during ventricular depolarization can be projected onto the sides of the Einthoven triangle to locate the mean QRS vector (Fig. 15-28). Key to understanding this analysis is the fact that a bipolar lead records only that portion of the electrical vector parallel to its lead axis (see Fig. 15-13).

The amplitudes of the vectors measured by leads I, II, and III (calculated by subtracting negative from positive deflections in the recordings shown along the bottom of Fig. 15-28) can be drawn as arrows along the sides of the Einthoven triangle. The largest vector is in lead II, which has the tallest QRS complex, because the angle of this bipolar lead most nearly parallels the axis of the dipole generated during ventricular depolarization.

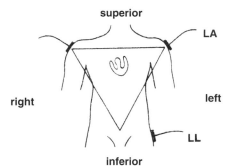

FIGURE 15-27 Einthoven triangle. In the frontal plane, the heart is assumed to lie in the center of an equilateral triangle, the corners of which are electrodes placed on the left arm (LA), right arm (RA), and left leg (LL).

In contrast, the smallest QRS is recorded in lead III because this lead is most nearly perpendicular to the dipole. This illustrates an important principle, that the smallest QRS complex, or the QRS complex in which upward and downward deflections are most nearly the same, is recorded in the lead oriented most nearly at a right angle to the mean QRS axis; these QRS complexes are often called *transitional* because they represent transitions between regions of electronegativity and electropositivity.

Vectors calculated using the Einthoven triangle are approximations because the triangle defined by the limb leads is not equilateral, the heart is not in its center, and the body is not a homogeneous volume conductor. Other ways to analyze these electrical vectors have been proposed, but as body shape varies among individuals, these offer little advantage over the Einthoven triangle.

UNIPOLAR LIMB LEADS

Three unipolar limb leads are conventionally recorded in the clinical ECG. Each measures the potential difference between an exploring electrode that is influenced by the cardiac dipole, and an "indifferent" electrode assumed to record zero potential. As noted above, the indifferent electrode used in electrocardiography is Wilson's *central terminal* (V), which is constructed by connecting the electrodes on the right arm (R), left arm (L), and left leg or foot (F) (Fig. 15-29). The first unipolar leads to be used, called *VR*, *VL*, and *VF*, recorded the potential differences between V (Wilson's central terminal) and the right arm, left arm, and left leg (F, foot), respectively. The central terminal was assumed to measure zero potential so that an upright deflection is inscribed when the exploring electrode is positive relative to the central terminal. In lead VF, for example, an upright deflection is recorded when the left leg electrode faces an approaching wave of depolarization; that is when the electrical vector is directed inferiorly.

The potentials recorded from leads VR, VL, and VF are very small because in each of these leads one electrode is connected to both sides of the recording device. Lead VF, for example, records the potential difference

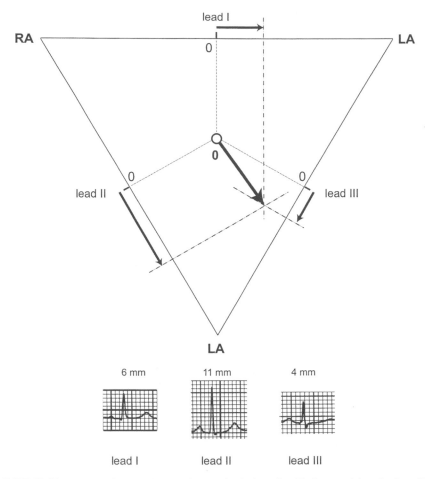

FIGURE 15-28 A normal mean QRS vector projected on the Einthoven triangle described in Figure 15-27. The QRS deflections in leads I, II, and III shown at the bottom of the figure are from the ECG in Figure 15-8. The tail of the vector, which represents "zero" potential, is the open circle at the center of the triangle, which is projected by the *dotted lines* to the midpoints of the three sides. The magnitudes of the mean QRS vector projected to each side of the triangle are determined by subtracting negative from positive deflections (numbers above the three leads at bottom). Perpendiculars drawn from the heads of the vectors projected along the sides of the triangle (*dashed lines*) intersect at the head of the mean QRS vector (*dark arrow within the triangle*). This vector is approximately +70°.

between the electrode on the left leg and Wilson's central terminal, which also is connected to the left leg. To increase the size of these recordings, Goldberger "augmented" the unipolar limb leads by disconnecting the lead that is on both sides of the circuit from the central terminal (Table 15-4); for example, in lead aVF (augmented VF), the leg electrode is disconnected from the V lead. A similar maneuver is used to construct leads aVR and aVL. While "augmentation" increases the size of the deflections, it means that these leads are not unipolar; thus, in aVF, the "central terminal" made

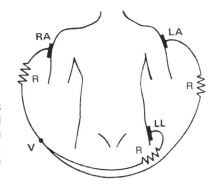

FIGURE 15-29 Wilson's central terminal (V) is constructed by connecting the three limb lead electrodes. Resistances are placed between each electrode and the central terminal to overcome effects of variable resistances between the electrodes and the skin.

by connecting the left and right arm electrodes does not record "zero" potential. This deviation from theory illustrates the empirical nature of the interpretation of electrocardiographic contour.

CHEST LEADS

The six chest leads in the conventional twelve-lead ECG (V_1–V_6) are unipolar leads that record the potential differences between Wilson's central terminal (V) and electrodes placed at six positions on the chest wall (Table 15-5). As in the unipolar limb leads, the central terminal is assumed to record "zero" potential, so an upright deflection is recorded when the electrode on the chest wall is in an area of electropositivity, which occurs when a wave of depolarization approaches this electrode.

TABLE 15-5 **Standard Unipolar Chest Leads**

Lead	Potential Difference Between	"Zero" Electrode
V_1	Fourth intercostal space just to the right of the sternum and the "V" lead	The "V" lead
V_2	Fourth intercostal space just to the left of the sternum and the "V" lead	The "V" lead
V_3	Midway between V_2 and V_4 electrodes and the "V" lead	The "V" lead
V_4	5th intercostal space at the midclavicular line and the "V" lead	The "V" lead
V_5	Left anterior axillary line horizontally to the left of V_4 and the "V" lead	The "V" lead
V_6	Mid-axillary line horizontally to the left of V_5 and the "V" lead	The "V" lead

In all cases, the "V" lead is made by connecting the right arm, left arm, and left leg electrodes.

The chest leads are useful in evaluating abnormalities arising in one or the other ventricle. Leads V_1 and V_2, which are placed over the anterior, right chest wall, are influenced by depolarization of the right ventricle (see below), while leads V_5 and V_6, over the left side of the chest, are normally dominated by left ventricular depolarization. However, because the left ventricle is so much thicker than the right, the potentials generated during left ventricular depolarization dominate the ECG; as a result, the potentials generated by right ventricular depolarization are often obscured, even in leads V_1 and V_2. The QRS complexes in leads V_1 and V_2 of the normal ECG are therefore inverted because their configuration is determined by depolarization of the left ventricle, which generates a vector that recedes from the anterior right side of the chest (see Fig. 15-8). The QRS complexes in V_5 and V_6 are normally upright because these leads record the wave of depolarization approaching the left ventricle.

NORMAL VECTORS

The angle of the mean QRS vector in the frontal plane is calculated using a convention that assigns an angle of 0° to a vector pointing to the left arm, +90° to a vector pointing to the foot, −90° to a vector directed superiorly, and ±180° to a vector pointing to the right arm. Each of the limb leads is assigned an angle, as shown in Table 15-6.

The normal mean QRS axis lies between −30° and +110° (Fig. 15-27); mean QRS vectors greater than +110° represent *right axis deviation*; those less than −30° are designated as *left axis deviation* (Fig. 15-30). More recently, some authorities have narrowed the range of normal QRS axis to between 0° and +90°; while this makes it easier to estimate "normal" axis, it increases the number of individuals who are stated to have an abnormal ECG. The problems created by this simplification are ameliorated in part because individuals with normal hearts can have an abnormal QRS axis, and the QRS axis is often normal in patients with heart disease.

TABLE 15-6 **Frontal Plane Angles Conventionally Assigned to the Limb Leads**

Lead	Vector Angle
I	0°
II	+60°
III	+120°
aVR	−150°
aVL	−30°
aVF	+90°

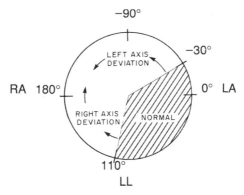

FIGURE 15-30 The angles of ECG vectors in the frontal plane are assigned values according to the convention shown here. A vector directed to the left is assigned an angle of 0°, and one directed to the right is said to have an angle of 180°. A vector directed inferiorly has an angle of +90°, and one directed superiorly has an angle of −90°. Normal mean QRS vectors range between −30° and +110°. Vectors with angles less than −30° exhibit left axis deviation, and those with angles greater than +110° exhibit right axis deviation.

The chest leads define the position of the cardiac dipole in the horizontal plane of the body. However, mean QRS vectors are not usually calculated in this plane; instead, attention is paid to the lead containing the "transitional QRS," where upward and downward deflections are most nearly equal. The transition from the inverted QRS normally seen in leads V_1 and V_2 to the upright QRS normally seen in leads V_5 and V_6 usually occurs in lead V_3 or V_4 (see Fig. 15-8).

Mean T-wave vectors, which can be calculated according to the same conventions used to estimate QRS vectors, are used to estimate the QRS-T angle (the angle between the mean QRS- and T-wave vectors). The latter, sometimes called the *ventricular gradient*, can help determine whether a T wave is normal or abnormal because T-wave vectors are usually concordant with the mean QRS vector; for this reason, a wide QRS-T angle implies that the T wave is abnormal.

CONCORDANCE OF QRS COMPLEXES AND T WAVES

The normal concordance of QRS and T (see Fig. 15-8) differs from the relationship shown schematically in Figures 15-14 to 15-18. This is because the last areas of the ventricles to depolarize are the first to repolarize, as illustrated in Figure 15-31. This figure differs from Figure 15-17 because repolarization normally proceeds in a direction opposite to that of depolarization, which causes the deflection inscribed during repolarization (the T wave) to be concordant with that inscribed during depolarization (the QRS complex). The direction of the T wave is determined largely by the long action potentials in the Purkinje fibers in the endocardium (see Chapter 14), which cause the first regions of the ventricle to depolarize to be the last to repolarize.

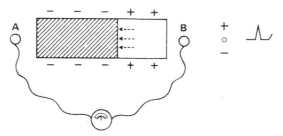

FIGURE 15-31   Strip of myocardium depicted in Figures 15-14 to 15-18 showing why T waves are normally concordant with the QRS complex. This is because repolarization begins in regions of the ventricles that were last to depolarize. This figure, which should be compared with Figure 15-17, shows that when repolarization proceeds in a direction opposite to that of depolarization, the deflections caused by depolarization and repolarization have the same polarity.

SOME ABNORMAL ELECTROCARDIOGRAMS

A few abnormal ECGs are included at this point to illustrate the clinical application of some of the principles discussed in this and earlier chapters, and to demonstrate how electrocardiographic abnormalities can be understood in terms of altered physiology.

INTRAVENTRICULAR CONDUCTION DELAY

The normal synchrony of right and left ventricular depolarization is lost when conduction in one of the bundle branches is blocked. Under these conditions, impulses transmitted from the atria still depolarize both ventricles, but activation of the "blocked" ventricle is delayed and follows an abnormal pathway. The result is an ECG abnormality called *bundle branch block*, in which the QRS complexes are prolonged and abnormal in contour. Activation of the blocked ventricle is delayed because of the longer path followed by the wave of depolarization, which must cross the interventricular septum to reach the blocked ventricle, and because the wave of depolarization is transmitted through ventricular myocardium, which conducts more slowly than the His–Purkinje system (Table 15-1). The abnormal pathway of ventricular activation in right and left bundle branch block causes characteristic abnormalities in the prolonged QRS complex. The T waves also are abnormal in bundle branch block because abnormal spread of the wave of depolarization alters the pattern of repolarization; for this reason, these are often called *secondary* T-wave abnormalities. *Primary* T-wave abnormalities, on the other hand, result from local abnormalities in repolarization.

RIGHT BUNDLE BRANCH BLOCK. Delayed conduction of the wave of depolarization into the right ventricle in right bundle branch block (Fig. 15-32) widens the QRS complex and generates a late wave of depolarization that is directed toward the blocked ventricle. In Figure 15-32, the duration of

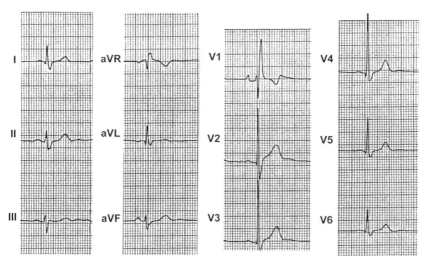

FIGURE 15-32 Right bundle branch block. The diagnosis is established by abnormal prolongation of the QRS complex in the limb leads to 0.14 sec and the tall, broad late R wave over the right ventricle (recorded in lead V_1). The broad late S waves in leads V_5 and V_6 arise from the same late QRS vector, which is directed away from the left ventricle.

the QRS complex (measured in lead II) is 0.14 sec, which is significantly prolonged (see Table 15-3). Delayed activation of the right ventricle is responsible for the broad late R' wave in lead V_1, which is recorded from the anterior right side of the chest. Leads V_5 and V_6, which are over the left side of the chest, contain broad S waves because the wave of depolarization responsible for delayed activation of the right ventricle is directed away from these leads. These changes can be summarized in the statement that the late portions of the wave of depolarization that activates the blocked right ventricle is propagated to the right and anteriorly; this is in accord with the normal anatomical position of the right ventricle, which lies to the right and anterior to the left ventricle.

LEFT BUNDLE BRANCH BLOCK. Interruption of the left bundle branch delays activation of the left ventricle so that, as in the right bundle branch block, the QRS complex is widened. In Figure 15-33, the QRS duration in the limb leads is 0.14 sec. The late QRS vector in the precordial leads is directed to the left (toward lead V_6), which accounts for the tall late peak in the notched R wave in lead V_6. Delayed depolarization of the left ventricle also explains the broad downward deflection of the later parts of the QRS complex in lead V_1, which occurs because the late wave of depolarization that activates the left ventricle recedes from the right precordium.

Fascicular Blocks (Hemiblocks)

Interruption of the anterior or posterior fascicle of the left bundle branch does not prolong the QRS complex because the left ventricle distal to the blocked fascicle is still activated by the rapidly conducting Purkinje

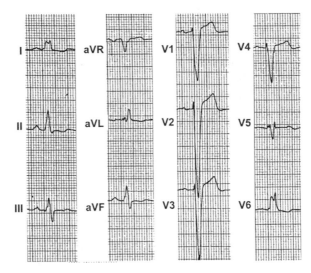

FIGURE 15-33 Left bundle branch block. The diagnosis of left bundle branch block is established by the prolongation of the QRS complex in the limb leads to 0.14 sec and the late R wave in lead V_6.

network. Instead, the fascicular blocks are characterized by abnormalities in the mean QRS vector.

LEFT ANTERIOR FASCICULAR BLOCK. The late electrical forces in left anterior fascicular block are deviated superiorly and to the left, toward the "blocked" region of the left ventricle. This causes left axis deviation but does not prolong the QRS.

The diagnosis of left anterior fascicular block is suggested in Figure 15-34 because lead II is the transitional lead, where positive and negative deflections are about equal. As lead II is assigned an angle of +60° (Table 15-6), if the two deflections were exactly equal, the mean QRS vector would be at right angles to +60°: either −30° (+60° minus 90°) or +150° (+60° plus 90°). The upright QRS in lead I and the inverted QRS in lead aVF tell us that the QRS axis must lie between 0° (toward the left arm) and −90° (away from the foot), which means that the QRS axis is about −30°. On careful examination, the downward QRS deflection in lead II is greater than the upward deflection, so the QRS axis is less than −30°, which meets criteria for abnormal left axis deviation. (There is some ambiguity in these criteria, as some authorities require a mean QRS axis of −45° or less for this diagnosis.)

LEFT POSTERIOR FASCICULAR BLOCK. Left posterior fascicular block is characterized by abnormal right axis deviation because the late unbalanced forces are deviated inferiorly and toward the right. In Figure 15-35, right axis deviation is suggested by lead I, where the downward deflection is greater than the upward deflection; this means that the mean QRS vector is directed toward the right arm. The upright QRS complexes in the inferior

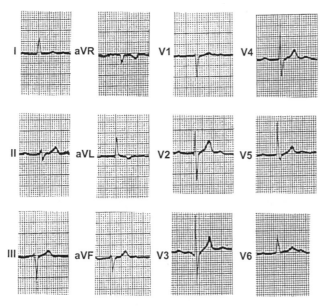

FIGURE 15-34 Left anterior fascicular block. Delayed conduction through the anterior fascicle of the left bundle branch explains the left axis deviation (mean QRS axis −40°).

leads (leads II, III, and aVF) tell us that the mean QRS axis is directed inferiorly rather than superiorly (Table 15-6). The net upward deflection (positive minus negative) in lead III, which is assigned an angle of +120° (Table 15-6) is approximately 14 mm, while that in lead aVF, which is assigned an angle of +90°, is approximately 12 mm, so the mean QRS

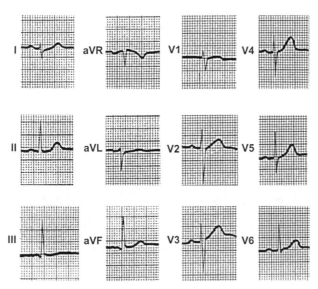

FIGURE 15-35 Left posterior fascicular block. Delayed conduction through the posterior fascicle of the left bundle branch explains the right axis deviation (mean QRS axis = +110°).

vector is more nearly parallel to lead III than to aVF. This tells us that the mean QRS vector is closer to $+120°$ than to $+90°$, which places this vector at an angle greater than $+105°$, which meets the criteria for abnormal right axis deviation (QRS $\geq +110°$).

Ventricular Hypertrophy

Electrocardiographic diagnosis of ventricular hypertrophy is difficult and has a poor predictive accuracy. The examples provided below, which focus on the QRS abnormalities, ignore additional criteria such as P-wave morphology and ST–T abnormalities. Ventricular hypertrophy generally— but not always—increases the voltage recorded by leads that "face" the hypertrophied ventricle; this causes tall R waves in lead V_1 in right ventricular hypertrophy (Fig. 15-36), and in lead V_6 in left ventricular hypertrophy (Fig. 15-37). These increases in QRS amplitude are due both to the increased mass and slowed conduction in the hypertrophied ventricle. Right and left ventricular hypertrophy are often associated with right and left axis deviation, respectively, but by themselves, abnormalities in the frontal plane QRS vector are not reliable criteria for these electrocardiographic diagnoses.

The abnormal ECGs in this chapter, which illustrate a few of the principles used in electrocardiographic interpretation, are provided to show how pathophysiological information obtained from the QRS complex can be used in the diagnosis of heart disease. These illustrations do *not* provide a realistic basis for the electrocardiographic diagnosis of cardiac disease, which is described in the many excellent textbooks of clinical cardiology and electrocardiography.

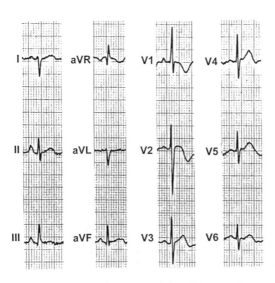

FIGURE 15-36 Right ventricular hypertrophy. The tall R wave in lead V_1 is due to abnormally large electrical forces directed toward the right ventricle. Unlike bundle branch block (Fig. 15-32), the QRS complex is not prolonged.

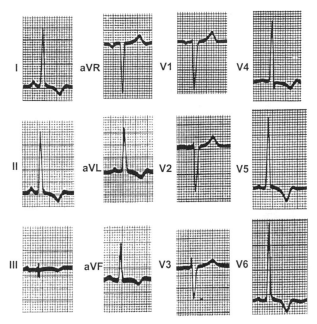

FIGURE 15-37 Left ventricular hypertrophy. The tall R waves in the left precordial leads (V₅ and V₆) are caused by abnormally large electrical forces directed toward the left ventricle. Unlike bundle branch block (Fig. 15-33), the QRS complex is not prolonged.

BIBLIOGRAPHY

The many different textbooks of electrocardiography have strengths and weaknesses. No single text is recommended because learning styles and tastes differ among students. Excellent and authoritative bibliographies are found in:

Friedman HH (1985). Diagnostic Electrocardiography and Vectorcardiography. Third Ed., NY, McGraw-Hill.

Gima K, Rudy Y (2002). Ionic current basis of electrocardiographic waveforms. A model study. Circ Res 90:889–896.

See also bibliographies to Chapters 13 and 14.

REFERENCES

James TN. Cardiac innervation: anatomic and pharmacologic relations. *Bull NY Acad Sci* 1967;43:1041–1086.

Lange PS, Er F, Gassanov N, et al. Andersen mutations of KCNJ2 suppress the native inward rectifier current I_{K1} in a dominant-negative fashion. *Cardiovasc Res* 2003;59:321–327.

Wenckebach KF, Winterberg H. Die unregelmässige Herztätigkeit. Leipzig: Wilhelm Engelmann, 1927.

Wu J, Wu J, Zipes DP. Early afterdepolarizations, U waves, and torsades de pointes. *Circulation* 202;105:675–676.

16

ARRHYTHMIAS

Cardiac arrhythmias were first noted in antiquity, when diagnosis was often based on the arterial pulse. Hippocrates observed that a slow pulse in elderly men heralded sudden death, and Galen predicted the imminent death of an otherwise healthy physician who had observed that his pulse was irregular. These and similar observations were systematized in the late 19th century, when smoked drum kymograph recordings of arterial and venous pulsations were used to define simple arrhythmias. Knowledge advanced rapidly at the beginning of the 20th century, when Einthoven's invention of the string galvanometer made it possible to record abnormalities of cardiac rate and rhythm in both experimental animals and patients. By mid-century, when many key features of clinical arrhythmias had been described (Katz and Pick, 1956), attention shifted to the physiological mechanisms that disturb impulse formation and propagation. Intracardiac recordings, which became available in the 1960s—along with advances in basic electrophysiology based on microelectrode recordings of intracellular potentials and, subsequently, on patch clamp measurements of the opening and closing of single ion channels—added further to the understanding of arrhythmogenic mechanisms. This understanding is now being extended by molecular biology, which has begun to characterize arrhythmogenic mechanisms in terms of the structures of specific voltage-gated ion channels (see Chapters 13–15).

A GENERAL CLASSIFICATION OF ARRHYTHMIAS

Normal heart rate is defined as 60 to 100 beats per minute (the phrase beats per minute is omitted in the remainder of this text), which was chosen because these limits correspond to 5 and 3 large (0.2 sec) "boxes" between QRS complexes in the standard ECG. Arrhythmias can occur when the heart beats too slowly (*bradycardias*) as well as when heart rate is too rapid (*tachycardias*) (Table 16-1). The causes of arrhythmias are generally described in terms of the structure where the arrhythmia is believed to have originated and the type of abnormality presumed to have altered the rhythm (Table 16-2).

It would seem logical that the causes of tachycardias are fundamentally different from those responsible for bradycardias, and that

TABLE 16-1 A Simple Classification of Clinical Arrhythmias

I. Bradycardias
   A. Sinus (SA) node
      1. Sinus bradycardia
      2. Sinoatrial block
   B. Atrioventricular (AV) node and bundle; atrioventricular block
      1. First-degree AV block
      2. Second-degree AV block
         a. Mobitz I (the Wenckebach phenomenon), usually block in the AV node
         b. Mobitz II, usually block in the AV bundle, bundle branches, and fascicles or in the distal His–Purkinje system
      3. Third-degree AV block
II. Tachycardias
   A. Premature systoles
      1. Atrial
      2. Junctional
      3. Ventricular
   B. Tachycardias
      1. Supraventricular
         a. Sinus
         b. Atrial
         c. Junctional
      2. Ventricular
   C. Flutter and Fibrillation
      1. Atrial
      2. Ventricular

---

mechanisms which cause extra depolarizations are the opposite of those that slow the heart. As is often the case, however, what seems obvious is wrong! Instead, many of the mechanisms responsible for bradyarrhythmias also cause tachyarrhythmias.

MECHANISMS RESPONSIBLE FOR BRADYARRHYTHMIAS

The most common causes of a slow pulse are *reduced pacemaker activity* (*chronotropy*) and *depressed conduction* (*dromotropy*). The former is caused by changes in the ionic currents responsible for sinoatrial (SA) node depolarization (see Chapter 14), while the latter, generally called *block*, occurs when conduction of the sinus impulse to the ventricles is impaired.

TABLE 16-2 A Simple Classification of Arrhythmogenic Mechanisms and Some Putative Electrophysiological Causes

I. Bradycardias
  A. Slowed SA node pacemaker activity
  B. Depressed (slowed) impulse conduction
    1. SA block
    2. AV block
      a. In AV node
      b. In AV bundle, bundle branches, or distal His–Purkinje system

II. Tachycardias
  A. Accelerated pacemaker activity
  B. Reentry
    1. Abnormal conduction (decremental conduction and unidirectional block)
    2. Inhomogeneities of the action potential characteristics
      a. Inhomogeneous resting potential
      b. Inhomogeneous depolarization
      c. Inhomogeneous repolarization and refractoriness
    3. Abnormal conducting structures
      a. Dual AV nodal conduction pathways
      b. Accessory pathway (bundle of Kent)
  C. Triggered depolarizations (afterdepolarizations)
    1. Early afterdepolarizations
    2. Delayed afterdepolarizations

Slowed Pacemaker Activity

The most common cause of slowing of the SA node pacemaker, called *sinus bradycardia*, is excessive parasympathetic (vagal) tone. Although a heart rate below 60 is by definition abnormal, sinus bradycardia is commonly seen in normal individuals in whom training has increased vagal tone. Hypothyroidism slows the sinus pacemaker, as do drugs, including β-adrenergic blockers and some L-type calcium channel blockers. Sinus bradycardia also can be caused by a condition, commonly seen in the elderly, that has the sibilant name *sick sinus syndrome*; because this syndrome can be accompanied by atrioventricular (AV) block and supraventricular tachycardias, it is sometimes called the *bradycardia–tachycardia syndrome*. When severe, sinus slowing can cause vasovagal syncope (the "swoon"), but rarely causes sudden death.

Abnormal slowing of "lower" pacemakers in the AV node or His–Purkinje system (AV bundle, bundle branches, fascicles) cannot cause

TABLE 16-3   **Major Sites of Conduction Block**

Site of Block	Usual Cause	Effect on the ECG
SA node	Structural or functional	Absent or delayed P waves
AV node	Functional	Prolonged PR interval or P waves not followed by QRS complexes
His–Purkinje system (AV bundle, both bundle branches; all three fascicles.)	Structural	Prolonged PR interval or P waves not followed by QRS complexes

a bradycardia as long as the ventricles are depolarized by impulses conducted from a normally functioning SA node. Failure of lower pacemakers is therefore apparent only if sinus rate is markedly slowed or conduction is blocked.

Depressed Conduction (Block)

The second cause of bradycardias, called *block*, occurs when impulse conduction is impaired. Depressed conduction can delay impulse propagation without altering the rate of ventricular beating, but when severe, this causes "dropped" (absent) beats. Three regions of the heart are especially vulnerable to block (Table 16-3); in two, the SA and AV nodes, conduction is normally slow and the safety factor low (Chapter 14). The third is the His–Purkinje system which, despite large action potentials and a high safety factor, is anatomically precarious because it includes critical conducting structures that are often small strands of tissue and so can be damaged or destroyed by disease.

SLOWING OF IMPULSE CONDUCTION. Conduction of the cardiac action potential depends on *ionic* and *electrotonic currents* that determine the *cable properties* of the heart (Figs. 16-1 and 16-2). The former include transverse currents that flow through plasma membrane ion channels and longitudinal currents that flow through gap junctions in the intercalated disc

FIGURE 16-1 Cable properties in a strand of cardiac muscle. Conduction (*from left to right*) depends on longitudinal extracellular electronic currents (*indicated by arrows*) between depolarized tissue (*shaded, left*) and resting tissue (*unshaded, right*), and ionic currents that flow transversely across the plasma membrane and longitudinally across the intercalated discs.

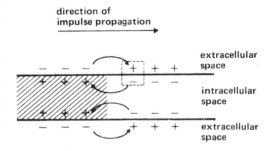

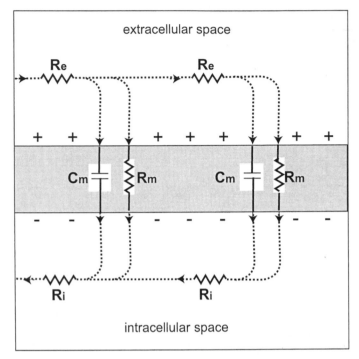

FIGURE 16-2   Current flow (*arrows*) across the region of the cardiac plasma membrane (*shaded*) within the small rectangle in Figure 16-1. Longitudinal currents are influenced by extracellular and intracellular resistances **Re** and **Ri**, respectively, while transverse current flow is determined by membrane resistance **(Rm)** and membrane capacitance **(Cm)**. Increased longitudinal resistance **(Re, Ri)** slows conduction, whereas increased membrane resistance **(Rm)** accelerates conduction.

(see Chapters 13 and 14). Block can be caused by excessive slowing of impulse conduction and therefore can result from abnormalities in any of the determinants of conduction velocity: action potential amplitude, rate of rise of the action potential, threshold, and internal and external electrical resistances (Table 16-4).

Two of the four determinants of conduction velocity listed in Table 16-4, *action potential amplitude* and *rate of depolarization*, are proportional to the inward, depolarizing currents responsible for the upstroke of the action potential. The third, *threshold*, reflects the ability of the depolarizing channels to be opened by an approaching wave of depolarization. *Electrical resistance*, the fourth determinant, is complex because longitudinal resistance (in the extracellular space and between the cytosol in adjacent cells) and transverse resistance (across the plasma membrane) have different effects on conduction velocity (see below).

Mechanisms that accelerate conduction include increased magnitude and more rapid appearance of the ionic currents that depolarize the plasma membrane, both shorten the time required for a wave of depolarization

TABLE 16-4 **Determinants of Conduction Velocity in the Heart**

Determinant	Structural and Functional Mechanism
Action potential amplitude	Number of open sodium or calcium channels in the plasma membrane
Rate of rise of the action potential	Number and rate of opening of sodium or calcium channels in the plasma membrane
Threshold	Amount of depolarization needed to open sodium or calcium channels in the plasma membrane
Electrical resistances	
Longitudinal	
Extracellular	Conductivity through the extracellular space
Intracellular	Number of open gap junction (connexon) channels in the intercalated disc, myocyte diameter
Transverse	Number of open plasma ion channels, membrane capacitance

to bring nearby resting tissue to its threshold. This is readily understood because larger action potentials initiate depolarizing currents further ahead of the wave front, while more rapid depolarization increases the rate at which the depolarizing currents reach resting tissue. The role of *threshold* is seen in the ability of a lowered threshold to extend the distance over which a propagated action potential can be initiated by an approaching wave of depolarization. The effects of *electrical resistances* on conduction velocity are complex because changes in longitudinal and transverse resistances have opposite effects. Decreasing internal resistance, which can occur when the gap junction channels in the intercalated disc are opened, *speeds* conduction by increasing longitudinal current flow (Fig. 16-2), whereas decreasing transverse resistance *slows* conduction by shunting current across the plasma membrane into the cell, which reduces the flow of longitudinal currents.

The determinants of conduction velocity can be equated to a row of falling dominoes (Fig. 16-3), where increasing the height of the dominoes, like increasing action potential amplitude, accelerates "impulse" transmission by allowing each falling domino to reach further ahead. Increasing the velocity at which each domino falls (as would occur if the dominoes were moved to the surface of Jupiter), like increasing the rate of depolarization, also accelerates transmission. If each domino were tipped slightly to reduce the energy needed to make it fall, the decreased mechanical threshold, like decreased threshold, would increase the velocity of propagation. Finally, placing the row of dominoes in a vacuum, like reducing longitudinal resistance, would increase conduction velocity by accelerating their rate of fall.

direction of
impulse propagation

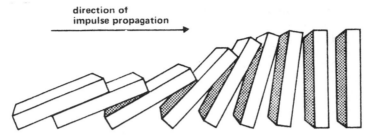

FIGURE 16-3 Propagation of an action potential viewed as a row of dominoes falling from left to right. Conduction is accelerated when the height of the dominoes is increased, each domino falls more rapidly, the inertia needed to tip each domino is decreased, or the resistance encountered as each falling domino is decreased.

Rapid conduction in the working cells of the atria, ventricles, and His–Purkinje system reflects the large number of sodium channels, which open rapidly and carry large depolarizing currents; conversely, the slower conduction velocity in the SA and AV nodes is due to the slower opening, lower conductance, and smaller number of the calcium channels that depolarize these cells. Refractoriness slows conduction by reducing the amplitude and rate of rise of action potentials (see Chapter 13). Closing of gap junction channels, which occurs in calcium-overloaded or acidotic hearts, slows conduction by increasing internal longitudinal resistance. Internal resistance also is high in cells with a small diameter. Extracellular fibrosis slows conduction by increasing resistance to longitudinal current flow outside of cells.

DECREMENTAL CONDUCTION AND BLOCK. Decremental conduction can occur when an action potential enters a region of the heart where conduction velocity is slowed (Fig. 16-4). If depression of the ability to generate a propagated action potential is so severe that the action potential ceases to serve as an effective stimulus to the excitable tissue ahead, conduction is blocked completely (Fig. 16-5). Decremental conduction is not always abnormal—for example, in the AV node, where cells have a small diameter, few gap junctions, and slowly rising calcium-dependent action potentials. These properties explain why conduction in the AV node is normally slow and why this structure is susceptible to block.

UNIDIRECTIONAL BLOCK. *Unidirectional block*, which is both common and clinically important, plays a role in the genesis of arrhythmias by disorganizing impulse propagation and causing conduction to fail. The term means what it implies: block of conduction, but in only one direction. Unidirectional block is a normal property of the AV node, where antegrade (forward) conduction from atria to ventricles is usually more rapid than retrograde (backward) conduction from ventricles to atria.

The classical model for unidirectional block is a strand of myocardial tissue compressed by a wedge-shaped wooden block, which causes an

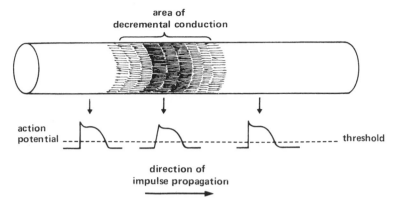

FIGURE 16-4 Decremental conduction in a region of slow conduction—for example, where the amplitude and rate of rise of the action potential are decreased (*shaded*). When an action potential transmitted in a strand of cardiac muscle encounters a region of decremental conduction (*top*), it becomes smaller and more slowly rising (*bottom*), but once the impulse has crossed the region of decremental conduction and emerges into normal tissue (*right*), a normal action potential is again generated, although after a delay. This behavior is a normal property of conduction through the AV node.

asymmetrically distributed impairment of conduction (Fig. 16-6) because when more pressure is applied to the tissue, conduction is more severely depressed. This is shown in (Figures 16-7 to 16-9), which illustrates how unidirectional block is produced in a 10-cm long strand of myocardium, and why conduction can fail in the retrograde direction (defined in these figures from right to left) but not in the antegrade direction (from left to right). The ability of different regions of the strand to initiate a regenerative response is plotted on the ordinate as the distance ahead that a propagated action potential can be initiated. Normal action potentials in the uncompressed

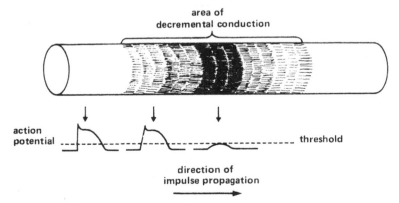

FIGURE 16-5 Conduction can be blocked completely in a strand of cardiac muscle containing a region of severe decremental conduction (*darkest shading*) in which action potentials are unable to bring the normal tissue ahead of the impulse to its threshold.

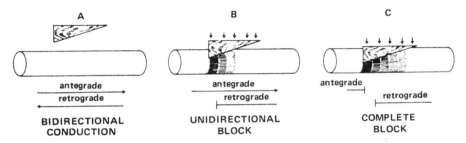

A   B   C

antegrade
retrograde

antegrade
retrograde

antegrade
retrograde

BIDIRECTIONAL
CONDUCTION

UNIDIRECTIONAL
BLOCK

COMPLETE
BLOCK

FIGURE 16-6   Unidirectional block produced by compression of a strand of cardiac muscle by a wedge-shaped wooden block (*darker shading indicates a greater degree of injury*).
A: Bidirectional conduction in the normal, uncompressed tissue. **B:** Moderate compression causes unidirectional block in which conduction can proceed from left to right
(defined here as the antegrade direction) but not from right to left (retrograde block).
C: Severe compression blocks conduction in both directions.

regions, from 0 to 2 cm and from 8 to 10 cm, can activate resting tissue up
to 2 cm ahead (Fig. 16-7), while between 2 and 3 cm, under the point of the
wedge, the strand is so severely damaged as to have completely lost the ability to initiate a propagated action potential. Action potentials in the less
depressed region, between 3 and 8 cm, can activate resting tissue but,
depending on the degree of compression, for only short distances ahead.

Action potentials initiated at 0 cm are conducted in the antegrade
direction (Fig. 16-8). Normal impulses in the uncompressed tissue, between
0 and 2 cm, generate a wave of depolarization that can cross the severely
depressed area between 2 and 3 cm. Although the latter cannot generate a
propagated impulse, electrotonic spread of current from the normal regions
can generate an action potential 2 cm ahead (arrow a in Fig. 16-8), which initiates an action potential at 4 cm. Although the tissue at 4 cm is depressed,

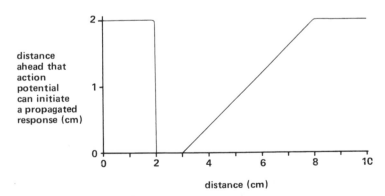

distance
ahead that
action
potential
can initiate
a propagated
response (cm)

distance (cm)

FIGURE 16-7   Distribution of the ability of the moderately compressed strand of cardiac
muscle (Fig. 16-6B) to generate a propagated action potential. Normal tissue (at 0–2 and
8–10 cm) can activate resting muscle up to 2 cm ahead. The ability of the tissue between
2 and 3 cm to initiate a propagated action potential is completely lost and is depressed
from 3 to 8 cm.

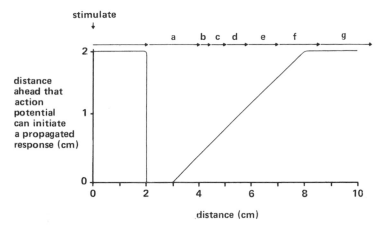

FIGURE 16-8 Antegrade conduction in the strand of cardiac muscle shown in Figure 16-7. An impulse entering from the left is able to cross the most severely depressed region, where the ability to initiate a propagated action potential has been lost, although antegrade conduction (left to right) is delayed.

it is able to depolarize tissue a short distance (0.4 cm) ahead, at 4.4 cm (arrow b); here the action potential is less depressed and therefore conducts 0.6 cm to the right, reaching the tissue at 5.0 cm (arrow c). At 5.0 cm, the ability to conduct is still less depressed, so the impulse continues to propagate to the right, gaining speed as it emerges from the depressed area until it reaches uncompressed tissue at 8 cm. Because conduction velocity is directly

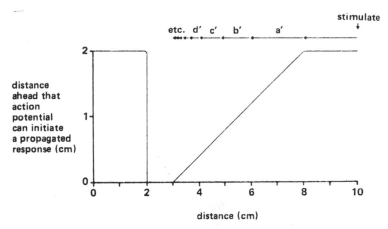

FIGURE 16-9 Retrograde block in the strand of cardiac muscle shown in Figure 16-7. An impulse entering from the right encounters increasingly impaired conduction, so the impulse becomes progressively less able to initiate an action potential. As the impulse approaches the most severely depressed tissue (from 2 to 3 cm), the responses become so small that they cannot excite the resting tissue ahead; as a result, retrograde conduction (right to left) is blocked.

proportional to the lengths of the arrows in Figure 16-8, the antegrade impulse reaches normal tissue to the right after a delay.

When retrograde condition is initiated by stimulating the tissue at 10 cm, rather than at 0 cm, the conduction abnormality is quite different (Fig. 16-9). At 8 cm, although the impulse encounters damaged tissue and conduction begins to slow, it is still conducted normally to the left and so depolarizes the tissue 2 cm ahead, at 6 cm, where action potentials can propagate only 1.2 cm (arrow a'). The next area to be depolarized is therefore at 4.8 cm (the head of arrow b'), where the action potential can conduct only 0.8 cm to reach the tissue at 4 cm (arrow c'). Here, the action potential conducts an even shorter distance (arrow d'). The speed of action potential propagation continues to decrease, as evidenced by the shorter arrows, until the impulse reaches the severely depressed area at 3 cm where, because propagated action potentials can no longer be generated, retrograde conduction is blocked.

Unidirectional block is common in diseased hearts—for example, in areas of ischemia or scarring where nonuniform depression of conduction velocity can be caused by heterogeneous refractoriness or resting depolarization. Asymmetrical fibrosis, which slows conduction by increasing longitudinal resistance, along with nonuniform reduction in the number of open gap junction channels and an asymmetrical increase in threshold, also can cause unidirectional block.

MECHANISMS RESPONSIBLE FOR TACHYARRHYTHMIAS

Tachyarrhythmias are generally described in terms of how they appear clinically (Table 16-1). A single early beat is a *premature systole*, and a series of premature systoles is a *tachycardia*. Very rapid regular activation of the atria or ventricles is called *flutter*, while disorganization of activation, where there is no effective beating, is *fibrillation*. Three mechanisms account for most tachyarrhythmias: accelerated pacemaker activity, reentry, and triggered depolarizations (Table 16-2). All can occur in many regions of the heart as a single premature systole or a sustained tachycardia.

Accelerated Pacemaker Activity

The most easily understood of the mechanisms responsible for premature systoles and tachycardias is accelerated firing of a pacemaker cell. This mechanism, which operates in the SA node to cause *sinus tachycardia*, also occurs in "lower" pacemakers, where it can cause a *junctional tachycardia* and *accelerated idioventricular rhythm*.

Reentry

The definition of a reentrant beat is simple: Reentry occurs when a single impulse traveling through the heart gives rise to two or more propagated responses. However, several mechanisms cause reentrant arrhythmias (Table 16-2).

ABNORMAL CONDUCTION (DECREMENTAL CONDUCTION AND UNIDIRECTIONAL BLOCK).
The ability of decremental conduction and unidirectional block to cause premature systoles and tachycardias can be seen at the junction between a Purkinje fiber and the ventricular myocardium (Fig 16-10a) or within a bundle of branched myocardial fibers (Fig. 16-10b). A premature systole can be initiated when a wave of depolarization reaches an area where

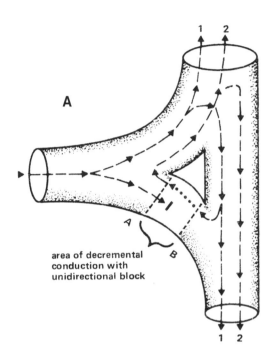

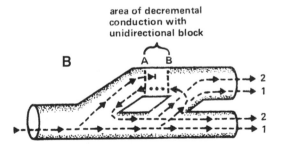

FIGURE 16-10 Reentry where a Purkinje fiber impinges on the ventricular myocardium (a) and within a branched strand of cardiac muscle (b). In both situations, a region of decremental conduction and unidirectional block (between **A** to **B**) prevents antegrade conduction, but if the impulse travels around the depressed area (1), it can be conducted slowly through the depressed region in the retrograde direction (*dotted line from* **B** *to* **A**). After a delay, the retrograde impulse can re-enter the myocardium proximal to the region of decremental conduction; if this occurs after the tissue proximal to the depressed area has recovered from the first impulse, the retrograde impulse can initiate a premature systole (2).

SUMMATION

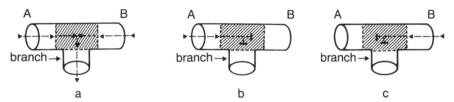

FIGURE 16-11   Summation. Weak impulses arriving simultaneously in a region of decremental conduction (*cross-hatched*) from opposite directions (**A** and **B**) can be summated to initiate a propagated action potential in an adjacent branch (**a**). However, if only one weak impulse enters the area of decremental conduction (**b**, **c**), it is not propagated into the branch.

antegrade conduction is blocked because the impulse cannot cross the depressed region (A in Fig. 16-10 a and b). However, if propagation through other regions of the heart brings the impulse to the distal end of the depressed area, it can be conducted in a retrograde direction through the area of unidirectional block (B in Fig. 16-10 a and b). This enables the impulse to reach the proximal end of the depressed area after a delay that, if it is long enough for the proximal tissue to recover its excitability, can allow the retrograde impulse to depolarize (re-enter) the proximal region and generate a premature systole. Passage of the retrograde impulse usually increases the refractoriness of the depressed area, which blocks conduction in both directions and terminates reentry, but this process can become repetitive so as to generate a sustained tachycardia.

Two phenomena, called *summation* and *inhibition*, are seen in areas of decremental conduction and unidirectional block. Summation occurs when two subthreshold impulses that alone cannot initiate a response act together to generate a propagated action potential (Fig. 16-11). Inhibition, which is seen when a nonpropagated (subthreshold) action potential blocks conduction of a subsequent impulse (Fig. 16-12), explains a phenomenon called *concealed conduction* (see below).

INHOMOGENEITIES IN THE ACTION POTENTIAL. Heterogeneous distribution of virtually any abnormality in the cardiac action potential can disorganize the spread of the wave of depolarization, therefore causing a reentrant arrhythmia.

Regional depolarization, a common substrate for reentrant arrhythmias, is especially important in the early minutes or hours following an acute myocardial infarction, when potassium loss from energy-starved cells reduces resting potential across the plasma membrane (see Chapter 17). Two mechanisms allow localized areas of resting depolarization to cause arrhythmias: inactivation of depolarizing sodium and calcium currents, and the spread of electrotonic currents, called *injury currents*, between partially depolarized and normal regions that can activate resting

INHIBITION

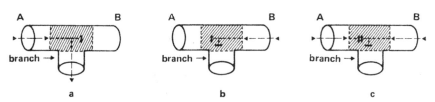

a   b   c

FIGURE 16-12   Inhibition. An impulse entering from one side (**A**) of a region of decremental conduction and unidirectional block (*cross-hatched*) is able to initiate a propagated action potential in an adjacent branch (**a**), whereas an impulse entering the region of decremental conduction from the other direction (**B**) is blocked (**b**). If the weaker impulse (from **B**) enters the region of decremental conduction immediately before the arrival of the stronger impulse (from **A**), the weaker impulse can prevent the branch from being activated (**c**).

cells (Fig. 16-13). Heterogeneities in the rate of rise and amplitude of the action potential, which can result from localized areas of ischemia or injury, and regional variations in refractoriness, also cause reentry.

Inhomogeneity of repolarization and refractoriness can initiate electrotonic current flow between regions of the heart that have repolarized at different times (Fig. 16-14); by delaying sodium and calcium channel reactivation, these heterogeneities can cause decremental conduction and unidirectional block. Inhomogeneity of repolarization is seen in regional ischemia, which can shorten and lengthen refractoriness (see Chapter 17), and in the severely damaged myocardium of patients with end-stage heart failure. Regional concentrations of mutated ion channels and local variations in the distribution of potassium channels, notably the stress-activated channels responsible for i_{to}, also can cause these inhomogeneities.

ABNORMAL CONDUCTING STRUCTURES. Abnormal conducting structures that link the atria and ventricles (see Chapter 15) can create electrical "short circuits" across the central fibrous body that cause reentrant supraventricular tachycardias. Most important are dual AV nodal conduction pathways and accessory pathways, which can generate *reciprocal rhythms* where impulses cross back and forth between the atria and ventricles.

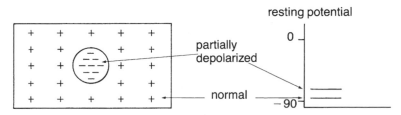

FIGURE 16-13   Inhomogeneous resting potential in which the potential at the surface of a group of partially depolarized cells (*center*) is more negative than that of the nearby normal tissue. These differences in resting potential can allow the depolarized cells to activate surrounding tissue.

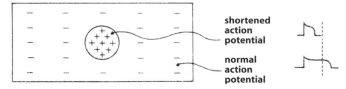

FIGURE 16-14 Inhomogeneous repolarization. Return to resting potential in a group of cells with abnormally short action potentials (*center*) can allow adjacent normal cells to depolarize the cells with the shorter action potential (*vertical dashed line, right*). A similar mechanism allows cells with abnormally long action potentials to reactivate nearby normal tissue.

DUAL AV NODAL CONDUCTION PATHWAYS. In some patients, AV conduction can be effected by two parallel pathways (Fig. 16-15). Because these pathways were initially believed to lie side-by-side within the AV node, they are called *dual AV nodal conduction pathways*, although it is now clear that the faster of the two pathways is frequently located in the lower right atrium outside of the AV node (Fig. 16-15). Because action potentials in the two pathways often have different durations and conduct at different speeds, they provide a substrate for reciprocal rhythms that cross back and forth between the atria and ventricles. This mechanism, in which antegrade impulses (from atria to ventricles) are propagated in one pathway and the retrograde impulses (from ventricles to atria) in the other, is the most common cause of the paroxysmal supraventricular tachycardias (see below).

ACCESSORY PATHWAYS, PRE-EXCITATION, AND THE WOLFF-PARKINSON-WHITE SYN-DROME. An accessory pathway (bundle of Kent), which is generally a strand of atrial myocardium located virtually anywhere along the AV junction, provides an electrical short circuit between the atria and ventricles (Fig. 16-16). Because accessory pathways are depolarized by sodium channel opening, and so conduct more rapidly than the AV node, impulses conducted from the atria through the accessory pathway reach the ventricles ahead of impulses conducted normally through the AV node (see Chapter 15).

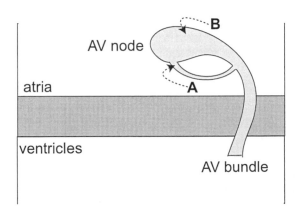

FIGURE 16-15 Dual AV nodal conduction pathways. The two pathways (**A** *and* **B**) can establish reentrant circuits that cause supraventricular tachycardias.

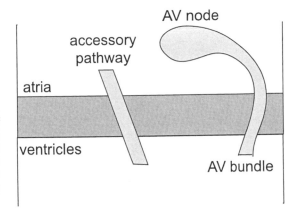

FIGURE 16-16 Pre-excitation. An accessory pathway (bundle of Kent), which is usually a strand of atrial tissue that crosses the fibrous skeleton of the heart (shaded), provides an abnormal conduction pathway linking the atria and ventricles.

Impulses conducted down an accessory pathway do not enter the ventricles by way of the His–Purkinje system and therefore initiate ventricular depolarization at an abnormal site, which alters the initial deflection of the QRS complex. This pathophysiology explains the clinical features of *pre-excitation* (the *Wolff-Parkinson-White syndrome* or *WPW*), which includes a short PR interval (<0.12 sec) and a distorted initial deflection of the QRS (called a *delta wave*) because it resembles the left half of a greek delta (Fig. 16-17).

Pre-excitation has recently been found in patients with hypertrophic cardiomyopathies caused by abnormalities in glycogen metabolism (see Chapter 18). The conduction abnormality is associated with gaps in the central fibrous body, possibly related to intracellular glycogen accumulation, through which strands of myocardium establish short-circuits between the atria and ventricles.

CIRCUS MOVEMENTS. Reentry was described as a "circus movement" by G. R. Mines in the early 20th century. Using a ring of excitable tissue (a

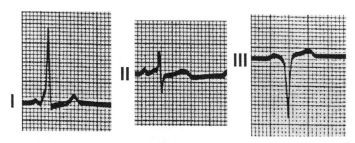

FIGURE 16-17 Pre-excitation (Wolff-Parkinson-White syndrome) recorded in the Einthoven bipolar leads. The PR interval is abnormally short (0.08 sec in lead I) because of rapid conduction through an accessory pathway, while the slurred upstroke of the QRS complex in lead I (the delta wave) is caused when this impulse initiates ventricular depolarization at an abnormal site.

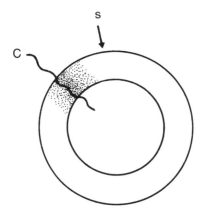

FIGURE 16-18 Initiation of a circus movement. When a ring of excitable tissue is lightly clamped (C) and stimulated alongside of the clamp (s), conduction is transiently blocked, so the wave of depolarization can propagate in only the clockwise direction. If the clamp is removed before the wave of depolarization returns to the area of block, the impulse continues to circle the ring.

jellyfish mantle), Mines caused unidirectional block by gently cross-clamping the ring and stimulating the tissue next to the clamp (Fig. 16-18). This allowed the resulting wave of depolarization to propagate in only one direction (clockwise in the example shown in Fig. 16-18) because conduction in the other direction was blocked by the clamp. If the clamp was removed before the impulse returned to the site of local block, the wave of depolarization traveled clockwise around the ring in a circus movement that continued until the tissue deteriorated and the circulating wave died out (Fig. 16-19).

Propagation of a circus movement can be interrupted if the leading edge of the wave of depolarization "catches up" with the refractory state left

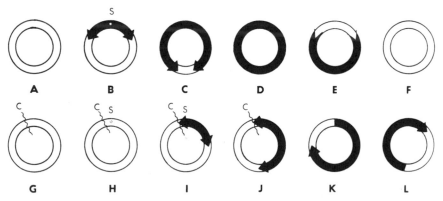

FIGURE 16-19 Initiation of a circus movement in a ring of excitable tissue containing an area of decremental conduction and unidirectional block. *Unshaded* areas are resting, *shaded* areas are activated. **Upper row:** Stimulation in the absence of block (S) depolarizes the ring in both directions (B,C), which leads to mutual cancellation of the two impulses (D) and failure to establish a circus movement. **Lower row:** When counterclockwise propagation is blocked, as in Figure 16-18, the stimulus (S) initiates a wave of depolarization that propagates only in the clockwise direction (I–K). If the impulse crosses the area of block (L), the wave of depolarization continues to circle the ring in the clockwise direction.

behind after its previous circuit, which extinguishes the circulating wave. This allows three mechanisms to stop a circus movement (Fig. 16-20). The first is to *depress conduction*—for example, by inactivating the channels that carry the inward currents propagating the wave of depolarization (*left*, Fig. 16-20a). The second is to *accelerate conduction* so that the wave of depolarization "catches up" with regions that are still refractory after the prior passage of the wave front (*left*, Fig. 16-20b). The third mechanism is to *prolong the refractory period*, which can extinguish the wave of depolarization when it reaches tissue that has not recovered from the prior passage of the impulse (*right*, Fig. 16-20c). A classical analogy is to view the impulse traveling around the circular pathway as a snake which, if its head catches up with its tail, bites itself, and dies. According to this analogy, depressing conduction is like killing the snake, while speeding the progress of its head or retarding the forward motion of its tail allows the snake to bite itself to death.

Triggered Depolarizations

Triggered depolarizations, which can result from early and late afterdepolarizations (see Chapter 14), cause premature systoles and tachycardias in the atria, His–Purkinje system, and ventricles. These are often the result of calcium overload, which explains why they differ from tachyarrhythmias caused by most other mechanisms listed in Table 16-2 that generally are suppressed by rapid stimulation. The latter phenomenon (called *overdrive suppression*), occurs because frequent depolarization

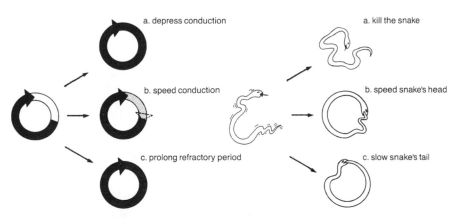

FIGURE 16-20 Three ways to stop the circus movement described in Figure 16-19. **Left:** The circus movement can be terminated if conduction is depressed **(a)**; if conduction velocity is accelerated so that the front of the impulse reaches the previously depolarized tissue during its refractory period **(b)**; or if prolongation of the refractory period allows the front of the wave of depolarization to reach the previously depolarized tissue before the latter has recovered from the preceding passage of the circus movement **(c)**. **Right:** These mechanisms can be viewed in terms of a snake traveling in a circle. The snake stops if it dies **(a)**, if its head reaches far enough ahead to bite its tail **(b)**, or if its tail lags behind so as to come within biting distance of the advancing head **(c)**.

increases sodium entry, which generates an outward repolarizing current by stimulating sodium efflux by way of the electrogenic sodium pump (see Chapters 7 and 14). The resulting increase in resting potential inhibits decremental conduction by reactivating sodium and calcium channels. In contrast, rapid electrical stimulation does not suppress calcium overload-induced afterdepolarizations. Instead, triggered depolarizations are made worse because more rapid stimulation increases calcium flux into the cytosol, which increases the depolarizing currents generated during calcium efflux from the cytosol by way of the Na–Ca exchanger (see Chapters 7 and 14).

CLINICAL ARRHYTHMIAS

The mechanisms and electrocardiographic features of several clinical arrhythmias, along with a few therapeutic principles, are detailed in the following pages to illustrate some clinical applications of the material covered above and in Chapters 13 to 15.

ABNORMALITIES OF THE SINUS NODE

The normal heart rate is determined by the frequency of depolarization of the SA (sinus) node pacemaker. By convention, a rate faster than 100 that originates in the SA node is a *sinus tachycardia*, while slowing of the SA node pacemaker to a rate less than 60 is a *sinus bradycardia*.

Sinus Tachycardia

The electrocardiographic characteristics of sinus tachycardia (Fig. 16-21) are normal QRS complexes preceded by normal P waves that occur at a rate greater than 100. P waves are normal because the tachycardia originates in the SA node, while the PR interval and QRS complexes are normal because the ventricles are depolarized normally by way of the AV node, AV bundle, and His–Purkinje system. (Atrioventricular and intraventricular conduction may be abnormal in sinus and other supraventricular tachycardias when heart rate is extremely rapid or the heart is diseased.)

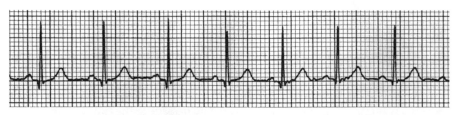

FIGURE 16-21 Sinus tachycardia (lead II). The rates of atrial and ventricular depolarization are approximately 120. Each QRS complex, which is normal, follows a normal P wave after a normal PR interval of 0.12 sec.

Sinus tachycardia typically begins and ends gradually, and is usually slowed by vagal stimulation; these characteristics distinguish this common—and usually benign—arrhythmia from paroxysmal supraventricular tachycardia (see below).

Increased sympathetic activity and reduced vagal tone, which occur normally during physical exercise and emotional stress, are the most important causes of sinus tachycardia (see Chapter 14); other causes include fever, anemia, hyperthyroidism, and stretch of the SA node (the Bainbridge reflex).

The maximum rate of exercise-induced sinus tachycardia is sometimes stated to equal 220 minus the patient's age, so a healthy 20-year-old is expected to achieve a sinus rate of 200, while maximum sinus rate during exertion by a 70-year-old is only 150. This relationship, however, is highly variable.

Sinus Bradycardia

By definition, sinus bradycardia occurs when the SA node pacemaker rate is less than 60. The ECG in sinus bradycardia therefore shows a slow heart rate in which normal P waves are followed by normal QRS complexes after a normal PR interval (Fig. 16-22). The most common causes of sinus bradycardia are increased parasympathetic (vagal) activity and decreased sympathetic activity (see Chapter 14). The tonic parasympathetic tone that normally slows the sinus pacemaker is increased by physical conditioning, which explains the resting sinus bradycardia characteristic of the "athlete's heart." Severe sinus bradycardia can cause vasovagal syncope, once called a *swoon*, and can be triggered by reflexes in patients with acute inferior or posterior myocardial infarction (see Chapter 17). Drugs that cause sinus bradycardia include β-*adrenergic receptor blockers* and some *L-type calcium channel blockers*. The former inhibit pacemaker activity indirectly by reducing the synthesis of cyclic AMP, while the latter act directly to inhibit calcium channel opening in the SA node. *Cardiac glycosides* slow the SA node by a central effect that increases parasympathetic activity.

Sinus Arrhythmia and Wandering Pacemaker

A perfectly regular sinus rate is not, as might be expected, a sign of a healthy heart; instead, small variations in cycle length, called *sinus*

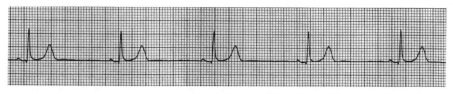

FIGURE 16-22   Sinus bradycardia (lead II). Normal QRS complexes follow normal P waves after a normal PR interval but at a rate of 45.

arrhythmia, are characteristically seen in normal individuals. This variability, which is caused by physiological oscillations in sympathetic and parasympathetic tone, is lost in patients with heart disease largely because of inappropriate overstimulation of the neurohumoral response (see Chapter 8). For this reason, clocklike regularity of the heart beat suggests that the normal fine tuning by the autonomic nervous system has been blunted. Decreased heart rate variability is one of the first signs of heart disease and tends to disappear with advancing age, so sinus arrhythmia actually is a sign of good health!

Changes in sinus rate that accompany normal respiration, called *respiratory sinus arrhythmia*, alter cycle length without affecting impulse propagation through the atria, AV node, and ventricles; for this reason, the only changes are in the firing rate of the SA node. (Fig. 16-23). Respiratory sinus arrhythmia occurs when stimuli arising in stretch receptors in the lung and chest wall alter the balance between sympathetic and parasympathetic influences on the SA node; heart rate accelerates during inspiration because of decreased vagal tone and increased sympathetic tone, while increased vagal tone and decreased sympathetic tone during expiration slow the SA node pacemaker.

Another common benign SA node arrhythmia is *wandering pacemaker*, which is characterized by changes in P-wave morphology (Fig. 16-24). This arrhythmia, which also can be related to respiration, is caused by shifts in the site of pacemaker activity within the SA node.

Sinoatrial Block

Heart rate can be slowed when impulses arising in the SA node fail to depolarize the atria (Fig. 16-25). This abnormality, called *SA block*, can

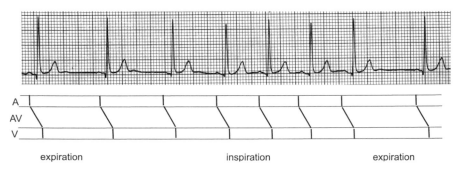

FIGURE 16-23 Respiratory sinus arrhythmia (lead II). Atrial and ventricular depolarization accelerate during inspiration and slow during expiration, but each QRS complex is preceded by a normal P wave and a normal PR interval. The arrhythmia is diagrammed below, using a "Lewis diagram;" the eponym recognizes Sir Thomas Lewis, a pioneer in electrocardiography. The *top line* represents the SA node, the *upper space* **(A)** the atria, the middle space **(AV)** the AV node, and the lower space **(V)** the ventricles. The downward angle of the lines represent the speed of impulse propagation. Each beat in this arrhythmia begins in the SA node and is conducted normally through the atria, AV node, and ventricles.

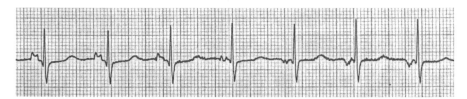

FIGURE 16-24 Wandering pacemaker (lead II). Heart rate in this series of sinus beats is regular, with cycle lengths between 0.69 and 0.72 sec. The marked changes in P-wave morphology can be explained by shifts in the location of the pacemaker within the SA node.

be difficult to distinguish from sinus bradycardia because depolarization of the SA node pacemaker cannot be recorded by the ECG (see Chapter 15). SA block can be caused by drugs and other factors that slow the SA node pacemaker (see above), by occlusion of the SA node artery, and by apoptosis, fibrosis, and degeneration of the nodal cells.

ABNORMALITIES OF ATRIOVENTRICULAR CONDUCTION

Abnormal conduction in the AV node can cause both bradyarrhythmias and tachyarrhythmias. The former are discussed below, while reentry in the AV junction, which can cause supraventricular tachycardias, is described later in this chapter.

The AV node has a low safety factor (see Chapter 14), so reduction in the size of its calcium-dependent action potentials is a common cause of AV block. However, not all impairment of AV conduction occurs in the AV node because diseases affecting the AV bundle, bundle branches, and fascicles, where conduction depends on sodium currents, also can inhibit conduction between the atria and ventricles. Although conduction abnormalities caused by depressed calcium-dependent conduction in the AV node and impaired sodium-dependent conduction in the His–Purkinje system are not readily distinguished by casual examination of the ECG, they occur in different patterns, have different causes and prognosis, and frequently require different treatment (see below).

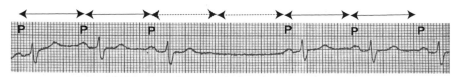

FIGURE 16-25 Sinoatrial block (lead II). P waves are regular throughout the record except after the third QRS complex, where a P wave is missing ("dropped"). The first P wave after the dropped beat occurs when it would have been expected had there been no interruption in the regular sinus P waves (*dashed arrows*), which indicates that the sinus impulse preceding the missing P wave failed to depolarize the atria because its exit from the SA node was blocked.

The terms *AV dissociation* and *AV block*, while often used inter-changeably, have different meanings. Atrioventricular *dissociation* refers to any condition that impairs impulse transmission from the atria to the ventricles, whereas AV *block* implies that the AV dissociation has been caused by abnormal conduction. For example, during a supraventricular tachycardia at a rate of 200, the normally low safety factor of the AV node often blocks every other P wave and so slows the ventricular rate to 100, therefore the abnormality is *2:1 AV dissociation* (two atrial beats for each ventricular beat). If, on the other hand, atrial rate is 100 and only half of the atrial impulses depolarize the ventricles, the condition is *2:1 AV block* because the normal AV node should be able to transmit 100 impulses each minute. This semantic distinction is useful in communicating the signifi-cance of AV conduction abnormalities.

First-, Second-, and Third-Degree Atrioventricular Block

Three degrees of AV block are recognized clinically: *first-degree AV block*, the mildest, is an abnormal delay in AV conduction that prolongs the PR interval; *second-degree AV block* is more severe because some, but not all, P waves fail to activate the ventricles; while in *third-degree AV block*, no impulses are conducted from the atria to the ventricles.

FIRST-DEGREE ATRIOVENTRICULAR BLOCK. First-degree AV block is readily identified by prolongation of the PR interval in an ECG where all P waves are followed by QRS complexes (Fig. 16-26). Although the delay between atrial and ventricular systole is increased, this abnormality has little or no effect on the pumping of the heart. Instead, the clinical significance of this arrhythmia is that it can herald the appearance of more severe AV block.

SECOND-DEGREE ATRIOVENTRICULAR BLOCK. Second-degree AV block, in which some but not all atrial impulses depolarize the ventricles, may or may not be accompanied by an irregular pulse. If, as in Figure 16-27, the sinus rate is regular at 96, but only one-half of the atrial impulses reach the ventricles, the pulse rate will be regular at a rate of 48. Without additional

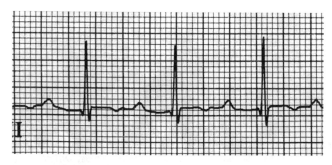

FIGURE 16-26 First-degree AV block (lead II). Each P wave is followed by a QRS complex, but the PR interval is abnormally prolonged to 0.26 sec.

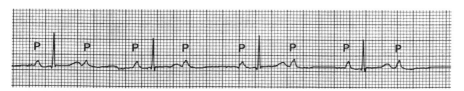

FIGURE 16-27 Second-degree AV block with 2:1 AV conduction (lead II). There are twice as many P waves (P) as QRS complexes, so every other atrial impulse is blocked.

information, such as analysis of the arterial and venous pulses or, more commonly, an ECG, it is not possible to tell whether the slow pulse is due to sinus bradycardia or to AV block. The obvious electrocardiographic feature of second-degree AV block is that some P waves are blocked ("dropped") because they are not followed by a QRS complex.

In uncomplicated second-degree AV block, all ventricular depolarizations are initiated by impulses propagated through the AV node; therefore all QRS complexes are preceded by a P wave, but because some atrial impulses fail to reach the ventricles, there are more P waves than QRS complexes. In 2:1 AV block, every other P wave is blocked (Fig. 16-27), but other ratios between P waves and QRS complexes are possible; in Figure 16-28, for example, every fifth P wave fails to reach the ventricles, so the rhythm is 5:4 AV block.

Changes in the PR interval that precede the blocked P waves are the basis for a classification of second-degree AV block that helps distinguish block in the AV node from the more dangerous form of AV block caused by impaired conduction in the His–Purkinje system.

MOBITZ I AND II SECOND-DEGREE ATRIOVENTRICULAR BLOCK. Mobitz I second-degree AV block occurs when the blocked P waves are preceded by progressive prolongation of the PR interval in a pattern called the *Wenckebach*

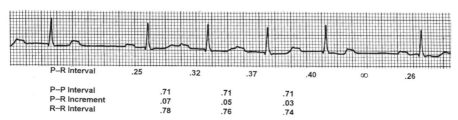

P–R Interval	.25	.32	.37	.40	∞	.26

P–P Interval	.71	.71	.71
P–R Increment	.07	.05	.03
R–R Interval	.78	.76	.74

FIGURE 16-28 Mobitz type I second-degree AV block demonstrating the Wenckebach phenomenon (lead II). Beginning with the second QRS complex, which is preceded by a PR interval of 0.25 sec, the PR intervals increase progressively until a P wave is completely blocked; this is the typical Wenckebach phenomenon. Because the PR prolongation occurs in decreasing increments, the intervals between successive QRS complexes (R–R intervals) shorten before the dropped beat; this causes a slight increase in ventricular rate, called *group beating*. The pause that follows the completely blocked P wave allows the AV junction to recover, which accounts for the shortened PR interval of the first cycle after the dropped beat.

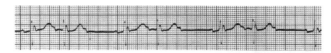

FIGURE 16-29 Mobitz type II second-degree AV block (lead V₁). In this example of 3:2 AV block, the PR interval before all of the conducted QRS complexes is 0.18 sec and does not increase prior to the dropped beats. The prolonged QRS complexes (0.14 sec) are probably a manifestation of the conduction system disease that caused the AV block.

phenomenon (Fig. 16-28). In the less common Mobitz II second-degree AV block, the Wenckebach phenomenon is absent because progressive PR prolongation does *not* precede the dropped beats (Fig. 16-29).

   Mobitz I second-degree AV block is commonly caused by physiological or pharmacological effects that slow AV node conduction, such as excessive vagal activity, a β-adrenergic receptor blocker, or a calcium channel blocker. For this reason, this form of second-degree AV block can be treated if a potentially reversible cause can be identified and eliminated; furthermore, when Mobitz I block worsens, progression is generally gradual (e.g., 4:3 block progressing to 3:2, then to 2:1 block). Because calcium channels in the AV node are inhibited by parasympathetic tone, Mobitz I AV block generally responds to a muscarinic receptor blocker like atropine. (Sympathetic stimulation, while logical, can cause dangerous side effects.)

   Mobitz II second-degree AV block is most often caused by anatomic lesions in the His–Purkinje system, so this form of AV block is unlikely to be alleviated by decreased vagal tone or drug therapy. Because Mobitz II block implies that conduction in the AV bundle, which depends on sodium-dependent action potentials, is "hanging by a thread," this form of AV block can progress suddenly, often without warning, to third-degree (complete) AV block (Fig. 16-30). For this reason, Mobitz II second-degree AV block is generally an indication for an electronic pacemaker.

   Not all patients with second-degree AV block in the AV node exhibit progressive prolongation of the PR interval before blocked P waves, and the Wenckebach phenomenon can be seen where the block is in the His–Purkinje system. An intracardiac electrogram (see Chapter 15) can

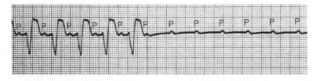

FIGURE 16-30 Mobitz type II AV block (monitor lead recorded in an ambulance). The PR interval in the conducted beats, where the QRS is prolonged, is about 0.20 sec. Sudden failure of atrial depolarization to activate the ventricles after the seventh P wave causes cardiac arrest. This is Mobitz II block because the PR interval does not increase before cessation of AV conduction. (Retouched).

help define the site of the block because block in the AV node prolongs the A–H interval, whereas block in the more distal conduction system prolongs the H–V interval (Fig. 16-31). These are sometimes called *supra-His* and *infra-His* block, respectively.

THE WENCKEBACH PHENOMENON. Progressive lengthening of the PR interval before the dropped beat in second-degree AV block, the *Wenckebach phenomenon*, is seen most commonly when block is in the AV node. Karl F. Wenckebach, a pioneer in the study of clinical arrhythmias, described this behavior in 1899 by recording carotid and jugular venous pulsations on a smoked drum kymograph. Sadly, and from a grammatical standpoint inexcusably, Professor Wenckebach has become a verb, as in: "The patient is Wenckebaching."

The features of the Wenckebach phenomenon are diagrammed in Figure 16-28, where the first PR interval after the blocked P wave (second from left) is 0.25 sec. The following three PR intervals are 0.32, 0.37, and 0.40 sec, after which the fifth P wave is blocked (PR = ∞). The progressive prolongation of the PR interval occurs by decreasing increments (listed below the ECG in Fig. 16-28), so that when sinus rate (P–P interval) is constant, the decreasing increments in PR interval cause a slight acceleration of ventricular rate. This phenomenon, called *group beating*, is documented at the bottom of Figure 16-28, where cycle length (R–R interval) shortens from 0.78 to 0.74 sec in the group of four QRS complexes.

There are two explanations for progressive prolongation of the PR interval after the dropped beats. The first, increasing depression of AV conduction due to repeated depolarization, can be caused when propagation of a series of impulses through the depressed AV node (or AV bundle) inactivates a progressively increasing fraction of the calcium (or sodium) channels. This increases the PR interval until, when too few depolarizing channels open to generate a propagated action potential, conduction fails, which is like killing the snake in Figure 16-20. The pause after the

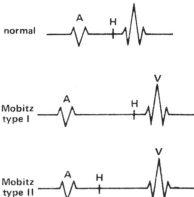

FIGURE 16-31 Intracardiac electrograms in AV block. **Top:** Normal. **Middle:** First-degree AV block with prolonged A–H interval and normal H–V interval indicating block in the AV node. **Bottom:** First-degree AV block with normal A–H interval and prolonged HV interval indicating block in the distal His–Purkinje system.

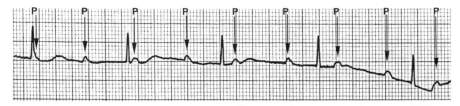

FIGURE 16-32 Third-degree AV block (complete heart block) (lead II). Although this ECG superficially resembles 2:1 AV block, there is no constant relationship between the P waves, which are regular at a rate of 102, and the QRS complexes, which are regular at a rate of 45. The atria and ventricles are therefore beating independently. The normal QRS duration (0.06 sec) indicates that the ventricles are activated by an AV junctional pacemaker above the bifurcation of the bundle of His.

dropped QRS allows depolarizing channels to recover, so the cycle starts again. The second explanation highlights the progressive shortening of the RP interval (the interval between the QRS complex and the following P wave). This is seen in Figure 16-28, where each increase in PR interval brings the next P wave closer to the preceding QRS complex. As a result, impulses conducted from the atria begin to reach the AV junction earlier during the relative refractory period left behind after the preceding beat, so these atrial impulses become blocked. According to the snake analogy, this would occur if, each time the serpent made its circle, the head came closer to the tail until the snake bit itself (Fig. 16-20c). Most evidence now favors the second explanation.

THIRD-DEGREE ATRIOVENTRICULAR BLOCK. Third-degree AV block, also called *complete AV block* or simply *heart block*, occurs when all conduction between the atria and ventricles is interrupted. Because the atria and ventricles beat independently in third-degree AV block, P waves and QRS complexes bear no relationship to each other (Fig. 16-32). When the atrial rhythm in complete heart block is under the control of the SA node, the atrial rate is regular and faster than the ventricular rate, which is controlled by a lower pacemaker. Third-degree AV block also can be diagnosed when ventricular rate is slow and regular in a patient with atrial fibrillation (Fig. 16-33).

The site of the lower pacemaker that controls ventricular systole in patients with third-degree AV block is suggested by the configuration of

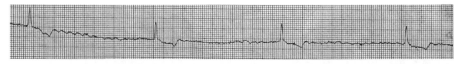

FIGURE 16-33 Third-degree AV block in a patient with atrial fibrillation (lead II). Diagnosis of the latter is based on the absence of P waves and undulations of the baseline. The QRS complexes are widened to approximately 0.12 sec and appear at a regular rate of 26, which indicates that the ventricles are depolarized by a pacemaker below the bifurcation of the bundle of His.

the QRS complex. Impulses generated by a wave of depolarization that reaches the ventricles from *above* the bifurcation of the bundle of His are conducted simultaneously into the two ventricles, therefore the QRS complex is narrow (Fig. 16-32), whereas QRS complexes initiated by a pacemaker *below* the bifurcation of the bundle of His are prolonged because activation of the two ventricles is no longer synchronous.

The consequences of third-degree AV block are determined mainly by the rate of ventricular beating. If the latter is normal or nearly normal, as can occur in congenital heart block, the functional impairment is usually minor and due mainly to loss of the atrial "primer pump" (see Chapter 11). When ventricular rates are very slow, however, cardiac output is reduced (see Chapter 12). Patients with intermittent third-degree AV block often experience syncopal episodes, called the *Stokes-Adams syndrome*; in these patients, complete failure of lower pacemakers can cause *asystolic cardiac arrest*.

Pathophysiology of AV Block

The clinical significance of AV block depends in part on whether it is in the AV node or the His–Purkinje system. This is because block in the AV node is usually an exaggeration of the physiologically slow conduction, which is often reversible, whereas block in the AV bundle, bundle branches, and fascicles is due most commonly to anatomical lesions that are generally irreversible. The latter occurs in two degenerative syndromes, called *Lenégre's disease* and *Lev's disease*. Lenégre's disease can be caused by degeneration or apoptosis of His–Purkinje cells in and below the AV bundle, or a cardiac sodium channel mutation. Lev's disease is usually due to fibrosis of the connective tissue skeleton of the heart or calcification of the mitral and aortic valve rings, both of which can damage the proximal regions of the His–Purkinje system in the upper part of the interventricular septum. Block in the His–Purkinje system also occurs in ischemic heart disease, where because of the extensive collateral circulation in the interventricular septum (see Chapter 1), this usually indicates that multivessel coronary artery occlusion has severely damaged the interventricular septum. The appearance of block in or below the AV bundle in a patient with acute myocardial infarction therefore has a bad prognosis, not only because of the danger that third-degree AV block might develop (which can usually be managed by an electronic pacemaker), but because it is a marker for extensive left ventricular damage.

BIFASCICULAR BLOCK, TRIFASCICULAR BLOCK, AND BILATERAL BUNDLE BRANCH BLOCK. Bundle branch block and fascicular blocks do not prevent atrial impulses from reaching the ventricles (see Chapter 15), but block in both bundle branches (*bilateral bundle branch block*) or all three fascicles (*trifascicular block*) cause AV conduction to fail. When counting fascicles, the right bundle branch is often viewed as a third fascicle (Table 16-5),

TABLE 16-5 **Fascicles and Fascicular Blocks**

I. Fascicular Blocks		
Conduction Blocked In	**Remaining Pathways**	**ECG Abnormality**
Left anterior fascicle	Right bundle branch + left posterior fascicle	Left axis deviation
Left posterior fascicle	Right bundle branch + left anterior fascicle	Right axis deviation
Right bundle branch	Left anterior + left posterior fascicle	Right bundle branch block
II. Bifascicular Blocks		
Conduction Blocked In	**Remaining Pathway**	**ECG Abnormality**
Left anterior fascicle + right bundle branch	Left posterior fascicle	Right bundle branch block + left axis deviation
Left posterior fascicle + right bundle branch	Left anterior fascicle	Right bundle branch block + right axis deviation
Left anterior + left posterior fascicle	Right bundle branch	Left bundle branch block
III. Trifascicular Block		
Conduction Blocked In	**Remaining Pathway**	**ECG Abnormality**
Left anterior + left posterior fascicle + right bundle branch	None	Third-degree AV block

so the combination of right bundle branch block with either left anterior fascicular block or left posterior fascicular block, called *bifascicular block*, distorts the QRS; however, because a single fascicle still conducts impulses from the atria to the ventricles, AV conduction is preserved. *Trifascicular block*, which is the combination of block in both fascicles of the left bundle branch along with right bundle branch block, impairs AV conduction so that this diagnosis is suggested when a patient with known bifascicular block develops a prolonged PR interval or higher degree of AV block.

The clinical impact of the conduction abnormalities listed in Table 16-5 depends on whether AV conduction is preserved through at least one fascicle. Neither left anterior and left posterior fascicular blocks, which alter the mean QRS axis but do not prolong the QRS, nor bundle branch block, which prolongs ventricular depolarization, delay the *onset* of ventricular depolarization; as a result, atrioventricular conduction is not impaired, and the PR interval is not prolonged.

ARBORIZATION BLOCK AND MASQUERADING BUNDLE BRANCH BLOCK. Conduction block in the distal Purkinje system, called *arborization block*, is often seen in end-stage heart failure where QRS complexes are markedly prolonged and distorted. An uncommon form of arborization block, called *masquerading bundle branch block*, can be diagnosed when the QRS is markedly prolonged and right axis deviation accompanies left bundle branch block or left axis deviation accompanies right bundle branch block; however, these criteria are rather vague and can overlap those for bifascicular block, so arborization block and masquerading bundle branch block are not commonly diagnosed. These concepts are assuming new importance because of the success of "cardiac resynchronization therapy" in alleviating symptoms and prolonging survival in patients with severe heart failure and a prolonged QRS complex (see Chapter 18).

PREMATURE SYSTOLES

Premature systoles, which can be generated in any region of the heart, are often called *extrasystoles*. The latter term, however, is a misnomer when premature systoles *replace* a beat of the atria or ventricle and therefore are not *extra* in that they do not add to the number of beats. Premature systoles also are referred to as *ectopic beats* because, except when they arise in the sinus node (which is rare), the impulse is generated at an abnormal (ectopic) site.

Atrial Premature Systoles

Atrial premature systoles are characterized by the early appearance of abnormal P waves followed by QRS complexes that resemble the QRS complexes in the rest of the ECG (Fig. 16-34). The QRS complexes are usually normal because most atrial premature systoles are conducted

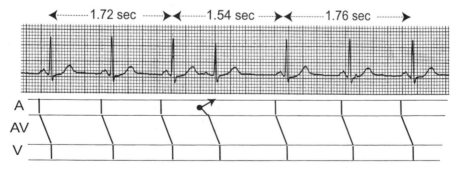

FIGURE 16-34 Atrial premature systole (lead II). The fourth P wave is premature and followed by a normal QRS complex after a normal PR interval. The intervals between the two sinus P waves immediately before and after the premature systole (1.72 and 1.76 sec) are greater than that between the two sinus P waves that "enclose" the premature systole (1.54 sec), which indicates that the atrial premature systole penetrated and reset the timing of the SA node as shown on the Lewis diagram.

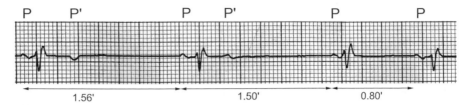

FIGURE 16-35 Blocked atrial premature systoles (lead II). The ECG begins with a diphasic sinus P wave that is followed, after a PR interval of 0.14 sec, by a slightly prolonged QRS complex. An inverted P wave (**P'**) that is superimposed on the T wave following this QRS is an atrial premature systole that, because it does not depolarize the ventricles, is *blocked.* The second QRS complex, which is initiated by another sinus P wave (**P**), is followed by a second blocked premature atrial systole (**P'**), after which the third and fourth QRS complexes are preceded by sinus P waves. The third QRS complex, which resembles the other QRS complexes, is preceded by a short PR interval (~0.11 sec) and so represents an "escape" beat (see below) caused by depolarization of a pacemaker in the AV junction. The absence of an inverted deflection on the T wave of the third QRS, and the constant appearance of sinus P waves (which occur at intervals of 0.80 sec and twice 0.78 and 0.75 sec) support the interpretation that the downward deflections after the first two QRS complexes (*labeled* **P'**) are premature P waves.

normally from the atria into the ventricles by the His–Purkinje system. The PR interval after an atrial premature systole also is normal unless atrial depolarization comes so early that it reaches the AV node before the latter has recovered from the preceding impulse, in which case the PR interval can be prolonged. If an atrial premature systole reaches the AV node during its absolute refractory period, no QRS complex will follow the premature P wave; this is called a *blocked atrial premature systole* (Fig. 16-35).

ABERRANT CONDUCTION AND SUPERNORMALITY. QRS complexes that follow atrial premature systoles can be abnormal if the wave of depolarization conducted through the AV node reaches one of the bundle branches before the latter has recovered from the preceding normal beat (Fig. 16-36). If an impulse conducted from an atrial premature systole is blocked in one of the bundle branches, most commonly the right where the refractory period is especially long, it causes a phenomenon called *aberrant conduction* where the QRS is prolonged. Because long diastolic intervals prolong both the action potential and refractory period (the interval–duration relationship described in Chapter 14), atrial or junctional premature systoles are more likely to be conducted with aberrancy when a short cycle follows a long cycle: This is the "Ashman phenomenon" (see Fig. 14-9).

Supernormal conduction (see Chapter 14), seen in a patient with intermittent right bundle branch block, occurred when an atrial premature systole shortened the QRS when it was conducted into the right bundle branch during its supernormal period (Fig. 16-37).

RESETTING OF THE SA NODE PACEMAKER. Atrial premature systoles are often propagated into the sinus node, where they reset the timing of the

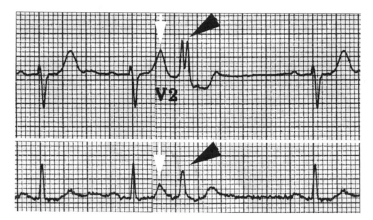

FIGURE 16-36 Atrial premature systole with aberrant ventricular conduction (lead V_2 *above*, lead II recorded simultaneously *below*). The second QRS complex is followed by a premature P wave that is superimposed on the T wave of the preceding ventricular beat, which explains the apparent peaking of this T wave (*downward white arrows*). The third QRS complex, which follows the premature P wave (*black arrowhead*), is prolonged to 0.12 sec and in lead V_2 has a contour typical of right bundle branch block. This prolonged QRS complex was probably caused by an atrial premature depolarization that was conducted aberrantly because, although it was initiated by a premature P wave, arrived at the bifurcation of the bundle of His before the right bundle branch had recovered from the preceding depolarization. (*Retouched.*)

subsequent sinus P waves (Fig. 16-38). This explains why the first normal P wave following the atrial premature systole in Figure 16-34 appears sooner than would be expected if the SA node had maintained its normal timetable. Atrial premature systoles also can be followed by a compensatory pause (see below).

Junctional Premature Systoles

Premature depolarizations in the AV junction, either in the AV node or the AV bundle above the bifurcation of the bundle of His, generate premature QRS complexes that are normal in contour because the ventricles are depolarized synchronously by impulses conducted through the two bundle branches. Whether or not the resulting *junctional premature systoles* are associated with a premature P wave depends on when and whether the wave of depolarization is propagated into the atria. P waves generated by junctional premature systoles are often called *retrograde P waves* because the premature impulses enter the atria from the AV node, which lies in the right atrium near the top of the interventricular septum, instead of from the SA node, which is located at the right atrial-superior vena caval junction. For this reason, the frontal plane vector generated by a normal P wave is directed inferiorly and to the left, while retrograde P waves generate vectors directed superiorly and often to the right (Fig. 16-39). As a result, typical retrograde P waves are inverted in lead II.

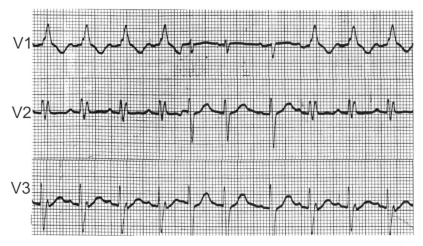

FIGURE 16-37 Supernormality in a patient with rate-dependent bundle branch block (leads V_1, V_2, and V_3 recorded simultaneously). The first four QRS complexes, which are sinus beats at a cycle length of 0.50 sec (P waves are clearly seen in lead V_2), are prolonged (QRS duration is 0.11 sec) and exhibit a right bundle branch block pattern. The fifth QRS complex, which is initiated by a premature P wave (the downward deflection on the T waves in leads V_1 and V_2) that shortens the interval between QRS complexes to 0.46 sec, has a normal duration of 0.06 sec. This can be explained if the impulse responsible for the fifth QRS reached the right bundle branch during its supernormal period. The QRS remains normal in the next beat (the sixth), where cycle length is again 0.46 sec. A third normal QRS (the seventh) then follows a long cycle (0.58 sec), which has allowed enough time for the right bundle branch to recover its excitability following the previous beat. The last three QRS complexes, where cycle length has returned to 0.50 sec, again exhibit a right bundle branch block pattern. Narrowing of the QRS and disappearance of the right bundle branch block pattern after the short cycles is attributable to supernormality.

Junctional premature systoles were once classified according to the relative timing of the retrograde P waves and QRS complexes; when the retrograde P wave preceded the QRS complex by <0.12 sec, the beat was called an *upper nodal* beat; when the P wave and QRS complex occurred at the same time, the beat was a *middle nodal* beat; and when

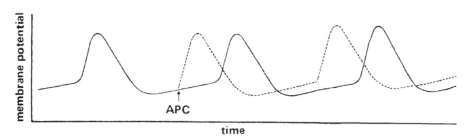

FIGURE 16-38 Resetting of the SA node pacemaker by an atrial premature systole. **Solid line:** Action potential of a pacemaker cell in the SA node that fires at regular intervals. **Dotted line:** Depolarization of the SA node pacemaker by an impulse conducted from an atrial premature systole (**APC**) advances the timing of the following SA node cycles.

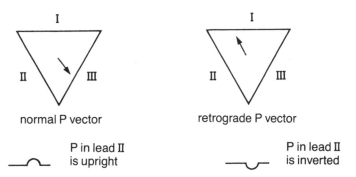

FIGURE 16-39 Normal and retrograde P waves. **Left:** A normal P wave in the frontal plane propagates to the left and inferiorly and so inscribes an upright deflection in lead II. **Right:** Retrograde P waves propagate superiorly, often to the right, and inscribe an inverted deflection in lead II.

the retrograde P wave followed the QRS complex, the beat was a *lower nodal* beat. These terms have fallen into disuse because it is now clear that the relationship between the QRS complexes and retrograde P waves in junctional premature systoles is determined by the relative rates of antegrade and retrograde conduction rather than where in the AV junction the premature systole originated. Junctional premature systoles that depolarize the atria before the ventricles generate a retrograde P wave that precedes the premature QRS complex (Fig. 16-40, above), whereas premature systoles that depolarize the ventricles before the atria give rise to P waves that follow the QRS complexes (Fig. 16-40, below). P waves are not seen if the premature impulse is not propagated into the atria, or if simultaneous depolarization of the atria and ventricles causes the P waves to be "buried" in the QRS complex.

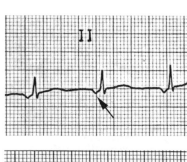

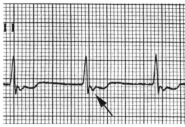

FIGURE 16-40 Retrograde P waves in junctional beats (lead II). These examples, taken from patients with accelerated junctional rhythms, show retrograde P waves (*arrows*) that precede (*above*) and follow (*below*) QRS complexes. Retrograde P waves can be absent (*not shown*) if they are buried in the QRS complex or if the impulses arising in the AV junction are not conducted to the atria.

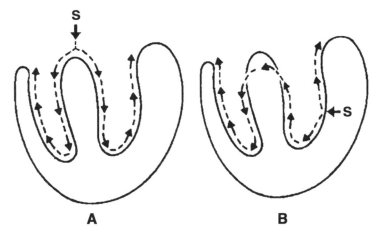

FIGURE 16-41 Mechanism of QRS prolongation by ventricular premature depolarization. **A:** A normal impulse conducted from above the bifurcation of the bundle of His depolarizes the ventricles simultaneously. **B:** An abnormal impulse that arises in either ventricle below the bifurcation of the bundle of His prolongs the QRS because of the increased length of the path of depolarization and slow conduction across the interventricular septum **(B). S:** Origin of the impulse that activates the ventricles.

Ventricular Premature Systoles

Premature impulses that arise below the bifurcation of the bundle of His give rise to QRS complexes that are abnormal because the normal synchrony of ventricular depolarization is lost (Fig. 16-41). For this reason, a premature QRS complex that differs from the normal QRS and is not preceded by a P wave is usually a ventricular premature systole (Fig. 16-42). This diagnosis cannot be made on the basis of QRS contour alone because the QRS complexes in bundle branch block and aberrancy, like those generated by ventricular premature systoles, are prolonged.

The timing of the P waves that appear after a ventricular premature systole generally differs from those that follow atrial or junctional premature

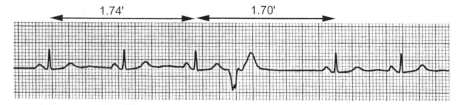

FIGURE 16-42 Ventricular premature systole (lead II). The fourth QRS complex, which is premature and not preceded by a P wave, is bizarre and wider than the normal QRS complexes in this record. The pause after the ventricular premature systole, called a *compensatory pause*, occurred because the subsequent SA node depolarization reached the AV junction during its refractory period. Because the cycle containing the ventricular premature systole was almost exactly twice the normal sinus cycle, the premature systole did *not* reset the SA node pacemaker.

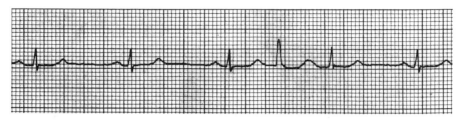

FIGURE 16-43 Interpolated ventricular premature systole (lead II). The third QRS, which is premature, is not preceded by a P wave and is prolonged, so it is ventricular in origin. As this premature systole occurs between two sinus beats, it is interpolated.

systoles. The latter, especially atrial premature systoles, are usually conducted into the SA node, where they shift the subsequent train of sinus beats ahead in time by resetting the sinus pacemaker (see above). Ventricular premature systoles, however, usually do not depolarize the SA node, although their conduction into the AV node often prevents the next sinus beat from depolarizing the ventricles; when this occurs, regular QRS complexes resume their normal schedule after a delay, called a *compensatory pause* (Fig. 16-42). The term *compensatory pause* is really a misnomer because the pause does not compensate for anything, except to allow the sinus beats to remain on the timetable they would have followed had there not been a premature systole. Some ventricular premature systoles occur between two sinus beats and so are *interpolated* (Fig. 16-43); in this case, the premature systole is a true extrasystole.

Ventricular premature systoles are common in individuals with normal hearts. A greater *frequency* of ventricular premature systoles means that they are more likely to be clinically significant. Even more important is their *complexity*; ventricular premature systoles that occur singly (Fig. 16-42 and Fig. 16-43) are generally of little consequence. *Multifocal ventricular premature systoles*, where the QRS complexes have different morphologies (Fig. 16-44), are of more ominous prognostic significance than unifocal ventricular premature systoles (i.e., having a single morphology). Ventricular premature systoles also are of more concern when they occur as *bigeminy*, where every other QRS is a ventricular premature systole (Fig. 16-45), or are *repetitive*, such as two ventricular premature

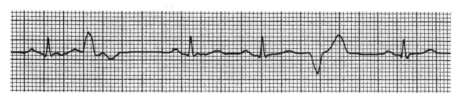

FIGURE 16-44 Multiform ventricular premature systoles (lead II). The second and fifth QRS complexes, which are premature, prolonged, bizarre, and not preceded by P waves, are multiform because of their different contours.

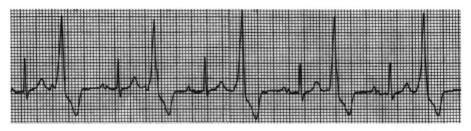

FIGURE 16-45 Ventricular bigeminy. QRS complexes alternate between sinus beats and ventricular premature systoles. (*Retouched.*)

systoles in a row (*couplets*) (Fig. 16-46) are less dangerous than three in a row (*triplets*), while a short run (*nonsustained ventricular tachycardia*) is generally a marker for significant risk of sudden cardiac death. Most dangerous is a run of ventricular premature systoles that lasts longer than 30 seconds, which is usually referred to as *sustained ventricular tachycardia*. Ventricular premature systoles that appear so early as to fall on the T wave of the preceding cycle, during the vulnerable period (see below) (the *R on T phenomenon*) (Fig. 16-47) can trigger ventricular fibrillation, especially in patients with heart disease.

TACHYCARDIAS

Tachycardias, which by definition occur when heart rate is sustained at rates greater than 100, are generally subdivided into *supraventricular* and *ventricular tachycardias*. Supraventricular tachycardias can originate in the SA node, atria, and AV junction, while the more dangerous ventricular tachycardias arise below the bifurcation of the bundle of His.

Supraventricular Tachycardias

Tachycardias arising above the bifurcation of the bundle of His can be classified according to their presumed site of origin or the presumed mechanism (Table 16-6A). Supraventricular tachycardias were initially classified as *sinus*, *atrial*, and *junctional* (or *nodal*) tachycardias on the

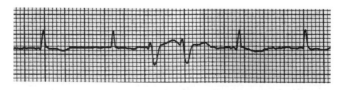

FIGURE 16-46 Ventricular premature systoles appearing as a couplet (lead II). The third and fourth QRS complexes, which are premature and prolonged, represent a couplet (two ventricular premature systoles in a row). The underlying rhythm in this patient is atrial fibrillation.

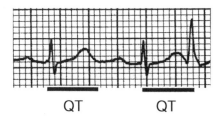

QT   QT

FIGURE 16-47   The "R on T" phenomenon (lead II). The third QRS, which is prolonged and differs from the other two QRS complexes, is a ventricular premature systole that falls at the end of the T wave of the preceding beat. This is confirmed because the QT intervals of the normal beats (*dark lines below the ECG*) are longer than the interval preceding the ventricular premature depolarization.

basis of electrocardiographic criteria such as P-wave morphology and the relationship between P waves and QRS complexes. This simple classification has become obsolete because modern therapy has made it essential to define the mechanism that causes the arrhythmia in each patient.

CLASSIFICATION BASED ON P-WAVE MORPHOLOGY AND THE PR INTERVAL. In *sinus tachycardia*, P-wave morphology is normal, and heart rate can be slowed by maneuvers that increase vagal activity. *Atrial tachycardia* is identified by abnormal (but not retrograde) P waves followed by normal QRS complexes after a normal PR interval, while in *junctional tachycardias*, the P waves are retrograde and either precede the QRS complex by an abnormally short interval (PR <0.12 sec) (Fig. 16-40, top) or occur during the ST segment (Fig. 16-40, bottom); however, P waves are not always seen.

CLASSIFICATION BASED ON MECHANISM. The simple electrocardiographic distinction between sinus, atria, and junctional tachycardias is being replaced with the mechanistic classification described in Table 16-6B. These mechanisms may not be apparent on the ECG, so today's "gold standard" is an invasive electrophysiological study that collects data from stimulating and recording electrodes placed in the heart.

At least eight different mechanisms can give rise to supraventricular tachycardias (Table 16-6B). *Reentry* can occur within the SA node, the atria, or between conduction pathways that include both the atria and ventricles. Reentrant tachycardias are usually paroxysmal, which means that they begin and end suddenly, and so represent a *paroxysmal supraventricular tachycardia* (*PSVT*). Supraventricular tachycardias also can be caused by accelerated *pacemaker activity* in the SA node (sinus tachycardia); *automatic tachycardias* also arise in the atria and AV junction. Some supraventricular tachycardias are attributed to *triggered activity* in the atria, but criteria to identify this mechanism are often unclear.

SINUS NODE REENTRY. This uncommon arrhythmia differs from sinus tachycardia in that it is generated by a reentrant circuit in the SA node,

TABLE 16-6 **Supraventricular Tachycardias**

A. Classification Based on P-Wave Morphology and the PR Interval		
Tachycardia	**P Waves**	**PR Interval**
Sinus	Normal	Normal or prolonged
Atrial	Abnormal	Normal or prolonged
Junctional	Retrograde	Short or absent
B. Classification Based on Mechanism		
Tachycardia	**Type of Mechanism**	**Specific Mechanism**
Sinus tachycardia	Increased pacemaker activity	Accelerated sinus pacemaker
Sinus node reentry	Reentry	SA node reentrant circuit
Automatic atrial tachycardia	Increased pacemaker activity	Ectopic atrial pacemaker
Atrial reentry	Reentry	Atrial reentrant circuit
Triggered atrial tachycardia	Triggered depolarizations	Triggered depolarizations in the atria
Automatic AV junctional tachycardia	Increased pacemaker activity	Ectopic His–Bundle pacemaker
AV nodal reentry	Reentry	Dual AV nodal reentrant circuit
Accessory pathway reentry	Reentry	Accessory pathway reentrant circuit

rather than accelerated depolarization of SA node pacemaker cells. The P waves in SA node reentry are normal, so this arrhythmia differs from sinus tachycardia in its paroxysmal behavior and termination by vagal maneuvers or electrical stimuli that interrupt the reentrant circuit.

AUTOMATIC ATRIAL TACHYCARDIAS. Automatic atrial tachycardias are characterized by abnormal P waves followed by a normal PR interval, unless the tachycardia is very rapid and normal decremental conduction in the AV node prolongs the PR interval. Unlike reentrant atrial tachycardias (see below), automatic atrial tachycardias usually do not begin suddenly and cannot be abolished by vagal stimulation or electrical defibrillation; for this reason, automatic atrial tachycardias are sometimes called *nonparoxysmal atrial tachycardias*.

Multifocal (or *chaotic*) *atrial tachycardias* (Fig. 16-48), which represent an important subset of the automatic atrial tachycardias, are characterized by irregular variations in both P-wave morphology and the

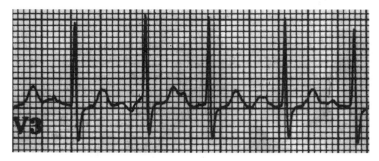

FIGURE 16-48   Multifocal atrial tachycardia (lead V₃). The rate is about 120 and slightly irregular; P-wave morphology changes throughout this record. (*Retouched.*)

PR interval. This arrhythmia is often seen in patents with pulmonary disease and can herald the appearance of atrial flutter or fibrillation.

ATRIAL REENTRY. Atrial reentry, like other reentrant arrhythmias, is generally paroxysmal. P waves in this uncommon tachycardia are abnormal, and the reentrant circuit can be interrupted by electrical stimulation of the atria. Unlike reentrant tachycardias that utilize a pathway that includes the AV node, where part of the reentrant circuit is calcium channel dependent, reentrant atrial tachycardias are not usually influenced by drugs that inhibit calcium channel opening.

AUTOMATIC AV JUNCTIONAL TACHYCARDIA. Junctional pacemakers, which are normally suppressed by the more rapid sinus pacemaker, can take control of the ventricles when the sinus node pacemaker slows or when impulse conduction from the sinus node is blocked. Under these conditions, discharge of these lower pacemakers generates *escape rhythms* at rates that are usually between 25 and 40 (see Chapter 15). Abnormal acceleration of a junctional pacemaker to a rate greater that 50 causes an automatic AV junctional tachycardia sometimes called an *accelerated junctional rhythm*; even though the rate of ventricular beating may not exceed 100, this is a tachyarrhythmia because the junctional pacemaker is firing more rapidly than normal.

The P waves in automatic AV junctional tachycardias, when they can be identified, are retrograde and can precede, follow, or be buried in the QRS complexes (see Fig. 16-40). These arrhythmias, which are usually nonparoxysmal, can be slowed, but not often terminated, by vagal stimulation and adenosine. Digitalis causes automatic AV junctional tachycardias by accelerating pacemaker activity in the AV junction; when slow (50–60), these junctional tachycardias are not necessarily a sign of digitalis toxicity, but because their rate increases as the dose of the cardiac glycoside is increased, acceleration of the tachycardia is a warning that too much drug is being administered. Rapid, digitalis-induced automatic AV junctional tachycardias can fail to activate the ventricles because these drugs have a centrally mediated vagal effect that inhibits AV conduction;

the resulting arrhythmia, which was once called *atrial tachycardia with block*, suggests digitalis toxicity.

AV NODAL REENTRY. AV nodal reentry, the most common cause of supraventricular tachycardia, is a reciprocal rhythm that utilizes the dual AV nodal conduction pathways described above (Fig. 16-25). These tachycardias, like other reentrant supraventricular tachycardias, are usually paroxysmal. The most common reciprocal circuit, in which conduction from atria to ventricles is via the slow pathway (Fig. 16-49B), is generally triggered when an atrial premature systole causes a wave of depolarization to enter the upper end of the AV node before the fast pathway has fully recovered from the preceding (normal) sinus beat. Because action potentials in the slower pathways in the AV node are generally briefer than those in the faster pathways, the atrial premature systole can enter the upper end of the AV node when the fast pathway is still refractory. As a result, the premature impulse is conducted through the slow pathway in the antegrade direction, from the atria toward the ventricles, and then returns to the atria in the retrograde direction via the fast pathway. Ventricular premature systoles, on the other hand, usually trigger tachycardias in which conduction from ventricles to atria is via the slow pathways (Fig. 16-49C).

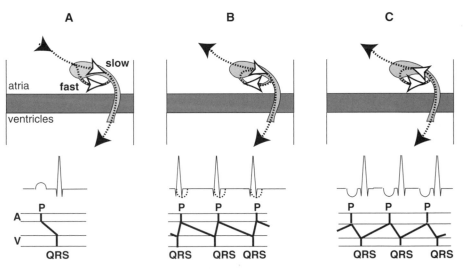

FIGURE 16-49 Supraventricular tachycardias caused by AV nodal reentry. A: Normal mechanism, in which the ventricles are depolarized from above the bifurcation of the bundle of His by an impulse transmitted by way of both the fast and slow pathways. B: Tachycardia in which impulses from a reentrant circuit in the AV junction (*open arrowheads*) are transmitted to the atria by way of the fast pathway and to the ventricles by the slow pathway (*black arrowheads*). This causes retrograde P waves to occur during or shortly after the QRS complexes (*below*) C: Less commonly, impulses reach the atria by way of the slow pathway and the ventricles by way of the fast pathway, which causes retrograde P waves to be inscribed just before the QRS in a pattern that resembles a short PR interval.

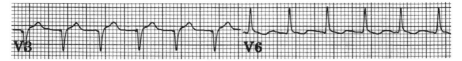

FIGURE 16-50 Supraventricular tachycardia without visible P waves (leads V_3 and V_6 recorded sequentially). The narrow QRS complexes, which appear at a regular rate of 150, are diagnostic of supraventricular tachycardia. The absence of retrograde P waves can be explained if the tachycardia had failed to depolarize the atria, or if the atria were depolarized at the same time as the ventricles.

Retrograde P waves are usually not seen during these tachycardias (Fig. 16-50) because impulses are transmitted to the atria via the fast pathway at about the same time as or shortly after the ventricles are activated by the slow pathway (Fig. 16-49B); as a result, P waves are either buried in the QRS complexes or appear immediately after ventricular depolarization on the ST segment (Fig. 16-51). When impulses reach the atria via the slow pathway and return to the ventricles via the fast pathway (Fig. 16-49C), retrograde P waves can be inscribed just before the QRS in a pattern that appears to be a short PR interval.

The "weak" point in these reentrant circuits is the AV node, which allows the arrhythmias to be terminated by inhibiting calcium channel–dependent conduction. This can be done using maneuvers that stimulate vagal activity or by administration of adenosine, a purinergic agonist that inhibits calcium channel opening. Cardiac glycosides, which have a central action that activates vagal outflow, also can be useful in treating these arrhythmias, as can calcium channel blockers and β-adrenergic blockers. Because all of these drugs can have undesirable effects, ablation has become the preferred treatment for these tachycardias.

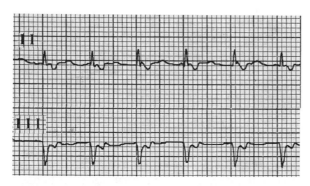

FIGURE 16-51 Supraventricular tachycardia with retrograde P waves (leads II and III recorded simultaneously). The narrow QRS complexes, which appear at a regular rate of 150, are diagnostic of supraventricular tachycardia. The small downward deflections on the ST segments are retrograde P waves, which indicates that this is a reciprocal tachycardia in which impulses travel from atria to ventricles by way of the slow pathway, and from ventricle to atria by way of the fast pathway.

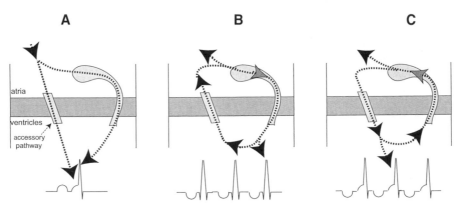

FIGURE 16-52 Supraventricular tachycardias in pre-excitation (Wolff-Parkinson-White syndrome). **A:** Normal sinus beat, in which an impulse transmitted by way of the accessory pathway initiates ventricular depolarization, causing the QRS complex to begin with a slurred upstroke, called a *delta wave*. Subsequent transmission of the impulse through the His–Purkinje system initiates the later QRS deflections. **B:** Tachycardia in which impulses are transmitted to the ventricles by the AV node and to the atria by way of the accessory pathway. This causes the delta waves to disappear and retrograde P waves to be inscribed just before the QRS complex. **C:** The less common tachycardia, where impulses reach the ventricles by way of the accessory pathway and the atria by way of the AV node. Delta waves are seen, and retrograde P waves occur shortly after the QRS complexes.

ACCESSORY PATHWAY REENTRY (WOLFF-PARKINSON-WHITE SYNDROME). Supraventricular tachycardias associated with pre-excitation (Wolff-Parkinson-White syndrome or WPW), which are usually paroxysmal, depend on a reciprocal circuit that involves the AV node and accessory pathway (Figs. 16-16 and 16-52). These tachycardias are generally initiated by an atrial premature systole that, because the atrial cells in the accessory pathways have a longer refractory period than those in the AV node, is conducted to the ventricles by way of the AV node and returns to the atria by way of the accessory pathway (Fig. 16-52B). This explains why QRS complexes recorded during supraventricular tachycardias in patients with pre-excitation usually do not begin with a delta wave. This behavior resembles the more common form of AV nodal reentry, where the antegrade limb is the slow pathway (Fig. 16-49B). Less commonly, where antegrade conduction is through the accessory pathway, delta waves are present (Fig. 16-52C); in the latter, P waves often cannot be identified because they fall on the QRS complex or ST segment.

Supraventricular tachycardias in patients with accessory pathways depend on both sodium- and calcium-dependent action potentials and therefore can be terminated when calcium channel opening is inhibited by vagal stimulation, adenosine, calcium channel blockers and β-blockers, or by antiarrhythmic drugs that block sodium channels. However, ablation therapy is now the preferred treatment, as it eliminates the need for medication and the occasional hospital visit if the arrhythmia recurs. Successful ablation therapy also eliminates a small but real risk of sudden death, which can occur if the patient develops atrial fibrillation. In pre-excitation, the ability of the accessory pathway to conduct impulses rapidly from the atria to the ventricles can allow atrial fibrillation, which itself is rarely lethal, to initiate ventricular fibrillation by transmitting the disorganized electrical activity from the atria to the ventricles.

Ventricular Tachycardia

The hallmark of ventricular tachycardia is a rapid series of widened QRS complexes (>0.12 sec) (Fig. 16-53) that are not preceded by P waves; if atrial activity is seen, the prolonged QRS complexes bear no fixed relationship to the P waves. The rates in ventricular tachycardias are similar to those of most supraventricular tachycardias, but the rhythm is often slightly less regular. Although all ventricular tachycardias have wide QRS complexes, not all wide QRS tachycardias are of ventricular origin because, as noted above, rapid heart rates in supraventricular tachycardias can cause aberrant conduction. The difficulty in distinguishing ventricular tachycardia from supraventricular tachycardia

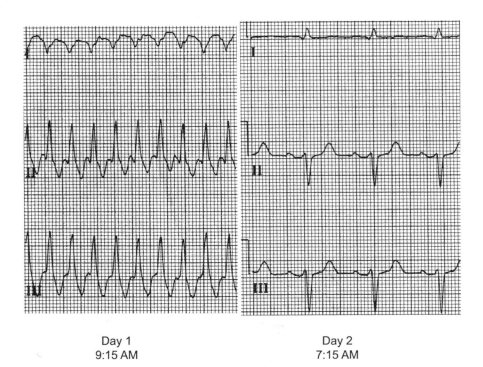

Day 1	Day 2
9:15 AM	7:15 AM

FIGURE 16-53 Ventricular tachycardia (leads I, II, and III). The QRS complexes recorded during the tachycardia on Day 1 are wider, begin differently, and have a different morphology compared with the QRS complexes recorded during sinus rhythm on Day 2. For these reasons, the first ECG is probably ventricular tachycardia.

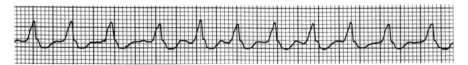

FIGURE 16-54   Wide QRS tachycardia (lead II). The rhythm is slightly irregular with an aver-age cycle length of approximately 0.38 sec, which corresponds to a ventricular rate of about 160; P waves cannot be identified. The irregular appearance of QRS complexes sug-gests that the underlying arrhythmia is atrial fibrillation, but this ECG also could represent ventricular tachycardia, or atrial tachycardia with pre-existing bundle branch block or aberrancy. For this reason, the rhythm is best described as a wide QRS tachycardia.

with prolonged QRS (Fig. 16-54) has led to the use of the term *wide QRS tachycardia*, which has the advantage of being descriptive without implying mechanism or suggesting therapy. This diagnosis indicates that more data are needed to distinguish between supraventricular and ven-tricular tachycardia.

The appearance of *fusion beats* or *captures* can establish a diagno-sis of ventricular tachycardia in a patient with a wide QRS tachycardia (Fig. 16-55). A fusion beat, which is evidenced by a narrow QRS com-plex, is initiated jointly by the normal wave of depolarization propagated into the ventricles by way of the His-Purkinje system and a focus within the ventricles; fusion beats therefore occur when the ventricles are depo-larized simultaneously from "above" by an impulse conducted through

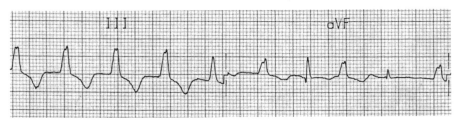

FIGURE 16-55   Ventricular tachycardia with fusion beats and captures (continuous recording of leads III and aVF; the two *vertical lines* mark the lead change). The first four QRS complexes (in lead III) are wide (0.12 sec) and occur at a cycle of about 0.56 sec, which corresponds to a rate of 107. The fifth QRS is slightly early (the preceding interval is 0.50 sec) and is narrower than the other complexes in this lead. The mechanism for the nar-rower QRS is apparent after the lead change, where the sixth QRS complex (now in lead aVF) is again wide, with a duration in this lead of 0.11 sec, and is followed by a beat with a narrow QRS (0.07 sec) after an interval of 0.52 sec. This beat, the seventh QRS, represents a "capture" in which a supraventricular impulse conducted through the AV junction has depolarized the ventricles. The eighth QRS complex is again wide while the ninth QRS, which follows the preceding QRS by 0.54 sec and has a contour midway between that of the wide QRS beats and the capture in lead aVF, is a *fusion beat* in which the ventricles are depolarized by both the ventricular focus and an impulse conducted from above the bifurcation of the bundle of His. The final (tenth) QRS in this record is another ventricu-lar beat. The appearance of captures and fusion beats demonstrates that the wide QRS beats are ventricular in origin.

FIGURE 16-56 Ventricular tachycardia with a typical capture (lead III). The first three QRS complexes, which are wide and not preceded by P waves, are ventricular in origin. The fourth QRS, which is narrower and preceded by an obvious P wave, is a capture.

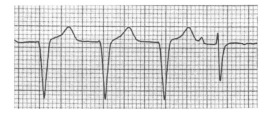

the AV node, and from "below" by an ectopic ventricular impulse. A typical capture, which occurs when a narrowed QRS is preceded by a P wave in a patient with a wide QRS tachycardia (Fig. 16-56), indicates that the origin of the tachycardia originated below the bifurcation of the bundle of His.

Ventricular tachycardias arise in regions with sodium-dependent action potentials, so they are not slowed by vagal stimulation, adenosine, or calcium channel blockers. Although β-blockers are useful in preventing ventricular tachycardias, the antiarrhythmic effect is due largely to their ability to reduce the arrhythmogenic effects of energy starvation and calcium overload, rather than a direct effect on the electrical properties of the ventricle.

Ventricular tachycardias can be *monomorphic*, where all of the QRS complexes are similar to one another, or *polymorphic*, when the contour of the QRS complexes is not all the same. Polymorphic ventricular tachycardia has a more ominous prognosis than monomorphic ventricular tachycardia. *Bidirectional tachycardias*, where QRS complexes alternate between an upward and downward direction, are seen in patients with calcium-overloaded hearts such as occurs with digitalis overdose and catecholaminergic polymorphic ventricular tachycardia (see below), and often herald ventricular fibrillation. Another special polymorphic ventricular tachycardia, called *torsades de points* (twisting of the points) (Fig. 16-57), is characterized by QRS complexes that undergo a slow transition between upward- and downward-directed complexes resembling the twisting of a sine wave. Torsades, which is probably triggered by afterdepolarizations, is seen in patients with long QT syndromes and calcium-overloaded hearts, and can be induced by drugs and drug combinations that prolong the QT interval.

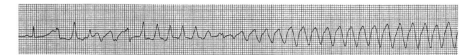

FIGURE 16-57 Torsades de points (monitor lead). The first QRS is a sinus beat with a very long QT (>0.50 sec) that is interrupted by a premature QRS, which falls on the T wave of the preceding cycle; the latter is followed by a sequence of ventricular premature beats that appears to "twist" around the baseline, which is the typical appearance of torsades.

Ventricular tachycardias can be automatic when the arrhythmia is initiated by a pacemaker in the His–Purkinje system below the bifurcation of the bundle of His. The latter usually fire at rates between 25 and 40, so their activity is not seen unless the impulses normally conducted by way of the His–Purkinje system are blocked. Ventricular pacemaker rates in the range between 60 and 100, which are not associated with the high mortality of more rapid ventricular tachycardias, are generally referred to as *accelerated idioventricular rhythms*, reserving the term *ventricular tachycardia* for the more rapid, and more dangerous, ventricular arrhythmia.

A special type of automatic ventricular rhythm, called *parasystole*, occurs when the regular discharge of an idioventricular pacemaker causes wide QRS complexes to appear at a regular rate; the timing of the sinus beats, in which QRS complexes are narrow and preceded by P waves, is independent of the slower, wide QRS beats (Fig. 16-58). Not all parasystolic impulses initiate a QRS complex because they cannot depolarize the ventricles when they occur during the refractory period following a sinus beat. In simple parasystolic rhythms, sinus impulses do not reset the parasystolic focus, so the wide QRS complexes in these parasystolic rhythms appear "on schedule" unless they reach the ventricles during their refractory period (Fig. 16-58). This was likened by my father to a wicked knight (the parasystole) who emerges from his castle on a strict schedule to raid the surrounding villages, unless his exit from the castle is blocked by the appearance of the king's men (the sinus QRS). Because the king's men cannot enter the castle, the knight maintains his strict schedule of attempted raids. Parasystolic rhythms do not always adhere to this simple behavior because electrotonic currents generated when a sinus beat

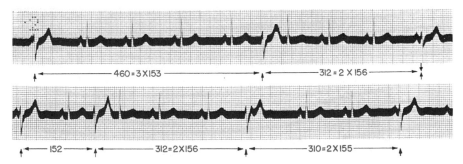

FIGURE 16-58 Parasystole (lead II). The intervals between the wide QRS complexes in this record are multiples of the cycle length of a parasystole that fires at a regular interval of 1.52 to 1.56 sec (small upward arrows), but is not depolarized by the sinus beats. Not all parasystolic impulses initiate a QRS because many occur during the refractory period of preceding sinus beats. The QRS at the end of the upper strip (small upward and downward arrows) is a fusion beat. Modified from Katz and Pick, 1956. (The thick lines in this and the other ECGs taken from this text, which were recorded by a string galvanometer, are shadows cast by the quartz string that moves up and down in response to small changes in potential.

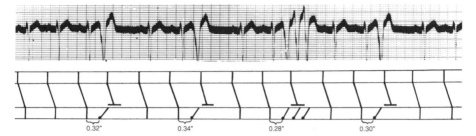

FIGURE 16-59   Salvo initiated by an "R on T." The third of the four ventricular premature systoles initiates a "salvo" (three ventricular premature systoles in a row); this premature QRS complex follows the preceding QRS by 0.28 sec and so falls during the T wave. The other premature QRS complexes, which do not initiate repetitive firing, occur later (0.30–0.34 sec) after the preceding sinus beat. The cycle lengths before the ventricular premature systoles are given on the Lewis diagram. (Modified from Katz and Pick, 1956.)

partially depolarizes the surrounding myocardium can both accelerate and delay discharge of the parasystolic pacemaker; this can cause parasystolic rhythms that, while marvelously complex, are highly regulated and so exhibit a predictable behavior (Jalife and Moe, 1981).

THE VULNERABLE PERIOD. Ventricular premature systoles that fall on the T wave of the preceding cycle ("R on T") (Fig. 16-47) can initiate a repetitive ventricular response, such as torsades (Fig. 16-57), a salvo (Fig. 16-59), or ventricular fibrillation. The later portion of the T wave therefore represents the *vulnerable period* (Fig. 16-60, see also Chapter 14), when the *ventricular fibrillation threshold* reaches its nadir. Even small electrical currents that reach the ventricles during the vulnerable period can cause sudden death.

Vulnerability is due largely to the tendency of impulses to become disorganized when they reach the ventricles during their relative refractory period, when repolarization is most heterogeneous. Because sodium channels are in different phases of recovery during the vulnerable period, the stage is set for inhomogeneities that cause decremental conduction and unidirectional block (see above). Earlier stimuli, during the S–T segment, fall during the absolute refractory period and cannot generate a propagated wave of depolarization, while stimuli that arrive after the end of the T wave find the ventricles fully recovered and able to generate large, rapidly rising action potentials that conduct rapidly and do not tend to become disorganized. Although the vulnerable period occurs at about the

FIGURE 16-60   The vulnerable period. Impulses that reach the ventricles during the middle and terminal portions of the T wave (*unshaded*) are most likely to initiate ventricular tachycardias and fibrillation.

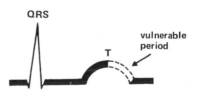

same time as the supernormal period, these two phenomena are not directly related.

FLUTTER AND FIBRILLATION

Regular depolarization of the atria at rates exceeding 250 to 350 or of the ventricles at rates of 150 to 300 causes an arrhythmia called *flutter*, while totally disorganized depolarization at even faster rates, where the fibrillating chamber resembles a bag of worms, is *fibrillation*. The importance of increased heart size in sustaining these arrhythmias was described in 1914 by W. E. Garrey, who noted that ventricular fibrillation is difficult to produce in a small isolated heart, like that of the cat, but hard to avoid in a large isolated heart, like that of the cow. To test the hypothesis that increased heart size favors fibrillation, Garrey did the very simple experiment of isolating a cow heart, causing it to fibrillate, and then cutting it into small pieces. As the mass of fibrillating tissue decreased, the pieces eventually ceased to fibrillate and instead either beat synchronously or stopped contracting altogether. This role of heart size explains both the increased risk of atrial fibrillation and the difficulty of restoring and maintaining sinus rhythm after cardioversion in patients with dilated atria. Increased ventricular size in patients with heart failure also predisposes them to serious arrhythmias.

Atrial Flutter and Fibrillation

Atrial flutter and fibrillation accelerate ventricular rate and abolish the ability of the atria to serve as a primer pump (Chapter 11). Although the hemodynamic consequences of these arrhythmias can be minor, especially in patients with normal hearts in whom the rate of ventricular beating is not increased, both are dangerous because stasis of blood in the fluttering or fibrillating atria often leads to clot formation. The latter can break off as *emboli* that travel from the right atrium to a pulmonary artery, and from the left atrium to a peripheral artery; both can be disastrous, especially when a systemic embolus blocks a cerebral artery therefore causing a stroke.

ATRIAL FLUTTER. Atrial flutter is a special form of reentry in which a wave of depolarization goes round and round in the right atrium. Atrial rates in this arrhythmia are usually close to 300, but normal decremental conduction in the AV node usually reduces the ventricular rate to 150 (2:1 AV dissociation), 100 (3:1 AV dissociation), or 75 (4:1 AV dissociation). In this way, the normal low safety factor in the AV node protects these patients from excessively rapid rates of ventricular beating. The ECG in atrial flutter usually shows a "saw tooth" pattern in the inferior leads, called *F waves*, that replace the normal P waves (Fig. 16-61). The QRS complexes in atrial flutter are normal unless there is aberrant conduction, bundle branch block, or another disorder of ventricular depolarization.

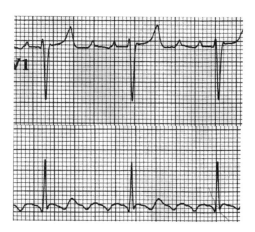

FIGURE 16-61   Atrial flutter with 4:1 AV dissociation (lead V$_1$ *above* and lead II *below*, recorded simultaneously). Atrial depolarization gives rise to regular saw-toothlike undulations of the baseline in lead II; these are typical F (flutter) waves. The atrial activity in lead V$_1$ resembles P waves, but these are the same flutter waves recorded in lead II. Because of the 4:1 AV dissociation, the ventricular rate is one-fourth that of the atria.

The reentrant circuit in atrial flutter typically lies within the right atrium, where impulses loop around the tricuspid valve ring, inferior vena cava, crista terminalis, and inferior vena cava in either a clockwise or, more commonly, a counterclockwise direction. However, other pathways can cause this arrhythmia. Because the circuit involves atrial myocardium, and so is maintained by sodium channel–dependent conduction, vagal stimulation and inhibition of calcium channel opening rarely abolish this arrhythmia, but both can slow the "ventricular response" by increasing block in the AV node. The treatment of choice is becoming ablation therapy, so because of the variability in the arrhythmogenic pathways, these patients require careful mapping of the reentrant circuit.

ATRIAL FIBRILLATION. The atrial rhythm in atrial fibrillation is disorganized, and the rate at which impulses pass through any point in the atria generally exceeds 400. The electrocardiographic manifestations of this activity are undulations in the baseline, called *f waves*, that are irregular in amplitude and frequency (Fig. 16-62). Ventricular rates in atrial fibrillation, like those in atrial flutter, are less than those in the atria; but unlike atrial flutter, the ventricular rhythm is usually irregularly irregular. The contour of the QRS complexes is normal (unless other abnormalities modify ventricular depolarization) because the ventricles are depolarized by impulses that arise above the bifurcation of the bundle of His.

In the early 20th century, two competing mechanisms were proposed to explain atrial fibrillation: rapidly discharging ectopic foci and one or more reentrant circuits in the atria. More recently, atrial fibrillation in many patients has been found to be caused by rapidly firing foci in the left atrium near the ostia of the pulmonary veins, which has made it possible to use radiofrequency ablation to destroy the arrhythmogenic sites.

When atrial fibrillation persists, the atria undergo changes similar to those that occur in chronically overloaded ventricles (see Chapter 18).

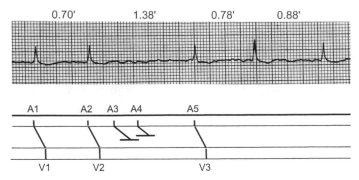

FIGURE 16-62 Atrial fibrillation (lead II). Rapid, disorganized atrial activity causes the irregular undulations of the baseline (*f waves*) that in some places occur at intervals less than 0.16 sec. The QRS complexes appear at irregularly irregular intervals, with cycle lengths ranging between 0.70 and 1.38 sec. These variations in ventricular cycle length cannot be explained simply by the timing of the arrival of f waves at the AV node, but instead reflect large changes in the apparent refractory period of the AV junction caused by concealed conduction. This is shown in the Lewis diagram, where the first three QRS complexes labeled V1 to V3 are diagrammed along with five atrial impulses, labeled A1 to A5. (For simplicity, most atrial impulses—which occur more frequently than shown here—are not included in the Lewis diagram.) Impulses A1 and A2, which are relatively far apart, are both conducted through the AV node to generate QRS complexes V1 and V2, but A3 occurred so soon after A2 that its passage through the AV node was blocked (*short horizontal line*). Conduction of A3 into the AV node then blocked the next impulse (A4). However, the next impulse (A5) entered the AV node much later after A4, so the AV node was able to recover from A4; as a result, A5 generated the third QRS complex (V3). The long pause in ventricular beating after V2 is explained by *concealed conduction*, in which A3 and A4 were conducted into the AV node, where they delayed the appearance of the next QRS complex (V3), but their conduction was *concealed* because they did not generate QRS complexes.

These changes, often called *atrial remodeling*, pose an important clinical problem as they tend to make it impossible to abolish the arrhythmia by using electrical cardioversion or drugs; these changes also make it difficult, and sometimes impossible, to maintain sinus rhythm when this can be restored in patients with long-standing atrial fibrillation.

CONCEALED CONDUCTION. Variations in the rate of ventricular beating in patients with atrial fibrillation are due in part to the irregular arrival of atrial impulses at the upper end of the AV node, but this cannot explain the marked differences in cycle length commonly seen in these patients. Instead, the variations in cycle length can be attributed to a mechanism called *concealed conduction* (Langendorf, 1948). This mechanism can be identified by close examination of the ECG shown in Figure 16-62, where intervals between QRS complexes (the "R–R interval") can exceed 1 sec, whereas intervals between f waves average about 0.15 sec. The short cycles demonstrate that the refractory period of the AV node is less than approximately 0.70 sec (the shortest R–R interval), so the long cycles, which exceed 1.3 sec, cannot be explained by random variations in the arrival of atrial impulses at the upper end of the AV node. Instead, the large differences in ventricular cycle lengths occur when atrial impulses enter, but do not cross, the AV junction. This mechanism, which is an example of "inhibition" (see Fig. 16-12), is called concealed conduction because many atrial impulses that enter the AV node do not reach the ventricles and their conduction is concealed, but the fact that conduction has occurred is evidenced by their ability to prevent subsequent impulses from reaching the ventricles.

Concealed conduction is readily demonstrated in the student laboratory when an isolated heart preparation, such as a turtle ventricle, is impaled with copper wires and stimulated electrically. At slow frequencies, each stimulus causes a contraction. When the rate of stimulation is increased gradually, the heart initially contracts in response to each stimulus; however, at higher rates, some stimuli fail to activate the heart. Further increases in stimulation frequency often causes "standstill," where no contractions occur. The failure of the heart to respond to the rapidly delivered stimuli is not due to irreversible damage because interrupting the train of stimuli allows slow stimulation again to cause contractions. The blocked stimuli, and the standstill at high rates of stimulation, are due to concealed conduction caused when rapidly delivered stimuli generate nonpropagated responses that, while unable to evoke visible contractions, cause a local refractory state that prevents subsequent stimuli from initiating contraction. The rapid stimuli are therefore conducted because they block subsequent stimuli, but their conduction is concealed, as no contractile responses are generated.

Ventricular Flutter and Fibrillation

Ventricular flutter and fibrillation are lethal arrhythmias that disorganize contraction in the ventricles to such an extent that the heart cannot sustain blood pressure or maintain cardiac output. The ECG in ventricular flutter resembles a sine wave (Fig. 16-63) that is probably caused by a large circus movement around the ventricles. In ventricular fibrillation (Fig. 16-64), chaotic oscillations of the baseline replace the QRS complexes.

There are two explanations for ventricular fibrillation (Chen et al., 2003). The first, sometimes called the *multiple wavelet hypothesis*, views the arrhythmia as occurring when a wave front breaks up into new wavelets. The other explanation, the *focal source hypothesis*, views ventricular fibrillation as a chaotic disorder that is maintained by a rotating spiral wave of depolarization called a *rotor*. The latter can be initiated

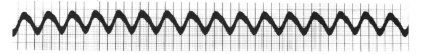

FIGURE 16-63 Ventricular flutter (lead II). The electrical activity of the ventricles resembles a sine wave; neither QRS complexes nor T waves can be made out. (From Katz and Pick, 1956.)

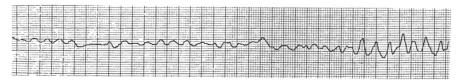

FIGURE 16-64 Ventricular fibrillation. Ventricular depolarization causes the rapid chaotic undulations in the baseline of this lethal arrhythmia.

when a wave front moving through the heart begins to slow at its edges (Fig. 16-65) or encounters an obstacle (Fig. 16-66), both of which cause the wave front to form spirals. As conduction slows at the edges of the front, the electrical vectors in the curved region are no longer parallel to the direction of propagation, which by increasing the curvature of the wave front causes the spirals to form rotors (Fig. 16-67). The tendency for rotor formation is increased by inhomogenetics in the density of the inward rectifier i_{K1} (Samie et al., 2001).

ION CHANNEL MUTATIONS. The discovery that mutations in cardiac ion channels and related proteins can cause ventricular tachycardia and fibrillation as well as other arrhythmias (Table 16-7, see Chapters 14 and 15) has opened a new era in the diagnosis and management of arrhythmias. The potential clinical impact of this molecular biology is illustrated by the Brugada syndrome (Fig. 16-68), which is emerging as a major cause of sudden death; some estimates put this syndrome second to only accidental death

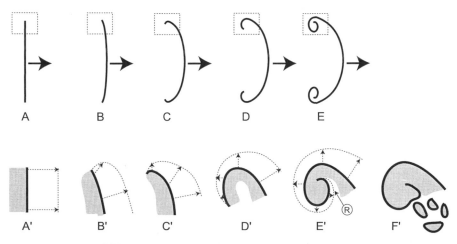

FIGURE 16-65 Postulated mechanism that causes ventricular fibrillation. When a wave of depolarization moving through the heart (A) slows at its edges, the front becomes curved (A–C) and eventually forms spirals (D). When the tips of the spirals move behind tissue that has already been depolarized, and so is refractory (circled R in E), the spirals can continue as "rotors" or break down into multiple disordered waves (F). The lower series of diagrams is an enlargement of the areas within the dashed rectangle in the upper series. Shaded areas are regions of slow conduction.

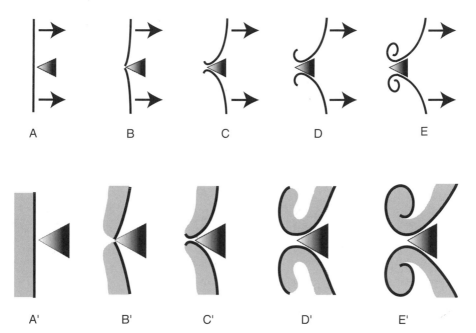

FIGURE 16-66 Postulated mechanism that causes ventricular fibrillation. When a wave of depolarization moving through the heart **(A)** encounters an obstacle, such as a scar (*triangle*), the center of the wave slows **(B–C)** and forms spirals **(D–E)** that can form rotors. The lower series of diagrams is an enlargement of the area near the obstacle in the upper series. Shaded areas are regions of slow conduction.

in causing mortality in young adults (Antzelevitch et al., 2005). The Brugada syndrome, which was first identified in 1992, can be caused by more than 80 mutations in the SCN5A gene that encodes the cardiac sodium channel; associated arrhythmias include polymorphic ventricular tachycardia and ventricular fibrillation as well as supraventricular arrhythmias.

ANTIARRHYTHMIC DRUGS

Virtually all antiarrhythmic drugs inhibit the opening or reactivation of voltage-gated ion channels. Although these drugs can abolish reentrant circuits by alleviating arrhythmogenic mechanisms like decremental

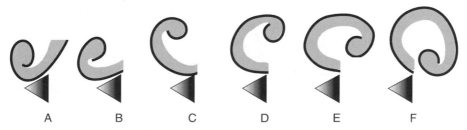

FIGURE 16-67 Rotor formation from the spiral wave in Figure 16-66E.

TABLE 16-7 **Some Arrhythmogenic Mutations in Voltage-Gated Ion Channels and Other Proteins**

Abnormal Structure	Gene	Mutated Protein	Clinical Syndrome
I_{Ks} channel			
	KCNQ1	KvLQT1	LQT1 syndrome
	KCNE1	MinK	LQT5 syndrome
	KCNQ1	KvLQT1	Familial atrial fibrillation
I_{Kr} channel			
	KCNH2	HERG	LQT2 syndrome
	KCNE2	MirP1	LQT6 syndrome
	KCNH2	HERG	Short QT syndrome
I_{Na} channel			
	SCN5A	hH1 (Nav 1.5)	LQT3 syndrome
	SCN5A	hH1 (Nav 1.5)	Brugada syndrome
	SCN5A	hH1 (Nav 1.5)	Lenégre's syndrome
I_{KI} channel			
	KCNJ2	Kir2.1	Andersen-Tawil Syndrome
Ankyrin	ANKB	ankyrin	LQT4 syndrome
Ryanodine receptor	RyR2	ryanodine receptor	CPVT 1
Calsequestrin	CASQ	calsequestrin	CPVT 2

Abbreviations: LQT: Long QT; CPVT: Catecholaminergic polymorphic ventricular tachycardia. Based on Priori (2004) and Clancy and Kass (2005). See also Chapter 14 and Table 15-2.

conduction, they not only modify ion channel function in the area where an arrhythmia originates, but also act in other regions of the heart. This complication makes it dangerous to administer several classes of these drugs.

Classification

The most widely accepted classification of antiarrhythmic drugs is that of Vaughan-Williams (1989) (Table 16-8), although other classifications have been proposed (Members of the Sicilian Gambit, 2001). Class I antiarrhythmic drugs block sodium channels, but subtle differences have led to their separation into three subclasses. Class IA agents, such as quinidine, procaineamide, and disopyramide, depress sodium channels and slow conduction in the atria, His–Purkinje system, and ventricles; because they also increase refractoriness and prolong action potential duration, they are especially useful in rapid tachycardias. Class IB agents,

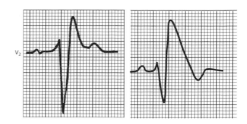

FIGURE 16-68   The Brugada syndrome. A single complex from lead V$_2$ in two patients with this syndrome show the characteristic pattern of ST-segment elevation, which resembles a broad R'.

like lidocaine, diphenylhydantoin, and mexilitine, have little or no effect on sodium channels in resting cells, but shorten the action potential and are potent inhibitors of sodium-dependent conduction in depolarized areas; the latter explains why Class IB drugs are effective in depressing conduction in ischemic areas of the heart. Class IC agents, like flecainide, propafenone, and moricizine, inhibit sodium channel opening but have less effect to prolong refractoriness.

TABLE 16-8   **Classification of the Antiarrhythmic Drugs**

Class and mechanism of action	Examples
I. Sodium channel blockade (inhibits i_{Na}), slows action potential upstroke	
IA. Inhibits i_{Na}, slows depolarization, prolongs refractoriness	Quinidine, procaineamide, disopyramide
IB. Little or no inhibition of depolarization at normal resting potential, shortens refractoriness in depolarized cells	Lidocaine, mexilitine, tocainide
IC. Inhibits i_{Na}, slows depolarization, minimal prolongation of refractoriness	Flecainide, propafenone, moricizine
II. β-adrenergic blockade (reduces activation of i_{CaL}), slows SA pacemaker and AV conduction	Propranolol, metoprolol, atenolol, timolol
III. Potassium channel blockade (inhibits i_K), prolongs refractoriness	Amiodarone, sotalol, bretylium, ibutilide, dofetilide
IV. Calcium channel blockade (inhibits i_{CaL}), slows SA pacemaker and AV conduction	
Dihydropyridines	Nifedipine, amlodipine, nitrendipine
Phenylalkylamines	Verapamil
Benzothiazepines	Diltiazem

The Class II agents are the β-adrenergic receptor blockers, which indirectly inhibit calcium channel opening by blocking their response to sympathetic stimulation (see Chapter 8). Class III agents, which include amiodarone, sotalol, bretylium, ibutilide, and dofetilide, inhibit repolarizing potassium current and therefore prolong the cardiac action potential; these drugs have little or no effect to inhibit depolarizing currents. The L-type calcium channel blockers are the Class IV agents; phenylalkylamines (e.g., verapamil) and benzothiazepines (e.g., diltiazem) slow the SA node pacemaker and inhibit conduction in the AV node, but dihydropyridines have only a minor effect on the heart.

The Modulated Receptor Hypothesis

Although all Class I agents inhibit sodium channel opening, the responses to different members of this class are affected by the state of the channel. These changes can be explained by the *modulated receptor hypothesis* (Hondeghem and Katzung, 1977), which considers an ion channel to be a "receptor" whose ability to bind a drug is modulated by voltage- and time-dependent changes in channel conformation (Fig. 16-69). These interactions can be characterized as reversible reactions in which each state of the channel binds to the drug with different rates of association and dissociation.

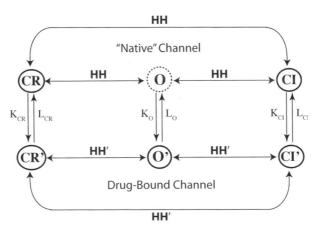

FIGURE 16-69 The modulated receptor hypothesis. Three states of a "native" ion channel (upper: **CR**: *closed, resting*, **O**: *open*, **CI**: *closed, inactivated*) can be characterized by transitions that reflect Hodgkin-Huxley kinetics as described in Chapter 13 (HH). Three inactive states of the channel after it has bound a drug that blocks channel opening (lower: **CR'**, **O'**, and **CI'**), which correspond to the three states of the native channel, also exhibit Hodgkin-Huxley kinetics (HH') but the rate constants of the transitions are different. Binding of the drug to the channel is defined by association constants (K_{CR}, K_O, and K_{CI}) and dissociation constants (L_{CR}, L_O, and L_{CI}). Of the six states shown, only the open state of the native channel (**O**, surrounded by dotted circle) allows the ion the cross the membrane.

Proarrhythmic Effects

A serious limitation in the clinical use of many antiarrhythmic drugs is their ability to worsen arrhythmias and cause sudden death. These proarrhythmic effects were so serious as to have caused the premature termination of major clinical trials (CAST INVESTIGATORS, 1989;

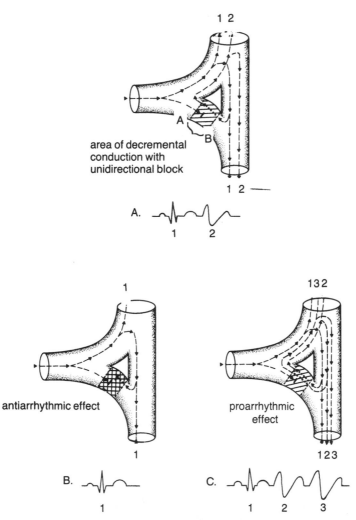

FIGURE 16-70 Antiarrhythmic and proarrhythmic drug effects in a region of decremental conduction and unidirectional block. **A:** Passage of a single impulse through the depressed tissue generates a single premature systole (see Fig. 16-10). **B:** An antiarrhythmic drug can abolish the reentrant circuit by further depressing conduction so as to convert the unidirectional block to bidirectional (complete) block. **C:** A proarrhythmic effect can occur if the drug slows conduction elsewhere in the reentrant circuit, which by delaying the return of an impulse to the depressed region provides sufficient time for the latter to recover its ability to propagate additional reentrant impulses.

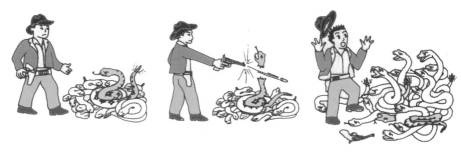

FIGURE 16-71 Allegory showing proarrhythmic effects of antiarrhythmic therapy. An attempt to survive in a snake pit (*left*) by shooting one threatening snake (*center*) can fail if the shot awakens a large number of previously dormant serpents (*right*). This situation is reminiscent of administering an antiarrhythmic drug that, although it eliminates one site for arrhythmia, increases the likelihood of sudden death by provoking other arrhythmogenic foci. (Modified from Katz, 1998.)

CAST II INVESTIGATORS, 1992). Most proarrhythmic effects of Class I agents are due to depressed conduction, which as noted above also is responsible for the antiarrhythmic effect; both are caused by inhibition of sodium channel opening. Proarrhythmic effects are less common in patients without structural heart disease but can be quite dangerous in patients with diseased hearts, where conduction is often depressed in areas outside of the arrhythmogenic focus. Figure 16-70 shows how a drug that, by depressing conduction in a region of decremental conduction and unidirectional block, can both prevent and cause a reentrant arrhythmia. A more general explanation for the proarrhythmic effect of an antiarrhythmic drug is provided by equating use of the drug to an attempt to survive in a snake pit by shooting one threatening snake, only to fail when the shot awakens a large number of previously dormant serpents (Fig. 16-71). This situation is like eliminating the threat posed by one arrhythmogenic mechanism only to increase the risk of sudden death by exacerbating other arrhythmogenic mechanisms.

BIBLIOGRAPHY

Chen P-S, Weiss JN. Runaway pacemakers in ventricular fibrillation. Circulation 2005;112:148–150.

Cosío FG, Martín-Peñato A, Pastor A, et al. Atypical flutter: a review. *PACE* 2003;26: 2157–2169.

Falk RH. Medical progress. Atrial fibrillation. *N Eng J Med* 2001;344:1067–1078.

Nattel S. New ideas about atrial fibrillation. *Nature* 2002;415:219–226.

Olgin JE, Zipes DP. Specific arrhythmias: diagnosis and treatment. In: Zipes DP, Libby P, Bonow RO, et al., eds. *Braunwald's heart disease*, 7th ed. Philadelphia: Elsevier Saunders, 2005:803–863.

Peters NS, Wit AL. Myocardial architecture and ventricular arrhythmogenesis. *Circulation* 1998;97:1746–1754.

Wagner CD, Persson PB. Chaos in the cardiovascular system: an update. *Cardiovasc Res* 1998;40:257–264.

Weiss JN, Chen PS, Wu TJ, et al. Ventricular fibrillation. New insights into mechanisms. *Ann NY Acad Sci* 2004;1015:122–132.

Wyse DG, Gersh BJ. Atrial fibrillation: a perspective. Thinking inside and outside the box. *Circulation* 2004;109:3089–3095.

Zipes D, Jalife F. *Cardiac electrophysiology. From cell to bedside*, 3rd ed. Philadelphia: WB Saunders, 2000.

REFERENCES

Antzelevitch C, Brugada P, Borggrefe M, et al. Brugada syndrome. Report of the second consensus conference. *Circulation* 2005;111:659–670.

CAST Investigators. The Cardiac Arrhythmia Suppression Trial Investigators. Preliminary report: effect of encainide and flecainide on mortality in a randomized trial of arrhythmia suppression after myocardial infarction. *N Eng J Med* 1989;321:406–412.

CAST II Investigators. The Cardiac Arrhythmia Suppression Trial II Investigators. Effect of the anti-arrhythmic agent moricizine on survival after myocardial infarction. *N Eng J Med* 1992;327:227–233.

Chen PS, Wu TJ, Ting CT, et al. A tale of two fibrillations. *Circulation* 2003;108:2298–2303.

Clancy CE, Kass RS. Inherited and acquired vulnerability to ventricular arrhythmias: cardiac Na^+ and K^+ channels. *Physiol Rev* 2005;85:33–47.

Garrey WE. The nature of fibrillary contraction of the heart. Its relation to tissue mass and form. *Am J Physiol* 1914;33:397–414.

Hondeghem L, Katzung BG. Time- and voltage-dependent interaction of antiarrhythmic drugs with cardiac sodium channels. *Biochim Biophys Acta* 1977;472:373–398.

Jalife J, Moe GK. Excitation, conduction, and reflection of impulses in isolated bovine and canine cardiac Purkinje fibers. *Circ Res* 1981;49:233–247.

Katz AM. Selectivity and toxicity of antiarrhythmic drugs: molecular interactions with ion channels. *Am J Med* 1998;104:179–195.

Katz LN, Pick A. *Clinical electrocardiography*. Part I: the arrhythmias. Philadelphia: Lea and Febiger, 1956.

Langendorf R. Concealed A-V conduction: the effect of blocked impulses on the formation and conduction of subsequent impulses. *Am Heart J* 1948;35:542–552.

Members of the Sicilian Gambit. New approaches to antiarrhythmic therapy. Emerging therapeutic applications of the cell biology of cardiac arrhythmias. *Circulation* 2001;104: 2865–2873;2990–2994.

Priori SG. Inherited arrhythmogenic diseases. The complexity beyond monogenic disorders. *Circ Res.* 2004;94:140–145.

Samie FH, Berenfeld O, Anumonwo J, et al. Rectification of the background potassium current. A determinant of rotor dynamics in ventricular fibrillation. *Circ Res* 2001;89: 1216–1223.

Vaughan-Williams EM. Classification of antiarrhythmic actions. In: Vaughan-Williams EM, Campbell TJ, eds. *Handbook of experimental pharmacology. Antiarrhythmic drugs.* Berlin: Springer-Verlag, 1989:45–57.

More complete descriptions of the clinical features of the topics discussed in this chapter are found in textbooks of electrophysiology, cardiology, and electrocardiography.

17

THE ISCHEMIC HEART

Because its high energy needs can be met only by oxidative metabolism (Chapter 2), the heart requires an uninterrupted supply of oxygen. For this reason, coronary artery occlusion causes an almost immediate loss of function and, within hours, death of the energy-starved cardiac myocytes. Ischemic cell death, called *myocardial infarction*, is a leading cause of death and disability in developed countries. Although this condition is often referred to as *ischemic heart disease*, the cause lies in the coronary arteries, so the myocardium is the victim and not the perpetrator; for this reason, the alternative names, *coronary heart disease, arteriosclerotic heart disease*, and *arteriosclerotic cardiovascular disease* seem more appropriate.

Conditions other than coronary occlusion can cause the heart to become energy-starved; these include aortic stenosis and pulmonary hypertension, in which pressure overload increases the oxygen requirements of the left or right ventricle to levels that exceed the amount that can be supplied by even a normal coronary circulation, and anemia, which reduces the oxygen-carrying capacity of the blood. *Angina pectoris* (literally strangling in the chest), the typical symptom in patients with an energy-starved heart, is therefore not diagnostic of ischemic heart disease, but instead indicates that the heart's demand for oxygen exceeds the amount supplied by the coronary circulation.

CORONARY OCCLUSIVE DISEASE

A detailed discussion of the pathophysiology of arterial occlusive disease, which is a major topic of *vascular biology*, is beyond the scope of the present text. It is appropriate, however, to note that coronary atherosclerosis, by far the most common cause of coronary occlusion, is the result of a chronic inflammatory process that evolves over many decades. Significant decreases in coronary flow generally appear late in the course of this process, usually when endothelial damage leads to the formation of platelet plugs and thrombi (clots) that occlude one or more major coronary arteries. In most cases, occlusion is initiated by disruption of a fibrous cap that separates soft lipid-filled atherosclerotic lesions within the arterial wall from the blood flowing through the lumen. This process, called *plaque rupture*, exposes collagen and other thrombogenic elements in the atherosclerotic lesion to the moving column of blood in the artery, which can occlude the diseased vessel by triggering platelet aggregation and thrombus formation. Coronary vasospasm, a less common cause of coronary occlusion, can be caused when vasoconstrictor peptides are released from activated platelets in arteries that may lack obvious atherosclerotic lesions.

Total occlusion of a major coronary artery generally causes *transmural ischemia*, where the entire thickness of the ventricular wall becomes ischemic. However, total occlusion of a similar artery in a patient with a well-developed collateral circulation may cause significant ischemia only in the subendocardium, which is less well perfused than the epicardium (see Chapter 1), and where wall stress is higher (see Chapter 11). Subendocardial ischemia also occurs when myocardial oxygen demand is increased in a patient with a partial coronary artery occlusion, which explains the characteristic electrocardiographic (ECG) finding of ST segment depression in a "positive" stress test (see below). Ischemia caused by interruption of coronary flow, either transmural or subendocardial, persists until the energy-starved tissue dies or perfusion is restored, whereas ischemia evoked by exertion is typically relieved by rest, which reduces myocardial energy demand.

ANGINA PECTORIS

The key to evaluating patients with ischemic heart disease is the clinical history, which in addition to suggesting the diagnosis, helps to illuminate the underlying pathophysiology and provides an essential guide to therapy. Angina pectoris, the typical symptom caused when cardiac energy demand exceeds energy supply, is a visceral pain that localizes poorly and is often difficult to describe. Most patients experience a heaviness or squeezing in the left chest, but others note a vague discomfort that may be mistaken for indigestion. Angina typically radiates to the inner arm, neck, or jaw but may be referred elsewhere—for example, to the site of an old arm or shoulder injury or the socket of a lost tooth. However, patients may not experience typical symptoms even after total coronary occlusion has caused a large myocardial infarction.

The symptoms of ischemic heart disease can appear in two patterns often described as "demand" angina and "supply" angina. *Demand angina*, as the name implies, occurs when the chest pain syndrome is provoked by increased cardiac work, such as during exercise. Demand angina almost always forces patients to stop exertion and is typically relieved promptly by rest, usually within a few minutes. The severity of demand angina can be quantified in terms of the amount of effort needed to provoke symptoms, most precisely by a stress test. In *supply angina*, which typically occurs without provocation, the imbalance between energy supply and energy demand is caused by a decrease in supply, so its appearance indicates that coronary flow has been suddenly reduced by a new occlusion or vasospasm.

One of the most important characteristics of angina pectoris is its stability; that is, whether the discomfort is staying the same, improving, or worsening. Angina can persist unchanged for years, when the coronary artery disease does not progress. Spontaneous improvement, which was often seen before procedures were developed to revascularize the heart, usually occurs when blood flow to underperfused regions is increased by enlargement of partially occluded coronary arteries, called *vascular remodeling*, or when collateral vessels develop. Angina that increases in severity, lasts longer, or is provoked by decreasing effort indicates that the underlying coronary disease is worsening.

Stable Angina

The pattern of symptoms in patients with *stable angina pectoris* is typically that of demand angina, where the chest discomfort is made worse when myocardial oxygen demand is increased—for example, by exertion or emotional upset. Although symptoms occur when myocardial cells become anaerobic, the substance or substances responsible for the chest discomfort remain unclear.

Stable angina generally has a benign prognosis because brief episodes of ischemia do not damage the heart. For this reason, the natural history of stable angina is determined largely by progression of the disease in the coronary arteries. Careful management of the risk factors for atherosclerosis, such as high LDL cholesterol, diabetes, hypertension, and overweight, as well as elimination of smoking, are therefore key to improving prognosis. When symptoms develop, treatment usually relies on β-blockers and vasodilators to reduce energy demand; nitrates, which act by decreasing preload and dilating intercoronary collaterals; and drugs, like aspirin, that prevent platelet aggregation and clotting in the diseased coronary arteries.

Vasospastic Angina

Angina in patients with coronary vasospasm typically occurs at rest, usually without a clear predisposing cause. This syndrome, also called *vasospastic angina*, *variant angina*, or *Prinzmetal's angina* (after Myron Prinzmetal), is dangerous because unlike demand angina, which can be relieved by rest, the ischemia continues until the constricted coronary artery dilates or the ischemic myocardium dies. In some patients, coronary vasospasm triggers arrhythmias that may be fatal; in others, the ischemia can last long enough to cause a myocardial infarction. The obvious goal of treatment is to relieve the coronary vasoconstriction, which can be done with variable success using combinations of nitrates, calcium channel blockers, and other drugs.

ACUTE CORONARY SYNDROMES: UNSTABLE ANGINA AND ACUTE MYOCARDIAL INFARCTION

Worsening of symptoms, called *acute coronary syndrome* or *instability*, usually follows one of three patterns. The least severe, *unstable angina*, occurs when symptoms worsen without evidence of myocardial cell death. The other two, which are accompanied by evidence of necrosis, are *non–ST elevation myocardial infarction (NSTEMI)* and *ST elevation myocardial infarction (STEMI)*. These were formerly called *transmural* or *Q-wave myocardial infarction,* and *subendocardial* or *non–Q-wave* or *nontransmural myocardial infarction*, respectively. Although all acute coronary syndromes result from increasing coronary occlusion, they differ in pathophysiology and prognosis and require different therapy (see below).

Unstable Angina

The pathophysiology of angina and its relationship to energy starvation explains the clinical history in patients with unstable angina, where the severity of the symptoms increases, the amount of effort needed to evoke the chest discomfort decreases, or angina appears at rest. The appearance of unstable angina usually indicates that the occlusive disease in the coronary arteries is worsening but also can be caused when a complicating condition, like anemia, impairs oxygen delivery to the heart. Unstable angina often follows a "stuttering" course caused when platelet plugs and thrombi in a newly damaged artery break up or dissolve and then reform.

Instability generally results from plaque disruption, where damage to the fibrous cap in a previously stable coronary artery atherosclerotic lesion exposes a thrombogenic surface that leads to the formation of platelet plugs and thrombi. Worsening of symptoms therefore has ominous prognostic implications and can herald a myocardial infarction or sudden cardiac death. For this reason, unstable angina is a medical emergency that requires prompt expert medical attention.

Acute Myocardial Infarction

Acute myocardial infarction occurs when coronary flow is reduced to levels so low as to cause myocardial cell death. Most clinical infarctions involve the left ventricle; right ventricular infarction can occur but is less common. Because the endocardium is especially vulnerable to energy starvation (see above), coronary occlusion causes endocardial myocytes to be severely injured and to die sooner than those in the epicardium.

The criteria now used to classify patients with myocardial infarction center on whether the ST segments in ECG leads facing the infarction are depressed or elevated. The distinction between NSTEMI and STEMI is determined largely by how much of the ventricular wall is injured or infarcted (see below).

β-adrenergic blockers reduce the energy demands of the heart and so can alleviate symptoms and improve prognosis when administered immediately after a coronary occlusion; their energy-sparing effects, although of little value in totally ischemic regions of the heart, can be quite beneficial in regions where perfusion is reduced but not totally abolished. Nitrates, calcium channel blockers, and other vasodilators are useful because they reduce afterload, which reduces energy demand; nitrates also decrease preload and selectively dilate collateral vessels. Aspirin and other platelet inhibitors, along with antithrombotic drugs like heparin, also improve prognosis. However, the most effective treatment for patients with STEMI is reperfusion of the ischemic myocardium either with thrombolytic agents or, preferably, primary angioplasty.

JEOPARDIZED MYOCARDIUM AND "ISCHEMIA AT A DISTANCE"

The consequences of coronary occlusion are influenced by collateral vessels that, by connecting large epicardial coronary arteries, allow more than one major coronary artery to supply a given region of the heart (Fig. 17-1). Collateral vessels generally develop when partial occlusion of a coronary artery reduces, but does not totally interrupt, blood flow to a region of the heart. Because this collateral circulation increases with

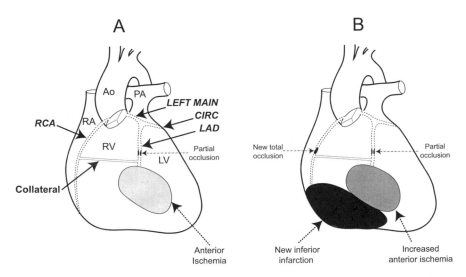

FIGURE 17-1 Ischemia at a distance. **A:** Anterior view of a heart where partial occlusion of the left anterior descending coronary artery (LAD) has stimulated the development of a collateral vessel linking the occluded artery to a normal right coronary artery (RCA). The anterior region of the left ventricle supplied by the partially occluded LAD can become ischemic (*light shading*) when the energy demands of the heart are increased. **B:** A new total occlusion of the RCA not only causes an inferior infarction (*black*), but also decreases blood flow to the anterior region that had previously received a dual blood supply (*dark shading*). This is because the RCA occlusion *jeopardized* the blood supply to this region, which came to depend entirely on the partially occluded LAD. The RCA occlusion therefore caused ischemia to appear in a region (the anterior wall) that is not normally supplied by this vessel, which is an example of *ischemia at a distance*. (CIRC, circumflex coronary artery; RA, right atrium; LA, left atrium; RV, right ventricle; LV, left ventricle; PA, pulmonary artery; Ao, aorta.)

advancing age, occlusion of a major coronary artery in young patients, who generally have few collateral vessels, usually causes a large infarct, whereas the same occlusion in an older patient with an extensive collateral circulation may cause only minor symptoms and sometimes no symptoms at all.

The role of collaterals can be understood by considering a patient with a large collateral vessel connecting a normal right coronary artery (RCA) to a partially occluded left anterior descending coronary artery (LAD), which together provide the anterior wall of the left ventricle with a dual blood supply (Fig. 17-1A). Occlusion of the RCA in this setting not only leads to necrosis of the inferior wall, which had received its entire blood supply from this vessel, but causes blood flow to the anterior wall to become *jeopardized* because the latter has become entirely dependent on the partially occluded LAD for its entire blood supply (Fig. 17-1B). Because the RCA occlusion has caused ischemia in a region that is outside of its normal distribution (the anterior wall), this situation is called *ischemia at a distance*. The common occurrence of jeopardized myocardium in patients with coronary atherosclerosis illustrates the importance of collateral blood flow and provides one reason why the clinical consequences of a coronary occlusion vary among patients (Habib et al., 1991).

INITIAL CONSEQUENCES OF CORONARY ARTERY OCCLUSION

Patients who sustain an acute myocardial infarction generally experience severe chest pain, loss of pump function, and arrhythmias. The hemodynamic complications depend largely on the amount of the left ventricle that has been infarcted, but the severity of the arrhythmias that accompany myocardial infarction does not correlate well with infarct size.

Two reflexes influence the clinical picture in acute myocardial infarction. Most important is the hemodynamic defense reaction (see Chapter 8), which is activated because these patients are generally in pain and terrified; this functional response also is stimulated when a large infarction causes blood pressure to fall. This neurohumoral response causes sympathetic simulation that worsens energy starvation in the ischemic myocardium by increasing heart rate and contractility, and by causing arteriolar vasoconstriction that increases afterload; other adverse effects of sympathetic stimulation include arrhythmias and sudden death. The second reflex, which is activated in patients with inferior and posterior left ventricular infarction, is a powerful vagal response (the von Bezold–Jarisch reflex, see below) that reduces blood pressure, slows the sinus node pacemaker, and can lead to AV block.

Hypoxia, like ischemia, causes energy starvation, but the consequences differ because coronary occlusion, in addition to interrupting oxygen supply to the heart, prevents the removal of metabolites and, by reducing the pressure within the coronary arteries supplying the left ventricle, attenuates the "garden hose effect" (see below).

Early Pump Failure

Interruption of coronary flow to the mammalian heart is followed almost immediately by a decrease in contractility and profound impairment of ventricular filling. The depressed contractility, which is accompanied by abbreviation of systole, causes the ischemic ventricular wall to bulge outward during systole because it cannot overcome the intraventricular pressure generated by the normally perfused myocardium. The resulting decrease in ejection increases the volume of blood in the ventricle at end-diastole, which because the heart lies within nondistensible pericardium, impairs filling.

THE GARDEN HOSE EFFECT. The early pump failure caused by coronary artery occlusion precedes a major fall in (ATP) content and other metabolic changes (Fig. 17-2). The most likely explanation for the rapid impairment of ejection is decreased sarcomere length caused by attenuation of the distending effect of intracoronary pressure (the *garden hose effect*, see Chapter 10) (Vogel et al., 1982; Koretsune et al., 1991).

METABOLIC ABNORMALITIES. Oxygen tension within the myocardium falls almost to zero within a minute after complete cessation of blood flow. This reflects the very high affinity of the respiratory chain for oxygen, which causes the ischemic myocardial cells to consume all of the available oxygen within a few minutes after the myocardium loses its blood supply; as a result, oxidative phosphorylation comes to a complete halt. Anaerobic energy production is increased in part by decreases in ATP and glucose-6-phosphate levels, increased ADP, AMP, and P_i levels, and sympathetic stimulation, which accelerates glycogen breakdown, glucose uptake, and glycolysis (see Chapter 2). Sympathetic stimulation also stimulates fatty acid release from triglycerides, but because these lipids cannot be oxidized in the ischemic heart, fatty acids and their derivatives accumulate (see below).

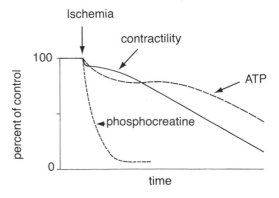

FIGURE 17-2 Time courses of the decline in contractility, ATP content, and phosphocreatine after the onset of ischemia. (Based on data from Williamson, 1966.)

The increased rate of anaerobic glycolysis in the ischemic heart is transient and ceases when NAD^+ levels fall to levels below those needed to reduce glyceraldehyde-3-phosphate, and conversion of pyruvate to lactate causes the heart to become acidotic. The latter inhibits glycolysis, contractile protein interactions (see Chapter 4), and many of the calcium fluxes that participate in excitation–contraction coupling and relaxation (see Chapter 7).

ATP levels fall rapidly after coronary occlusion but initially do not become low enough to deprive the substrate-binding sites of the contractile proteins and ion pumps of their energy source; this is because the normal cytosolic ATP concentration is 5 to 10 mM, whereas most substrate-binding sites are saturated at ATP concentrations less than 1 μM. Attenuation of the allosteric effects of high ATP concentrations can increase diastolic stiffness by inhibiting the dissociation of actin and myosin (see Chapter 4), and reduce contractility and impair relaxation by slowing ion pumps, ion exchangers, and passive ion fluxes through membrane channels (see Chapter 7) (Table 17-1). Reduction in the allosteric effect of ATP also inhibits the sodium pump (see Chapter 7), which has several adverse consequences that include a rise in cytosolic sodium, that impairs relaxation by reducing calcium efflux by way of the Na–Ca exchanger, and reduced potassium influx that inactivates calcium and sodium channel opening by decreasing resting membrane potential. These

TABLE 17-1 **Effects of Diminished Allosteric Effects of ATP on Myocardial Contraction and Relaxation**

Process	Immediate Consequence	Mechanical Effect
Actin–myosin interactions	Loss of "plasticizing" effect; reduced dissociation of thick and thin filaments	Negative lusitropic, contracture (rigor)
Plasma membrane Ca channels	Reduced Ca influx into the cytosol	Negative inotropic
Plasma membrane Ca pump	Reduced Ca efflux from the cytosol; increased intracellular Ca	Negative lusitropic, contracture
Plasma membrane Na pump	Reduced Na efflux; increased intracellular Na; decreased Ca efflux by the Na–Ca exchanger; increased intracellular Ca	Negative lusitropic, contracture
Sarcoplasmic reticulum Ca channels	Reduced Ca release during systole; less Ca release for binding to contractile proteins	Negative inotropic
Sarcoplasmic reticulum Ca pump	Reduced Ca uptake during diastole; failure to remove Ca from contractile proteins	Negative lusitropic, contracture

effects decrease cardiac output and blood pressure and, by slowing impulse conduction, set the stage for arrhythmias.

The most important effects of ATP depletion are due to a decrease in the free energy of ATP hydrolysis, which reduces the energy made available by hydrolysis of the terminal phosphate bond in ATP, which is proportional to the ATP/ADP ratio. Because even a slight fall in ATP concentration causes a disproportional increase in ADP concentration, energy starvation can reduce the free energy of ATP hydrolysis to levels that slow both the calcium pump of the sarcoplasmic reticulum (Tian and Ingwall, 1996) and cross-bridge cycling (Tian et al., 1997a,b).

ACIDOSIS. Acidification of the ischemic heart is due largely to lactate formation and hydrolysis of ATP; the latter releases inorganic phosphate, a weak acid that liberates hydrogen ions at the pH found in the cytosol of cardiac myocytes. Some of these protons are absorbed when phosphocreatine hydrolysis releases creatine, which is a weak base, but the net effect is to acidify the ischemic heart. In addition to slowing glycolysis (see Chapter 2), protons interfere with many of the reactions involved in contraction and relaxation when they compete with calcium for binding sites on a number of channels, pumps, and exchangers (see Chapters 4 and 7). Acidosis also can cause arrhythmias by slowing conduction, which occurs when protons close gap junctions in the intercalated disc (see Chapter 13) and inhibit the opening of voltage-gated ion channels (see Chapter 16).

POTASSIUM. The large amounts of phosphate released by hydrolysis of ATP and phosphocreatine in the ischemic heart reduce the calcium sensitivity of the contractile proteins and may form calcium phosphate complexes that trap calcium within the sarcoplasmic reticulum. Because phosphate, along with lactate, readily crosses the plasma membrane, when these anions appear in ischemic cells, they pour into the extracellular space. To maintain electrical neutrality when these anions leave the cell, they are accompanied by potassium, the major intracellular cation. This causes a large potassium efflux that, by reducing the ratio $[K^+]_i/[K_+]_o$, decreases the Nernst potential for potassium (see Chapter 14). The latter, which depolarizes the ischemic myocardial cells, has several effects, all of them bad. Depolarization slows conduction, which leads to reentrant arrhythmias, depresses excitability, and has a negative inotropic effect that contributes to the early pump failure. Because the depolarization caused by coronary artery occlusion is inhomogeneous, it generates *injury currents* that are a major cause of lethal arrhythmias (see Chapter 16).

ELECTROCARDIOGRAPHIC ABNORMALITIES IN THE ISCHEMIC HEART

Coronary artery occlusion causes characteristic ECG abnormalities and a variety of arrhythmias, many of which are quite dangerous. The latter are often exacerbated by reflexes that are activated in patients who experience an acute myocardial infarction.

Injury Currents and ST Segment Shifts

Depolarization of ischemic myocardial cells establishes differences in resting potential that allow current to flow between the normally perfused and ischemic regions of the heart. These currents, called *injury currents*, cause diagnostic ST segment shifts on the ECG that help distinguish between subendocardial ischemia, which depresses the ST segment, and transmural ischemia, which causes ST elevation. The mechanisms by which injury currents cause these characteristic ST segment shifts are complex because ST segment devaluations cannot be distinguished from changes in the TP segment. This is because there is no "zero" in the clinical ECG, where the baseline, by convention, is assumed to be the potential difference recorded during the TP segment (see Chapter 15). For this reason, diastolic injury currents, which displace the TP segment, are interpreted as ST segment shifts; TP depression becomes ST elevation, and TP elevation becomes ST depression (Fig. 17-3).

ST SEGMENT ELEVATION IN TRANSMURAL ISCHEMIA. The major cause of ST segment elevation in leads facing a region of transmural injury is a diastolic injury current caused when ischemia depolarizes the resting myocardium. This reduces the positive charge at the surface of the ischemic cells so that during diastole, leads that face the ischemic region are in a region of electronegativity. According to electrocardiographic convention (see Chapter 15), this depresses the TP segment (Fig. 17-3A) which, because the TP segment is viewed as the baseline, is interpreted as ST elevation. During systole, when the entire heart is depolarized, the potential difference between the normally perfused and ischemic regions is decreased. This reduces the injury current and so normalizes the TP segment (and therefore the ST segment as well). There are other explanations for ST elevation in acute transmural ischemia; these include potential differences caused by action potential abbreviation and slow conduction in the ischemic region.

The ST segment elevation in patients with transmural ischemia usually disappears within 24 to 48 hours after the infarction. This can result from two very different mechanisms: the underperfused myocardium is no longer ischemic, which occurs when reperfusion allows the ischemic cells to recover, or acidosis and calcium overload in the ischemic cells increase internal resistance by closing connexon channels in the gap junctions (see Chapter 13).

ST SEGMENT DEPRESSION IN SUBENDOCARDIAL ISCHEMIA. Subendocardial ischemia causes ST segment depression when a layer of perfused myocardium separates the partially depolarized endocardium from the epicardial surface of the heart (Fig. 17-3B). Because normally perfused epicardial cells are more positively charged during diastole than cells in the ischemic subendocardium, an ECG lead facing the ischemic region records TP segment elevation that, for the reasons given above, is interpreted as ST segment depression.

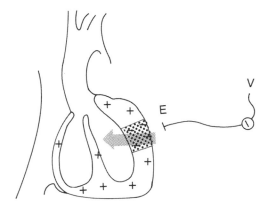
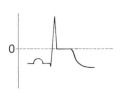

A. Transmural Ischemia

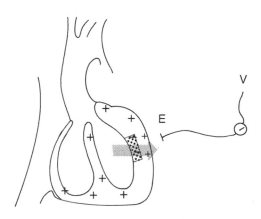
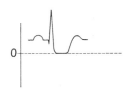

B. Subendocardial Ischemia

FIGURE 17-3 Injury currents caused by transmural and subendocardial ischemia. The ECG (*right*) records the potential difference between an electrode (**E**) that faces the surface of the ischemic region and a central terminal (**V**) that is defined as "zero." The ischemic region is *shaded*, and the surface potentials shown are those during diastole. **A**: Transmural ischemia, which depolarizes the ischemic myocardium, causes a diastolic injury current in which the lead facing the ischemic region is in an area of electronegativity. This causes an electrical vector directed away from the lead (*shaded arrow*). By convention, this lead inscribes a downward deflection that causes TP segment depression. During systole, when the normal myocardium also becomes depolarized, the injury current is reduced, which returns the TP segment toward baseline. By convention, TP depression during diastole is interpreted as ST segment elevation. **B**: Subendocardial ischemia causes a diastolic injury current in which the lead facing the ischemic region is in an area of electropositivity, which causes an electrical vector directed toward the lead (*shaded arrow*). By convention, this lead inscribes an upward deflection that causes TP segment elevation that, for the reasons given in **A**, is interpreted as ST segment depression.

ST segment depression is commonly seen in *demand ischemia*—for example, during exercise—because energy starvation is most severe in the endocardium, where energy demands are highest and blood supply most precarious. ST depression also is seen in left ventricular hypertrophy, even when the coronary arteries are normal, because of the vulnerability of the subendocardium to energy starvation.

Abnormal Q Waves and Myocardial Cell Death

The appearance of abnormal Q waves is a useful electrocardio-graphic "marker" for transmural cell death in the left ventricle (Fig. 17-4). These initial downward deflections appear in leads facing the infarct because the infarcted regions, which had normally transmitted a wave of depolarization toward the lead, have become electrically silent. A useful way to view abnormal Q waves is to visualize the electrically silent myocardium as a "window" through which a lead can "look" into the left ventricular cavity, where downward QS complexes are normally recorded. The latter is readily understood because ventricular depolarization begins in the endocardium, which causes all of the electrical vectors in the ventricular wall to be directed away from the cavity (see Chapter 15); as a result, an electrode catheter placed in the cavity of the normal left ventricle records a downward deflection. Abnormal Q waves also occur when viable myocardium is replaced by scar tissue—as in a ventricular aneurysm or when a tumor invades the wall of the ventricle—and therefore are not diagnostic of infarction.

Although abnormal Q waves suggest transmural infarction, and the absence of Q waves in patients with acute myocardial infarction suggests subendocardial infarction, pathological findings do not always confirm these electrocardiographic diagnoses. For this reason, these patterns, which

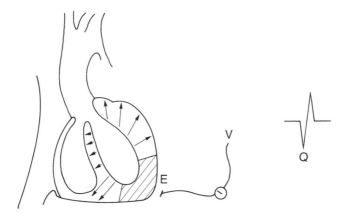

FIGURE 17-4   Abnormal Q waves. A lead facing a transmural infarction, which is electrically "silent," records a downward initial QRS deflection because depolarization of the noninfarcted myocardium generates electrical vectors that are directed away from this lead.

came to be called *Q-wave infarction* and *non–Q-wave infarction*, are now referred to as *ST elevation myocardial infarction* (STEMI) and *non–ST elevation myocardial infarction* (NSTEMI). This distinction is useful clinically because, as might be expected, the prognosis of a non–Q-wave infarction is better than that following a Q-wave infarction. Furthermore, clinical trials have shown that because the benefits of reperfusion outweigh the risks in STEMI but not NSTEMI, these two syndromes must be treated differently.

Electrocardiographic Localization of a Myocardial Infarction

The presence of abnormal Q waves and ST segment shifts in leads that face ischemic regions of the left ventricle are useful in localizing an infarction (Table 17-2) and can help to identify the infarct artery. Occlusion of the left anterior descending coronary artery is usually responsible for anterior and anteroseptal infarctions, while occlusion of the right coronary or circumflex coronary arteries generally causes inferior and posterior infarctions. However, electrocardiographic criteria for infarct localization often fail to correlate with the pathological findings.

A more important distinction based on the location of an infarct is that between *anterior* infarctions, which tend to be larger, and *inferoposterior* infarctions, which are frequently associated with the von Bezoldt–Jarisch

TABLE 17-2 Electrocardiographic Localization of Myocardial Infarctions

Localization	Leads in Which Abnormal Q Waves are Found
ANTERIOR	
Anteroseptal	V_1, V_2
Anterior	V_2, V_3, V_4
Anterolateral	I, aVL, (V_4), V_5, V_6
Extensive Anterior	I, aVL, V_1–V_6
INFEROPOSTERIOR	
Inferior	II, III, aVF
Posterior	R in V_1*
Inferolateral	II, III, aVF, (V_5), V_6
Posterolateral	R in V_1*, V_6 (V_5)
Inferoposterior	R in V_1*, II, III, aVF

*The abnormally tall R wave in lead V_1 would, in a lead placed on the patient's back, be recorded as a Q wave. Because posterior leads, called V_7 and V_8, are rarely used, the diagnosis of posterior infarction is usually made in lead V_1, where an abnormally tall initial R wave is equivalent to the inverted Q wave that would have been recorded in leads V_7 and V_8.

reflex (see below). A useful but not very precise index of the extent of left ventricular damage is the number of leads that show electrocardiographic abnormalities, especially Q waves.

"Evolution"

A key feature of the ECG changes in myocardial infarction is their *evolution*, which refers to dynamic changes that can continue for several days and sometimes for weeks. The initial abnormality, which appears within a few minutes after the onset of symptoms, is a marked increase in the amplitude of the T waves in leads facing the infarction. These tall T waves, called *hyperacute* T waves, often merge with the elevated ST segments in a pattern that resembles a tombstone (Fig. 17-5). A likely cause of the increased T-wave amplitude is the high extracellular potassium level that results from potassium efflux from the ischemic cells (see above); elevated serum potassium (hyperkalemia) also causes tall T waves, but with a somewhat different contour.

Hyperacute T waves usually last only a few hours and disappear both after reperfusion, and when the infarct artery is not reopened and the myocardium remains ischemic. The ST segment elevations rapidly return to normal if the ischemic myocardium is reperfused while it is still viable, but ST segment normalization requires 1 to 2 days when the infarct artery remains occluded. If an infarction is transmural, Q waves appear after a few hours (Fig. 17-6) and generally persist when the infarction is large. After a small infarction, however, Q waves often diminish in size and can disappear as the necrotic area shrinks and forms a scar.

T wave evolution, a much more puzzling electrocardiographic finding, describes a slowly deepening T-wave inversion in leads facing the ischemic region (Fig. 17-6) that can progress for several days and sometimes weeks when patients are improving clinically. T-wave evolution in ischemic heart disease is not a marker for cell death, but instead is caused by changes in the ion channels in regions of the heart that remain viable

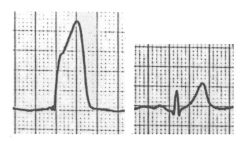

FIGURE 17-5 Hyperacute T wave (lead V_4). The first record, obtained from a patient two hours after experiencing the onset of severe chest pain, shows a large hyperacute T wave that, along with the markedly elevated ST segment, resembles a tombstone. The second record was obtained two hours later, after administration of streptokinase had lysed the clot obstructing his coronary artery and the patient had become pain-free.

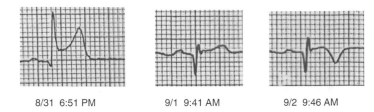

8/31 6:51 PM   9/1 9:41 AM   9/2 9:46 AM

FIGURE 17-6   Evolution of an acute inferior myocardial infarction (lead aVF). The first record (8/31) was obtained in the emergency room while the patient was experiencing chest pain. The subsequent records, taken one day apart, show typical evolution. On the second day (9/1), resolution of the ST segment elevation indicates that the injury current had disappeared, while the new Q wave indicates that the inferior wall of the left ventricle had become infarcted. On the third day (9/2), the appearance of a symmetrically inverted ("coved") T wave is typical of T-wave evolution. The infarct artery was not opened because neither thrombolytic therapy or primary angioplasty was available at the time this patient was seen.

after an episode of severe ischemia. Similar T-wave evolution is seen after severe tachycardia (*post-tachycardia T-wave syndrome*), transient bundle branch block, and pacing; like T-wave evolution after infarction, all can progress for several days or weeks after the initiating event. These stress-induced repolarization abnormalities, sometimes called *T-wave memory* (Rosenbaum et al., 1982), result from stretch- or stress-induced molecular changes that include decreased expression of Kv4.3, which prolongs the action potential by reducing i_{to1}; changes in i_{CaL} channel kinetics; and redistribution of Cx43 in the gap junctions of the intercalated disc.

ARRHYTHMIAS

Sudden death, a common occurrence in patients following a coronary occlusion, can be caused by a number of mechanisms, including cardiac rupture and pulmonary embolism; however, the most common cause is an arrhythmia. The appearance of these arrhythmias is not closely correlated to the extent of ischemia, so patients with minimal cardiac damage can die suddenly within a few minutes or hours after the onset of an acute myocardial infarction. Although most arrhythmias are the direct result of myocardial ischemia, reflexes frequently increase the risk of sudden death during the first few days after an infarction. Norepinephrine released at sympathetic nerve endings by the hemodynamic defense reaction (see Chapter 8) tends to disorganize conduction, and a powerful vagal response called the *von Bezold–Jarisch reflex*, is evoked when ischemia stimulates receptors on the inferior and posterior walls of the left ventricle. Arrhythmias that occur weeks, months, and even years after the acute infarction are generally initiated by reentry in the scarred ventricle (see Chapter 16) and by new ischemic events caused by worsening of the underlying coronary artery disease. Because of this changing substrate, use of drugs to prevent sudden death in these patients is like chasing a moving target. This became apparent many years ago, when patients successfully resuscitated from ventricular fibrillation in the first hours after a myocardial infarction were found to have little increased risk of a late arrhythmic death, which indicates that different pathophysiological mechanisms are responsible for early and late arrhythmias.

Arrhythmias Associated with Myocardial Infarction

Several pathophysiological mechanisms cause arrhythmias after a coronary occlusion. The tachyarrhythmias that appear within a minute after total occlusion of a coronary artery are caused when injury currents are generated by the ischemic myocytes, whose plasma membranes are depolarized. These are sometimes followed several hours later by accelerated idioventricular rhythms most likely caused by increased pacemaker activity in ischemic His–Purkinje cells. If the ischemic myocardium is reperfused, calcium overload–induced transient depolarizations can initiate dangerous arrhythmias. Later on, after recovery from the acute event, arrhythmias are usually caused by reentry in damaged or scarred regions of the heart. Bradyarrhythmias can be caused by vagal reflexes, in which case they are almost always transient, or by structural damage to the atrioventricular (AV) conduction system.

TACHYCARDIAS. In the first minutes after a coronary artery becomes occluded, when potassium efflux depolarizes the plasma membrane of the ischemic myocytes (see above), diastolic potential differences between the normal and ischemic regions of the ventricle generate injury currents that are the most important cause of early sudden death. Partial depolarization also inactivates sodium channels, which results in small, slowly conducting action potentials that provide the substrate for decremental conduction and unidirectional block (see Chapter 16). Acidosis and calcium overload also favor reentry in energy-starved cardiac myocytes by closing gap junction channels in the intercalated disc. Other causes of reentry include local changes in action potential duration, both shortening and prolongation, which cause inhomogeneities of repolarization. Because these initial arrhythmogenic mechanisms subside in the first hours after coronary occlusion, when the ischemic cells die, the risk of sudden death decreases rapidly after the acute infarction.

Triggered activity generates dangerous arrhythmias during or immediately after an occluded coronary artery is reopened—for example, after successful thrombolytic therapy or primary angioplasty, or when a clot in an infarct artery lyses spontaneously. Brief episodes of an *idioventricular rhythm* at rates between 60 and 100 are sometimes seen 18 to 36 hours after an acute myocardial infarction; in many cases, the accelerated ventricular pacemaker is unmasked by slowing of the sinus rate when the patient falls asleep. These rhythms are generally benign.

Patients with healed myocardial infarctions also are at risk for arrhythmias, due largely to heterogeneities in the damaged ventricles caused by scarring or persistent ischemia; these arrhythmias are most common in patients with left ventricular dysfunction or heart failure (see Chapter 18). Although atrial fibrillation occurs in patients with ischemic heart disease, this arrhythmia is not common unless left ventricular failure has caused atrial dilatation or there has been an atrial infarct.

BRADYARRHYTHMIAS: SINUS BRADYCARDIA AND AV BLOCK. Bradyarrhythmias can be caused by both functional and anatomical mechanisms. This is a very important distinction because functional AV block is almost always transient, whereas AV block caused by infarction of the conducting system is usually irreversible.

FUNCTIONAL (REFLEX) BRADYARRHYTHMIAS. Identification of the role of the *von Bezold–Jarisch reflex* in patients with inferoposterior infarction (Costantin, 1963) led to a major advance in the management of acute myocardial infarction. This reflex, which occurs when ischemia activates stretch receptors in the inferior and posterior walls of the left ventricle, triggers a powerful parasympathetic reflex and inhibits sympathetic activity, which together cause sinus bradycardia and AV block. The hallmark of the latter is Mobitz I second-degree AV block and the Wenckebach phenomenon (see Chapter 16). Reflex vagal discharge also evokes a visceral response that causes nausea and vomiting and can lead to severe hypotension by dilating peripheral resistance vessels. Patients with this reflex can appear to be near death in the first hours after what may be only a small infarction, but improvement is usually rapid because the reflex soon ends, and patients often make an excellent recovery.

Appreciation of the von Bezoldt–Jarisch reflex reduced mortality in patients with inferoposterior infarction; the once routine use of vasoconstrictors and sympathomimetic drugs to treat hypotension caused by reflex vasodilatation was quickly abandoned, as these drugs are dangerous and often ineffective. Instead, volume repletion more safely brings blood pressure toward normal, while atropine, a muscarinic blocker, usually restores sinoatrial (SA) and AV node function without the hazards associated with β-adrenergic stimulation. If an electronic pacemaker is required, it is usually needed only temporarily because the reflex is transient and ends when the ischemic tissue either dies or is reperfused.

BRADYARRHYTHMIAS CAUSED BY STRUCTURAL ABNORMALITIES. Sinus bradycardia and SA block can be caused by occlusion of the SA node artery, which accompanies atrial infarction. Because the SA node artery is usually a branch of the right coronary artery, these arrhythmias most commonly accompany inferoposterior infarction. Sinus slowing caused by this mechanism, which is less common than reflex bradycardia, is generally transient.

The most dangerous bradyarrhythmias after myocardial infarction result from structural damage to the AV conduction system, which can cause Mobitz II second-degree AV block (see Chapter 16). This arrhythmia implies a high risk of irreversible third-degree AV block and therefore is an indication for a permanent electronic pacemaker. Because the AV bundle and parts of the bundle branches run in the interventricular septum, and so receive a dual blood supply from the left anterior descending and posterior descending coronary arteries (see Chapter 1), infarctions that damage these conducting structures indicate that the patient has multivessel coronary artery disease. For this reason, block of conduction in the His–Purkinje system, including new bundle branch block, identifies patients with large infarctions who, if they recover, are likely to develop heart failure.

CELL DEATH

Myocardial cell death begins 15 to 40 minutes after the heart's blood supply is cut off completely, and about 6 hours later, few viable cells remain in the ischemic region. This progression resembles a wave of necrosis that begins in the endocardium, where energy requirements are greatest, and spreads outward through the wall of the left ventricle toward the epicardium. The timetable depends on collateral flow and is slower in patients with a well-developed collateral circulation.

The histological appearance of the infarcted myocardium depends on whether or not the tissue has been reperfused (Fig. 17-7). Regions where blood flow to the dying myocytes has not been restored form pale, acellular infarcts by a process sometimes called *mummification* (Bouchardy and Manjo, 1971/1972); the dying cells undergo autolysis because inflammatory cells cannot gain access to the tissue downstream from the occluded coronary artery. A much more violent process takes place when irreversibly damaged ischemic cells are reperfused, which causes a hemorrhagic infarct (Reimer and Jennings, 1991). Under these conditions, uncontrolled calcium entry causes contraction band necrosis, where the hypercontracted cardiac myocytes literally tear themselves apart; because blood can reach this region, the process attracts inflammatory cells. Late reperfusion has some benefits even when injured cells cannot be salvaged.

Ischemic myocardial cells can die in either of two ways, by necrosis or by apoptosis; the former is an uncontrolled, explosive process that leads to fibrosis, whereas apoptotic cell death is a highly regulated process that is not associated with inflammation.

Necrosis

The hallmark of necrosis is plasma membrane damage (see Chapter 9), which allows intracellular proteins, such as transaminases, creatine phosphokinase, and troponin components, to leak into the bloodstream. This explains why increased circulating levels of these molecules are useful in the

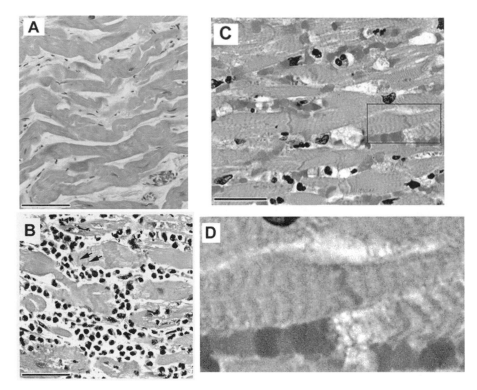

FIGURE 17-7 Histology of acute myocardial infarction. **A.** Pale acellular infarction, approximately 12 hours old, in a patient whose infarct artery was not reperfused; inflammatory cells are absent and the myocytes, which are relaxed, appear "wavy". **B.** Reperfused infarction showing hypercontracted myocytes surrounded by inflammatory cells and erythrocytes, a few myocytes contain contraction bands (arrows). **C.** Another region of the heart shown in **B**: the transverse striations are contraction bands. **D.** Enlargement of the area in **B** that is enclosed by the rectangle. H & E stain, 200x. Scale bar = 100 μm. Photomicrographs provided by Drs. Margaret A. French and Nora R. Ratcliffe.

diagnosis of myocardial infarction. Many factors contribute to membrane damage, including free radicals, fatty acids, increased lipase and protease activity, osmotic stress, and calcium overload.

In the normal heart, the free radicals generated when electrons pass along the respiratory chain are neutralized at the time they are transferred to molecular oxygen and combined with protons to form water (see Chapter 2). In the ischemic heart, however, the lack of oxygen prevents electrons from being transferred harmlessly to form water, which leads to the release of highly reactive oxygen free radicals. ATP hydrolysis provides another source of free radicals. This occurs when ADP is converted to ATP and AMP by *adenylyl kinase* (see Chapter 2) after which the AMP is dephosphorylated to form adenosine. The latter is deaminated to yield inosine, which is then converted to hypoxanthine, and finally to xanthine in a reaction that generates superoxide radicals. Free radicals also can be generated in the ischemic heart by catecholamine breakdown, arachidonic acid metabolism, and the catalytic activity of lipases and proteases. Inflammatory cells that are attracted to damaged regions of the heart release cytokines that also generate free radicals.

When long-chain fatty acids, their CoA and carnitine derivatives, and lysophosphatides accumulate in energy-starved hearts, the detergent effects of these amphipathic compounds can alter membrane structure and function. It is not clear, however, whether enough of these substances accumulate in the ischemic myocardium to cause irreversible damage. Activation of lipases and proteases after prolonged ischemia also may contribute to membrane damage. Osmotic overload has been suggested to contribute to plasma membrane rupture because large numbers of small molecules appear in the cytosol of ischemic myocardial cells; these include ADP and P_i generated by ATP hydrolysis, creatine and P_i formed from phosphocreatine, and glucose-1-phosphate released by glycogenolysis.

Calcium overload, an important consequence of energy starvation, inhibits oxidative phosphorylation when calcium accumulates in the mitochondria (see Chapter 2). Calcium overload also activates a number of energy-consuming reactions (see Chapter 7), the most important of which are contractile protein interactions that can cause cardiac myocytes to tear themselves apart; this is a major cause of reperfusion injury and explains the appearance of the hypercontracted state called *contraction band necrosis* (Fig. 17-7).

A fascinating cause of calcium overload is the *calcium paradox*, in which reintroduction of calcium into the fluid surrounding cells that have been exposed to very low extracellular calcium concentration leads to contracture and cell death. The calcium paradox can result from plasma membrane damage that follows prolonged exposure to low extracellular calcium; it is more likely, however, that the excessive calcium uptake occurs when this cation enters the cytosol in exchange for the large amount of sodium that had accumulated in the cells when extracellular calcium was low.

APOPTOSIS. Although necrosis is the major mechanism that leads to myocardial cell death after prolonged ischemia, apoptosis (see Chapter 9) also occurs after reperfusion of severely ischemic myocardium (Eefting et al., 2004; Foo et al, 2005). Inflammation is usually not seen in apoptotic tissue because the dying cells are broken down into small membrane-contained fragments that are engulfed by phagocytes (see Chapter 9). A major cause of this programmed cell death appears to be cytochrome C release into the cytosol from damaged mitochondria.

The effectiveness of thrombolysis and primary angioplasty in reperfusing ischemic regions after coronary artery occlusion, along with evidence that inhibition of apoptosis can reduce infarct size in animal models where ischemia is followed by reperfusion, suggests that antiapoptotic therapy could be valuable in these patients.

Protection of the Ischemic Myocardium and Infarct Size Reduction

During open heart surgery, where it is difficult to perfuse the arrested heart, ischemic damage can be minimized by slowing the rate of energy utilization. This is usually accomplished by cooling the heart after it has been arrested in diastole with a *cardioplegic solution*. The latter generally contain potassium, which stops the heart, along with substrates, antioxidants, and drugs that inhibit calcium entry.

Human coronary arteries are "end arteries" (Hirzel et al., 1977), which limits the delivery of cardioplegic and other agents to the ischemic tissue in a patient who has had a complete coronary occlusion. However, substances able to preserve myocyte viability can reach the ischemic region by way of the bloodstream in patients with collateral vessels. In the last analysis, of course, the most effective way to reduce infarct size is to restore coronary flow.

PRECONDITIONING, STUNNING, AND HIBERNATION

Most regions of the myocardium in patients with chronic ischemic heart disease are either adequately perfused or have become infarcted and replaced by scar. In some patients, however, perfusion of some regions can be impaired so severely as to cause injury but not myocardial cell death. This can initiate three processes: *preconditioning*, *stunning*, and *hibernation*. Preconditioning, which occurs after episodes of ischemia that do not last long enough to kill cells, increases the resistance of the myocardium to subsequent, more prolonged episodes of ischemia. Stunning is a state of depressed mechanical function that can follow a brief period of ischemia, while hibernation describes poorly functioning regions of chronically underperfused but viable myocardium that can regain the ability to contract when coronary flow is re-established.

Preconditioning

Preconditioning, which is caused by brief episodes of ischemia that do not irreversibly damage the myocardium, delays the onset of cell death after a subsequent, more prolonged episode of ischemia. This process occurs in two phases, *classical* or *early* preconditioning that appears within minutes, and a *delayed* or *late* process, sometimes called the *second widow of protection* (or *SWOP*), that begins after approximately 24 hours and lasts for about three days. Both are mediated by a remarkable diversity of signaling systems.

Classical preconditioning can be initiated when adenosine, norepinephrine, bradykinin, opiods, and other extracellular messengers bind to G protein–coupled receptors that activate G_i-mediated responses, as well as by nonreceptor-mediated responses to free radicals, calcium, hypothermia, stretch, and other stimuli. Most, if not all, of these signals exert their preconditioning effects by activating protein kinases, including protein kinase C, mitogen-activated protein kinases (MAP Kinases) tyrosine kinases, and PI3-kinases (see Chapter 9). Plasma membrane and mitochondrial $i_{K.ATP}$ channels participate in this process, but the effector mechanisms that cause protection are not well understood.

Delayed preconditioning is no less complex than the classic process. Triggers include adenosine, bradykinin, nitric oxide, prostanoids, opioids, and other substances, while signal transduction is mediated by protein kinase C, tyrosine kinases, and probably all three classes of MAP kinases. Effector mechanisms include increased expression of heat shock proteins, antioxidant enzymes, and mitochondrial $i_{K.ATP}$ channels.

Stunning

Stunning refers to a state of depressed contractile function that, like preconditioning, follows brief episodes of ischemia. The negative inotropic effect of stunning, which does not involve cell death and so is completely reversible, can last as long as several weeks. This reversibility distinguishes stunning from infarction, where function is lost irreversibly.

Stunning can be caused by oxygen free radicals, notably •OH, and nitric oxide, but it is not clear whether free radical scavengers can prevent, or reverse, stunning. Other possible pathogenic factors include abnormal calcium fluxes, reduced subendocardial blood flow, and damage to the myofilaments, mitochondria, and/or extracellular matrix.

Hibernation

Hibernation occurs when heart muscle is chronically underperfused but receives enough blood to maintain its viability. The result is a regional wall motion abnormality that is often very difficult to distinguish from an infarct. Unfortunately, the pathophysiology of hibernation remains poorly understood.

Although hibernation is not common, it is important that this syndrome be recognized in patients with left ventricular dysfunction and, especially, heart failure. Although revascularization does not always lead to significant improvement, a correct diagnosis followed by successful angioplasty or bypass surgery can sometimes restore virtually normal cardiac function in patients with what had been viewed as a hopeless prognosis.

CONCLUSION

The emphasis of this chapter, which highlights the effects of ischemia on the heart, should not obscure the fact that ischemic heart disease is caused by disease of the coronary arteries. For this reason, although patients can gain considerable benefit from appropriate management of the cardiac abnormalities, in the last analysis, prevention and treatment of this common condition will depend on advances in vascular biology.

BIBLIOGRAPHY

Armstrong SC. Protein kinase activation and myocardial ischemia/reperfusion injury. *Cardiovasc Res* 2004;61:427–436.

Bolli R, Marban E. Molecular and cellular mechanisms of myocardial stunning. *Physiol Rev* 1999;79:609–634.

Braunwald E. Unstable angina. An etiological approach to management. *Circulation* 1998;98:2219–2222.

Camici PG, ed. Repetitive stunning. *Heart Failure Rev* 2003;8:125–180.

Cobbe SM, Poole-Wilson PA. The time of onset and severity of acidosis in myocardial ischemia. *J Mol Cell Cardiol* 1980;12:745–760.

Davies MJ. Stability and instability: two faces of coronary atherosclerosis. The Paul Dudley White lecture. *Circulation* 1996;94:2013–2020.

Depre C, Taegtmeyer H. Metabolic aspects of programmed cell survival and cell death in the heart. *Cardiovasc Res* 2000;45:538–548.

Eisen A, Fisman EZ, Rubenfire M, et al. Ischemic preconditioning: nearly two decades of research. A comprehensive review. *Atherosclerosis* 2004;172:201–210.

Gettes LS, Cascio WE. Effect of acute ischemia on cardiac electrophysiology. In: Fozzard H, Haber E, Katz A, et al., eds. *The heart and cardiovascular system*, 2nd ed. New York: Raven Press, 1991:2021–2054.

Heusch G. Hibernating myocardium. *Physiol Rev* 1998;78:1055–1085.

Ingwall JS. *ATP and the heart*. Boston, MA: Kluwer, 2002.

Kloner RA, Bolli R, Marban E, et al. Medical and cellular implications of stunning, hibernation and preconditioning. *Circulation* 1998;97:1848–1867.

Kloner RA, Jennings RB. Consequences of brief ischemia: stunning, preconditioning, and their clinical implications. Part 1. *Circulation* 2001;104:2981–2989.

Kloner RA, Jennings RB. Consequences of brief ischemia: stunning, preconditioning, and their clinical implications. Part 2. *Circulation* 2001;104:3158–3167.

Pathberg KW, Rosen, MR. Molecular determinants of cardiac memory and their regulation. *J Mol Cell Cardiol* 2004;36:195–204.

Pfeffer MA, Braunwald E. Ventricular remodeling after myocardial infarction. Experimental observations and clinical implications. *Circulation* 1990;81:1161–1172.

Ross R. Atherosclerosis—an inflammatory disease. *N Eng J Med* 1999;340:115–126.

Yeghiazarians Y, Braunstein JB, Askari A, et al. Unstable angina pectoris. *N Eng J Med* 2000;342:101–114.

Yellon DM, Downey JM. (2003). Preconditioning the myocardium: from cellular physiology to clinical cardiology. *Physiol Rev* 2003;83:1113–1151.

For more complete discussions of ischemic heart disease and vascular biology, readers should consult textbooks of medicine and cardiology.

REFERENCES

Bouchardy B, Manjo G. A new approach to the histological diagnosis of early myocardial infarcts. *Cardiology* 1971/1972;56:327–332.

Costantin L. Extracardiac factors contributing to hypotension during coronary occlusion. *Am J Cardiol* 1963;11:205–217.

Eefting F, Rensing B, Wigman J, et al. Role of apoptosis in reperfusion injury. *Cardiovasc Res* 2004;61:414–426.

Foo RS-Y, Mani K, Kitsis RN. Death begets heart failure in the heart. *J Clin Invest* 2005;115:565–571.

Habib GB, Heibig J, Forman SA, et al. Influence of coronary collateral vessels on myocardial infarct size in humans. Results of phase I Thrombolysis in Myocardial Infarction (TIMI) trial. *Circulation* 1991;83:739–746.

Hirzel HO, Sonnenblick EH, Kirk ES. (1977). Absence of a lateral border zone of intermediate creatine phosphokinase depletion surrounding a central infarct 24 hours after acute coronary artery occlusion in the dog. *Circ Res* 1977;41:673–683.

Koretsune Y, Corretti MC, Kusuoka H, et al. Mechanism of early ischemic contraction failure. Inexcitability, metabolite accumulation or vascular collapse. *Circ Res* 1991; 68:255–262.

Reimer KA, Jennings RB. Myocardial ischemia, hypoxia, and infarction. In: Fozzard H, Haber E, Katz A, et al., eds. *The heart and cardiovascular system*, 2nd ed. New York: Raven Press, 1991:1875–1973.

Rosenbaum MB, Blanco HH, Elizari M, et al. Electronic modulation of the T wave and cardiac memory. *Am J. Cardiol* 1982;50:213–222.

Tian R, Ingwall JS. Energetic basis for reduced contractile reserve in isolated rat hearts. *Am J Physiol* 1996;270:H1207–H1216.

Tian R, Nascimben L, Ingwall JS, et al. Failure to maintain a low ADP concentration impairs diastolic function in hypertrophied rat hearts. *Circulation* 1997a;96:1313–1319.

Tian R, Christe ME, Spindler M, et al. Role of MgADP in the development of diastolic dysfunction in the intact beating rat heart. *J Clin Invest* 1997b;99:745–751.

Vogel WM, Apstein CS, Briggs LL, et al. Acute alterations in left ventricular diastolic chamber stiffness. Role of the "erectile" effect of coronary arterial pressure and flow in normal and damaged hearts. *Circ Res* 1982;51:465–476.

Williamson JR. Glycolytic control mechanisms. II. Kinetics of intermediate changes during the aerobic-anoxic transition in perfused rat heart. *J Biol Chem* 1966;241:5026–5036.

18

HEART FAILURE

Heart failure is a lethal rapidly progressing syndrome that, in the 1980s, had a 5-year survival of less than 50% (Ho et al, 1993); this is similar to that for stage III breast cancer (metastases to the chest wall or internal mammary lymph nodes). However, definitions of heart failure traditionally focus on the abnormal hemodynamics, highlighting the accumulation of blood behind a failing ventricle and the low cardiac output. In the 1960s, when contractility was found to be depressed in failing hearts, and in the 1980s, when it became clear that relaxation also is impaired, attention was drawn to abnormalities in the heart muscle. Efforts to correct these abnormalities stimulated the development of drugs that improve hemodynamics and increase contractility, which seemed to be a rational way to treat these patients. In the 1980s, large, randomized clinical trials began to examine the effects of therapy and, to the surprise of almost everyone, drugs with beneficial short-term effects often worsened long-term prognosis. These counterintuitive findings made it clear that factors other than poor pump function and depressed contractility are of critical importance in this syndrome. They also indicate that any useful definition of heart failure must expand the traditional focus on impaired pump function and depressed myocardial contractility to include the molecular changes that damage the failing heart. This text defines heart failure as *a clinical syndrome in which heart disease reduces cardiac output, increases venous pressures, and is accompanied by molecular abnormalities that cause progressive deterioration of the failing heart and premature myocardial cell death.*

HEMODYNAMIC ABNORMALITIES

The heart, which is a biological pump that moves blood from a region of low pressure (the veins) to one at higher pressure (the arteries), can be compared with a mechanical pump that moves water out of a leaky basement into a garden hose (Fig. 18-1). Failure of the pump can cause the basement to flood and reduce flow out of the hose, which in heart failure are analogous to increasing venous pressure and decreasing cardiac output, respectively. To make this a more "realistic" model of clinical heart failure, the defective pump also must deteriorate rapidly.

A 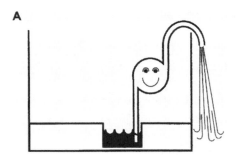 B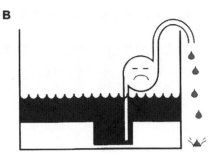

FIGURE 18-1   The failing heart as a defective pump in a leaky basement. **A:** The heart can be viewed as a pump that moves water from a leaky basement into a hose. **B:** Failure of the pump can cause inadequate emptying of the basement, which then floods (high venous pressure or "backward failure"); inadequate flow of water into the hose (low cardiac output or "forward failure"); or both. (From Katz, 2000.)

The clinical manifestations of heart failure are, of course, more complex. In the first place, the heart is two pumps—the right and left ventricles– that operate in series. For this reason, when blood backs up behind one ventricle, it becomes more difficult for the other ventricle to eject, and when less blood is pumped out of one ventricle, less returns to the other. Furthermore, the heart is a reciprocating pump, where phases of filling alternate with phases of ejection, so impaired emptying reduces filling, and impaired filling reduces emptying. This is because when less blood is ejected, the increased volume of blood remaining in the heart at the end of systole reduces its ability to fill during the next diastole (see Chapter 12); conversely, when filling is reduced, the heart cannot eject a normal volume.

A simple way to characterize the clinical consequences of heart failure is to define the reduced ejection of blood into the aorta and pulmonary artery as *forward failure*, and the reduced return of blood from the veins to the heart as *backward failure*. Patients with heart failure also can be classified in terms of whether the primary abnormality involves the left or right ventricle. This suggests that there are four types of heart failure (Table 18-1), but this is an oversimplification because filling is a major determinant of ejection, ejection is a major determinant of filling, and the two ventricles operate in series.

Backward and Forward Failure

The concepts of forward and backward failure are useful in characterizing the causes of heart failure because some diseases directly impair filling, and others directly impair ejection. Causes of backward failure of the left heart include mitral stenosis, where the narrowed valve impedes the return of blood to the left ventricle, and hypertrophic cardiomyopathy, where severe concentric hypertrophy reduces the capacity of the left ventricle to fill. Pericardial tamponade and constrictive pericarditis, whose

TABLE 18-1 **Hemodynamic Patterns of Heart Failure**

Site of Failure	Type of Failure	Major Hemodynamic Consequence
Right heart	Forward	Reduced ejection into pulmonary artery—low cardiac output
Right heart	Backward	Increased systemic venous pressure
Left heart	Forward	Reduced ejection into aorta—low cardiac output
Left heart	Backward	Increased pulmonary venous pressure

hemodynamic effects are due largely to right atrial compression, cause backward failure of the right heart. Forward failure of the left heart occurs when ejection is inhibited by a mechanical obstruction such as aortic stenosis, when diffuse myocardial disease reduces systolic shortening as occurs in the dilated cardiomyopathies, and when a portion of the left ventricle is replaced by scar after a large myocardial infarction. The most common causes of forward failure of the right heart are pulmonary hypertension and pulmonic stenosis.

Although the distinction between forward and backward failure is useful in understanding signs and symptoms (see below), it is of no value in describing the abnormal hemodynamics because impaired filling reduces ejection and impaired ejection reduces filling, and to the same extent. Application of the concepts of backward and forward failure to clinical heart failure also is difficult because these hemodynamic patterns are modified by circulatory effects of the neurohumoral response (see Chapter 8); for example, fluid retention, which increases preload, worsens backward failure (Fig. 18-2) and the increased afterload caused by peripheral vasoconstriction reduces ejection, and therefore worsens forward failure (Fig. 18-3). Therapy also modifies these patterns; for example, vasodilators

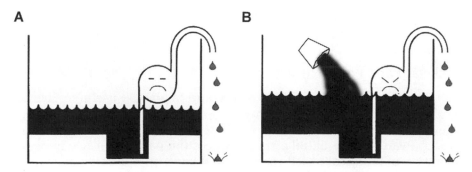

FIGURE 18-2 Effect of fluid retention. If the failing heart is viewed as a defective pump in a leaky basement (Fig. 18-1), fluid retention worsens the flooding.

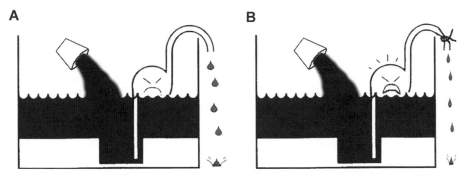

FIGURE 18-3 Effect of vasoconstriction. If the failing heart is viewed as a defective pump in a leaky basement (Fig. 18-1), vasoconstriction increases the work of the pump and decreases its forward output.

improve forward failure because the reduced afterload increases ejection. Similarly, when diuresis depletes circulating blood volume, the lower venous pressure alleviates backward failure; excessive diuresis, however, can reduce preload to such an extent as to worsen forward failure.

The clinical manifestations of forward failure are sometimes equated erroneously with depressed contractility (decreased inotropy) and those of backward failure with impaired relaxation (decreased lusitropy). However, the link between these hemodynamic patterns and abnormalities involving contraction and relaxation is tenuous. Furthermore, the manifestations of forward and backward failure are influenced by interactions between the peripheral circulation and the diseased heart (see below), so the severity of forward or backward failure, defined as reduced cardiac output and increased venous pressure, respectively, provides little information regarding the extent of depressed contractility or impaired relaxation.

Systolic versus Diastolic Dysfunction and Systolic versus Diastolic Heart Failure

In some patients with heart failure, the major underlying problem is impaired ejection, while in others, the underlying cause is impaired filling. Unfortunately, the terms used to describe these different pathophysiologies are often used imprecisely; for example, systolic and diastolic *heart failure*, which refer to different subsets of patients with heart failure, are often equated to systolic and diastolic *dysfunction*, which refer to different pathophysiologic mechanisms. Confusion also arises when forward and backward failure are equated to systolic and diastolic heart failure, respectively, as well as when a low cardiac output is interpreted to mean that a patient has systolic heart failure and a high venous pressure to mean that the problem is diastolic heart failure. These interpretations, of course, ignore the fact that a heart unable to fill normally cannot empty normally, and a heart unable to empty normally cannot fill normally.

SYSTOLIC AND DIASTOLIC DYSFUNCTION. *Systolic dysfunction*, which describes abnormalities of ventricular ejection, can be caused by biochemical abnormalities that impair cardiac myocyte shortening, when part of the ventricular wall is replaced by scar after a myocardial infarction, or by a structural abnormality like aortic stenosis. *Diastolic dysfunction*, which describes the pathophysiology of impaired ventricular filling, can be caused by cardiac myocyte abnormalities that slow relaxation, by diseases that reduce cavity volume, or by hemodynamic abnormalities like mitral stenosis and pericardial tamponade that mechanically impede ventricular filling.

Systolic and diastolic dysfunction cannot be identified on the basis of stroke volume or venous and arterial pressures, so the distinction requires additional data. Systolic dysfunction is suggested by reduced + dP/dt, ejection rate, or systolic compliance (the end-systolic pressure–volume relationship, see Chapter 11), while diastolic dysfunction is suggested when –dP/dt, ventricular filling rate, or diastolic compliance (the end-diastolic pressure–volume relationship) is reduced.

SYSTOLIC AND DIASTOLIC HEART FAILURE. Distinctions between systolic and diastolic heart failure are usually based on the ejection fraction (EF) and so are often called *heart failure with low EF* and *heart failure with preserved EF*, respectively. However, EF is the ratio between stroke volume, a *physiological* measurement, and end-diastolic volume, an *architectural* measurement, so that this ratio cannot be used to quantify either ventricular function or ventricular architecture.

The major reason why EF is decreased in most patients with systolic heart failure is increased end-diastolic volume rather than reduced stroke volume. This is especially true in older patients, where any decrease in stroke volume is limited by the normally low cardiac output in the elderly; for example, cardiac index (cardiac output normalized for body surface area) at age 70 is approximately 2.5 $l/min/m^2$, which is only slightly greater than that in moderate to severe heart failure, where stroke volume is 1.6 to 2.3 $l/min/m^2$ (Baim and Grossman, 2000). All this may seem puzzling to those who do not deal with these issues on a regular basis, but it should be clear that because both types of heart failure decrease stroke volume, the distinction between systolic and diastolic heart failure depends mainly on ventricular end-diastolic volume. However, there are exceptions; for example, high output failure, where EF is preserved by the increased stroke volume caused by an arteriovenous fistula or by vasodilatation in patients with conditions like anemia and thiamine deficiency (beriberi heart disease).

Systolic heart failure in developed countries is most often caused by myocardial infarction; less common causes include dilated cardiomyopathies and myocarditis (Table 18-2). Dilated cardiomyopathies appear to be familial in one-fourth to one-third of patients (Keeling et al., 1995; Grünig et al., 1998; Baig et al., 1998); however, the frequency with which

TABLE 18-2 **Some Common Causes of Systolic and Diastolic Heart Failure**

Systolic Heart Failure (heart failure with low EF)
Eccentric hypertrophy (increased cavity volume)
Global: Dilated cardiomyopathies, viral or toxic myocarditis
Regional: Myocardial infarction
Diastolic Heart Failure (heart failure with preserved EF)
Concentric hypertrophy (reduced cavity volume)
Hypertrophic cardiomyopathy, hypertensive heart disease

viral infection causes this syndrome is controversial. The left ventricular wall motion abnormality in systolic heart failure can be either diffuse (global) or regional. *Global* wall motion abnormalities are caused by conditions such as idiopathic dilated cardiomyopathy and myocarditis, where shortening is impaired uniformly throughout the ventricle, whereas a *regional* wall motion abnormality is usually seen after a myocardial infarction has destroyed part of the left ventricle (see Chapter 17).

Diastolic heart failure is most commonly seen in patients with concentric left ventricular hypertrophy, in whom wall thickness has been increased by a chronic increase in systolic stress. The underlying etiologies are usually hypertension and the decreased aortic compliance that accompanies aging. Less common causes include hypertrophic, restrictive, and infiltrative cardiomyopathies.

It is important to recognize that systolic and diastolic *dysfunction* are not always the causes of systolic and diastolic *heart failure*, respectively. For example, it is not unusual to see an elderly patient in whom a sudden increase in arterial blood pressure has reduced left ventricular ejection so much as to cause acute left heart failure. This often occurs in patients whose EF under basal conditions is normal or even slightly *increased* because of moderately severe concentric left ventricular hypertrophy. The appearance of acute left heart failure when increased afterload impairs ejection by a heart that under basal conditions seems to be normal is a common picture in diastolic heart failure.

Right and Left Heart Failure

The clinical picture in most patients with heart failure is dominated by the signs and symptoms of left ventricular failure; this is especially true in developed countries, where the major etiologies of heart failure are coronary and hypertensive heart disease (Table 18-3). Patients with dilated cardiomyopathies also suffer mainly from left heart failure. Right heart failure, which is less common, occurs most often in patients with congenital heart disease and *cor pulmonale*; the latter can be caused by chronic lung disease, multiple pulmonary emboli, or primary pulmonary hypertension.

TABLE 18-3 **Some Common Causes of Heart Failure**

Etiology	Right/Left Heart Failure	Systolic/Diastolic Heart Failure	Global/Regional Wall Motion Abnormality
Myocardial infarction	Left	Systolic	Regional
Dilated cardiomyopathy/ myocarditis	Left	Systolic	Global
Hypertensive heart disease	Left	Diastolic	Global
Hypertrophic cardiomyopathy	Left	Diastolic	Often regional
Valvular/ congenital	Depends on structures affected	Depends on structures affected	Global
Cor pulmonale	Right	Both	Global

Right heart failure can come to dominate the clinical picture in patients with left heart failure when the chronically elevated left atrial pressure causes pulmonary arterial hypertension. The latter, which occurs when increased pulmonary venous pressure leads to vasoconstriction and proliferative changes in the pulmonary arterioles, reduces blood flow through the lungs and so alleviates the symptoms caused by elevated left atrial pressure, although it substitutes right heart overload for left heart failure. This pathophysiology is described by Paul Wood (1954) in one of the outstanding clinical papers of the 20th century.

Circulatory Failure, Heart Failure, and the Descending Limb of the Starling Curve

It is essential to distinguish between *circulatory failure*, which can cause signs and symptoms resembling those seen in heart failure, and *heart failure*, where the same clinical picture is the result of heart disease. Circulatory failure can occur when intravenous infusion of large amounts of saline increases systemic and pulmonary venous pressures to levels that produce many of the signs and symptoms of backward failure, or when hemorrhage lowers cardiac output to levels seen in forward failure; both can occur when the heart is normal. Renal or hepatic disease also can cause fluid retention that mimics backward failure. For these reasons, not all patients with fluid retention, high venous pressure, or low cardiac output can be assumed to have heart failure.

Between the 1920s and the 1960s, students were often taught that the failing heart operates on the descending limb of the Starling curve (see

Chapters 6 and 11), even though Starling himself had made it clear that the heart cannot achieve a steady state when increasing chamber volume decreases its ability to eject. Although this essential relationship is not lost in patients with heart failure, these curves often become flatter.

Signs and Symptoms of Heart Failure

The clinical picture in heart failure consists of *signs*, which are objective manifestations of depressed cardiac performance, and *symptoms*, which are abnormalities perceived by the patient. The consequences of increased venous pressure are readily understood because transmission of this pressure upstream behind a failing ventricle elevates capillary pressure, which increases the hydrostatic forces that cause fluid to be transudated across the capillary endothelium into the tissues. The result is edema in the lungs of patients with left heart failure; and peripheral edema, ascites (fluid in the peritoneal cavity), and pleural effusions in right heart failure. Fatigue, the major symptom associated with decreased cardiac output, is due mainly to a skeletal muscle myopathy (see below).

BACKWARD FAILURE. Backward failure of the left heart causes shortness of breath (dyspnea) largely by increasing the work required to ventilate the congested lungs; this occurs when the elevated pulmonary venous pressure causes the lungs to become stiff and inelastic, like a water-logged sponge. In contrast to the normal work of breathing, which is rarely perceived, the increased respiratory effort caused by interstitial edema in the lungs cannot be ignored and leads to dyspnea. This symptom is exacerbated by weakness of the respiratory muscles (see below). Arterial hypoxia, caused by ventilation–perfusion mismatch and impaired oxygen exchange in the edematous pulmonary interstitium, probably plays only a minor role in cardiac dyspnea.

Cardiac dyspnea, unlike the dyspnea caused by pulmonary disease, generally becomes more severe when the patient lies down (*orthopnea*) because elevation of the legs drains blood out of the leg veins and so increases central blood volume. *Paroxysmal nocturnal dyspnea* occurs after the patient has been recumbent for several hours, during which time slow resorbtion of fluid from the dependent tissues in the body (mainly the legs) expands blood volume; after a few hours, this can increase pulmonary venous pressure to an extent that the patient awakens with dyspnea.

When high pulmonary venous pressure increases transudation across the pulmonary capillaries, the fluid first appears in the interstitium, from which it is carried to the systemic veins via lymphatic vessels. If the rate of transudation is rapid, and exceeds the rate at which the fluid can be removed by the lymphatics, the interstitium becomes edematous; because of the effects of gravity, the edema appears mainly in the lower lobes of the lung, where on an ordinary chest X-Ray it causes thin horizontal lines, called *Kerley B lines*, to appear in the lower lung fields. When a large amount of fluid accumulates in the interstitium, it can interfere with gas exchange between the pulmonary capillaries and the alveoli; because oxygen is much less soluble in water than carbon dioxide, the most prominent effect is arterial hypoxia.

When backward failure of the left heart becomes severe, fluid enters the air spaces. This can result in râles, which are crackling sounds described by Hippocrates as like the "seething of vinegar"; because of the effects of gravity, râles appear initially at the lung bases. In very severe left heart failure, fluid can flood the airspaces, which leads to pulmonary edema that can literally drown a patient. Some protection against this catastrophe occurs when vasoconstriction and a proliferative response in the pulmonary arteries reduces venous return to the left heart; however, this converts left heart failure to right heart failure (see above).

Backward failure of the right heart causes fluid to be transudated into the soft tissues (edema) and body cavities (anasarca), causing a syndrome that was once called *dropsy*. Examination of the jugular venous pressure provides an accurate bedside measurement of right atrial pressure and so can be used to quantify the severity of backward failure of the right heart. Estimation of left atrial pressure, however, is indirect and generally requires that clinical findings be supplemented with the results of tests like the chest X-ray and ECG, and sometimes direct catheter measurement.

FORWARD FAILURE. Fatigue has emerged as one of the most common and troublesome problems in heart failure. This symptom, which is attributed to forward failure, is not a direct consequence of reduced perfusion of skeletal muscle, but instead is caused by a skeletal muscle myopathy that is accompanied by biochemical changes similar to those associated with fatigue. The causes of this myopathy are complex and include disuse, inflammation, apoptosis, changes in fiber type and myosin isoform shifts, and loss of mitochondria and oxidative enzymes. The latter impairs ATP regeneration from fats, which leads to an increased glycolytic rate that accelerates the appearance of acidosis during exercise. Cytokines, notably TNF-α, appear to play an important causal role in this myopathy.

Interplay between the Failing Heart and the Peripheral Circulation

Changes in the peripheral circulation have important effects on the performance of the failing heart and therefore influence the clinical state of these patients. Two peripheral changes that exacerbate the hemodynamic abnormalities in patients with heart failure are initiated by the neurohumoral response (see Chapter 8); these are fluid retention, which increases preload and so worsens backward failure (Fig. 18-2), and vasoconstriction, which increases afterload and so worsens forward failure (Fig. 18-3). Therapy also can modify the hemodynamics of heart failure. Diuretics reduce congestion by alleviating fluid overload, while vasodilators, which reduce afterload, facilitate ejection and improve energetics in the failing heart. This interplay can be illustrated by Guyton diagrams (see Chapter 12) and pressure–volume loops (see Chapter 11).

INTERPLAY BETWEEN VENOUS RETURN AND CARDIAC OUTPUT. The interplay between the heart and the circulation can be described by plots of the influence of atrial pressure on venous return and cardiac output (see Chapter 12). Impaired ejection modifies this interplay when the decreased stroke volume reduces cardiac output, which worsens forward failure, and when increased filling pressure worsens backward failure (Fig. 18-4). Fluid retention can improve forward failure because increased preload moves the failing heart up its Starling curve; however, the more important consequence is to worsen backward failure by causing a further increase in venous pressure.

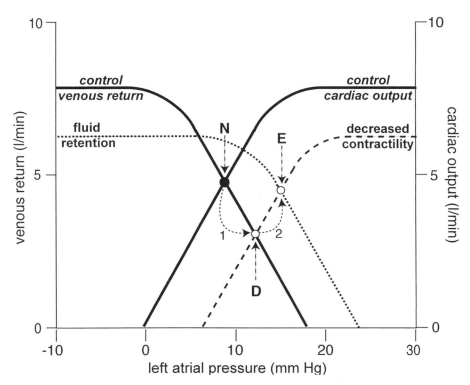

FIGURE 18-4 Guyton diagram showing curves relating atrial pressure to venous return and cardiac output. Control curves are shown by *solid lines*. Decreased contractility (*dashed line*) shifts the relationship between atrial pressure and cardiac output to the right and downward, which increases filling pressure and reduces cardiac output (arrow 1, from point **N** to point **D**). Fluid retention caused by the neurohumoral response shifts the relationship between atrial pressure and venous return to the right (*dotted line*), which increases cardiac output but at the expense of increased filling pressure (arrow 2, from point **D** to point **E**).

PRESSURE–VOLUME LOOPS. Each pressure–volume loop is constrained by an end-systolic pressure–volume relationship, which is a *Starling curve* that defines the inotropic state of the ventricle, and an end-diastolic pressure–volume relationship that defines its lusitropic state (Fig. 18-5). The interplay between the heart and circulation are determined by the preload, which determines the point along the end-diastolic pressure–volume relationship at which systole begins, and by afterload, which for simplicity is defined as the pressure at which the aortic valve opens and ejection begins.

Decreased contractility, which occurs rapidly after an acute myocardial infarction and more slowly in a patient with dilated cardiomyopathy, shifts the end-systolic pressure–volume relationship downward and to the right (Fig. 18-5A). Because ejection is reduced, end-systolic (residual) volume increases, so addition of a constant venous return to this increased end-systolic volume increases end-diastolic volume in the next cycle (Fig. 18-5B). This simple hemodynamic adjustment increases preload which, according to Starling's law of the heart, increases stroke volume.

THE NEUROHUMORAL RESPONSE. Two important hemodynamic adjustments are effected by the neurohumoral response (see Chapter 8). *Vasoconstriction*, which initially results from the α-adrenergic effects of sympathetic activation, and later from regulatory effects of angiotensin II, endothelin, and vasopressin, increases afterload. This response, which increases aortic pressure and reduces stroke volume (Fig. 18-5C), is usually detrimental in patients with heart failure because it reduces cardiac output and increases cardiac energy expenditure (see Chapter 12). *Salt and water retention by the kidneys*, the other consequence of the neurohumoral response, increases preload and so shifts the end-diastolic point upward and to the right along the end-diastolic pressure–volume relationship (Fig. 18-5D). According to Starling's law, this increases stroke volume, but it is at the expense of an increased filling pressure.

Two other components of the neurohumoral response increase contractility and facilitate filling; both result from β-adrenergic stimulation of the heart. The inotropic response, which shifts the end-systolic pressure–volume relationship upward and to the left (Fig. 18-5E), along with the chronotropic response to β-stimulation, increases the ability of the failing heart to eject at a given end-diastolic volume and afterload. The lusitropic response shifts the end-diastolic pressure–volume relationship downward and to the right (Fig. 18-5F), which improves backward failure by reducing end-diastolic pressure; this response improves forward failure when the increased end-diastolic volume increases ejection (Starling's law of the heart).

EFFECTS OF THERAPY. Because the neurohumoral response has both beneficial and deleterious effects (see Chapter 8 and Table 8-2), therapy that reverses these responses is both beneficial and deleterious (Table 18-4). Vasodilators lower blood pressure, which by unloading the failing ventricle reduces energy demand and increases cardiac output. However, by

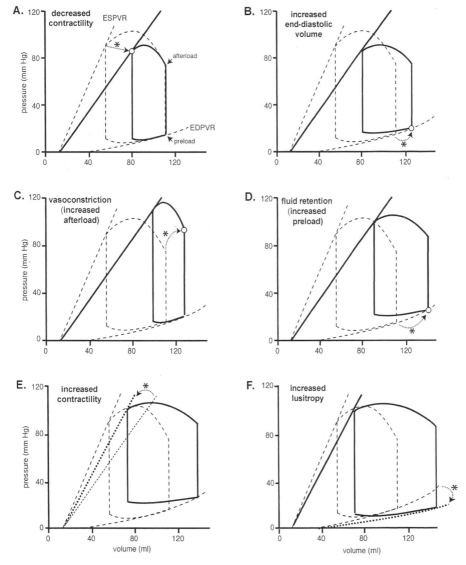

FIGURE 18-5 Left ventricular pressure–volume loops in heart failure. Curves for the non-failing heart are shown by *dashed lines*. Changes are indicated by a dotted arrow and asterick **A**: Depressed contractility shifts the end-systolic pressure–volume relationship to the right and downward (*solid curve*), which if afterload remains constant causes the end-diastolic point (*open circle*) to move to a higher volume thereby reducing stroke volume. **B**: Reduced ejection increases end-diastolic pressure and volume (*open circle*), which according to Starling's law increases stroke volume; this is apparent when the *solid curves* in **A** and **B** are compared. **C**: Vasoconstriction increases afterload (*open circle*), which moves the end-systolic point to the right and upward, thereby increasing pressure but reducing stroke volume; this is apparent when the *solid curves* in **B** and **C** are compared. **D**: Fluid retention increases preload (*open circle*), which increases stroke volume but at the expense of increased end-diastolic pressure and volume; this is apparent when the *solid curves* in **C** and **D** are compared. **E**: Increased contractility (*dotted line*) increases stroke volume, which is apparent when the *solid curves* in **D** and **E** are compared. **F**: Increased lusitropy (*dotted line*) also increases stroke volume, which is apparent when the *solid curves* in **E** and **F** are compared. (ESPVR, end-systolic pressure–volume relationship; EDPVR, end-diastolic pressure–volume relationship.)

TABLE 18-4 Some Beneficial and Deleterious Effects of Therapy in Heart Failure

Therapy	Beneficial Effect	Deleterious Effect	Consequence
Vasodilators	Decreased afterload		Increased cardiac output
	Decreased energy demand		Slowed deterioration
		Decreased blood pressure	Decreased perfusion of brain, heart
		Decreased blood pressure	Neurohumoral stimulation
		Further activation of the neurohumoral response	
Diuretics	Decreased diastolic pressure		Decreased venous pressure
	Decreased wall stress		Slowed deterioration
		Decreased preload	Decreased cardiac output
β-Adrenergic blockade	Decreased energy demand		Slowed deterioration
	Antiarrhythmic effects		Less sudden death
		Decreased ejection	Decreased cardiac output
		Decreased filling	Decreased cardiac output
		Decreased heart rate	Decreased cardiac output

lowering blood pressure, vasodilators reduce perfusion of the brain and heart and, by activating the baroreceptor response, further intensify the neurohumoral response. Diuretics, which decrease wall stress and venous pressure, also lower cardiac output. Modern diuretics are so effective in eliminating salt and water and reducing congestion that the older term *congestive heart failure* (CHF) is being replaced by *heart failure*. However, by reducing preload, diuretics decrease ejection (Starling's law of the heart), so that excessive diuresis can cause backward failure to be replaced with forward failure. The negative inotropic effect of β-blockers reduces ejection, which along with their ability to slow the heart reduces cardiac output; however, these detrimental effects are overridden by a beneficial proliferative response (see below). Cardiac glycosides, the first drugs to be used to treat this syndrome, increase myocardial contractility; however, many of the beneficial effects of these drugs are due to a centrally mediated counterregulatory response that slows ventricular rate and reduces afterload.

BIOCHEMICAL AND BIOPHYSICAL ABNORMALITIES IN THE FAILING HEART

Heart failure is associated with abnormalities in the myofibrillar proteins and most of the structures involved in excitation–contraction coupling. These abnormalities, which impair both contraction and relaxation, result from both functional responses, notably those initiated by energy starvation, and proliferative responses that, by modifying gene expression, alter the size, shape, and composition of the heart.

Energy Starvation

The controversy as to whether the failing heart is in an energy-starved state is an old one and goes back at least to the 1930s, but it is only recently that analytic tools like nuclear magnetic resonance (NMR) spectroscopy were able to show conclusively that ATP and phosphocreatine levels are significantly reduced in overloaded and failing hearts. This causes a state of energy starvation that is especially severe in the subendocardial regions of the left ventricle, where a combination of high wall stress and low perfusion can cause myocyte necrosis.

Energy starvation in the failing heart results from an imbalance between energy consumption, which is generally increased, and energy production, which is usually decreased. In systolic heart failure, energy utilization is increased when dilation of the ventricle and thinning of its walls increase systolic wall stress—for example, when infarction of part of the left ventricle overloads the remaining myocardium. Energy utilization in diastolic heart failure can be increased by the high afterload caused by hypertension and decreased aortic compliance, both of which are common causes of this syndrome. Valvular and congenital heart disease increase energy expenditure by increasing cardiac work.

Mechanisms that reduce energy production in failing hearts include decreased capillary density and increased intercapillary distance, both of which impair substrate diffusion. The greater diameter of hypertrophied cardiac myocytes also increases the distance over which oxygen must diffuse and so can cause the core of the enlarged fibers to become hypoxic. A more important mechanism is reduced fatty acid oxidation, which decreases the amount of ATP generated from these energy-rich substrates. Early reports that mitochondrial volume is decreased in the failing heart have not been confirmed in more recent studies; instead, evidence now points to impaired mitochondrial function caused by reduced synthesis of oxidative enzymes. The latter is due to an abnormal proliferative response that is mediated in part by reduced expression of PPARα, which plays a key role in mitochondrial biogenesis (see Chapter 2). The reduced ability of the failing heart to regenerate high energy phosphates is exacerbated when the phosphocreatine shuttle (see Chapter 2) is slowed by a decrease in creatine phosphokinase content; an isoform switch that replaces the M isoform of creatine phosphokinase with the B isoform facilitates ADP rephosphorylation but provides only a limited compensation for the reduced content of this enzyme.

Mitochondrial dysfunction has several additional adverse effects; lipid accumulation caused by reduced fatty acid oxidation may contribute to necrosis by damaging membranes, while release of reactive molecules, notably cytochromes and reactive oxygen species, can lead to apoptosis. Accelerated glycolysis caused by impaired oxidative phosphorylation leads to acidosis (see Chapter 2), which inhibits many processes involved in excitation–contraction coupling, contraction, and relaxation (see Chapters 4 and 7). Among the most important of the latter is an increase in cytosolic calcium, which initiates a number of vicious cycles that lead to myocyte necrosis (Fig. 18-6).

Mechanisms by which a fall in ATP concentration can impair cardiac performance are detailed in Chapter 17. Lack of substrate for the energy-consuming reactions responsible for contraction and relaxation, the most obvious, is important only in dying hearts where ATP concentration reaches levels low enough to deplete high-affinity sites of this substrate. Reduction in the allosteric effects of higher ATP concentration, and especially a decrease in the free energy of ATP hydrolysis, play a more important role in depressing contraction and slowing relaxation in the failing heart.

MOLECULAR ABNORMALITIES

The maladaptive effects of chronic overloading are due in part to the fact that adult human cardiac myocytes are terminally differentiated cells with little or no capacity to proliferate (see Chapter 9). Although a limited capacity for mitosis can be seen when adult cardiac myocytes are subjected to severe stress, these attempts to proliferate are abortive because the new cells do not form connections with neighboring cells that allow them to participate in ejection; instead, they form buds that become surrounded by fibrous tissue (Ring, 1950). This inability to generate functional myocytes means that the overloaded heart can only enlarge existing myocytes. However, this is an unnatural response that, while initially adaptive, has maladaptive consequences that eventually come to dominate the response to chronic overload.

The adaptive nature of overload-induced hypertrophy was recognized in the 18th century, when cardiac enlargement, like skeletal muscle hypertrophy in an athlete, was noted to increase the heart's ability to do work. Two forms of enlargement, now called *concentric* and *eccentric*

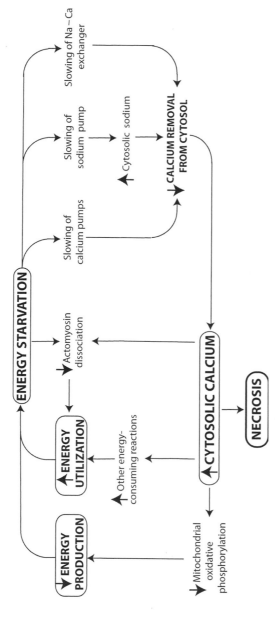

FIGURE 18-6 Energy starvation, by increasing cytosolic calcium, contributes to several vicious cycles that can cause cardiac myocyte necrosis. Energy starvation impairs calcium removal from the cytosol by inhibiting the Na–Ca exchanger, the sodium pump, and the calcium pumps of the sarcoplasmic reticulum and plasma membrane. The resulting increase in cytosolic calcium inhibits actomyosin dissociation, which in addition to impairing relaxation increases energy utilization and so worsens the energy starvation. Oxidative phosphorylation also is inhibited when some of the increased cytosolic calcium is taken up by the mitochondria, which decreases energy production. Worsening of the calcium overload amplifies these vicious cycles and can lead to necrosis of the energy-starved cells.

hypertrophy, were described in the early 18th century. The latter, also referred to as *dilatation*, was quickly recognized to have a very poor prognosis, whereas concentric hypertrophy was initially viewed as an adaptive response that could delay the appearance of dilatation. By the end of the 19th century, however, it had become clear that concentric hypertrophy also has adverse long-term consequences. More recently, a third type of cardiac hypertrophy, the exercise-induced *physiological hypertrophy* seen in trained athletes, was identified and found to differ markedly from the hypertrophy induced by a chronic hemodynamic overload. The most important differences between pathological and physiological hypertrophy are that the latter is neither associated with progressive deterioration of the heart nor accompanied by reversion to the fetal phenotype (see below).

Osler (1892) described three phases in the hypertrophic response of the heart to overload (Table 18-5). The first, *development*, alleviates symptoms because the enlarged heart is better able to meet the increased load. The clinical improvement continues in the second phase, which Osler called *full compensation*, but ends with *broken compensation*, a third, maladaptive, phase where degeneration and weakening of the heart muscle worsen symptoms and cause the death of the patient. Meerson (1961), who was the first to use modern methods to study overload-induced myocardial degeneration in animal models, proposed three phases similar to those of Osler (Table 18-5).

The ability of overload-induced hypertrophy to worsen prognosis in human heart failure was overlooked throughout most of the 20th century and did not come into focus until the late 1980s, when clinical trials showed that survival in heart failure averages less than 5 years after the onset of symptoms. At the same time, progressive dilatation of the failing ventricle (now called *remodeling*) came to be recognized as a major cause of clinical deterioration. These observations, which indicated that the deleterious effects of hypertrophy are so damaging that they can be viewed as a "cardiomyopathy of overload" (Katz, 1990), again drew attention to the architectural, cellular, and molecular consequences of maladaptive cardiac hypertrophy.

Myocardial Cell Death

Myocardial cell death is a calamity because the heart has little or no ability to replace its terminally differentiated myocytes. Furthermore, myocyte loss increases the work that must be done by the surviving myocytes and so establishes a vicious cycle in which cell death increases overload, which intensifies the hypertrophic response, which accelerates cell death, which increases overload, and so on.

Both necrosis and apoptosis can lead to cardiac myocyte death in the failing heart. Causes of necrosis include energy starvation (see Chapter 17) and possibly membrane damage caused by fatty acid accumulation (see above). Energy starvation is especially important because it increases cytosolic calcium and therefore establishes several vicious cycles that

TABLE 18-5   Three Stages in the Response to a Sudden Increase in Afterload

---

Phase 1

Osler: Development; Meerson: Transient breakdown

Clinical: Symptomatic left ventricular dysfunction after mild overload; acute left ventricular failure and cardiogenic shock after severe overload

Pathophysiology: Left ventricular dilatation, pulmonary congestion, low cardiac output, early hypertrophy

Phase 2

Osler: Full compensation; Meerson: Stable hyperfunction

Clinical: Class I–II heart failure

Pathophysiology: Improved symptoms, resolved pulmonary congestion, increased cardiac output, established myocardial hypertrophy

Phase 3

Osler: Broken compensation; Meerson: Progressive cardiosclerosis

Clinical: Class III–IV heart failure

Pathophysiology: Worsening congestion, hemodynamic deterioration, continued hypertrophy with progressive ventricular dilatation, myocardial cell death, fibrosis

---

increase energy demand and impair energy production (Fig. 18-6). Apoptotic cell death also is increased several-fold in end-stage heart failure, so this normally infrequent cause of cell death contributes to progression in this syndrome. Potential proapoptotic mechanisms include oxygen free radicals and cytochromes released from abnormal mitochondria (see above), and the ability of the signaling systems that mediate the hypertrophic response to stimulate pathways that cause programmed cell death (see Chapter 9). The latter can be activated by such stimuli as cell deformation, increased cytosolic calcium, and elevated levels of cytokines, like TNF-α, in patients with severe heart failure.

Architectural Changes

A large number of architectural phenotypes can be found in human hearts (Fig. 18-7; Table 18-6). Those that appear and then disappear during embryonic development are not abnormal, nor is the physiological hypertrophy induced by training. However, the phenotypes that appear when the heart is chronically overloaded are pathological because they are accompanied by maladaptive changes that include progressive dilatation, reversion to the fetal phenotype, myocyte death, and fibrosis, all of which are associated with arrhythmias. Furthermore, eccentric and concentric hypertrophy, rather than impaired contractility and relaxation, are generally the most important causes of abnormal cardiac performance in patients with chronic heart failure (Fig. 18-8).

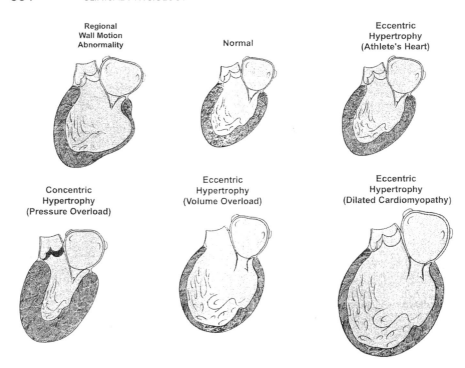

FIGURE 18-7 Five architectural patterns of cardiac hypertrophy and a normal left ventricle (*center of top row*). The eccentric hypertrophy seen in the "athlete's heart" (*top right*), an example of physiologic hypertrophy, differs from the pathological eccentric hypertrophy in dilated cardiomyopathies, where ejection is decreased (*bottom right*), and that caused by chronic volume overload (*bottom center*) where ejection is increased. Myocardial infarction causes a regional wall motion abnormality (*top left*) when the noninfarcted regions of the ventricle undergo eccentric hypertrophy. All differ from the concentric hypertrophy caused by chronic pressure overload (*bottom left*). (From Katz, 2000.)

Pathological hypertrophy was initially divided into two phenotypes: concentric hypertrophy, where cavity volume is reduced and wall thickness is increased, and eccentric hypertrophy, where the heart is dilated and its walls thinned. These architectural patterns, however, fail to tell a complete story. For example, the pathological eccentric hypertrophy caused by a chronic volume overload is very different from the eccentric hypertrophy found in familial dilated cardiomyopathies (see below), and both differ from the physiological dilatation seen in the "athlete's heart." Similarly, the concentric hypertrophy caused by a chronic pressure overload, such as hypertension and aortic stenosis, differs from that in patients with hypertrophic cardiomyopathies. These and other differences reflect the diverse changes in cellular structure and molecular composition that accompany the many types of cardiac hypertrophy.

Cellular Changes

The possibility that abnormal myocyte size and shape contribute to the abnormal architecture in overloaded hearts was suggested more than

TABLE 18-6 **Examples of Different Cardiac Myocyte Phenotypes**

Normal embryonic phenotypes
Normal adult phenotypes
  Working myocardial cells
    Atrial myocardium
    Ventricular myocardium
  Specialized cells
    Nodal cells
    His–Purkinje cells
Physiologic hypertrophy phenotype
  The "athlete's heart": Exercise-induced hypertrophy
Pathological phenotypes
  Eccentric hypertrophy
    Volume overload (e.g., aortic and mitral regurgitation)
    Myocyte damage (e.g., viral or toxic myocarditis)
    Myocyte stretch caused by myocardial infarction
    Dilated cardiomyopathies
  Concentric hypertrophy
    Pressure overload (e.g., aortic stenosis, hypertension)
    Hypertrophic cardiomyopathies

40 years ago, when Grant et al. (1965) postulated that eccentric hypertrophy (dilatation) occurs when sarcomeres are added to cardiac myocytes in series, which cause the cells to become longer, whereas parallel addition of sarcomeres in concentric hypertrophy causes the myocytes to become thicker (Fig. 18-9). This insight has been confirmed by studies of the size and shape of cardiac myocytes isolated from hypertrophied human hearts; in concentric hypertrophy, myocyte size is increased largely by a greater cross-sectional area, whereas cell length is increased in myocytes isolated from eccentrically hypertrophied hearts (Gerdes et al., 1994). These different cardiac myocyte phenotypes probably occur because diastolic stretch causes new sarcomeres to be added at the ends of these cells, which increases cell length, whereas increased systolic stress causes new sarcomeres to be added throughout the myocytes, which increases their width (Russell et al., 2000).

Different patterns of cellular hypertrophy have been shown to be controlled by different signaling pathways; for example, cardiotrophin-1 (a cytokine) induces cell elongation in neonatal cardiac myocytes, whereas an α-adrenergic agonist (phenylephrine) causes the cells to become thicker (Wollert et al., 1996). Furthermore, different mitogen-activated protein kinases (MAP Kinases) are activated when cardiac myocytes are stretched during diastole and during systole (Yamamoto et al.,

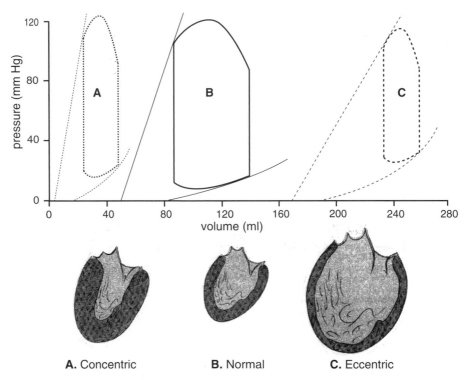

A. Concentric   **B.** Normal   **C.** Eccentric

FIGURE 18-8   Effects of changing cardiac phenotype (*below*) on the pressure–volume loop (*above*). **A**: Concentric hypertrophy; **B**: normal; **C**: eccentric hypertrophy. Note that in eccentric and concentric hypertropy, the major cause of reduced stroke volume are not decreases in contractility (the end-systolic pressure–volume relationship), but instead are the architectural changes in the ventricle (below). (Based on data of Kass, 1988.)

2001). The latter findings provide a clue as to why different architectural phenotypes are induced by pressure overload (e.g., the concentric hypertrophy seen in aortic stenosis) and volume overload (eccentric hypertrophy in aortic insufficiency), and provide evidence that increased systolic stress and increased diastolic stretch activate different cytoskeletal signaling pathways.

Increased sarcomere length was once suggested to contribute to dilatation, but it is now clear that sarcomere length remains normal in both eccentric or concentric hypertrophy. Another early explanation for ventricular dilatation, side-to-side slippage between adjacent cardiac myocytes, probably occurs in *acute* dilatation, when it contributes to the infarct expansion that can occur immediately after a large myocardial infarction. In contrast, the slowly progressing dilatation (remodeling) seen in chronic systolic heart failure results from a combination of myocyte elongation and myocyte death.

Eccentric hypertrophy (remodeling)

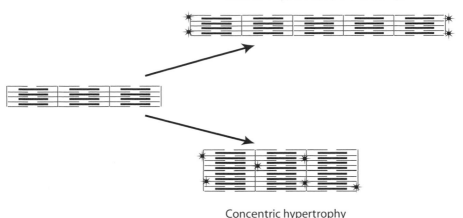

Concentric hypertrophy

✳Site of sarcomere addition.

FIGURE 18-9 Cellular basis for eccentric and concentric hypertrophy. Eccentric hyper-trophy (dilation) occurs when sarcomeres are added in series at the ends of cells, whereas in concentric hypertrophy, sarcomere addition occurs throughout the cell.

Molecular Changes

The possibility that heart failure is accompanied by molecular abnormalities in the contractile proteins was suggested almost 50 years ago, when the molecular weight of cardiac myosin was reported to increase threefold in an animal model of heart failure (Olson et al., 1959); however, subsequent studies showed that these data were flawed. The first solid evidence of a molecular change in failing hearts was published in 1962, when Alpert and Gordon found that myofibrils isolated from failing hearts have a low ATPase activity. This abnormality, which pro-vided a potential explanation for the depressed contractility in these patients, opened a new field of research that led to the discovery of molecular changes in most of the myofibrillar proteins as well as changes in several metabolic enzymes and many of the membrane proteins that participate in both the extracellular and intracellular calcium cycles (Table 18-7).

The molecular and ultrastructural changes that accompany cardiac hypertrophy are not due simply to an overall stimulation of myocyte growth, but instead result from highly regulated growth responses that are tailored to specific types of load. For example, pressure overload and chronic volume overload cause different pathological hypertrophic responses, both of which are accompanied by increased expression of fetal gene programs (reversion to the fetal phenotype), whereas expression of adult genes is increased in physiological hypertrophy.

TABLE 18-7 **Some Molecular Alterations in Hypertrophied or Failing Hearts**[§]

A. Contractile Protein Isoform Shifts	
Protein	**Heart Failure**
Myosin heavy chain	Expression of low ATPase (β) isoform[*]
Myosin light chain	Isoform shift[*]
Actin	Isoform shift[*]
Troponin I	No change or decreased expression
Troponin T	Isoform shift[*]
Troponin C	No change
Tropomyosin	No change
B. Sarcoplasmic Reticulum Proteins	
Protein	**Heart Failure**
Calcium pump ATPase (SERCA)	Decreased content[*]
Phospholamban	Decreased content[*] (less than for SERCA2a)
Calcium release channel (ryanodine receptor)	Probably decreased, altered function
FKBP12.6 (calstabin)	Impaired function (calcium leak)
Calsequestrin and calreticulin	Normal
C. Plasma Membrane Proteins	
Protein	**Heart Failure**
Transient outward potassium channels (i_{to})	Decreased activity
Inward rectifying potassium channels (i_{K1})	Decreased activity
L-type calcium channels	Normal or decreased[*] content
Na–Ca exchanger	Increased content[*]
Sodium pump	Decreased content, isoform shift[*]

[§]The changes listed in this table represent an arbitrary overview of the molecular abnormalities that have been reported in overload-induced hypertrophy and heart failure; not all have been found in humans and all experimental models. Published findings also disagree because of differences in etiology and the severity of the syndromes studied.
[*]Reversion to the fetal phenotype.

CONTRACTILE PROTEINS. The best-known molecular change in the failing heart is increased expression of the slow (β) myosin heavy chain isoform, which reduces contractility by decreasing maximal shortening velocity (see Chapters 4 and 6). In contrast to this change in phenotype, which is an example of reversion to the fetal phenotype, training-induced physiological hypertrophy (the athlete's heart) causes the *opposite* change; greater expression of the fast (α) myosin heavy chain isoform, which increases ATPase activity and contractility (Scheuer and Buttrick, 1987). Even in pathological hypertrophy, the extent of the myosin heavy chain isoform shift depends on the nature of the overload—for example, overexpression of the slow β-isoform is less in chronic volume overload than in chronic pressure overload (Calderone et al., 1995).

Chronic overload causes isoform shifts to occur in other myofibrillar proteins, including the myosin light chains, troponin T, and actin. Isoform shifts also have been found in cytoskeletal proteins, including titin, α-actinin, myosin-binding protein C, microtubules, and fibronectin. These isoform shifts, along with changes in the contents of several myofibrillar proteins, depress contractility and reduce the calcium-sensitivity of the contractile process. The latter cannot be attributed to changes in troponin C, the calcium-binding protein of the thin filament which is highly conserved, but instead to allosteric effects caused by the troponin T isoform shift.

SARCOPLASMIC RETICULUM. Relaxation is impaired and contractility depressed in the failing heart by reduced contents of three major sarcoplasmic reticulum proteins that participate in the intracellular calcium cycle; these are the calcium release channel, calcium pump ATPase, and phospholamban (Table 18-7). There is, however, no convincing evidence for isoform shifts involving these membrane proteins. The reduced content of the calcium pump ATPase provides another example of reversion to the fetal phenotype because the sarcoplasmic reticulum is poorly developed in embryonic hearts, which depend mainly on the extracellular calcium cycle (see Chapter 7).

THE PLASMA MEMBRANE. Changes in the plasma membrane in overloaded and failing hearts include decreased expression of the potassium channels that carry i_{to}, which by reducing the transient outward current contributes to arrhythmogenic inhomogeneities of repolarization by prolonging the cardiac action potential. The density of the inward rectifying potassium channels that carry i_{K1} also is decreased in pathological hypertrophy, which by reducing resting potential increases the susceptibility of failing hearts to ventricular fibrillation (see Chapter 16). It is not clear whether the number of L-type plasma membrane calcium channels remains the same or decreases, but there is widespread agreement that expression of the Na–Ca exchanger is increased. When the latter transports calcium from the cytosol into the extracellular fluid, it generates an inward current during the vulnerable period of the action potential. This arrhythmogenic current, which is a major cause of late afterdepolarizations (see Chapter 14), is increased further when energy starvation and inotropic agents increase cytosolic calcium (see Chapter 16) and probably represents the most important cause of sudden cardiac death in patients with heart failure.

FIBROSIS AND DEPOSITION OF CONNECTIVE TISSUE. Severe heart failure is accompanied by fibrosis of the walls of the heart that occurs when fibroblasts and other connective tissue cells are stimulated to increase the production of matrix proteins (see Chapter 9). However, fibrosis also is secondary to cardiac myocyte necrosis. In addition to the increased collagen content, the type of collagen changes in the failing heart. During the initial response to overload, the more elastic embryonic type III collagen is synthesized preferentially, whereas when the overload becomes chronic, type III collagen is replaced by type I collagen, which has a higher tensile strength (Chapman et al., 1990; Marijianowski et al., 1995). One reason why physiological hypertrophy lacks adverse long-term effects is that it is not accompanied by abnormal fibrosis (Weber and Brilla, 1991).

Extracellular matrix proliferation in the chronically overloaded heart has both maladaptive and adaptive consequences. The increased connective tissue content impairs filling, can injure myocardial cells, and by slowing impulse conduction provides a substrate for arrhythmias. However, connective tissue proliferation also slows progressive dilatation; many of the reported beneficial effects of "cardiomyoplasty," where the *latissiumus dorsi* muscle is wrapped around the failing heart, appear to be due to fibrosis in the skeletal muscle. A similar fibrotic response may contribute to the inhibition of remodeling reported after injection of stem cell preparations into the walls of infarcted or failing hearts. The latter findings have stimulated efforts to inhibit remodeling by placing a plastic mesh around failing hearts.

Stimuli That Cause Hypertrophy

Several signaling pathways mediate the hypertrophic response (Fig. 18-10). Although most participate in both adaptive and maladaptive growth responses, some pathways appear to favor physiological hypertrophy, while others mediate pathological concentric hypertrophy and progressive dilation (remodeling). Because of extensive cross-talk between proliferative signaling pathways (see Chapter 9), it is difficult to assign a specific function to one or another signaling mechanism; it has recently become clear, however, that different signaling systems can favor either physiological or pathological hypertrophy.

The pathways summarized in Figure 18-10 are divided into five groups that appear to evoke different types of hypertrophy; these are (1) PI3K/PIP$_3$/Akt pathways, (2) G protein–coupled receptor (GPCR) pathways, (3) mitogen-activated protein kinase (MAPK) pathways, (4) cytokine-activated pathways, and (5) histone deacetylases (HDACs).

PI3K/PIP₃/AKT PATHWAYS. Insulin, insulin growth factor (IGF), and growth hormone (GH) evoke proliferative responses when they bind to receptor tyrosine kinases that activate phosphoinositide 3'-OH kinase (PI3K), a serine/threonine kinase that phosphorylates a membrane lipid called *phosphatidylinositol trisphosphate* (PIP₃). When phosphorylated, the latter activates *Akt* (also called *protein kinase B* or *PKB*), another serine/ threonine kinase, that induces *physiological* hypertrophy by activating mTOR (mammalian target of rapamycin), a regulator of protein synthesis, and inhibiting glycogen synthetase kinase 3 (GSK-3), an inhibitory serine/ threonine kinase. However, these signaling pathways also can induce *pathological* hypertrophy.

G PROTEIN–COUPLED RECEPTOR PATHWAYS. Mediators of the hemodynamic defense reaction, such as β-adrenergic receptor agonists, angiotensin II (Ang II), and endothelin, stimulate cellular responses when they bind to G protein–coupled receptor pathways (GPCR) and activate heterotrimeric G proteins (see Chapter 8). For example, β-adrenergic agonist–binding to $G_{\alpha s}$ activates adenylyl cyclase (AC) to form cyclic AMP (cAMP), an intracellular messenger that activates protein kinase A (PKA). In addition to its many functional effects (see Chapter 8), PKA phosphorylates several nuclear transcription factors that stimulate proliferative signaling. Binding of angiotensin II, endothelin, vasopressin, and other extracellular messengers to their GPCR stimulates proliferative signaling by activating $G_{\alpha q}$, which along with $G_{\beta \gamma}$ activates phospholipase C (PLC). The latter releases two intracellular messengers: diacylglycerol (DAG) and inositol trisphosphate (InsP₃). DAG activates protein kinase C (PKC), which phosphorylates nuclear transcription factors, while InsP₃ releases small amounts of calcium that activate calcium/calmodulin kinase (CAMK), which phosphorylates additional nuclear transcription factors. Calcium also activates a protein phosphatase called *calcineurin*, which dephosphorylates and activates *NFAT (nuclear factor of activated T cell)*, which activates additional transcription factors *MEF2C* and *GATA4*. The predominant response to these GPCR-mediated signals is *pathological hypertrophy*.

MITOGEN-ACTIVATED PROTEIN KINASE PATHWAYS. MAP kinases can be activated by cell deformation and binding of peptide growth factors to receptor tyrosine kinases. Many MAP Kinase pathways are mediated by a monomeric G protein called *RAS*, but MAP Kinase pathways also can be activated by additional signaling cascades, such as Jak/STAT. The three major MAP Kinase pathways described in Chapter 9, extracellular receptor-mediated kinases (ERK) and two stress-activated pathways, c-Jun kinase (JNK) and p38 kinase (p38K), are all activated by overload. Like the GPCR-activated pathways, the major response to MAP Kinase activation is *pathological* hypertrophy.

CYTOKINE PATHWAYS. Ligand-bound cytokine receptors regulate proliferative signaling by releasing an inhibitory effect of IκB that allows the

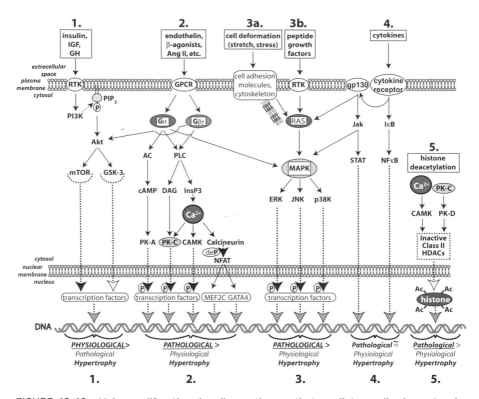

FIGURE 18-10   Major proliferative signaling pathways that mediate cardiac hypertrophy divided arbitrarily into five groups. Reading from *left* to *right*, these are the (1) PI3K/PIP₃/Akt pathways, (2) G protein–coupled receptor (GPCR) pathways, (3) mitogen-activated protein kinase (MAPK) pathways, (4) cytokine-activated pathways, and (5) histone deacetylases (HDACs). The major response to the PI3K/PIP₃/Akt pathways is *physiological* hypertrophy, whereas the major response to the GPCR and MAPK pathways is *pathological* hypertrophy; cytokines appear to mediate both *physiological* and *pathological* hypertrophy. The PI3K/PIP₃/Akt pathway is activated when insulin, insulin growth factor (IGF), and growth hormone (GH) bind to receptor tyrosine kinases (RTK); the cascade involves phosphorylation of phosphatidylinositol trisphosphate (PIP₃) by phosphoinositide 3′-OH kinases (PI3K), which activates a protein kinase called Akt or protein kinase B. The latter activates a regulator of protein synthesis called mammalian target of rapamycin (mTOR) and inhibits an inhibitory serine/threonine kinase called glycogen synthetase kinase 3 (GSK-3); the major response to these two regulators is physiological hypertrophy. GSK-3 also participates in the signaling pathways that lead to pathological hypertrophy. Mediators of the hemodynamic defense reaction, such as β-adrenergic receptor agonists, angiotensin II (Ang II), and endothelin, activate mainly pathological hypertrophy when the activated GPCR interacts with the heterotrimeric G proteins to activate Gₐ and G_βγ, which control a number of signaling pathways (see Chapter 9). Activated GPCRs interact with the heterotrimeric G proteins. Binding of β-adrenergic agonists to Gₐₛ activates adenylyl cyclase (AC) to form cyclic adenosine monophosphate (cAMP), which stimulates protein kinase A (PKA) to phosphorylate several nuclear transcription factors. Other isoforms of Gₐ, notably Gₐq, along with G_βγ, activate phospholipase C (PLC) to form diacylglycerol (DAG) and inositol trisphosphate (InsP₃). DAG activates protein kinase C (PKC), which phosphorylates additional nuclear transcription factors. Calcium released from intracellular stores by InsP₃ activates PKC and calcium/calmodulin kinase (CAMK),

transcription factor NFκB to move to the nucleus, where it stimulates gene transcription (see Chapter 9). Cytokines also activate proliferative responses when gp130-mediated signaling pathways stimulate *janus kinase (Jak)*, a protein kinase that activates both a transcription factor called *signal transducer and activator of transcription (STAT)* and stress-activated MAP kinases. Cytokine-activated proliferative signaling pathways appear to participate in both *physiological* and *pathological* hypertrophy; it is not clear which is the predominant response in failing hearts, but adverse effects of gp130 knockout in mice and anticytokine therapy in humans may be due in part to inhibition of adaptive hypertrophy.

HISTONE DEACETYLASE PATHWAYS. An additional mechanism that regulates cardiac hypertrophy is provided by histone acetyltransferases (HATs) that stimulate gene transcription when histone acetylation "unwinds" the DNA strands. Proliferative signaling is therefore increased by inhibition of histone deacetylation (HDAC). This occurs when CAMK and PKC phosphorylate class II HDACs in the heart, which by inhibiting histone deacetylases, allow transcription factors like MEF2 to stimulate *pathological* hypertrophy.

ARRHYTHMIAS AND SUDDEN DEATH

Arrhythmias, which account for more than one-half of the deaths in patients with heart failure, are due in part to cardiac enlargement and fibrosis, which slow conduction and disorganize the spread of the wave of depolarization. Additional arrhythmogenic mechanisms include reduced resting potential, which is caused when the sodium pump is

---

both of which phosphorylate nuclear transcription factors. Calcium also activates calcineurin, a protein phosphatase that dephosphorylates and activates nuclear factor of activated T cell (NFAT), which activates the transcription factors MEF2C and GATA4. Pathological hypertrophy also can be stimulated when peptide growth factors bind to RTKs, and when cell deformation activates various cytoskeletal molecules; many of these pathways are mediated by RAS, a monomeric G-protein, which stimulates MAPK pathways; the latter include extracellular receptor-mediated kinases (ERK) and two "stress-activated" pathways, c-Jun kinase (JNK) and p38 kinase (p38K), all of which phosphorylate nuclear transcription factors. Ligand-bound cytokine receptors activate gp130-mediated signaling pathways by stimulating janus kinase (Jak); the latter activates a transcription factor called signal transducer and activator of transcription (STAT) as well as MAP kinases. Cytokine-bound receptors also regulate proliferative signaling when they release an inhibitory effect of IκB on the transcription factor NFκB. Cytokines appear able to induce both *physiological* and *pathological* hypertrophy. Calcium and protein kinase C also stimulate hypertrophy by inactivating class II histone deacetylases (HDACs), which by increasing histone acetylation reduces an inhibitory effect on DNA transcription. (*Thin solid arrows*, signaling pathways; *dotted arrows with solid arrowheads*, phosphorylations (P) and dephosphorylations (deP) that activate transcription factors; *dotted arrows with open arrowheads*, phosphorylations (P) and acetylations (AC) that inhibit transcription factors; *dotted arrows with shaded arrowheads*, factors that regulate transcription.)

inhibited by energy starvation (see Chapter 7), and by a reduced number of i_{K1} channels (see above). Acidosis and elevated intracellular calcium also are arrhythmogenic because they close gap junctions (see Chapter 13), which slows conduction by increasing intracellular resistance (see Chapter 14). The decreased density of i_{to} channels described above is arrhythmogenic because the resulting action potential prolongation causes inhomogeneities of repolarization (see Chapter 16). However, the most important cause of sudden death appears to be the inward current generated by the electrogenic calcium efflux mediated by the Na–Ca exchanger (see Chapters 7 and 10). This arrhythmogenic ion flux, which initiates afterdepolarizations and triggered activity (see Chapter 16), is increased in heart failure by reversion to the fetal phenotype, which increases the dependence of hypertrophied hearts on the extracellular calcium cycle (see above), and by energy starvation and inotropic drugs, both of which cause cytosolic calcium overload and so increase calcium efflux by way of the sodium–calcium exchanger.

FAMILIAL CARDIOMYOPATHIES

The importance of molecular abnormalities in clinical heart failure became apparent in 1990, when myosin heavy chain mutations were found in hypertrophic cardiomyopathy (Geisterfer-Lowrance et al., 1990). A remarkable variety of inherited abnormalities is now known to cause hypertrophic and dilated cardiomyopathies (Table 18-8). Most hypertrophic cardiomyopathies are associated with contractile protein abnormalities (see Chapter 4), while many dilated cardiomyopathies are caused by changes in cytoskeletal proteins (see Chapter 5). However, mutations in other proteins can cause both hypertrophic and dilated cardiomyopathies, and different mutations in a single protein can cause both of these architectural phenotypes.

The frequent association of familial dilated cardiomyopathies with conduction system defects suggests that underlying cytoskeletal protein mutations disrupt linkages between ion channels and regulatory proteins (see Chapters 5 and 13). Hypertrophic cardiomyopathies that are accompanied by intracellular glycogen accumulation are often associated with pre-excitation (Wolff-Parkinson-White syndrome, see Chapter 16), which occurs because these mutations cause gaps in the central fibrous body, a connective tissue insulator that normally separates the atria and ventricles (see Chapter 1). These gaps allow impulses to be conducted abnormally through myocardial tissue from the atria to the ventricles.

IMPLICATIONS OF THERAPEUTIC SUCCESSES AND FAILURES

Several types of therapy have been used to manage patients with heart failure. Until the late 1980s, all were directed at improving the

TABLE 18-8 **Some Causes of Familial Cardiomyopathies in Humans**

Hypertrophic Cardiomyopathies

Myofibrillar protein mutations

β-myosin heavy chain, regulatory myosin light chain, essential myosin light chain, troponin T, troponin I, troponin C, α-tropomyosin, cardiac actin

Cytoskeletal protein mutations

titin, myosin-binding protein C, LIM protein, T cap

Mutations in nuclear-encoded metabolic proteins (with intracellular glycogen accumulation)

AMP-activated protein kinase; Danon's disease: lysosome-associated membrane protein-2 (LAMP); Pompe's disease: lysosomal acid α-1,4-glucosidase; Fabry's disease: lysosomal hydrolase α-galactosidase

Membrane protein mutations

Calcium release channel (ryanodine receptor)

Other

Nkx2.5

Dilated Cardiomyopathies

Myofibrillar protein mutations

β-myosin heavy chain, troponin T, troponin I, troponin C, α-tropomyosin, cardiac actin

Cytoskeletal protein mutations

Z-line–related

titin, cypher/ZASP (cypher/Z-band alternatively spliced PDZ-motif protein), telethionin, T cap, desmin

Dystrophin-related

β-sarcoglycan, δ-sarcoglycan, dystrophin, dystrobrevin,

Desmosome-related (arrhythmogenic right ventricular dysplasia)

plakoglobin, desmoplakin, plakophilin-2

Nuclear

emerin, lamin A/C

Other

metavinculin

Membrane protein mutations

Phospholamban, SUR2A (K_{ATP} channel)

---

hemodynamic abnormalities; these include diuretics, which reduce pre-load; vasodilators, which reduce afterload; and inotropes, which increase contractility. Despite improving short-term symptoms, however, most vasodilators and virtually all inotropes worsen long-term prognosis.

TABLE 18-9   Therapy That Improves Prognosis in Patients with Heart Failure

Drugs that increase nitric oxide (NO) production
Nitrates
Drugs that inhibit angiotensin II actions
Inhibition of angiotensin II production: Angiotensin–converting enzyme (ACE) inhibitors
Inhibition of angiotensin II binding to its receptors: Angiotensin II receptor blockers (ARBs)
Drugs that inhibit β-adrenergic receptor activation
β-blockers
Drugs that inhibit aldosterone actions
Cardiac resynchronizing therapy (CRT)
Left ventricular assist devices (LVADs)

At the time this chapter was written, prognosis in systolic heart failure had been shown to be improved by drugs that inhibit the neurohumoral response either directly or by a counterregulatory action (Table 18-9). These include nitrates, which increase nitric oxide production; angiotensin-converting enzyme (ACE) inhibitors and angiotensin II receptor blockers (ARBs), which inhibit regulatory angiotensin II actions; β-adrenergic receptor blockers; and drugs that reduce aldosterone binding to its receptors. Two devices also prolong survival: cardiac resynchronization therapy (CRT), which reduces heterogeneities of conduction and contraction, and left ventricular assist devices (LVADs) that unload the failing heart.

Nitrates, ACE inhibitors, and angiotensin II receptor blockers were first used to treat heart failure because they are vasodilators that can reduce preload and afterload. However, the long-term benefits of these drugs cannot be attributed to this functional effect because most other vasodilators fail to improve survival, and many worsen a prognosis. Instead, the ability of nitrates, ACE inhibitors, and angiotensin II receptor blockers to prolong survival appears to be due to inhibition of the maladaptive proliferative signaling that leads to progressive dilatation (remodeling). The beneficial effect of β-blockers, which because of their negative inotropic effect had been almost universally viewed a decade earlier as contraindicated, were discovered accidentally; it is still not clear whether their benefits are due to their energy-sparing effect, their ability to inhibit remodeling, or both. Many were surprised when spironolactone, an aldosterone antagonist that had been used for decades as a potassium-sparing diuretic, was found to improve prognosis; however, it is not clear whether this long-term benefit results from reduced fibrosis or inhibition of maladaptive hypertrophy. Cardiac resynchronization therapy was introduced to minimize the electrical heterogeneities caused by the increased time required to depolarize the left ventricle in patients with end-stage heart failure and a prolonged QRS complex, while left ventricular assist devices (LVADs) are used mainly as a "bridge" to keep severely ill patients alive long enough to receive a heart transplant. It is now clear, however, that the benefits of *all* of the drugs and devices listed in Table 18-9 are due, at least in part, to inhibition of maladaptive proliferative signaling, as evidenced by their ability to slow, and sometimes reverse briefly, remodeling and reversion to the fetal phenotype.

Treatment of Systolic and Diastolic Heart Failure

Virtually all of the trials that established the therapeutic benefits described in Table 18-9 included only patients with a low EF (systolic heart failure), where progressive dilatation is a major cause of the poor prognosis. Unfortunately, much less is known about the growing population of patients, mostly elderly, who have heart failure without progressive left ventricular dilatation (diastolic heart failure). It is by no means clear that strategies to improve prognosis in patients with systolic heart failure will have a similar survival benefit when used to treat patients who have diastolic heart failure; in fact, little or no reduction in long-term mortality has been seen in studies in which some of these drugs were used to lower blood pressure in patients with hypertension, a leading cause of heart failure with preserved EF. One reason why therapy that improves prognosis in systolic heart failure may not have the same benefit in diastolic heart failure is that, *by definition*, progressive dilatation does not contribute to the clinical deterioration in the latter. Until this and other questions are answered by appropriately designed clinical trials, management of diastolic heart failure will remain among the most important unresolved challenges in dealing with this syndrome.

A FINAL COMMENT AND A SPECULATION ABOUT THE FUTURE

There is no better way to conclude this text than with this discussion of heart failure, which documents the clinical relevance of virtually *all* of the material covered in the preceding pages. Energy production and energy utilization, the contractile proteins and cytoskeleton, the extracellular and intracellular calcium cycles, functional and proliferative signaling, the electrical activity of the heart, and of course, cardiovascular hemodynamics are all of practical importance in understanding and treating this syndrome. The increasing clinical relevance of these topics, which only a few years ago were often viewed as arcane basic science that was of little or no help in managing patients, clearly demonstrates how modern biology is closing the "gap" between bench and bedside (see Preface).

Our present understanding of heart failure and its treatment also provides a glimpse into the future. Most relevant are the insights now emerging from the role of polymorphisms in determining responses to therapy; for example, β-blockers are of less benefit in African American patients who have a low-activity β-receptor (Small et al., 2002; Perez et al., 2003), patients who express a polymorphism that increases nitric oxide synthesis have a better prognosis than those without the more active gene (McNamara et al., 2003), and patients who have the more active isoform of the angiotensin–converting enzyme require higher doses of ACE inhibitors than those with the less active isoform (McNamara et al., 2004). These findings, along with a rapidly improving ability to identify patients who are likely to have adverse reactions to specific drugs, indicate that we are on the threshold of an era of "individualized" medicine, where therapy can be tailored to the pathophysiology in the *individual* patient rather than to the *average* patient in a large population.

The idea of individualized therapy is not new, however. More than 2000 years ago, when discussing the "absolutes," Aristotle wrote in his *Nicomachean Ethics* (I.vi.14–16):

> . . . it is not easy to see . . . how anybody will be a better physician . . . for having contemplated the absolute idea. In fact, it does not appear that the physician studies even health in the abstract: he studies the health of the human being—or rather of some particular human being, for it is individuals he has to cure.

BIBLIOGRAPHY

Akazawa H, Komuro I. Roles of cardiac transcription factors in cardiac hypertrophy. *Circ Res* 2003;92:1079–1088.

Arad M, Seidman JG, Seidman CE. Phenotypic diversity in hypertrophic cardiomyopathy. *Hum Mol Genet* 2002;11:2499–2506.

Arad M, Maron BJ, Gorham,JM, et al. Glycogen storage diseases presenting as hypertrophic cardiomyopathy. *N Engl J Med* 2005;352:362–372.

Barger PM, Kelly DP. Fatty acid utilization in the hypertrophied and failing heart: molecular regulatory mechanisms. *Am J Med Sci* 1999;318:36–42.

Bonne G, Carrier L, Richard P, et al. Familial hypertrophic cardiomyopathy. From mutations to functional defects. *Circ Res* 1998;83:580–593.

Bueno OF, Molkentin JD. Involvement of extracellular signal-regulated kinases 1/2 in cardiac hypertrophy and cell death. *Circ Res* 2002;91:776–781.

Bugaisky L, Gupta M, Gupta MG, et al. Cellular and molecular mechanisms of hypertrophy. In: Fozzard H, Haber E, Katz A, et al., eds. *The heart and cardiovascular system*, 2nd ed. New York: Raven Press, 1992:1621–1640.

Colucci WS. *Atlas of heart failure. Cardiac function and dysfunction*, 4th ed. Philadelphia: Current Medicine, 2005.

Dorn GW II, Force T. Protein kinase cascades in the regulation of cardiac hypertrophy. *J Clin Invest* 2005;115:527–537.

Eichhorn EJ, ed. *Cardiology clinics. New insights into dilated cardiomyopathy*. Philadelphia: Saunders, 1998.

Finck BN, Kelly DP. Peroxisome proliferator-activated receptor α (PPARα) signaling in the gene regulatory control of energy metabolism in the normal and diseased heart. *J Mol Cell Cardiol* 2002;34:1249–1257.

Fitts RH. Cellular mechanisms of muscle fatigue. *Physiol Rev* 1994;74:49–94.

Foo RS-Y, Mani K, Kitsis RN. Death begets failure in the heart. *J Clin Invest* 2005;115:565–571.

Frey N, Katus HA, Olson EN, et al. Hypertrophy of the heart. A new therapeutic target. *Circulation* 2004;109:1580–1589.

Gerdes AM, Capasso JM. Editorial review: structural remodeling and mechanical dysfunction of cardiac myocytes in heart failure. *J Mol Cell Cardiol* 1995;27:849–856.

Gerdes AM. Cardiac myocyte remodeling in hypertrophy and progression to failure. *J Card Fail* 8[Suppl 6]:S264–S268.

Giordano FJ. Oxygen, oxidative stress, hypoxia, and heart failure. *J Clin Invest* 2005;115:500–508.

Goldsmith EC, Borg TK. The dynamic interaction of the extracellular matrix in cardiac remodeling. *J Cardiac Failure* 2002;8:[Suppl]:S314–S318.

Gomes AV, Potter JD. Molecular and cellular aspects of troponin cardiomyopathies. *Ann N Acad Sci* 2004;1015:214–224.

Graham RM, Owens WA. Pathogenesis of inherited forms of dilated cardiomyopathy. *N Eng J Med* 1999;341:1759–1762.

Gustafsson AB, Gottlieb RA. Mechanisms of apoptosis in the heart. *J Clin Immunol* 2004;23:447–459.

Hosenpud JD, Greenberg BH, eds. *Congestive heart failure. Pathophysiology, diagnosis, and comprehensive approach to management*, 2nd ed. New York: Springer, 2000.

Hoshijima M, Chien KR. Mixed signals in heart failure: cancer rules. *J Clin Invest* 2002;1098:849–855.

Huss JM, Kelly DP. Mitochondrial energy metabolism in heart failure: a question of balance. *J Clin Invest* 2005;115:547–555.

Ingwall JS, Weiss RG. Is the failing heart energy starved? On using chemical energy to support cardiac function. *Circ Res* 2004;95:135–145.

Kalsi KK, Smolenski RT, Pritchart RD, et al. Energetics and function of the failing human heart with dilated or hypertrophic cardiomyopathy. *Eur J Clin Invest* 1999;29:469–477.

Katz AM. Evolving concepts of heart failure: cooling furnace, malfunctioning pump, enlarging muscle. Part I. Heart failure as a disorder of the cardiac pump. *J Card Fail* 1997;3:319–334.

Katz AM. Evolving concepts of heart failure: cooling furnace, malfunctioning pump, enlarging muscle. Part II. Hypertrophy and dilatation of the failing heart. *J Card Fail* 1998:4: 67–81.

Keller DI, Carrier L, Schwartz K. Genetics of familial cardiomyopathies and arrhythmias. *Swiss Med Weekly* 2002;132:401–407.

Kelly DP. Peroxisome proliferator-activated receptor α as a genetic determinant of cardiac hypertrophic growth: culprit or innocent bystander? *Circulation* 2002;105:1025–1027.

Libera LD, Vescovo G. Muscle wastage in chronic heart failure, between apoptosis, catabolism and altered anabolism: a chimaeric view of inflammation? *Curr Opin Clin Nutr Metab Care* 2004;7:435–441.

Lips DJ, deWindta LJ, van Kraaij DJW, et al. Molecular determinants of myocardial hypertrophy and failure: alternative pathways for beneficial and maladaptive hypertrophy. *Europ Heart J* 2003;24:883–896.

Mancini DM, LaManca J, Henson D. The relation of respiratory muscle function to dyspnea in patients with heart failure. *Heart Failure* 1992;8:183–189.

Mann DL, ed. *Heart failure: a companion to Braunwald's heart disease*. Philadelphia: Saunders, 2004.

McKinsey TA, Olson EN. Toward transcriptional therapies of the failing heart: chemical screens to modulate genes. *J Clin Invest* 2005;115:538–546.

Miller AJ. *Lymphatics of the heart.* New York: Raven Press, 1982.

Morita H, Seidman J, Seidman CE. Genetic causes of human heart failure. *J Clin Invest* 2005;115:518–526.

Norman M, Simpson M, Mogensen J, et al. Novel mutation in desmoplakin causes arrhythmogenic left ventricular dysplasia. *Circulation* 2005;112:636–642.

Packer M, Cohn JN. Consensus recommendations for the management of heart failure. *Am. J Cardiol* 1999;83[Suppl 2a];1A–38A.

Poole-Wilson PA, Colucci WS, Massie BM, et al. *Heart failure. Scientific principles and clinical practice.* New York: Churchill Livingstone, 1997.

Ross RS. The extracellular connections: the role of integrins in cardiac remodeling. *J Card Fail* 2002;8:[Suppl]:S326–S331.

Rumyantsev PP. Interrelations of the proliferation and differentiation of processes during cardiac myogenesis and regeneration. *Int Rev Cytol* 1977;51:187–273.

Saffitz JE, Kléber AG. Effects of mechanical forces and mediators of hypertrophy and remolding of gap junctions in the heart. *Circ Res* 2001;94:585–591.

Selvetella G, Hirsch E, Notte A, et al. Adaptive and maladaptive hypertrophic pathways: points of convergence and divergence. *Cardiovasc Res* 2004;63:373–380.

Small KM, Wagoner LE, Levin AM, et al. Synergistic polymorphisms of beta1- and alpha2C-adrenergic receptors and the risk of congestive heart failure. *N Engl J Med* 2002;347:1135–1142.

Swynghedauw B. Molecular mechanisms of myocardial remodeling. *Physiol Rev* 1999;79:215–262.

van Empel VP, De Windt LJ. Myocyte hypertrophy and apoptosis: a balancing act. *Cardiovasc Res* 2004;63:487–499.

Wilson JR. Exercise intolerance in heart failure. Importance of skeletal muscle. *Circulation* 2004;91:559–661.

Yano M, Ikeda Y, Matsuzaki M. Altered intracellular Ca^{2+} handling in heart failure. *J Clin Invest* 115:556–564.

Additional discussions are found in textbooks of medicine and cardiology.

REFERENCES

Alpert NR, Gordon MS. Myofibrillar adenosine triphosphatase activity in congestive heart failure. *Am J Physiol* 1962;202:940–946.

Baig MK, Goldman JH, Caforio ALP, et al. Familial dilated cardiomyopathy: cardiac abnormalities are common in asymptomatic relatives and may represent early disease. *J Am Coll Cardiol* 1998;31:195–201.

Baim DS, Grossman W. *Grossman's cardiac catheterization, angiography and intervention.* Philadelphia: Lippincott Williams & Wilkins, 2000.

Calderone A, Takahashi N, Izzo NJ Jr, et al. Pressure- and volume-induced left ventricular hypertrophies are associated with distinct myocyte phenotypes and differential induction of peptide growth factor mRNAs. *Circulation* 1995;92:2385–2390.

Chapman D, Weber KT, Eghbali M. Regulation of fibrillar collagen types I and III and basement membrane type IV collagen gene expression in pressure overloaded rat myocardium. *Circ Res* 1990;67:787–794.

Geisterfer-Lowrance AAT, Kass S, Tanigawa G, et al. A molecular basis for familial hypertrophic cardiomyopathy: a β cardiac myosin heavy chain gene missense mutation. *Cell* 1990;62:999–1006.

Gerdes AM, Kellerman SE, Malec KB, et al. Transverse shape characteristics of cardiac myocytes from rats and humans. *Cardioscience* 1994;5:31–36.

Grant C, Greene DG, Bunnell IL. Left ventricular enlargement and hypertrophy. A clinical and angiocardiographic study. *Am J Med* 1965;39:895–904.

Grünig E, Tasman JA, Kücherer H, et al. Frequency and phenotypes of familial dilated cardiomyopathy. *J Am Coll Cardiol* 1998;31:186–194.

Ho KKL, Anderson KM, Kannel WB, et al. Survival after the onset of congestive heart failure in Framingham heart study subjects. *Circulation* 1993;88:107–115.

Kass DA. Evaluation of left-ventricular systolic function. *Heart Failure* 1988;4:198–205.

Katz AM. Cardiomyopathy of overload. A major determinant of prognosis in congestive heart failure. *N Eng J Med* 1990;322:100–110.

Katz AM. *Heart failure. Pathophysiology, molecular biology and clinical management.* Philadelphia: Lippincott Williams & Wilkins, 2000.

Keeling PJ, Gang Y, Smith G, et al. Familial dilated cardiomyopathy in the United Kingdom. *Br Heart J* 1995;73:417–421.

Marijianowski MMH, Teeling P, Mann J, et al. Dilated cardiomyopathy is associated with an increase in the type I/type III collagen ratio: a quantitative assessment. *J Am Coll Cardiol* 1995;25:1263–1272.

McNamara DM, Holubkov R, Postava L, et al. Pharmacogenetic interactions between angiotensin-converting enzyme inhibitor therapy and the angiotensin-converting enzyme deletion polymorphism in patients with congestive heart failure. *J Am Coll Cardiol* 2004;44:2019–2026.

McNamara DM, Holubkov R, Postava L, et al. Effect of the Asp298 variant of endothelial nitric oxide synthase on survival for patients with congestive heart failure. *Circulation* 2003;107:1598–1602.

Meerson FZ. On the mechanism of compensatory hyperfunction and insufficiency of the heart. *Cor et Vasa* 1961;3:161–177.

Olson RE, Piatnek DA. Conservation of energy in cardiac muscle. *Ann NY Acad Sci* 1959; 72:466–478.

Osler W. *The principles and practice of medicine.* New York: Appleton, 1892.

Perez JM, Rathz DA, Petrashevskaya NN, et al. β1-adrenergic receptor polymorphisms confer differential function and predisposition to heart failure. *Nat Med* 2003;9:1300–1305.

Ring PA. Myocardial regeneration in experimental lesions of the heart. *J Path Bact* 1950;62: 21–27.

Russell B, Motlagh GHG, Ashley WW. Form follows function: how muscle shape is regulated by work. *J Appl Physiol* 2000;88:1127–1132.

Scheuer J, Buttrick P. The cardiac hypertrophic responses to pathologic and physiologic loads. *Circulation* 1987;75[1 Pt 2]:I63–168.

Small KM, Wagoner LE, Levin AM. Synergistic polymorphisms of beta1- and alpha2C-adrenergic receptors and the risk of congestive heart failure. *N Engl J Med* 2002;347: 1135–1142.

Weber KT, Brilla CG. Pathological hypertrophy and cardiac interstitium. Fibrosis and the renin-angiotensin-aldosterone system. *Circulation* 1991;83:1849–1865.

Wollert KC, Taga T, Saito M, et al. Corticotrophin-1 activates a distinct form of cardiac muscle cell hypertrophy. Assembly of sarcomeric units in series via gp130/leukemia inhibitory factor receptor-dependent pathways. *J Biol Chem* 1996;271:9535–9545.

Wood P. An appreciation of mitral stenosis. *Br Med J* 1954;1:1051–1063,1113–1124.

Yamamoto K, Dang QN, Maeda Y. Regulation of cardiac myocyte mechanotransduction by the cardiac cycle. *Circulation* 2001;103:1459–1464.

INDEX

Page numbers followed by f indicate figures; page numbers followed by t indicate tabular material.